D0908946

PSYCHIATRIC ASPECTS OF HEADACHE

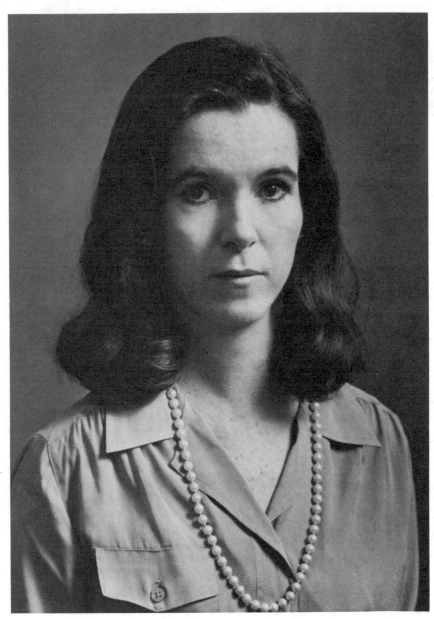

Sheila Morrissey Adler, Ph.D.
1941–1986

PSYCHIATRIC ASPECTS OF HEADACHE

Charles S. Adler, M.D., F.A.P.A.

Chief, Division of Psychiatry, Rose Medical Center
Clinical Assistant Professor of Psychiatry
University of Colorado School of Medicine
Denver, Colorado

Sheila Morrissey Adler, Ph.D.

Clinical and Developmental Psychology
Denver, Colorado

Russell C. Packard, M.D., F.A.A.N.

Director, Headache Management and Neurology Center of Pensacola
Chief, Section of Psychiatry, Sacred Heart Hospital
Pensacola, Florida

With Contributors

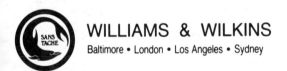

WILLIAMS & WILKINS
Baltimore • London • Los Angeles • Sydney

Editor: Nancy Collins
Associate Editor: Carol Eckhart
Copy Editor: Stephen C. Siegforth
Design: Alice Sellers/Johnson
Cover Design: JoAnne Janowiak
Illustration Planning: Wayne Hubbel
Production: Raymond E. Reter

Copyright © 1987
Williams & Wilkins
428 East Preston Street
Baltimore, MD 21202, U.S.A.

All rights reserved. This book is protected by copyright. No part of this book may be reproduced in any form or by any means, including photocopying, or utilized by any information storage and retrieval system without written permission from the copyright owner.

Accurate indications, adverse reactions, and dosage schedules for drugs are provided in this book, but is is possible that they may change. The reader is urged to review the package information data of the manufacturers of the medications mentioned.

Printed in the United States of America

Library of Congress Cataloging in Publication Data

Main entry under title:

Psychiatric aspects of headache.

    Includes bibliographies and index.
    1. Headache–Psychosomatic aspects. I. Adler, Charles S. II. Adler, Sheila Morrissey. III. Packard, Russell C. [DNLM: 1. Headache–psychology. WL 342 P974]
RB128.P79 1987   616.07'2   86-24689
ISBN 0-683-00056-X

87 88 89 90 91 10 9 8 7 6 5 4 3 2 1

On the tenth of November 1986, while attending an international meeting on headache in London, Doctor Sheila Morrissey Adler died most unexpectedly. Only two weeks before departing for England, she and her husband had celebrated the completion of this volume's final manuscript, a project that had absorbed them for close to ten years. Although only 45 years old when she died, and despite the presence of a, severe, nonprogressive muscular dystrophy, present since birth, Doctor Adler had attained international prominence in the fields of headache, self-regulation, and psychology. All who knew Sheila Adler will remember her as she would wish to be remembered: not for her handicap, but for her remarkable determination in overcoming it, to love generously, work creatively, and reach out warmly and gregariously to comfort the distressed of spirit, wherever she met them, whatever their station. She was the sparkling, driving impetus, impelling and fashioning this book to its completion—in the words of Rilke, becoming the "crystal cup that shatters even as it rings." More than her final victory over fate, this book is her very child. It is with joy and with pride that we dedicate it to her.

Foreword

Psychiatric Aspects of Headache represents the most comprehensive compendium of germaine information about the complex problems of headache patients. The editors and their contributors, a world famous group of clinicians and researchers, clarify our thinking about pain and its problems, the myriad manifestations of specific headache syndromes, the psychobiological aspects of stress and stress management, and the treatment of various type of headaches in relationship to development perspectives. They describe in a scholarly and lucid fashion, with case examples, the precise details and conceptual models of what can be loosely called "headache."

Of special interest are the psychological manifestations of the patient as well as the patient/physician interaction. Certainly a superior contribution to our knowledge is the description of the attributes of personal reactions to pain, and the development of understanding the meaning of symptoms and their relationship to personality development and their psychodynamic and psychological aspects is especially laudatory. The neurobiological contributions to the understanding of stress disorders and their relation to depression as well as the chronobiological aspects of human experience are signal contributions to enhancing the treatment of headache patients.

The therapeutic influences of various specific therapies as well as the psychotherapeutic interventions and special somatic therapies as both "state of the art." Indications for treatment vary in health and disease: the role of headache as "sickness" as well as in the states of "wellness" is a new fresh view in the specialty of psychiatry. The authors' clinical experience and scientific knowledge adequately document without speculation our current knowledge. The utilization of the biopsychosocial model allows the view from the domain of biological and biomedical perspectives as well as from the psychosocial perspective. Integration of these various perspectives provides a cohesive treatment plan for the patient. This effort to organize knowledge in a systematic way, attempting to discover patterns of relationships among phenomena, also helps to explain events. Modern psychiatry ranges from the molecular to large and complex social systems and therefore generates questions of great magnitude: Those who attempt to integrate these two create enormous dissonance to proponents of each system. The bravery and courage of those who have attempted this integration is a major contribution to the integration of psychiatry and medicine.

The contributions of the late Sheila Morrissey Adler to these chapters bespeaks the extraordinary loss to scholarship we shall all feel with her passing.

Shervert H. Frazier, M.D.
General Director/Psychiatrist in Chief
McLean Hospital
Belmont, Massachusetts
Professor of Psychiatry
Harvard Medical School
Boston, Massachusetts

Preface

This book was written to fill what its authors/editors perceived to be a substantial gap in the literature of headache. It is therefore directed towards an unusually broad and diverse readership: neurologists, internists, family practitioners, orthopedists, psychoanalysts, psychiatrists, psychologists, social workers, psychophysiologists, psychopharmacologists, researchers, students or scholars in any of the health sciences, and even astute, educated, or simply curious lay persons (be they headache sufferers or otherwise). It is a project that we have approached, for obvious reasons, with humility, reassuring and remotivating ourselves with the following thought: One has to start somewhere. Hopefully, its contents will suffice, perhaps even endure. Yet time works against all knowledge. Still, it is impossible to predict what progress may ultimately be stimulated by a beginning, any beginning. Even an irritating grain of sand can, over the years, evolve into a lustrous pearl if it provokes a hearty response from the oyster.

But, to return to the original point: Can we truly address so many audiences and still be effective? We believe we can, and that, furthermore, we must. Headache restricts itself to no single specialist's domain, however one might wish it otherwise, and headache patients come as a unit, indivisible into muscles, arteries, bones, bloodstream, brain, or mind. They are only unified by their pain and its location. This is also true of the psychologically influenced headache patient, whether that influence be contributary or resultant.

The authors firmly recognize that psychiatry and psychology are not relevant to all chronic headache patients. Yet the experienced clinician is as cognizant as the man on the street that emotion and headache interact with considerable frequency. To argue at length over the exact proportion would be not merely pedantic, but would deter us from our true task and challenge: to combine forces and understand that interaction when it does occur in a way that will enable us to help these persons reduce their deep distress.

Finally, the sheer number of patients with chronic head pain demands such a book, demands that the problem be looked at from all angles, and asserts that "attention must be paid!" It can be seen that the authors of this book *have* paid attention, as they are professionals who have devoted their careers to observing headache patients. Their diversity of background reflects the chimeral nature of headache as well as the polyglot composition of both national and international organizations springing up to study and treat this black symptom of multitudinous disorders.

As most headache patients are seen by generalists, neurologists, or internists, this book is first of all geared to be both understandable and practical for them. Some sections delve in a more specialized way into the questions and needs of mental health professionals involved with headache patients. (For the chronic patient with significant psychological overlay, the interested psychiatrist, who has combined medical, psychological, and neurological training, is currently considered to be an insufficiently tapped resource as a primary headache physician.)

Our appreciation for their help in preparation of this book goes to the patient and skillful staff at Williams & Wilkins, as well as to Stanley Weiss, M.D., Thomas Brown, Ph.D., Lauren Starnes Duncan, J.D., Ms. Gretchen Packard, Ms. Sally Thompson, Ms. Rose Franzien, and to the many others who contributed their work, their encouragement, and their forthright critiques.

Charles S. Adler
Sheila Morrissey Adler
Russell C. Packard

Contributors

CHARLES S. ADLER, M.D., F.A.P.A.
Chief, Division of Psychiatry
Rose Medical Center
Clinical Assistant Professor of Psychiatry
University of Colorado School of Medicine
Denver, Colorado

SHEILA MORRISSEY ADLER, Ph.D.
Clinical and Developmental Psychology
Denver, Colorado

R. SCOTT BENSON, M.D.
Clinical Assistant Professor of Psychiatry
University of Florida School of Medicine
Director, Adolescent Unit
West Florida Hospital Pavillion
Private Practice, Child Psychiatry
Pensacola, Florida

DIETRICH BLUMER, M.D.
Chairman, Department of Psychiatry
Henry Ford Hospital
Detroit, Michigan
Professor of Psychiatry
University of Michigan School of Medicine
Ann Arbor, Michigan

FRANK BROWN, Ph.D.
Private Practice, Clinical Psychology
Pensacola, Florida

GEORGE W. BRUYN, M.D., D.Sc.
Chairman, Department of Neurology
Academic Hospital
Professor of Neurology
State University, Leiden
Leiden, The Netherlands

MACDONALD CRITCHLEY, C.B.E., M.D., F.R.C.P., Hon. F.A.C.P.
President Emeritus
World Federation of Neurology
Consultant Neurologist
The National Hospital
London, England

JAMES D. DEXTER, M.D.
Professor and Chairman
Department of Neurology
University of Missouri School of Medicine
Columbia, Missouri

SEYMOUR DIAMOND, M.D.
Director
Diamond Headache Clinic
Adjunct Professor of Pharmacology
The Chicago Medical School
North Chicago, Illinois

JOHN EDMEADS, M.D., F.R.C.P. (C), F.A.C.P., F.A.A.N.
Editor-in-Chief, *Headache*
Head, Division of Neurology
Sunnybrook Medical Center
Professor of Medicine (Neurology)
University of Toronto
Toronto, Ontario, Canada

ARNOLD P. FRIEDMAN, M.D., F.A.C.P., F.A.A.N., L.F.A.P.A.
Chairman, Research Group on Headache and
  Migraine
World Federation of Neurology
Consultant, Neurological Associates of Tucson

Adjunct Professor of Clinical Neurology
University of Arizona School of Medicine
Tucson, Arizona

JANE ROBERTS GILL, M.S.W., C.S.W.
Senior Clinical Social Work Supervisor
The Headache Research Foundation
The Headache Centre at Faulkner Hospital
Boston, Massachusetts

JOHN R. GRAHAM, M.D., M.A.C.P.
Chairman, Board of Trustees
The Headache Research Foundation
Lecturer on Medicine
Tufts University School of Medicine
Boston, Massachusetts

MARY HEILBRONN, Ph.D.
Research Coordinator
Henry Ford Hospital
Detroit, Michigan

CHASE PATTERSON KIMBALL, M.D., F.A.P.A.
President
International College of Psychosomatic Medicine
Professor of Psychiatry and Medicine, and
  Director, Consultation-Liaison Service
The University of Chicago School of Medicine
Chicago, Illinois

LEE KUDROW, M.D.
Director
California Medical Clinic for Headache
Encino, California

ROBERT S. KUNKEL, M.D., F.A.C.P.
Head, Section on Headache
Department of Internal Medicine
The Cleveland Clinic
Cleveland, Ohio

NINAN T. MATHEW, M.D., F.R.C.P. (C)
Director
Houston Headache Clinic
Clinical Associate Professor of Neurology
University of Texas School of Medicine
Houston, Texas

JOSE L. MEDINA, M.D., F.A.C.P.
Director
Chicago Headache Center and Neurology
  Services
Staff Neurologist, Cook County Hospital
Associate Professor of Neurology
The Chicago Medical School
North Chicago, Illinois

PATRICK O'CONNELL, M.D., F.A.P.A.
Private Practice of Psychiatry
Pensacola, Florida

FRED OVSIEW, M.D.
Associate Attending Physician
Northwestern Memorial Hospital
Associate in Psychiatry and Neurology
Northwestern University Medical School
Consultant in Neuropsychiatry
The University of Chicago School of Medicine
Chicago, Illinois

RUSSELL C. PACKARD, M.D., F.A.A.N.
Director
Headache Management and Neurology Center
  of Pensacola
Chief, Section of Psychiatry
Sacred Heart Hospital
Pensacola, Florida

JOEL R. SAPER, M.D., F.A.C.P.
Director
Michigan Headache and Neurological Institute
Clinical Associate Professor of Medicine
  (Neurology)
Michigan State University School of Medicine
Ann Arbor, Michigan

WILLIAM G. SPEED III, M.D., F.A.C.P.
Director
Speed Headache Associates, P.A.
Associate Clinical Professor of Medicine
The Johns Hopkins University School of
  Medicine
Baltimore, Maryland

EGILIUS L.H. SPIERINGS, M.D., Ph.D.
Director
The Headache Research Foundation
Assistant Professor of Neurology
Tufts University School of Medicine
Boston, Massachusetts

A. DIXON WEATHERHEAD, M.D., F.R.C. Psych.
Senior Staff Psychiatrist
Department of Psychiatry
The Cleveland Clinic
Cleveland, Ohio

MARCIA WILKINSON, D.M., F.R.C.P.
President
International Headache Society
Honorary Director
The City of London Migraine Clinic
London, England

Contents

Foreword vii
    SHERVERT H. FRAZIER, JR., M.D.

Preface ix

Contributors xi

SECTION 1. PERSPECTIVES ON HEADACHE

1. A Historical Perspective on Psychiatric Thinking about
   Headache 3
       CHARLES S. ADLER, M.D.
       SHEILA MORRISSEY ADLER, PH.D.
       ARNOLD P. FRIEDMAN, M.D.

2. The Inscrutability of Pain, with Particular Reference to Migraine
   and to Headache 22
       MACDONALD CRITCHLEY, M.D.

3. Differing Expectations of Headache Patients and Their
   Physicians 29
       RUSSELL C. PACKARD, M.D.

4. The Headache Patient and the Doctor 34
       JOHN R. GRAHAM, M.D.

5. Psychodynamics of Head Pain: An Introduction 41
       CHARLES S. ADLER, M.D.
       SHEILA MORRISSEY ADLER, PH.D.

SECTION 2. ASSESSMENT OF THE HEADACHE PATIENT

6. First Things First: The Physical Workup 59
       ROBERT S. KUNKEL, M.D.

7. Mythology in the Management of Headache 64
       JOHN EDMEADS, M.D.

8. Evaluating the Psychological Factors in Headache 70
       CHARLES S. ADLER, M.D.
       SHEILA MORRISSEY ADLER, PH.D.

9. The Psychiatric Aspects of Headache in Children 84
       R. SCOTT BENSON, M.D.

10. **Symptom Formation and the Meaning of Diagnostic and Therapeutic Procedures to the Patient**. 92
    CHASE PATTERSON KIMBALL, M.D.
    FRED OVSIEW, M.D.

11. **Multiple Headaches in Cases of Multiple Personality Disorder** 101
    RUSSELL C. PACKARD, M.D.
    FRANK BROWN, PH.D.

SECTION 3.   PSYCHIATRIC ASPECTS OF SPECIFIC HEADACHE SYNDROMES

12. **Clinical and Psychodynamic Aspects of Tension Headache**. 111
    CHARLES S. ADLER, M.D.
    SHEILA MORRISSEY ADLER, PH.D.

13. **Chronic Headaches and the Dysthymic Pain Disorder: Profile and Treatment of a Variant of Depressive Disease** 124
    DIETRICH BLUMER, M.D.
    MARY HEILBRONN, PH.D.

14. **The Migraine Patient: Descriptive Studies** 131
    CHARLES S. ADLER, M.D.
    SHEILA MORRISSEY ADLER, PH.D.

15. **The Migraine Patient and the Migraine Attack: Clinical Studies** 142
    CHARLES S. ADLER, M.D.
    SHEILA MORRISSEY ADLER, PH.D.

16. **Psychodynamics of Migraine: A Developmental Perspective**. 158
    CHARLES S. ADLER, M.D.
    SHEILA MORRISSEY ADLER, PH.D.

17. **Psychiatric and Mental Presentations of the Migraine Prodrome, Aura, and Attack** 181
    GEORGE W. BRUYN, M.D., D.Sc.

18. **Conversion Headache** 194
    A. DIXON WEATHERHEAD, M.D.

19. **Psychiatric Aspects of Posttraumatic Headaches** 201
    WILLIAM G. SPEED, III, M.D.

20. **Psychometric and Descriptive Aspects of Cluster Headache**. 207
    LEE KUDROW, M.D.

21. **Psychodynamics of Cluster Headaches** 212
    CHARLES S. ADLER, M.D.
    SHEILA MORRISSEY ADLER, PH.D.
    JOHN R. GRAHAM, M.D.

SECTION 4.   PSYCHOBIOLOGY OF STRESS AND HEADACHE

22. **The Physiology and Biochemistry of Stress in Relation to Headache** 237
    EGILIUS L.H. SPIERINGS, M.D., PH.D.

23. **The Relationship between Headache Syndromes and Sleep** 254
    JAMES D. DEXTER, M.D.

24. **Depression and Headache: A Pharmacological Perspective**. 259
    SEYMOUR DIAMOND, M.D.

25. Cyclical Migraine: Its Relationship to Depression and Its Treatment with Lithium. 275
JOSE L. MEDINA, M.D.

26. Medication Compliance among Headache Patients 280
RUSSELL C. PACKARD, M.D.
PATRICK O'CONNELL, M.D.

27. Drugs and Headache: Misuse and Dependency 289
NINAN T. MATHEW, M.D.

SECTION 5.   TREATMENT

28. An Overview of Treatment Options for the Psychologically Influenced Headache Patient 301
JANE ROBERTS GILL, M.S.W., C.S.W.

29. The Patient with Acute Migraine: Definitive Support 306
MARCIA WILKINSON, D.M.

30. Psychotherapy and the Headache Patient. 313
CHARLES S. ADLER, M.D.
SHEILA MORRISSEY ADLER, PH.D.

31. From Theory to Technique: A Psychotherapeutic Miscellany for Headache 332
CHARLES S. ADLER, M.D.
SHEILA MORRISSEY ADLER, PH.D.

32. Perspectives from a Headache Center with an Inpatient Unit 340
JOEL R. SAPER, M.D.

33. The Psychological Use of Biofeedback and Other Self-Regulatory Techniques in Headache Treatment. 349
CHARLES S. ADLER, M.D.
SHEILA MORRISSEY ADLER, PH.D.
RUSSELL C. PACKARD, M.D.

Index. 369

SECTION ONE

Perspectives on Headache

A Historical Perspective on Psychiatric Thinking about Headache

CHAPTER ONE

CHARLES S. ADLER, M.D.
SHEILA MORRISSEY ADLER, PH.D.
ARNOLD P. FRIEDMAN, M.D.

To understand a science, it is necessary to know its history.

AUGUST COMTE

Those who do not remember the past are destined to repeat it.

GEORGE SANTAYANA

What has been recorded through the ages about headache is persuasive on one point: even those who *do* remember the past are destined to repeat it. Although repetition is inevitable, for those who have understood history, the repetitions are likely to contain elements of progress. So, in pursuit of such progress, let us confront medicine's history of understanding the psychology of headache, be it grand or comic. This chapter will reveal it as both with, it is hoped, the empathy we would wish future generations to have when looking back on our own endeavors.

This section will explore mankind's changing understanding of the role of mind and emotion in headache's symptoms, causes, and therapies. To do this, we will also have to look at our growing understanding of what mind and emotion are, and of their relationship to the body. By exposing the roots of our present knowledge, we may thus suggest the direction in which that knowledge has been evolving.

Any endeavor—such as understanding and treating headache—undertaken in a particular age, place, and culture inevitably entwines with this greater context. By looking at the psychology of headache, we may therefore catch a glimpse, not only of medicine's odyssey, but also of society's. Perhaps this will make our quest more enjoyable—and more familiar.

Because migraine—especially classical—leaves more distinctive footprints, its path through history is easier to track. Table 1.1 will show that today's migraine sufferer has cause to feel a kinship with the great as well as the humble in history. In the text, we will also show that the physician in search of effective treatment for intractable head-

3

TABLE 1.1
SOME FAMOUS MIGRAINEURS

Julius Caesar	Thomas Jefferson	Ulysses S. Grant
Saint Paul	Friedrich Nietzsche	Peter Tchaikovsky
Father of St. Luke	Immanuel Kant	Alfred Nobel
John Calvin	Edgar Allan Poe	Leo Tolstoy
Queen Mary Tudor	Frederic Chopin	Tzarina Alexandra
Blaise Pascal	Charles Darwin	Sigmund Freud
First Duke of Marlborough	Karl Marx	Virginia Woolf
Carolus Linnaeus	Louis Carroll	Princess Margaret

aches—but who has been stymied—has cause to feel a bond with generations of frustrated head healers.

PSYCHE AND SOMA

Contemplating the mind/body relationship was probably an activity known to our remote ancestors, in that the origin of consciousness can in many ways be equated with the evolution of consciousness of the "self." In every age, the search to understand the true relationship between mind and body, self and nonself, has undoubtedly gained impetus from the symptom of pain, which inevitably raises the question: "Whence comes the torment?"

The Greeks gave us the words *psyche*—formally meaning breath, but also used to signify the energy in living things—and *soma*, meaning body. They combine to form "psychosomatic." Throughout history these Siamese twins have wrestled each other for dominance in the recurring tides of theory, yet never has one been able to hold its temporary advantage; and this is foreordained by their inherent relationship.

Descartes gave voice to one position, "I think, therefore I am", which is "not different from the belief of the common man, held onto from infancy, often in contradiction to later formed beliefs, that his psyche precedes his embodiment and will survive his body's disintegration" (1). This is also the position taken in Genesis, "In the beginning was the word," *followed* by the creation, secondarily, of matter.

Awareness of "soma" generated an alternate view of the relationship:

The Greeks . . . tried to dignify matter and raise it to a position of equality with spirit, even to the eminence of pre-existence. Their atomists believed that from the clashing of original atoms came all—an idea personally reducible to 'I am; therefore I think.' Which is preeminent, spirit or matter, mind or body? How to heal depends, to a certain extent, on the resolution of that question (1).

Even today the twins still grope for position, as though unfazed by several millenia's thought. The current American Psychiatric Association *Diagnostic and Statistical Manual of Mental Disorders (DSM III)* (2) has replaced the old diagnosis of "psychophysiological disorder" with "psychological factors affecting a physical condition." (Migraine and tension headaches are considered to fall into this category). One can read in these changes the continuing battle for primacy.

Equally fascinating have been our attempts through the ages to treat headache. There is evidence dating back to prehistoric times, revealing a fascinating mixture of the logical and the intuitive, the hopeful and the proven. Attempted treatments have included primitive surgeries, religious rituals, charms, herbs, and exorcisms (3)—and to this day, none of these approaches has died out entirely. Because the dominant headache treatment in any era reflected that era's beliefs about the etiology of head pain—and consequently of the mind/body relationship—we will review the history of theory and treatment together.

PSYCHOSOMATIC THOUGHT: ITS PRIMAL MOORINGS

A thesis of this chapter is that each age's capacity to treat headache was limited by the sophistication with which it could appreciate the relationship between mind, body, and outside world. This appreciation has evolved to a degree that has been fully recognized only recently, in Julian Jaynes' *The Origin of Consciousness in the Breakdown of the Bicameral Mind* (4).

Jaynes' exposition clarifies that inherent limits were imposed upon medical thought in given eras by the level to which consciousness had evolved. The importance and complexity of the work cannot be sufficiently reflected in this short essay. (Please note that the terms subjective and objective are used differently in this chapter than they are in Jaynes.)[1]

During psychological development, the individual must first learn to distinguish him-

---

[1] Though both usages are lexically correct, Jaynes' use of the two terms better suits his purposes of cognitive paleontology, while our definitions are more familiar to current psychiatry and may, therefore, be clearer for purposes of this chapter. How do they differ? Jaynes uses "subjective" to refer to an awareness of inner mental processes, that which evolved in man over the last 5000 years. His "objective" refers to the less advanced form of reflex mental activity that preceded such awareness. This chapter uses these words in a different—almost opposite—fashion. "Subjective" here means mental functioning in which inner perceptions are accepted at face value, without validation against "outside" criteria. Thus, projections, illusions, and hallucinations would all be included. Awareness of self may or may not exist. Our "objective" thinking only occurs in persons with self-awareness, however, because it attempts to differentiate self-generated percepts from externally generated ones. It uses external, theoretically impartial checks to validate the "reality basis" of thoughts and perceptions.

self from the primary homogeneous matrix of existence and experience. He subsequently learns the more subtle distinction between experiences which are primarily mental and those which are primarily somatic.

The axiom that ontogeny recapitulates phylogeny is as true for psychological development as it is for physiological. One therefore sees that modes of understanding are similar, though not identical, in the young child, the young culture (i.e., primitive, tribal), and early civilization. In all three, awareness of the self is first not at all, and then only incompletely, differentiated from awareness of the outside world. Impulses, wishes, and fears that should be identified as intrapsychic are instead perceived to be motives or actions, sometimes benevolent, but usually not, of enemies, spirits, demons, or supernatural forces. Jaynes reminds his readers of the mentation evidenced in the *Iliad*, where vividly hallucinated machinations of the gods blended into an uninterrupted stream of awareness which also encompassed personal passions and actual battles with the enemy.

In primitive societies, as in early civilizations, illness is typically seen as punishment sent from afar (5). It is also often viewed that way by children who are sick or in pain. [Before a certain age, children not only picture death as external, but also see it merely as the result of bad luck (that might be avoided) rather than as integral to biology (6). Many shows on television prolong this fantasy for adults.]

In all these situations, unwanted impulses and fears are either projected onto the environment in the form of brooding and vengeful spirits, or are not distinguished from it in the first place. When these were believed to be the causes of illness the most sensible treatment—the treatment of choice—was to appease or to counterattack them. The shaman, high priest, or medicine man would perform a rite to convince the patient that a stronger, protective, and forgiving spirit was being called forth. Both parties entered into trances and other altered states of consciousness to intensify these perceptions. Sometimes medications were used to further this cause, as in the peyote ceremonies of Northern Peru (5). Charms, ceremonies, and intricate rituals drew upon the culture's most authoritative symbols of power to augment the patient's faith that malevolent spirits would be vitiated.

Sometimes the sick person was encouraged to identify with the healer. At other times he was given to believe that the healer temporarily took on his suffering, or reproached the evil forces responsible for it. Appeasement of those forces through sacrifice or self-punishment was yet another way to deal with illness. We should note with humility that the curandera of Mexico today approaches illness much as these ancient healers did and, depending upon a patient's underlying pathology and emotional development, is sometimes more effective than the modern allopathic physician. Superstition, like placebo, can be effective.[2]

TREATMENT OF HEADACHE THROUGH THE AGES

The first thing history teaches is this: headaches are more than epiphenomena of a stressful modern society. Their pulsatile thread is firmly rooted in biology, for it ex-

---

[2] The emotional help obtained in these rituals should be differentiated from today's scientifically based psychotherapy, even though at times it too uses nonspecific methods. To do otherwise would be like comparing the trepanation with flint instruments performed 10,000 years ago to release the "evil spirits" presumed to cause headaches to the modern neurosurgeon's use of this technique to relieve headaches of subdural hematoma.

These earliest times are also sometimes characterized as having a holistic orientation. However tempting it may be to idealize the past, its "psychosomatic" orientation probably differed sharply from that concept as currently understood. Today, mind and body are viewed as continuously interacting entities. In early societies mind and body had not yet developed strong, independent identities that would then be able to interact.

tends back to the beginnings of recorded history. Three thousand years before Christ a Sumerian poet bewailed his "sick" and "blinding" headache (7), and implored the gods for an afterlife free of pain. The first recorded treatment for headache also comes from Sumer: the elaborate Incantation of Eridu. The ceremony required a wise woman, hair of a virgin kid, and sanctified water, and it encouraged a Sumerian's headache to ascend to heaven (3).

NEOLITHIC HEADACHES

Trepanning of the skull was practiced in both Mediterranean areas (2000–3000 B.C.) and later in South America. In the first millenium A.D., Peruvian healers dripped coca juice (from which cocaine is derived) into incisions to serve as a local anesthetic. Considering the cure, Stone Age man might have hesitated before mentioning his headache to a hunt mate.

FROM THE CRADLE

The next rung on civilization's ladder is Mesopotamia. Tiu was the spirit responsible for headache, and the chant from Sumer noted above was his antidote (7). The following Mesopotamian verse (8) thunders its eloquent warning across 5000 years to inform us that the chant was not always successful:

Headache roameth over the desert: blowing like the wind,
Flashing like lightning, it is loosed above and below;
It cutteth off him who feareth not his god:
Like a reed,
Like a stalk of henna it slitteth his sinews.
It wasteth the flesh of him who hath no protecting goddess;
Flashing like a heavenly star, it cometh like the dew;
It standeth hostile against the wayfarer, scorching him like the day.
This man it hath struck, and
Like one with heart disease, he staggereth;
Like one bereft of reason he is broken;

Like one which has been cast into the fire he is
*   shrivelled;*
Like a wild ass . . . his eyes are full of cloud;
On himself he feedeth, bound in death;
Headache whose course, like the dread
*   windstorm, none knoweth,*
None knoweth its full time or bond.

In this quote not only is the *cause* of headache external, but its very *location* (and perhaps the location of a migraine aura, i.e., the lightning, the star) is outside the person. (To be yet more precise, inner and outer are not really distinguished from one another.)

Jaynes refers to this same passage to illustrate not headache, but the agonized state of early ("bicameral") man in the process of losing contact with the command hallucinations that guided and sustained him—which, indeed, were his substitute for many of modern man's ego functions. Seen that way, this is the earliest association between an inner sense of "loss" and headache.

DYNASTIC EGYPT

The ancient Egyptians also believed death and disease came from outside; indeed, the "breath of death" had a specific route into the body—through the left ear (9). Especially during earlier dynasties, illness was believed to be due to angry wishes of gods or people, living or dead.

The Egyptians' failure to adequately separate psyche from soma is seen in their preoccupation with death. Corpses were outfitted to quite literally follow the spirit into an afterlife and were even equipped with sailing vessels (should the deceased be wealthy enough) and provisions to give the body sustenance in that life.

In other ways, however, concerning things they could see directly, the Egyptians were a practical people. Therefore in *The Edwin Smith Surgical Papyrus* (9) dealing with the treatment of visible wounds, rational, cause-and-effect, commonsense treatments were advocated. On the other hand, disorders that were internal or appeared for unobvious reasons, which would include head-

aches, might be treated either directly (drugs, poultices, massage) or indirectly (rituals and rites). The physician who chose to use a spell might address the troubled organ directly: — "Oh, failing eyes . . ." (1).

Thus although a basis for therapeutics founded in experience was being formed in one area, a similarly reasoned comprehension of psychological phenomena eluded the Egyptians. This dichotomy is easy to understand: its vestiges can be heard underlying the cryptic remarks of many a modern-day house officer.

ASSYRIANS, BABYLONIANS, HEBREWS

The Babylonians and Assyrians relied heavily on magic too: each of 6000 complaints had its own demon whom an exorcist could specifically address and urge to leave the patient's body. Pain was punishment for moral or ritual error or was the result of sorcery or of the hand of a ghost escaped from an unburied body (1). Because the patient, through some sin he had committed, might have been responsible for the pain, he was "disgraced, and urged to look into his soul and examine his sins until the charms of the priest freed him from sickness. Disease was thought of as having a cause within the patient" (1). This last belief appears to have been only partial: although the *reason for the illness* coming was within the patient, the *illness itself* came from outside, as punishment.

To the ancient Hebrews, also, illness was the price paid for having offended God, although for them all 6000 demons were combined into a single deity at once both wrathful and benevolent. Illness was punishment for having disobeyed or angered him.

'I kill, and I make alive; I wound, and I heal',
God warned (Deuteronomy 32:39), and other
healers in the form of doctors were scorned.
For group sin there was the group punish-
ment. . . . for the sin of individual failure to
obey God there was the punishment of individ-
ual disease (1).

But by the second century B.C. the Jews had become a pragmatic people as well:

By then the sick among the Jews were urged to pray and then go to a doctor, for the Lord created doctors too. Physicians of Maccabean times would often whisper the ancient promise into the ear of a patient as he swallowed his medicine (1).

GREEKS

Before the Greek civilization faded it had sounded the major themes in psychosomatics which successive generations would primarily augment with variations, harmonies, and counterpoints. Evil spirits were, not surprisingly, still around—called the Keres by the Greeks—and one line of thought blamed health troubles on them. It was in this vein of thought that Aristotle surmised that the evil entity causing headache was wont to settle in the stomach, from which location it sent "humors" to the brain. But this "Homeric" view of mind-body interactions was to be profoundly challenged by the Greeks in three innovative ways: Asclepian, Hippocratic, and Platonic.

Asclepius

The first major Greek influence on psychosomatics was that of Asclepius, preceding Hippocrates by almost a millenium. The Greeks deified Asclepius as son of Apollo, god of medicine, and successor to Imhotep, Egypt's greatest physician. Although by the Golden Age of Greece Asclepius was but a faded memory, he had spawned a large priestly following and an empire of temples bearing his name.

The approach of these priests to the sick was more intuitive than objective, more psychological than physiological. It was introspective, and strongly tied to religious practices of the time. Even centuries later, patients who were treatment failures at the hands of Hippocratic physicians often found their way to the temples of Asclepius (5). Headache sufferers might well have been a sizeable part of that group.

The priests of Asclepius used the power of suggestion to faciliate the brain's self-healing capacities. Patients often arrived at the temple after a long and dangerous journey. Their stay began with a ceremonial fasting and cleansing, accompanied by prayer, and a tour of the temple's display of "testimonials." A rough analogue of the modern history and physical was then obtained. When the supplicant was deemed ready, the priest-physician led him to sacred ground, often through a maze of underground corridors. The patient then entered what was known as "the sleep of incubation," sometimes sleeping inside the skin of a recently sacrificed animal. This altered mental state facilitated contact with fantasies, emotions, and images, probably of hallucinatory intensity. In the healing dream that ensued, the god Asclepius would often appear

as a man, child, snake, or dog; he would touch the sick part of the patient's body and then disappear. The patient would wake up healed and have his dream decoded by an interpreter (9).

Sometimes the priest-physician talked to the "dreaming" patient; sometimes he did so while dressed in the robe of a god (to speed the healing along).

From the asclepion at Epidaurus comes the following account (10) of how incubation worked with one headache sufferer:

Agestratos suffered from insomnia on account of headaches. . . . He fell asleep and . . . thought the god . . . taught him wrestling. . . . He departed cured . . . competed at the Nemean games and was victor in wrestling.

Thus the Asclepian priests emphasized introspective and intuitive forces that could guide the patient toward health. In their procedures they took an active role in ministering to the sick, but primary healing powers still resided in the gods of the patient as revealed through facilitated hallucination.[3] Patients

---

[3] The "healing" process was quintessentially bicameral; the role of the priest-physician was to augment regression into that older cognitive system and then integrate its "messages" with the more evolved consciousness of the awakened state.

with psychogenic or psychological features to their illness were probably those most likely to be helped.

Hippocrates

The most dramatic challenge to the traditional gods-and-magic medical orientation came from the school of thought founded by Hippocrates on the Isle of Cos. Its difference and its strength came from its commitment to objectivity. The Hippocratic physicians analyzed, observed—indeed, experimented with—the external, objective world, and included in that world the human body. Kolb (11) considers these the first truly scientific steps in biology. Alcmaeon, for example, actually dissected the brain and, observing that all sense organs were connected to it, inferred that the brain was the seat of reason. And *Hippocrates* himself described both patients with migraine and its visual aura:

In the corpus hippocratum, the brain was recognized to be the source of the emotion: 'And men ought to know that from nothing else but thence come joys, delights, laughter, and sports and sorrows, despondency, and lamentations. . . . And by the same organ we become mad and delirious and fears and terrors assail us, some by night and some by day and dreams and untimely wanderings and cares that are not suitable and ignorance of present circumstances, destitude and unskillfulness. All these things we endure from the brain when it is not healthy.' This point of view, that all illness, including psychiatric disturbance, is based solely on disordered physiology has dominated western medicine ever since (5).

Hippocrates rejected outright the idea that gods were the primary cause of mental disease. "If you cut into a head with a bad smell and too moist a brain,' Hippocrates pointed out in *Sacred Disease,* "you plainly see that it is not a god but disease that hurts a body" (1). Observable environmental influences (winds, water supply, temperature, etc.), rather than mystical ones, were recognized as primary in the cause and progression of illness.

Although some observers have considered Hippocrates' approach to treatment the start of an unbalanced "medical model" from which emotional factors were rudely excluded, this view is probably influenced more by where the approach has brought us today than by where it began. First, the case for making objectivity an ideal had to be argued emphatically to counter the dominant prevailing mode of thinking, one that hardly differentiated events from the feelings, beliefs, and expectations experienced in connection with them. This shift from a confused amalgam of objective and subjective to observational, inductive, and primarily objective methods was dramatic. It needed to be defended as well as cherished. Even today, the *New York Times* sits on the newsrack next to tabloids extolling astrology; one can only imagine the situation in Hippocrates' time!

Furthermore, Hippocrates was not oblivious to the influence of emotions:

Physical or fluid imbalance could be caused by emotional upset, too. Hippocrates reported that fear produced sweat and that shame brought on palpitations of the heart; he urged young physicians to look at patients with kindly expressions and never with impatience since impatience could inhibit the return of health. . . . It was Hippocrates who wrote 'in order to cure the human body it is necessary to have a knowledge of the whole of things' (1).

Thus, Hippocrates actually recognized psychosomatic interactions to a greater degree than those who would today, in his name, repudiate or de-emphasize them.

Plato

Plato and his mentor, Socrates, also raised the rational to new heights, and even turned its light on subjective experience. Plato considered mind and body as separate. His reflections moved him to divide the mind into opposing elements. Two such elements were the "rational" and the "instinctual" (11). Their competing claims might be harmonized by means of "*dialogues*" aimed at allowing reason to gain ascendancy. These dialogues have been called precursors of the conflict model of psychoanalytic psychotherapy—yet they differ, because "the analytic dialogue deals directly with the emotions while the philosophical dialogue attempts to discard them" (5).

Does the Platonic approach have a psychosomatic perspective too? Yes. "As it is not proper to cure the eyes without the head, nor the head without the body, so neither is it proper to cure the body without the soul"—Socrates (1).

ROMANS

Saint Luke, physician, disciple, and son of a classical migraineur recognized that migraine had psychological aspects and treated it with a form of counseling.

In medicine, as in so many other things, the Romans widely dispersed what the Greeks had handed them and advanced it slightly. Headache diagnoses are now roughly differentiated, thanks to Aretaeus of Cappadocia. He divided what was probably migraine ("heterocrania") from other acute headaches ("cephalagia"), and from chronic ones ("cephalea") (12). Another Roman physician, Cornelius Celsus, noted the constitutional nature of heterocrania (migraine), and ascribed the following symptoms to it:

There is much torpor, heaviness of the head, anxiety, and weariness. For they flee the light; the darkness soothes their disease: nor can they bear readily to look upon or hear anything disagreeable . . . (12).

Soranus of Ephesus described visual disturbances in heterocrania, and named them scotomata (13).

Representative of Roman medical thinking was the physician Galen who, in the second century A.D., set a benchmark unequaled for centuries. Like Hippocrates, Galen considered the brain to be the center of reason, sensation, and emotion. He thought the physical realities of a person ultimately determined thoughts and feelings, and were, therefore, primary. Yet, he also believed, like the Asclepian priests, that clarifying talk helped many patients find symptomatic relief (1). In this regard he displayed a surprising level of psychosomatic sophistication:

Galen reported that he began treating one case of depression with two causative possibilities in mind: the physical cause of the overbalance of black bile, and the psychic cause of inordinate desire. An erratic pulse in his woman patient at the mention of the dancer Pylades caused him to choose the second alternative (11).[4]

Regrettably, Galen considered the primary cause of hemicrania to be black bile irritating the brain (13).

The word pain itself derives from the latin *poena*, literally meaning "penalty" or "punishment." Presumption of a causal relationship between divine displeasure and suffering had far from died out. This view is substantiated both by what followed the reign of Rome and by a treatment proposed by no less august a Roman than Pliny the Elder: draping a hangman's noose over the aching head. This symbolic confession/submission continued in folk remedies for headache into the 19th century, where it reappears in the Appalachian Mountains, the hangman's noose symbolically replaced by a flour sack (3).

A second remedy advocated by Pliny was to tie lichens scraped from the head of a statue to the sufferers neck, using red string (his philosophy was presumably better than his physic). His contemporaries advocated applying other herbal remedies directly to the dolorous head. This belief, that a substance's pain relieving power increased with its proximity to the pain, was sophistry disguised as pharmacology, as its superficially logical hy-

---

[4] This was actually a controlled experiment, because deliberate mentioning of other men's names was first shown not to affect the pulse.

pothesis was divorced from empirical confirmation.

MIDDLE AGES

In the 12th century, the Abbess Hildegard of Bingen set down in an illuminated manuscript her interpretation, consonant with her time and calling, of what is widely considered to have been a migraine aura:

"I saw a great star all splendid and beautiful, and with it an exceeding multitude of falling sparks which with the star followed southward . . . and suddenly they were all annihilated, being turned into black coals . . . and cast into the abyss so that I could see them no more . . . all these I see not with the outward eye . . . but within my spirit, my eyes being open."

Since she believed these recurring visual phenomena to be divinely inspired, one can imagine her resentment had any physician "cured" them! (7, 11).

Perhaps the rapid philosophical advances in understanding mind/body relationships made by leading thinkers of the Classical period perplexed less educated Romans or frightened more superstitious ones; in any case, such progress was unable to hold the high ground indefinitely. Following the fall of Rome the so-called Dark Ages brought regression towards childlike, primary process explanations of pain, and treatment again took to the roads of exorcism and magic.

Primitive treatments were often advocated. In 10th century Arabia, for example, one headache remedy involved applying a hot iron to the head (3), an intervention which undoubtedly distracted the patient from his original distress! A Moorish treatment sprang from their theorem that, by using a specific ritual, illness could be transferred to someone else. For headache, the ritual was to beat a lamb or goat senseless, thus transferring the pains to the unfortunate animal (7).

As a palliative for the anger underlying many headaches this remedy may have proved more effective than uplifting.

These treatments were used, even though during the dark ages, the Greco-Roman tradition of scientific medicine was largely preserved and expanded in Arabic countries. The physician-philosopher Avicenna expressed thoughts about headache both sophisticated and practical in his 11th century classic, *The Canon of Medicine* (14):

It is asked 'Are symptoms to disease as shadow is to object?' The answer is that the two are associated but not inseparable . . . the term 'symptom' refers to phenomena, some of which are really the direct consequence of the disease, while others are only indirectly its results. . . . A symptom may be at the same time a malady. Thus headache is an effect of fever, but may also last so long as to amount to a 'disease'. . . . Pain such as headache may simply be a symptom. . . . But, to the patient, it is the thing; it is the malady. Little does it concern the patient that there is an underlying cause to be treated if the practitioner proves unable to relieve his pain. Furthermore, persistent pain impairs vitality; in this sense a pain is a disease.

In Avicenna's treatments for pain he recommended "walking about gently for a considerable time . . . aggreeable music—especially if it inclines one to sleep (like the mothers' lullaby to her child in pain)" and "being occupied with something very engrossing, which removes the severity of pain."

In Europe, the Middle Ages were a time of diminished regard for the physician, coincident with an increasing, and ultimately all-consuming, prominence of Church and clergy. Good and bad things happened to people as a result of the will of God, which could be influenced by prayer or by a person's spiritual state. Religious centers and shrines became gathering points for the ill, who wished to draw on their reputed power to heal. Relics of saints and wooden slivers said to be fragments of the true cross were viewed as amulets that might put one in more direct touch with God's healing power. (This idea occasionally resulted in profitable commerce in these items.) Headache treatment was caught up in and ran with the tide.

St. Gregory, Bishop of Tours, wrote enthusiastically on the treatment of headaches through pilgrimage to religious shrines. He recounted instances of miraculous cures, and bore personal witness that he had been promptly relieved of a severe headache by pressing his head to the railing around the tomb of St. Mark (3).

Just as God's influence might enter a person to heal, Satan might claim the soul of the unrepentant, transforming the latter into witch or warlock. Possession was a spiritual emergency requiring exorcism. Even several centuries after the Middle Ages, a young French nun was described (7) as being freed by exorcism from several Satanic Princes who held sway over different portions of her head.

This return to a belief that most illness results from external forces, which had to be fought off or won over, reflected renewed confusion over the boundary between self and nonself, and precluded progress in psychosomatic thinking. Instead, the era was preoccupied with discovering ways to remove bad things from the person (sin, Satan, excess or unbalanced humors) and to introduce good things into him (virtue, healing spirits, or herbal concoctions to which testimonial or custom had ascribed healing powers.)

A certain concreteness of outlook was evidenced in the ministrations of the Middle Ages. For example, Pliny's remedy of plant growth from a statue's head was revived and transformed; the dried moss was now taken from actual human skulls and put in direct touch with the problem area by being powdered and inhaled as snuff. An early manuscript, "The Letter of the Vulture" (7), recommended placing vulture brains mixed with oil in the nose to expel various head ailments. (Eventually the panacea from the New World, tobacco, also taken as snuff, would be advocated for headaches.)

Techniques for removing "bad" things were often equally concrete: for a problem headache the chief medical advisor to the French Court (7) recommended using "dried spanish flies" to induce blisters, which could then be drained of their serous humor. Cupping and bleeding were also popular to draw off offending humors. Such practices, though less harmful than the Neolithic procedure of sawing a hole in the skull, were motivated by a similar wish for purgation. Perhaps the search to vanquish a malign biochemical entity at the root of each headache type embodies these yearnings today.

THE RENAISSANCE

If the Renaissance was a garden flowering with art and green with new ideas, its weeds were a resurgent belief in demonology. These beliefs frequently reached their choking roots toward the mentally ill. Persons with unexplainable physical disorders and pains might also have had to convince their neighbors that these were unrelated to witchcraft or possession.

Medicine was still basically undifferentiated from religion and, with the exception of a few individuals, went along with these formulations. Nevertheless at the same time medicine was taking tentative steps in another direction—towards establishing, at least in some areas, a more separate identity.

Thus Paracelsus, one of the most influential—and controversial—physicians of the Renaissance period, viewed practitioners this way:

There are two kinds of doctors; those who heal miraculously, and those who heal through medicine . . . the physician has to accomplish that which God would have done miraculously, had there been but enough faith in the sick man (15).

[Later, Von Helmont would express, in a stronger voice, a similar view: "Let the divine inquire only concerning God, the naturalist concerning nature." It was a position that led to his arrest for heresy (15).]

Another giant of the Renaissance was Vesalius (15), who reintroduced the serious study of anatomy into medicine. His refinement of methods of autopsy evoked increased regard for the body as a proper area of inquiry for determining the causes of suffering.

The body's surface also attracted more attention in attempts to correlate behavioral characteristics with physiognomy. The thesis of Gian Battista Della Porta (9), widely disseminated in his time, was that a man's physical resemblance to a particular animal could be extrapolated to predict his behiavoral attributes (e.g., cautiousness or aggression). The naivete of this thesis may disguise its historical importance as another step toward recognizing how fully man is related to other species of animal, a conclusion whose final enunciation would have to await Darwin's *The Descent of Man* (16).

The long period during which mankind primarily viewed itself subjectively began its decline during the Renaissance. A preoccupation with the spiritual was to ever so slowly metamorphose into a preoccupation with the material. Blind adherence to subjectivity was gradually replaced by an oftentimes blind adherence to objectivity. The change was not sudden, however, as Galileo was to learn to his great discomfort, nor was it total.

SEVENTEENTH CENTURY

Pascal (11) marked migraine's footsteps not by what he wrote but by where, on the paper, he wrote it: crescent-shaped sections of manuscript pages were left blank, corresponding to the shape of a scotoma. As if to confirm this, doodles in the margin resembled the zigzag pattern of teichopsia.

The pendular movement between these extremes of thought reached its nadir in the 17th century. The resulting balance revived thinking about mind/body interactions. Much of that thought went into trying to discover the particular organ that mediated between emotions and bodily humors; after much de-

liberation Descartes (17), for example, concluded body and soul interact at the pineal gland. This theory was provided direct though specious confirmation by Wepfer (18), whose autopsy of a young murderess revealed a calcified pineal gland "in keeping with her stone-hearted deed."

Although Descartes' conclusion about the pineal gland has aged poorly,[5] the often-maligned Cartesian dualism, in which mind and body are separated, has much to be said for it. It began to differentiate the thinking (to which the laws of subjectivity and even of primary process could apply) from the being (to which only objective physical, chemical, and biological laws would be found to apply). This distinction is true whether a person is because he thinks, or whether he thinks because he is—and it is even true if both positions are moot.

Resistance to the new objectivity was hard to sustain. The philosopher Bishop Berkley tried with logical argument to prove that, because one can only know things subjectively, one must assume that nothing beyond the subjective exists; but the reaction of most people to these solopsistic discourses was similar to that of Dr. Samuel Johnson who, kicking at a stone in the road, exclaimed, "Thus do I disprove Bishop Berkley"; and Berkley's reasonings did not slow the sweep toward objectification.

Church and tradition were powerful, however, their wisdom and influence not to be brushed aside. Working out the balance between religion and what was to become, eventually, defined as science, was not easy and still continues. It is as though an undeclared compromise gave religion dominion over subjective sources of knowledge, while science primarily focused on supposedly objective ones. Medicine has ties to each. Because objective study of mind must unavoid-

---

[5] Descartes made many more enduring, though less notorious, contributions to psychosomatics. For example, he is considered to have espoused the existence of a "physiological unconscious" (17).

ably encompass both perspectives, psychology has often appeared to each side as unhealthily tainted by the influence of the other.

During this particular era the clinical approach to psychological aspects of headache was undoubtedly pulled to and fro by these competing points of view. In 1683 the great neuroanatomist Thomas Willis (11, 19) published an interesting case history of a patient with chronic headaches:

Some twenty years since, I was sent for to visit a most noble lady . . . sick with an almost continual headache, at first intermitting: she was of a most beautiful form, and a great wit, so that she was skilled in the liberal arts, and in all forms of literature, beyond the condition of her sex, and as if it were thought too much by nature, for her to enjoy so great endowments without some detriment, she was extremely punished with this disease. . . . But although this distemper, most grievously afflicting this noble lady, above 20 years (when I saw her) having pitched its tent near the confines of the brain, had so long besieged its regal tower, yet had not taken it: for the sick lady . . . found the chief faculties of her soul sound enough.[1]

Note in Willis' description the familiar theme of the headache being external to, even at odds with, the headache sufferer, and of its having been visited upon her, not by the gods now, but instead by a personified "nature," seemingly out of envy or as punishment.

AGE OF ENLIGHTENMENT

Carolus Linnaeus was a physician migraineur. His intense concern with minutiae was evidenced by his seminal organization of taxonomy. One curious problem attributed to Linnaeus, and perhaps a migraine symptom, was a recurring hallucination that his own double was shadowing him and mimicking his movements (11). This is called autoscopy, a rare phenomenon appearing

[1] Reprinted with permission of Wissenschaftliche Verlagsgesellschaft mbH, Stuttgart, West Germany.

in the literature of both psychiatry and neurology.

The 18th century French psychiatrist Pinel (9) anticipated later theories of psychosomatic functioning when he affirmed that it was the passions, not the pineal, that linked mind to body. In general, however, the excitement generated by man's new capacities to understand cause-and-effect relationships overshadowed any incipient interest in psychosomatic approaches. Thus, in his monumental work on pathological anatomy, Morgagni (20) described diseased organs as the specific seats of specific diseases. With regard to headache, he elaborated an argument to prove that, contrary to prevailing opinion, worms do not pass into the living brain through the nose, where they had been thought to grow and cause both brain putrefaction and head pain:

What then? You will say; shall we believe that no little animal, no soot, no snuff was ever found within the cavity of the skull? Indeed, I suspect that whoever asserts in his writings his having really seen such things, was certainly imposed upon, either by tricks of some juggler, by chance, or by his own incautiousness. For you know how deceitful the hands of jugglers are . . .

Yet, Morgagni does not dispute the possibility of worms in the frontal sinuses as a cause of pain, and cites examples such as this:

In a like manner the learned Heuchelius, when he saw two little worms like weevils coming forth by the same way (nostrils), and freeing the patient from the most violent tortures of the head, judg'd that they (the very minute egg of the insect) had been perhaps drawn up into the cavities of the nose, by incautiously smelling to flowers: for the young of these animals are frequently harbour'd there and it is not uncommon for us, to apply them close to our nostrils, while we make a full and strong inspiration.

He also described an early case of what is almost surely cluster headache:

I remember when I was a young man, I had a patient among my companions, in the place of my birth, by name Lawrence Bagattrini, who had been seiz'd not long before with an external, but very violent hemicrania, which returned every day at the eleventh hour, according to the method of reckoning the hours among the Italians. Whatever I did, had either no effect at all, or at least only that of shortening and alleviating the pain, for it still return'd at the same hour; and if any little error, or irregularity, was committed, it return'd with its former vehemence. Having for many days us'd all other remedies in vain, I at length got the better of the disorder, by means of a slight decoction of the woods; which gently agitating and impelling the circulating juices, threw the patient into sweats, and relieved him of his disorder. And Allonius testifies, that the same method succeeded with him also, in intolerable hemicranias, that return'd every day, at a certain hour.

Morgagni laid the groundwork for Virchow's ultimate conclusion in the following century that "There are . . . only diseases of organs and of cells" (21). While such positions would ultimately be applied with a dogmatism, their revolutionary stand was urgently needed at the time. The "big picture" of man in his universe had been focused on so exclusively and for so long that medical knowledge had become mummified in precedent, mysticism, unsupported generalizations, and unchallenged perspectives. In contrast, small organelles were now being observed for the first time, and cause-and-effect relationships never before imagined were inexorably becoming documented. Scientifically imprecise techniques, including psychosomatic ones, threatened this movement and were rejected, were viewed as too closely aligned to miracle cures of the past. Mesmer's demonstration of the power of hypnosis, for example, was scorned. Instead, medical enthusiasm pursued the detailed understanding of partial processes that could be isolated from the whole and firmly understood.

It was in this scientific climate that William Heberden (22), in his seminal *Commentaries on the History and Cure of Diseases*, cautiously emphasized how little was known about headache:

The nature of headaches is extremely obscure. Their manifest causes are very various, and often contrary to one another . . . Among the more tractable headaches, the same means, for no obvious reason, have had such opposite effects in relieving and exasperating similar pains, that it must be left to more enlightened posterity to lay down a certain method of cure; it not being always easy to satisfy ourselves in determining which is the most probable.

Heberden has still less to say about psychological influences:

Anxiety and perturbation of spirit, noise, fatigue of mind or body, too much light, the air of a room heated by a crowd of people, indigestion, and the acts of sneezing and coughing, have almost a certain and universal effect of making headaches worse.

Note that it is not the social encounter with the roomful of people, but their effect upon ambient temperature that is focused on as the causative agent.

As we have seen before, the mind/body persuasions of the age are reflected in its practice of medicine, and its practice of medicine is reflected in its treatment of headache.

NINETEENTH CENTURY

Migraineur Charles Darwin had a sensitive nature in many ways as familiar to his contemporaries as was his genius. Throughout his childhood, Charles assumed an almost permanent posture of apology for not measuring up to his overbearing father's expectations. As an adult he shunned crowds, and was almost incapable of relaxation (7).

Throughout the 19th century medical "objectivity" continued to consolidate its gains, mindful of religious sensibilities, yet less cowed by them. The time was not right for an attempt to synthesize the new discoveries with subjective approaches of the past, however. Even the objectifiable findings of Darwin, Pasteur, and Lister had to fight their battles for acceptance from the low ground. Thus

In the 19th Century the mind-body schism

spread to its furthest division. . . . Indeed, the thoroughly somatic or materialistic tenor of the times was shown by such scientists as Thomas Huxley (1825–1895), who believed that mental processes in themselves had no causal significance but were simply the product of somatic activity (1).

Of course, some workers paid attention to psychosomatic relationships—indeed, the term "psychosomatic" was coined in this century, [though there is disagreement over whether its author was Heinroth (1, 5, 9) or the poet Coleridge (23)].

In 1873 Liveing (24) published a scholarly work bringing together much of what was known about migraine. In it he noted that the disorder could be attributed in some measure to general mismanagement or faulty habits of life.

An article by Teed (25) in the *Journal of Nervous and Mental Diseases* 3 years after Liveing gives a flavor of late 19th century American attitudes toward migraine. Teed, himself a physician, had very personal observations, having suffered from this disorder for more than 40 years.

In investigating the causes of migraine, we find that attacks are limited to certain persons. . . . Those that suffer from it, or others of their family, manifest a peculiar mobility of the nervous system. . . . The first cause, therefore, arises from the natural constitution of the individual, under which the neurine may become so imperfect as to become thrown into commotion by such extremely slight causes . . . .

The treatment of this disorder is on the whole, most unsatisfactory . . . while the remedies recommended are legion, the curative efforts are directed towards the wrong portion of the causation. . . . The periphery receives attention, while the centre is neglected, or the only endeavor is to remove the central disturbance, i.e. the pain, immediately, and then trust to chance for its remaining absent for a longer or a shorter time, until the next attack . . . the list of remedies for migraine that have been reported as successful would of itself fill a volume. And yet the attacks return . . . .

But the man of business cannot leave his business; the literary man cannot leave his studies, nor the professional man his work; their daily bread depends on their following different pursuits; the fashionable lady will not relinquish the excitement of society, the hard working woman has no time to lay herself up; and yet in all of these and in a hundred other conditions of life, the physician is required to control these attacks . . . .

Migraine is often the result of some injurious habits, and these habits are the particular delight, and give direction to the life of the patient; thus it becomes almost impossible to break them off; and this gives the great difficulty in the treatment.

The work of Gowers is generally considered to be a high point in the ascendence of neurology during the 19th century, and his teachings set the tone for neurological writings well into this century. It is therefore surprising to note that, despite his genius in other areas, he discouraged attention to psychosomatic correlations. In his 1888 edition of *A Manual of Diseases of the Nervous System* (26), he presents his case quite clearly, and it is quintessentially materialistic:

In the study of diseases of the brain we are concerned only with cerebral processes. Unfortunately, however, the chief terms available are those of psychology, and we are obliged, therefore, to speak of mental processes when all that we need speak of, and are indeed justified in speaking of, are cerebral processes. However undesireable such a confusion may be, it is practically unavoidable.

In his section on migraine (17 pages in length) Gowers is true to his stated intentions: not a psychological word can be found. In the section on headache he clearly distinguishes real—organic—headache from "head pressure and other cephalic sensations." Of the latter, corresponding roughly to what we would today call tension headache, he remarks that

It may be called 'headache' or 'pain,' but however intense it is, inquiry shows that the sensation has not the character of actual pain, either acute or dull.

He considers that

Many of the slighter, continuous headaches associated with nervous weakness are largely maintained by attention, as is the case to an even greater degree with the cephalic sensations . . .

As a result

The only method of treatment that is effective is to make the patient realize the unimportant nature of the sensations, and try to neglect them by directing his attention to other subjects . . . he should persistently endeavor to 'snub' rather than to cultivate them. . . . Unfortunately the mental condition of some patients makes it impossible for them to thus ignore their sufferings; they continue to attend to the sensations, doubt the assurances of physicians who assert the unimportant nature of the sufferings, and seek the advice of others . . . his best chance of recovery is to keep away from doctors altogether.

TWENTIETH CENTURY

The noted neurologist (he did important work in cerebral palsy) and psychiatrist Sigmund Freud also had migraine. His headaches, sometimes frequent, were especially likely on Sundays. About these "weekend headaches": Freud was continually troubled by the anti-Semitic atmosphere he believed present in Vienna, and his reflections suggested that feelings about the "Christian Sabbath" triggered attacks.

Freud

Toward the end of the 19th century, widespread use of medical hypnosis documented the power of psychological forces to affect disease. The medical world's increasingly organic orientation was captured instead by the new chemical anesthesias (5). Nevertheless, the attention of at least one neurologist, a certain Sigmund Freud, was compellingly drawn to Charcot's demonstrations of hypnosis, and they planted the seeds of his later theories on

conversion hysteria. Freud realized not only that the mind could dramatically affect the body, but that it did so routinely, systematically, and for definite reasons; he would later show many of these reasons to be analyzable. The ultimate implications of this for both understanding and treating headaches are well known. However, this required him to first elucidate the concept of an unconscious (in some ways, actually, to resurrect it from the time of the Greeks), with its hidden needs, conflicts, and symbols.[6]

Freud and his followers studied free verbal productions systematically and objectively to understand the structures and organizing principles of the mind, just as Darwin had collected beaks of finches to see if there was biological method in their varied shapes. And just as Darwin learned from the bones of extinct species the genesis of current ones, Freud found that a patient's early memories could shed light on his current problem. From these explorations, the pathogenetic role of active unconscious complexes became apparent. These concepts finally fixated many of the more mysterious causes and instigators of physical distress within the recesses of the patient's own psyche. The concept of the unconscious allowed people to claim "ownership" of these forces while appreciating why they seemed as alien and inaccessible as the distant gods and spirits of the past.

What were Freud's thoughts on headache? During the period when his migraines were most troublesome Freud was intensely involved in his self-analysis, assisted by his good friend and physician, Wilhelm Fleiss. Fleiss also had migraine, yet was convinced

---

[6] Indeed, much of Freud's work consisted of a revival, integration, and redefinition of ideas formulated earlier but not synthesized into a unified theory. For example, as early as the 16th century, Juan Luis Vives (17) described the importance of psychological associations "delineating their evidence through 'similarity, contiguity, and opposites.' " He has been credited with being the first "to fathom the emotional issues underlying some associations, and the retrieving of long forgotten experiences through processes of association."

his headaches were related to an elusive nasal condition. As a result, he repeatedly had minor surgical procedures done on his nose in hopes of curing the headaches—to little avail. According to Schur (27) (Freud's physician in later years), these shared headache symptoms increased Freud's identification with Fleiss; it was an identification which, because of loyalty towards his friend, initially inhibited Freud from fully applying his insightfulness to psychological aspects of migraine. Yet his correspondence shows an increasing conviction of its relevance, especially as a trigger. In a letter he warns Fleiss:

Dearest friend . . . you are having severe headaches and are anticipating further surgery; this might sound gloomy and disagreeable if I did not fully share your expectation that the course you have taken [more nasal surgery] will free you from headaches. Just promise me one thing right now, and that is not to forget the factor which immediately precedes the knot[ty problem] "headache", and which is of a purely nervous nature . . . we shall write or talk about this further.

Schur concludes

On the basis of his correspondence with Fleiss we may assume that during the decade of their close relationship many of Freud's migraine attacks were in fact precipitated by intense stress, especially in his self-analysis. After the analysis had freed him from overt symptoms . . . and above all (of) his trans-ferencelike conflicts, the migraine attacks were of no great import and Freud's interest in migraine as a psychosomatic symptom consequently receded. However, during the years I acted as his physician, he still had migraine on the days of the Fohn.

Sigmund Freud: neurologist, psychoanalyst, migraineur. Were he alive, how might he have integrated the knowledge gained in these three roles with the scientific advances of today?

Modern Pioneers

Recognition that symbolic unconscious conflicts were the basis of conversion reactions was such an important theoretical advance

that *all* types of psychophysiological events were soon hooked onto this one bandwagon. Therefore, some theoreticians (28) tried to understand such psychologically influenced disorders as ulcerative colitis and peptic ulcer—and even, on occasion, fever and hemorrhage—as conversion symptoms symbolically expressing conflicts through the autonomic nervous system. In time, work by Cannon (29) and by Selye (30) showed that endocrine and autonomic nervous system responses to intense emotions distinguished psychophysiological disorders from symptoms mediated by the voluntary nervous system (conversion reactions).

Flanders Dunbar (31) and later Alexander (32), systematically correllated personality styles with illness. Alexander's work emphasized the *unconscious similarities* between patients with the same psychologically influenced disorder. His group distinguished conflicts stimulating the parasympathetic nervous system, which they considered a result of strong, unexpressed dependency needs, from those expressed through the sympathetic nervous sytem, which more typically related to conflicts stimulating aggression and fear. They saw psychosomatic breakdown as the result of a patient with a predisposing genetic vulnerability of a tissue, organ, or system encountering a situation that specifically reactivated old needs and conflicts. Manifest disease, therefore, came from the interaction between physical and emotional, historical and situational factors.

Between 1940 and 1960 it was observed (28) that many medical illnesses first appeared at times of psychosocial stress, and that remissions often coincided with a reduction in that stress. This was also a period when researchers monitored subjects physiologically while discussing topics designed to activate specific conflicts or affects.

In this way virtually every tissue and organ of the body innervated by the autonomic nervous system and available for observation or intubation, or accessible to electronic recording from surface or depth electrodes in unanesthesized humans was shown to be capable of considerable functional variability in reaction to a wide variety of provocative experimental

manipulations (From "Changing Theoretical Concepts in Psychosomatic Medicine," from *American Handbook of Psychiatry*, vol IV, edited by Silvano Arieti and Morton F. Reiser. Copyright 1975 by Basic Books Inc. Reprinted by permission of the publisher.)

Harold Wolff and Stuart Wolff—names well known in headache research—are also important names in general psychosomatics. They emphasized the significance of the physiological concomitants of defensive reactions—adaptive or maladaptive ones. Two of Wolff's students, Grace and Graham (33), proposed that it is the specific, long-standing attitude with which a person approaches life, accentuated at times of strain, that determines his most vulnerable organ system. Margolin (34) evolved the concept that the physiology itself can undergo a stress-induced regression to the point where it resembles the functional state present at a time of unsolved and forgotten conflict.

In the late 1960s, physiological recordings were shared with patients in the hope that this knowledge would allow them to influence it. It did, and clinical biofeedback was the result. Important for headache was the use of thermal feedback for migraine by Sargent et al. (35) and the introduction of electromyographic feedback for tension headache by Budzynski, Stoyva, and Adler (36).

The tone of this recent theoretizing is different from that of centuries past. Theories are stated in such a way that it is clear that they could be bolstered or overturned by evidence. Most importantly, their view of the mind is a scientific one, and the relationship between cerebral, somatic, social, emotional, and existential moorings is finally—we hope—correct.

CONCLUSION

Our century has seen a mushrooming of psychosomatic thought and the formulation of verifiable hypotheses about interactions between mind and body. We have seen the power of scientific medicine grow to a point at which it should now be secure enough to look back, we hope with only slight trepidation, towards the subjective.

The promise of psychiatry is its potential to view subjectivity objectively. Despite these centuries of progress, the subjective remains an infinitely complex and elusive kingdom in its own right and one that stubbornly defies definition by statistics, however urgent the wish or pure the motivation. Besides, human nature still yearns for magic, the simple explanation, and the panacea.

Freud's ambitious "project for a scientific psychology," in which he attempted to construct a purely biological model of mental processes, eludes us still, and we must cultivate patience while awaiting its day of completion. Each time the subjective resists domination—even domestication—by objectivity, fears arise in the scientific community. These fears relate not only to the collective memory of demonology in the Middle Ages and witch hunts in the Renaissance, but also to personal, immediate experiences each of us had in childhood, when parents seemed omniscient and reindeer flew through the air bearing gifts. Even in so cut-and dried an approach as biofeedback many patients view the instrument as a magical talisman that will confer to them secret powers over their bodies (rather than as a neutral tool to help them modestly influence psychosomatic interactions). Thus, there is still cause to fear that medicine might retreat from dealing with the subjective at all.

The fundamental psychological postulate of modern medicine is that the body and its functions can be understood in terms of physical chemistry, that living organisms are physio-chemical machines, and the ideal of the physician is to become an engineer of the body (31).

In large measure, psychiatry itself seems to be turning away from psychological appoaches, perhaps on the one hand sharing its medical colleagues' frustration at being unable to adequately subjugate the subjective and, on the other, wishing to be partners in the current exponential growth of man's capacity to subordinate the material world.

The question that remains unanswered is whether the recently reawakened awareness of the emotional components of illness will prove just a momentary shudder in the pendulum's continuing swing up toward materialism, or whether that pendulum is indeed slowing or even returning toward center. The key to its answer may well lie in the capacity of those exploring psychophysiologic interactions—such as those that occur with headaches—to tolerate frustration. To position oneself in this field means foregoing the "certainty" (all-encompassing, but not necessarily correct) that denizens of the 12th century had about causality, and it likewise means foregoing the "certainty" (correct, but so limited and partial that it often lacks value) of the biochemist.

Tolerating the insecurity of this middle road is our severest challenge. It is especially hard to dampen that moment of pride at finally elucidating the pathophysiology of headache by focusing on the possible limitations of that knowledge for understanding or influencing a patient's general welfare. It will not be helpful to us, as it was not helpful to the Egyptians before us, to divide knowledge against itself, or to value only its more easily measured segment. Indeed, the more we know about propensities toward irrationality, the more we can guarantee that it will not, for purposes of wish fullfillment, be unwittingly infused into our perceptions of nature's more obscure phenomena.

Many of the symptoms seen in headache work are only final links in a long causal chain; the origins of that chain are hidden deep within the brain, the mind—in the very sense of self. In our hearts we know how long it will take to follow the links of that chain to its primal mooring, and we know this is not an easy time frame to accept in an era of instant gratification. But the rewards of pursuing that long-range goal will be no less than a comprehensive theory of medicine, one incorporating both psychological and physiological realities of man. Although our generation may not reach that goal, perhaps some future one that does will look back and, with kind remembrance, note that we were the ones who targeted it in our sights and committed our resources to it.

In the meantime we must be pragmatists. We must use the objective when we know it and deal with the subjective as best we can. This is especially difficult in the face of the subjectivity of pain and its relief. In our slow progress toward understanding, neither can we afford to be intolerant of the patient, despite his often bewildering mixture of hope and eclecticism:

It is not uncommon, Bruner observes, to see a woman with a migraine headache first bind her brow with the leaf of a wild arum lily as did her Indian predecessors; then consult a curandera to have the causative hex lifted as did her Spanish ancestors in the Dark Ages; and finally go to a modern quack in the next village to have herself injected because, 'injections are good' (7).

It is astonishing how successful we have been at treating headache without even fully knowing what pain is or being able to accurately define how drugs and other interventions relieve it. The fact that we nonetheless often can efficiently block the pain of headache is, perhaps, as close as we dare come, in the present day, to magic.

REFERENCES

1. Kaplan HI: History of psychosomatic medicine. In Kaplan HI, Freedman AM, Sadock BJ (eds): *Comprehensive Textbook of Psychiatry III.* Baltimore, Williams & Wilkins, 1980, pp 1843–1853.

2. American Psychiatric Association: *Diagnostic and Statistical Manual of Mental Disorders,* ed 3. Washington, DC, American Psychiatric Association, 1980.

3. Friedman AP, Frazier, SH: *The Headache Book.* New York, Dodd, Mead, 1973, p 9.

4. Jaynes J: *The Origin of Consciousness in the Breakdown of the Bicameral Mind.* Boston, Houghton Mifflin, 1976.

5. Buckly PJ: An historical perspective on psychological treatment of medical illnesses. In Karsu

TB, Steinmuller RI (eds): *Psychotherapeutics in Medicine*. New York, Grune & Stratton, 1978, pp 1–11.

6. Adler CS: The meaning of death to children. *Arizona Med* March: 266–276, 1969.

7. Friedman AP: The headache in history, literature, and legend. *Bull NY Acad Med* 48:661–81, 1982.

8. Dudley R, Rowland W: *How to Find Relief from Migraine*. New York, Beaufort Books, 1982, p 17.

9. Breasted JH (ed): *The Edwin Smith Surgical Papyrus*. Chicago, University of Chicago Press, 1930, p 213.

10. Anderson EG: A mosaic of medical history. *Private Pract* April:67, 1985.

11. Critchley M: Migraine: From Cappadocia to Queen Square. In Smith R (ed): *Background To Migraine*. London, Alellign Henmann Medical Books, 1967, pp 28–38.

12. Kolb LC: *Modern Clinical Psychiatry*, ed 9. Philadelphia, Saunders, 1977, pp 3–9.

13. Bille B: Migraine in school children. *Acta Paediatr* 51(Suppl 136):13–14, 1962.

14. Avicenna: *The Canon of Medicine of Avicenna* (translated by OC Gruner. London, Luzac, 1930.

15. Osler W: *The Evolution of Modern Medicine*. New Haven, CN, Yale University Press, 1921, pp 140–163.

16. Darwin C: *The Descent of Man*. Norwalk, CN, Easton Press, 1979.

17. Schneck JM: *A History of Psychiatry*. Springfield, IL, Charles C Thomas, 1960, pp 50–51.

18. Isler H: Johann Jakob Wepfer (1620–1895): Discoveries in headache. *Cephalalgia: Int J Headache* 5(Suppl 3):424–425, 1985.

19. Isler H: *Thomas Willis 1621–1675: Doctor and Scientist*. New York, Hafner, 1968.

20. Morgagni GB: *The Seats and Causes of Diseases*, vol 1. London, Johnson & Payne, 1769, pp 3–17.

21. Virchow R: *Cellular Pathology*. London, John Churchhill, 1860.

22. Heberden W: *Commentaries on the History and Cure of Diseases*. London, T. Payne, 1802, p 97.

23. Levy NB: The giving-up-given-up complex. In Simons RC, Pardes H (eds): *Understanding Human Behavior in Health and Illness*. Baltimore, Williams & Wilkins, 1977.

24. Liveing E: *On Megrim, Sick Headache, and Some Allied Disorders*. London, J. & A. Churchhill, 1873.

25. Teed JL: On migraine. *J Nerv Ment Dis* 3:241–352, 1976.

26. Gowers WR: *A Manual of Diseases of the Nervous System*. Philadelphia, P. Blakiston & Son, 1888, pp 531, 1171–1196.

27. Schur M: *Freud: Living and Dying*. New York, International Universities Press, 1972, pp 78, 98–100.

28. Reiser MF: Changing theoretical concepts in psychosomatic medicine. In Arieti S, Reiser MF (eds): *American Handbook of Psychiatry*, vol IV, ed 2. New York, Basic Books, 1975, pp 477–500.

29. Cannon WB: *The Wisdom of the Body*. New York, Norton, 1932.

30. Selye H: *The Physiology and Pathology of Exposure to Stress*. Montreal, Acta, 1960.

31. Dunbar F: *Emotions and Bodily Changes*. New York, Columbia University Press, 1954.

32. Alexander F: *Psychosomatic Medicine: Its Principles and Applications*. New York, Norton, 1950.

33. Grace WJ, Graham DT: Relationship of specific attitudes and emotions to certain bodily diseases. *Psychosom Med* 14:243–251, 1952.

34. Margolin SG: Genetic and dynamic psychophysiological determinants of pathophysiological processes. In Deutsch F: *The Psychosomatic Concept in Psychoanalysis*. New York, International Universities Press, 1953, pp 3–36.

35. Sargent J, Walters D, Green E: Psychosomatic self-regulation of migraine headaches. *Semin Psychiatry* 5:415–428, 1973.

36. Budzynski TH, Stoyva J, Adler CS: Feedback-induced muscle relaxation: application to tension headache. *J Behav Ther Exp Psychiatry* 1:205–211, 1970.

The Inscrutability of Pain, with Particular Reference to Migraine and to Headache

CHAPTER
TWO

MACDONALD CRITCHLEY, M.D.

INTRODUCTION

The head pains in migraine offer an opportunity for mulling over the nature and meaning of painful experiences in general. Migraine is a common disorder, afflicting, it is believed, at least 10 percent of the community. It has been known to medical men longer than any other disorder with the exception of epilepsy. More than 2000 years ago it was clearly described, and since then there have been scores of brilliant accounts of the symptomatology, many supplied by physicians who were themselves migraineurs. During the past 30 years an upsurge in interest in this subject has taken place throughout the world, and yet, despite much physiological and pharmacological research, the advance in basic knowledge has been disappointing. During the past century speculation as to the cause of the migrainous diathesis and even about the actual source of the pain has roamed far and wide. Within living memory, indeed, the *fons et origo morbi* has shifted from the liver and bile ducts to the cerebrum.

Again, one can seriously inquire whether the power to relieve an attack of migraine has materially improved over the years, and whether prophylaxis has become more effec-

tive. Our memories do not go back far enough, so that comparisons are not possible. That there is a gap in our ability to shorten the attacks and to reduce their frequency has given support to a considerable gallimaufry of incursions into alternative medicine. This would never be so if we were in firm possession of a panacea.

Migraine is by no means the sole variety of headache. For reasons we do not understand, the head constitutes a *locus minoris resistentiae,* and headache must surely be one of the commonest complaints that induces a person to seek medical advice. Some have ventured to explain this clinical fact by reference to the concept of the body image, pointing out that the focus of personal indentity lies, most of the time, somewhere in the forepart of the cranium. This may be so, but the hypothesis is not supported by the realization that pain in the small of the back is an even commoner complaint than headache.

The cause of headache in a particular patient may prove to be trivial and no threat to the organism; on the other hand, headache may be a warning of a pathological calamity, such as meningitis or tumor, or of an intractable and enduring condition such as Paget's disease of the skull. Diagnosis is not helped by any correlation between intensity and gravity. A patient with an intracranial growth may be walking around and working despite his headache.

THE NATURE OF PAIN

Philosophers have had a great deal to say about the nature of pain and in particular about its function. Much of it is nonsense and based upon superstition as sanctimonious as it is cruel. Has pain, irrespective of its site, any teleological meaning, any purpose? In the past, biologists have tended to regard the role of pain as protective, betraying the presence of injurious influences, or of disease. Thus Herbert Spencer (1) pronounced: "pain is the correlation of some species of wrong—some kind of divergence from that course of action which perfectly fills all requirements." Presumably he was trying to say "pain means that something is the matter."

Though short, the memory of pain may condition behavior. Richet (2) said that pain is one of the bases of intelligence, because the existence of pain determines the conduct of all beings above the rank of pure automata. Some have gone further, and claimed that suffering has stimulating powers of immense therapeutic value; that it may constitute a positive virtue and in some persons act as a spur to work. Charles Bell (3), who should have known better, said that pain "is the companion and the guardian of human life." One hundred fifty years ago an eminent surgeon proclaimed that pain was a wise provision of nature, and patients ought to suffer pain while their surgeons were operating; that they were all the better for it and recovered better.

Some theologians, like some savages, have proclaimed pain to be a cleansing experience, and that its victims undergo a state of spiritual purification.

If pain is a "vigilant sentinel," to use a common cliche, then it must be rated a highly inefficient one, erratic and unreliable. Some deadly disorders, slowly or rapidly advancing, run their sinister course without the victim having suffered a moment's "pain" in the true sense of the word. On the other hand, certain intense and incurable pains serve no ostensible purpose; they are meaningless. As examples one can enumerate tic douloureux, the postherpetic neuralgias, and certain "central" pains, like those occurring in phantom limbs or the hemialgia of thalamic disease.

Surely pain is more malefic than protective; Nietzsche (4) spoke of "the senselessness of suffering." As Sir James Young Simpson, the pioneer of chloroform anaesthesia, put it: "All pain is *per se,* and especially when in excess, destructive, and even ultimately fatal in its action and effects. It exhausts the principle of life. It exhausts both the system and the part. Mere pain *can* destroy life" (5). Albert Schweitzer, too, was in no doubt about any alleged atoning effect: "Pain is a more terrible lord of mankind than even death itself" (6).

ON THE NATURE AND DESCRIPTION OF HEADACHE PAIN

Is it conceivable that migraine is an exception, and that it may fulfill some purpose or bring some cryptic benefit to the victim? The only possible advantage might be in the role of a feedback (in the strict sense of that much-abused word). Could it be that when stress of an emotional, mental, or physical kind reaches a critical level, an attack of migraine might intervene and bring a temporary halt to such a potentially noxious influence? If so, one would expect to find within the community a negative correlation between migraine and the various ailments we currently regard as stress disorders, e.g., peptic ulcer, coronary disease, rheumatoid arthritis, ulcerative colitis. At present, we simply do not know how to answer this quite straightforward question. Surely this would be a rewarding investigation well within the scope of community physicians, general practitioners, and immunologists. I have often made this suggestion, but so far no one has taken it up.

Still, within the ambit of the philosophy

of pain is the matter of the intensity and character of headache. When a patient proclaims he is suffering from a head pain the doctor must accept the statement as a subjective truth. There are no physical signs specific for pain. However, when the headache is migrainous, subtle objective signs may be present. A localized area of the scalp is tender, as is one eyeball. Tenderness is a subjective symptom, but it is confirmed if the patient winces or recoils when the allegedly tender area is stimulated, as by applying pressure. As a rule the eyelids droop. The artery in the temple may be more conspicuous on the side that aches. Pulsations are more bounding, and the vessel is sensitive to the touch. Local applications, either ice cold or hot, bring temporary relief.

When one seeks to ascertain the severity of any pain and its character, the physician relies upon two factors: the behavior of the victim and his description of the symptom. During an intense bout of migraine the patient seeks to stay immobile, either flat in bed or sitting propped up. Patients differ in their choice of posture, but tend to avoid movement. They do not toss or turn the head if they can avoid so doing. Never do they thump the skull or bang it against the wall, like some headache victims. When an intense restlessness is coupled with a complaint of severe pains in the head, one can usually exclude the principal states characterized by intense pains: subarachnoid bleeding, acute meningitis, the headache that follows air encephalography or even lumbar puncture, and some cases of migraine. The suspicion of underlying psychological disorder becomes uppermost.

The patient's statements usually are our only clue to the character of the pain (pressing, pounding, throbbing) and its force. It is within the latter category that the physician is in most doubt. Not only do degrees of severity exist in the case of migrainous headaches, but, more particulary, the choice of language complicates the issue. Some patients habitually employ superlatives and describe as agonizing or excruciating a headache that, judging by the patient's ability to carry on as usual, can scarcely be very severe.

A serious language problem may complicate an interview with an educationally underprivileged patient, or one from another culture. Among some groups the word "pain" is rarely employed. In others, odd metaphors may be used that bewilder the English-speaking doctor. Thus patients from the Caribbean may speak of "weakness" in the head (or on the "top-flat," "noggin," "dome," or "biscuit"). Again, among some primitive peoples, one can elicit no information in reply to a straightforward question such as "Do you ever get headaches?" To a Zulu, such a direct inquiry would be offensive, and no reply would be forthcoming. A physician experienced in the verbal taboos of such a culture might adopt a roundabout method of questioning. One has only to cross the Tweed to realize that a "sore head" represents what is conventionally called a headache elsewhere.

SENSITIVITY TO PAIN

Quite apart from the choice of words to describe severity, there probably exists a true continuum of sensitivity to pain. At one extreme are the hypersensitives who react severely to actual pain and who suffer greatly from even the mere anticipation of pain. By contrast, there are those who seem to possess a relative indifference to pain and for whom it holds no dread. The physical and mental correlates of this continuum are obscure.

Although long-continued pain carries in its wake feelings of despondency, deep melancholia may lie outside the picture. As Hippocrates (7) taught, physical and moral pain are in some ways antagonistic. Few take their lives because of sheer agony. Furthermore, many depressives elect to destroy themselves by methods that are potentially most unpleasant. Interviews with a number of failed suicides have indicated to me that slashing of the wrists or incompetent cutting of the throat were not attended by physical pain at the time.

Physicians realize, of course, that there is a clinical curiosity known as congenital insensitivity to pain. It is a rarity, mysterious in nature. By the time adolescence is reached there are numerous scars of cuts, burns, and fractures, all of which occurred at an earlier date, outside the awareness of the subject.

There are also some otherwise normal persons who admit or even boast that they have never "known what it is to have a headache." Severe blows to the head may produce dizziness or syncope, but not pain. And yet their tissues are not analgesic. Aftermath of alcoholic excess is marked by a hangover in which headache plays no part. Febrile illness, even such commonly painful ailments as sandfly fever and dengue, run their courses without headache.

The study of pain-insensitive patients, or the more commonly encountered patients with a limited form of nonsensitivity, may further our efforts to understand their antithetical counterparts suffering from chronic pain, including headache. It is a physiological axiom that one way to understand a function is to observe the effect of its absence. It is difficult to conceive any anatomical explanation for congenital insensitivity to headache, such as an absence of nerve fibers around the intra and extracranial blood vessels, because we know of no precedent in human morphology that is relevant. Although I have repeatedly called attention to this anomalous condition and urged that the subject be seriously investigated, we remain in the dark.[1]

PAIN OF PSYCHOGENIC ORIGIN

Patients with various psychological disorders not infrequently complain of pain, especially headache. It is then that one hears bizarre descriptions of pain, sometimes associated with odd similes. Probing on the part of the physician often leads to the conclusion that the patient is really referring to a cephalic sensation not quite identical with what is generally understood by "pain." The sensation may prove to be more in the nature of an uncomfortable pressure on top of the head, or a tight band around the cranium, or a sense of fullness or tension within the skull. Feelings of such types are usually not assuaged by even heavy doses of the ordinary analgesic drugs. On the other hand they may respond to antidepressants or tranquilizers. A therapeutic response of this kind is often a useful aid to differential diagnosis.

A true hypochondriac may employ extravagant terminology and speak of a distressing sensation as though the scalp or even the cortex were being eroded by acid or by insects. The use of the term "as if" renders unlikely the existence of a hallucinatory state.

Then there is the vexing question as to whether "psychogenic" pain has any existence at all. In essence, this is something of a quibble. It is dangerous to speak of, or to visualize, any such entity as an imaginary pain. Pain is a subjective experience, and although one might challenge the patient's evaluation of its intensity, it would be unsafe to question its actual existence.

Yet pain, either focal or generalized, may be induced by suggestion, as, for example, by hypnosis. Similarly, powerful emotion may inhibit (if only temporarily) the pains due to injury in the excitement of sport or battle. During states of ecstasy pain may be swamped or even replaced by a pleasurable experience, as evidenced by the martyrology of religion or the self-immolation of fakirs.

Suffering brings in its train a number of mental concomitants, especially if protracted and severe. Oddly enough, depression, as we have seen, is not profound. The ability to obtain pleasure through pain is suggestive of a psychotic state. This is to be distinguished, however, from pain suffered for a cause, which in a different sense glorifies it and provides gratification.

---

[1] Physicians in charge of pain clinics might learn much from questioning those sinister beings whose odious job it is to deliberately inflict pain on others. The period from 1930 to 1950 has probably witnessed more proficient torturers than at any time since the Middle Ages.

René Leriche (8), whose contributions to our ideas about the nature of pain were both original and stimulating, wrote: "Physical pain is not a simple affair of an impulse traveling at a fixed rate along a nerve. It is the resultant of a conflict between a stimulus and a whole individual." How does that conflict show itself? Much depends upon whether the pain is frequent, in which event the sufferer is at least spared the dread as to its possible significance. A sudden, unexpected pain brings with it considerable anxiety as to its nature and import; a sense of impending death may arise. Blissful calm is a myth, because irritability is an understandable accompaniment. Severe pain is demoralizing. It swamps the whole sensorium and concentrates thought to the exclusion of all other feeling. The sense of time is prolonged to an unconscionable degree. Somatic symptoms associated with enduring pain include anorexia, constipation, loss of weight, and sleeplessness.

The more complex psychological side effects of abiding pain arouse the most interest. Complicating and nonspecific in essence, they differ from one victim to another. Often they are quite difficult to describe. Hence the truth of the saying, "If you wish to probe the secrets of nature, read what poets and novelists have had to say." As professionals in manipulating words, nonmedical writers are in a strong position to elucidate what is almost ineluctable, that is, those transcendental pain experiences that baffle the linguistic capacity of less literate sufferers.

It would not be appropriate to quote passage after passage, though this would be easy. One description at least may be taken as exemplifying the intricacy of the matter. Regarding the birth of her second child, Nina Van Pallandt (9) wrote:

I had two breaths of gas. As the pain grew less I seemed to look into an incredible warm yellow light which became whiter and brighter as I was lifted and floated, slowly spinning, upwards. My body stretched, expanded and dissolved into this now unbearable but beautiful blinding white light. An explosion—a death. It was as if, in one split second, I was

totally part of the universe. In the next instant I heard a cry. "Es una niña," ["It's a girl"] the doctor said.

The color imagery with the use of the words "yellow" and "white" is particularly interesting, for it suggests that the writer might have been a potential synesthetic. It is by no means unknown for patients in the throes of an agony to become aware of shapes and, particularly, of colors. The phenomenon is one that lies midway between a vivid image and an actual hallucination. I have described a similar experience occurring in mechanics who sustained powerful electrical shocks (10). Perhaps the earliest reference to this "synalgia" was made by Homer when, in the *Iliad,* he wrote about "arrows, the harbingers of black pains."

For impressive accounts of the distress experienced in a severe attack of migraine, Pamela Hansford Johnson (herself a victim) was unsurpassed. Other extraordinary descriptions of pain are found in the writings of Jack London, who was subjected to torture; Hugh Walpole, for whom pain was an almost masochistic preoccupation; Moritz Jokai, who wrote convincingly about a psychogenic topalgia arising as a manifestation of guilt; Marcel Proust, who dealt with pain in his sleep; and Emma Goldman, in her description of the transmission of pain from a victim to a sympathizer. Special mention is deserved of the incredible diary of torment kept by Alphonse Daudet, entitled *La Doulou;* it describes incomparably the generalized tabetic pains that he endured while incapacitated during the last years of his life.

Whether there is any limit to the sensation of pain is a question raised by H. G. Wells. Does a steady increase in the violence of the stimulus automatically evoke a parallel heightening in the intensity of the pain? Or is there a limit or plateau of feeling? Wells suggested that if pushed beyond a certain point nociceptive agents may even prove pleasurable. This is rather borne out in the case of a Naval officer who managed to escape death from drowning (11). After his rescue he said that, as he tried to inhale while submerged, he had felt an intense, viselike pain in the chest, increasing with each breath. Later, however, his anguish abated. "I appeared to be in a pleasant dream, although I had enough willpower to think of friends at home, and still retain vivid recollections of the clearness of the sight of the Grampians, familiar to me in boyhood, which was brought to my view. Before finally losing consciousness, the chest pain had completely disappeared, and the sensation was actually pleasant."

Although it is commonly acknowledged that the experience of pain is in the brain, not the periphery, this fact is often disregarded in practice. However on occasion an episode will reaffirm this in most dramatic fashion. Take, for example, the following account of a patient of mine seen in 1935:

A male, age 57, at the age of 35 had sustained a crushing injury to the right foot. Though no bones were broken, the resulting pain was severe. Twelve months later, after months in the hospital, the foot was amputated just above the ankle joint on account of the persisting pain. The pain, however, continued not only in the stump but also in the phantom. Two months later a second amputation was carried out in the upper third of the thigh, but with no effect on the pain. A year after that, the stump was explored and the ends of the severed nerves freed and sectioned at a higher level. Because this measure was ineffectual, the sciatic nerve was then exposed and divided in two places. No benefit followed. Nine years after the original trauma, a posterior rhizotomy of the lumbosacral plexus was performed, and because this operation did not help, a chordotomy was conducted in the upper dorsal region. Even this measure failed to assuage the pain. . . . When seen 22 years after the original accident, the patient was still complaining of severe and immutable pain in the stump.

THE GROSS AND SCOPE OF A MIGRAINE CLINIC

Long experience in conducting two migraine and headache clinics has shown me the value of this type of specialized medical provision. Benefit accrues to both migraineurs and migrainologists.

Sufferers from chronic headaches have the advantage of detailed clinical study followed, if need be, by advanced investigative techniques. Not surprisingly, differential diagnosis every now and again discloses an unsuspected brain tumor, a state of malignant hypertension, or a problem that is of purely emotional origin.

Such a clinic also affords the opportunity for drug trials of various remedies in an endeavor to find something a little more effective and a little less toxic than available hitherto. This function, I suggest, ranks lowermost in the role of the clinic. Some such clinics also make provisions for treating patients in the throes of an acute attack. The victim is allowed to rest and relax in quietude, even to be mildly sedated, while any needed studies are carried out on the clinical state or its chemistry.

However, the importance of an adequately staffed migraine and headache clinic may be potentially even greater to the wellbeing of the community. As a matter of experience it can be asserted that the bulk of those attending suffer from some variant of migraine, complicated by an overlay of nonorganic character. Hence, evaluation of each patient may be far from simple. In the same way, management and treatment are complicated matters. Migraine, one finds, is sometimes a way of life, and all too often a veritable *via dolorosa*. Diagnosis must not only be shrewd, but must be seen by the patient to be shrewd and penetrating. The platitudinous term "diagnosis," let us remember, does not entail merely the act of attaching a label to someone's symptoms. By definition, the Greek expression "to diagnose" means to attain knowledge permeating right through the patient and his problem, and of necessity implies understanding not only the nature of the trouble but also its essence, cause, probable outcome, and methods used in its alleviation.

Having ruled out the likelihood of grave intracranial mischief, the doctor must discuss with the patient sympathetically, searchingly, and at length the clinical niceties of the case. As Dr. Samuel Johnson said, "questioning is not the mode of conversation among gentlemen" (12). Nor, for that matter, should it be among doctors; but at the same time neither should the interview be a monologue on the part of the patient. Now and again the doctor must pose a question, because patients do not always realize the relative significance of individual symptoms. Otherwise some key points may be glossed over, or others totally forgotten. Occasional interventions on the part of the doctor also demonstrate that he is still alert and interested. They even manifest warmth, and serve to oil the wheels of consultation.

The personal history must be traced back, and every detail needs to be elicited, not only to shed light on the present disorder, but also to illumine the sufferer himself. This will mean close inquiry into innermost social, dietetic, domestic, and environmental circumstances. Such probings are likely not only to elucidate which factors trigger an attack, but also to reveal what determines whether a patient will be in a good patch or a bad one at any particular period.

There is no substance to the objection that such a manner of working is grossly time consuming. It is not a question of how much time can be spared for an individual patient, but of how many patients in such circumstances can be adequately dealt with in a single session. The answer may well be only very few. This means more doctors must be on hand at the clinic, because this kind of approach may be required during follow-up visits as well as in the initial consultation.

Such, I submit, is the master plan for coping with a forbearing clientele, victims of a recurring torment that, without shortening one's days, racks one with pain and threatens to disrupt domestic happiness, professional advancement, and social enjoyment. Thank heaven if we might yet avoid the faceless horror of officialdom, where "your name is a number: your story a 'case': your need a 'request'. Your hopes . . . 'will be filed . . . fill up this form . . . come back next week' " (13).

REFERENCES

1. Spencer H: *The Data of Ethics*, 1900.
2. Richet C: *Transactions of the 3rd International Congress on Psychology*, 1896.
3. Bell C: *The Hand*. London, William Pickering, 1833.
4. Nietzsche FW: The genealogy of morals. In Kaufmann EW (ed): *The Portable Nietzsche*. New York, Viking Press, 1953.
5. Simpson JY: *Remarks on the Superinduction of Anaesthesia in Natural and Morbid Parturition*. Boston, William B. Little, 1848, p 13.
6. Schweitzer A: *On the Edge of the Primeval Forest*, 1900.
7. Hippocrates: *Aphorisms*, 1900, Vol 2, p 46.
8. Lericke R: Surgery of pain. Baltimore, Williams & Wilkins, 1939.
9. Van Pallandt N: *Nina*. London, Robert Hale, 1974.
10. Critchley M: Neurological effects of lightning and of electricity. *Lancet* 1:68–72, 1934.
11. Critchley M: Psychological aspects of shipwreck survivors. In Critchley M (ed): *The Black Hole and Other Essays*. London, Pitman, 1964, p 192.
12. Boswell J: *Boswell's Life of Johnson*. Edinburgh, William P. Nimmo, 1873.
13. Menotti GC: *The Counsul*, 1900.

CHAPTER THREE

Differing Expectations of Headache Patients and Their Physicians

RUSSELL C. PACKARD, M.D.

For centuries, man has been concerned with pain and how to relieve or eliminate it (1). it has been said that the most common demand made by patients is for pain relief (2), and one of the most common painful conditions that physicians are faced with is headache.

By tradition and training, physicians prescribe medication or treatment based on a presumed diagnosis. This diagnostic process, discussed in Section II of this volume, is an important first step in establishing a relationship with headache patients. Several authors have discussed the physician-patient relationship as the key to successful treatment of patients with headache (3–5). Chapter 4 of this volume discusses many factors important for establishing this therapeutic alliance. The present chapter will explore another important aspect of physician-patient relationships, and one that is often overlooked: the patient's actual expectations, and how well or poorly they correlate with what physicians believe headache patients want.

The patient with a headache obviously visits the physician for a particular reason, and this reason needs to be discovered. It must be kept in mind that every patient is an individual with his own concerns, fears, questions—and expectations. If the physician can learn about these fears and concerns, answer the patient's questions, and prescribe a successful treat-ment, both parties will usually be satisfied. However, it is not uncommon when treating patients with headache (or other patients presenting with pain) for something to go awry in this process; the headache persists, "the medicine doesn't work." This may cause the physician to try other medicines, order further studies, or call in a consultant (6). If the process continues, some physicians will begin to feel frustrated, helpless, or even angry as the patient continues to call and fails to improve (7, 8). The patient may also begin to grow frustrated or angry and search out other physicians or treatment fads.

Several things can cause the physician-patient relationship to break down or even fail to be properly established. These include poor communication and physician prejudice toward headache patients; or the patient may have a personality disorder or display poor compliance with the prescribed therapeutic regimen. Frequently, however, it occurs because the patient's expectations are never properly clarified or discussed, or they are not consistent with the physician's.

STUDIES OF PATIENT AND PHYSICIAN EXPECTATIONS

There have actually been few studies of expectations of headache patients per se, and even fewer regarding physician expectations. In a survey conducted in 1976 at a London migraine clinic, patients described qualities they thought would be most desirable in clinic doctors (9). These included a thorough understanding of migraine, sympathy, friendliness, and a willingness to listen patiently and with care. They were also interested in having a place to which they knew they could go when they had headaches, and clearly preferred consultations longer than 15 minutes.

In a study performed in 1979, this author surveyed 100 headache patients presenting to a general neurology clinic, in order to explore the reasons for which they were coming to the doctor (10). In addition, 50 physicians were asked why they thought headache patients were seeking their help. Both physicians and patients rated the importance of 12 factors, including expectations of pain relief. Findings from this study are summarized in Tables 3.1 and 3.2.

Table 3.1 compares the factors physicians and patients most often selected as the top three. Both groups selected pain relief and an explanation of what was causing the headache with a high frequency. However, physicians tended to rate pain relief in the top three more often (96%) than did patients

(69%). Physicians also thought patients wanted medications more often than the patients did (68% to 20%, respectively). The patients showed greater interest in receiving an explanation about medication (32%) than in receiving the medications per se, something the physician group failed to mention at all.

Although an explanation of the cause of the pain was desired almost as often as its relief, Table 3.2 reveals a great difference in how it was selected. In comparing only those factors selected first, it can be seen that two-thirds of the physicians thought patients were primarily seeking pain relief, but only one-third of the patients wanted pain relief first and foremost. Patients were more interested in having the pain explained to them, or in factors not recognized at all by the physicians. These included getting an eye exam, a neurological exam, or finding a doctor willing to follow them.

Most patients expected some pain relief following their visit. Nearly one-third (31%) stated that they had expected "total relief," while 67% expected only "some relief."

As a result of this study the author recognized both the importance of determining patient expectations and their usefulness in

TABLE 3.1
PHYSICIAN-PATIENT COMPARISON
FACTORS MOST OFTEN SELECTED IN TOP THREE

	PHYSICIANS (50)	PATIENTS (91)
Pain relief	96%	69%
Explanation	68%	77%
Medication	68%	20%
Explain medication	0%	32%
Time for questions	68%	20%
Doctor to follow	20%	26%
Neurological exam	6%	31%
Treatment (other)	2%	18%
Eye exam	2%	11%
Skull x-rays	2%	8%
Psychiatric evaluation	0%	3%
Group	0%	0%

TABLE 3.2
PHYSICIAN-PATIENT COMPARISON
FACTORS MOST OFTEN SELECTED FIRST

	PHYSICIAN GROUP (50)	PATIENT GROUP (100)
Pain relief	66%	31%
Explanation	22%	46%
Medication	6%	0%
Neurological exam	0%	7%
Doctor to follow	0%	4%
Eye examination	0%	4%
Explain medication	0%	3%
Time for questions	2%	3%
Treatment (other)	2%	1%
Skull x-rays	0%	1%
Psychiatric evaluation	0%	0%
Group	0%	0%

planning treatment. Another study was therefore designed along similar lines, and the data from it will be presented in this chapter.

As part of the intake process at a headache clinic, patients were asked to fill out a general medical history form and a headache history form before being seen by the physician-director. On the headache history form, data were obtained from 100 consecutive patients about whether they expected total, nearly total, or only some pain relief. Another portion of the form asked patients to rank four factors in order of importance: an explanation of the cause of their headache problem, pain relief, tests, and time for questions. The results are presented in Tables 3.3. and 3.4.

In Table 3.3, 68% of the patients ranked "relief of pain" first, with 28% ranking "explanation of cause" as most important. Both relief of pain and explanation of cause frequently scored (96%) in the first two choices. Having time for questions or getting tested were seen as considerably less important. Approximately two-thirds of the entire patient group ranked factors of importance in the following order:

1. Pain relief;
2. Explanation of cause;
3. Time for questions;
4. Tests.

It is important to note that, even though pain relief is ranked high (higher than in the previous study), almost one-third of the headache clinic patients were more concerned about knowing about the cause of their headache, and seeking pain relief was secondary.

TABLE 3.4
EXPECTATIONS OF PAIN RELIEF

NEUROLOGY CLINIC		HEADACHE CLINIC	
Total	31	Total	56
Some	67	Nearly total	34
None	2	Some	10
	100		100

The headache clinic survey also asked about the degree of expected (or hoped-for) pain relief. The answers are summarized in Table 3.4, and compared with neurology clinic responses. These questions about degree of relief were presented differently in the two studies, thus giving somewhat different results. In the neurology clinic survey the choices were "a bit," "all or none"/"total or some," whereas the headache clinic question was presented as "total, nearly total, or some."

Patients seeking total relief ranged from 31% in the neurology clinic sample to 56% in the headache clinic sample. It is noteworthy that 90% of the headache clinic population sample were expecting or hoping for total or nearly total relief.

Several important differences can be seen between this and the earlier study—the most notable being the higher expectation for pain relief than was found in the previous study. These differences may reflect differences in populations studied and in survey methods. The neurology clinic group had a larger selection of factors to choose from and rank in order of importance. Having more factors detected wider areas of patient concern than was possible in the headache clinic

TABLE 3.3
FACTORS RANKED BY 100 HEADACHE CLINIC PATIENTS AS
MOST IMPORTANT

	1ST	2ND	3RD	4TH
Relief of pain	68	24	4	4
Explanation of cause	28	60	9	3
Time for questions	3	8	67	22
Tests	1	8	20	71

study. For example, 23% of patients ranked as "most important" areas not even on the headache clinic list (e.g., an eye exam, a doctor to follow them, x-rays, a neurological exam).

The patient populations were also different. The neurology clinic group consisted either of active duty military personnel or their dependents, whereas the second group was drawn from a private practice. Whether the attitude of headache patients differs in these two settings is an interesting question for speculation, i.e., were patients coming to the military neurology clinic because it was available without cost? Does cost affect the patient's expectations? Conversely, does a patient coming to a headache clinic have higher and perhaps more unrealistic expectations or hopes? Or do these patients, because they are paying, expect something in return?

One further observation: The author at one point directly questioned 25 patients about the kind of relief they were expecting or hoping for. These patients filled out a general history form but not a headache history form. Not one stated that he expected "total relief." Most responses were on the order of "anything," "just something—anything," or "I just want to be more comfortable." In following this small group of patients, however, the author found that many later returned, complaining that "the headache isn't gone." This suggests that patients may be somewhat more at ease in expressing their hopes, fears, and expectations on paper than verbally, where they might be more guarded. This reticence was less obvious with other questions (such as whether the patient was concerned about having a brain tumor, a frequently unexpressed fear of patients presenting with headache).

DISCUSSION

In the evaluation and management of patients with headache, it is important to clarify and deal with the expectations of patients; it is equally important to be aware of our own expectations as physicians. From a review of the various surveys it is clear that patients come with many different concerns and expectations, and that these may or may not be similar to our own. There may also be important differences in what the patient reveals depending upon how the information is obtained. For instance, patients may not verbalize their internal hopes, fears, wishes, or expectations as clearly or directly as they do when filling out a written form. Bana et al (11) have noted that patients tended to report more details about their headaches to a computer terminal than to the physician. At other times, patient expectations may initially be unclear because of anxiety about the "meaning" of the headaches. To the layman, the terms "head" and "brain" are often synonymous (12).

The importance of defining expectations becomes apparent if we consider the following situation. If we as physicians assume or expect that a headache patient is coming to us for relief of pain or for medication, our goal will be to provide these. If, however, the patient mainly wants to know what is wrong, or is worried about his eyes, or simply wants a doctor willing to follow him for headaches, our pill may well be doomed to failure, and we may miss our greatest opportunity for providing relief: a simple explanation and reassurance.

Clarifying what are reasonable expectations for pain relief is extremely important. In both surveys, a large proportion of patients expected total or nearly total relief. The search for total pain relief is often like the unending search for perfection (13).

Patients (or physicians) seeking total pain relief are usually doomed to failure. This failure may then lead to a breakdown in the physician-patient relationshp and to the patient seeking other physicians and treatments. Because total relief of long-standing head pain is so rarely achieved, it should not be the only goal of treatment. Physician and patient should instead attempt to define more realistic goals such as a decrease in headache frequency and/or severity.

CONCLUSIONS

This chapter suggests that clarifying and defining expectations can be important in evaluating and managing patients with headache. For those physicians or clinics primarily treating headache problems, a written form enquiring about these expectations might prove useful. For the general practitioner, querying the patient directly about his expectations and clearly describing treatment goals for the patient is similarly important. Frequently, the simplest things can be the most helpful in establishing a good physician-patient relationship and in clarifying "hidden expectations." A brief explanation of the cause of the headache will usually be appreciated and can enhance the relationship immensely. Even for patients primarily seeking pain relief, this is a frequent underlying concern. Giving the patient an opportunity to ask questions and explaining all medications and treatments prescribed is especially useful in this age of patient enlightenment. A few extra moments spent on these factors during the initial session can enhance the entire treatment process and eliminate many potential problems in the future.

REFERENCES

1. Dalessio DJ (ed): General consideration of pain. In *Wolff's Headache and Other Head Pain,* ed 3. New York, Oxford University Press, 1972, p 3.
2. Engel GL: Psychogenic pain and the pain prone patient. *Am J Med* 26:899–918, 1959.
3. Friedman AP: Migraine headache. *JAMA* 222:1400–1402, 1972.
4. Packard RC: Psychiatric aspects of headache. *Headache* 19:370–374, 1979.
5. Saper JR: *Headache Disorders.* Boston, John Wright, 1983, p 8.
6. Goodwin DW: Psychiatry and the mysterious medical complaint. *JAMA* 209:1884–1888, 1969.
7. Packard RC: Emotional aspects of headache. *Neurol Clin* 1:445–457, 1983.
8. Adler G: The physician and the hypochondriacal patient. *N Engl J Med* 304:1394–1396, 1981.
9. Rose, FC: The migraine clinic at Charing Cross Hospital. *Hemicrania* 7:2–5, 1976.
10. Packard RC: What does the headache patient want? *Headache* 19:370–374, 1979.
11. Bana DS, Laviton A, Slack WV: Use of computerized database in a headache clinic. *Headache* 21:72–74, 1981.
12. Kolb LC: Psychiatric and psychogenic factors in headache. In Friedman AP, Merritt HH (eds): *Headache, Diagnosis and Treatment.* Philadelphia, Davis, 1959, pp 259–289.
13. Spiro HM: Pain and perfectionism—the physician and the pain patient. *N Engl J Med* 294:829–830, 1976.

CHAPTER
FOUR

The Headache Patient and the Doctor

JOHN R. GRAHAM, M.D.

The purpose of this chapter, basic to the goal of this book, is to discuss the relationship between physicians and patients—especially headache patients. Over the years, the "doctor-patient relationship" has received a lot of attention and has become somewhat of a "sacred cow" for the medical profession. Like many other "sacred cows," however, the attention it receives is frequently superficial and comes in the form of "lip service." Some who readily render this "lip service" really do not believe that this cow gives milk. Others may agree that the cow produces milk but add that they "don't have the time to milk her." This introductory chapter will discuss the nature of this relationship, its quality and value, some details of its cultivation, and the lean years of therapeutic famine that may result when no genuine attention is paid to it. Such considerations are important in the management of patients suffering from many illnesses, but they are especially vital in dealing with headache patients, in whom very often the problems of the person become entangled with the symptomatology of the disease.

THE THERAPEUTIC ALLIANCE

The term "therapeutic alliance" might best be substituted for the cold words "doctor-patient relationship." An alliance is formed by two or more people who join together for mutual friendly cooperation—in this case for the medical care of one by the other. The terms of the alliance or, really, the spirit in which it is made, have a lot to do with ultimate success or failure in treatment.

A patient who enters a "warm climate," in which his physician is genuinely interested in him as a person and his total welfare as well as his current illnesses, will probably develop a therapeutic alliance or relationship with his physician characterized by mutual trust and respect in both personal and medical matters. This promotes a sense of freedom of expression and confidence in which the patient feels free to tell everything about himself and his symptoms, and the doctor uses all of this information, medical and personal, to solve the problems this person is having. If the patient encounters a cool, crisp, rigid search by the physician looking only for the exact details of the disease, the patient may feel that his partner in this alliance is concerned only with the disease and very little with him.

Some illnesses and disorders do not require elaborate therapeutic alliances between patient and doctor for successful treatment. But there are few visits made by patients to physicians in which the patient does not come away with some feeling about what the doctor was like as a person, as well as whether his scientific therapy was effective.

In each encounter of this sort, even if only for minor medical treatment, another stone is added to the edifice of both the doctor's and the patient's "character." "Gee, he's a nice guy," says the patient about the physician who showed some personal interest—or, alternatively, "Boy, he's a cold fish!" Meanwhile, the doctor may be reacting with inwardly phrased feelings such as "What a neurotic!" or "She's going to give me lots of trouble." If even in these brief encounters for a hormone shot or an Ace bandage the terms of the alliance are being observed and tested, how much deeper an exploration will they receive when the patient presents with a major problem? Headache patients often arrive at the office with a mixture of physiological and psychological factors in which a mutual therapeutic alliance becomes paramount in successful treatment.

Psychiatrists often develop a strong alliance with their patients and consider it a vital part of therapy. Other medical practitioners tend to forget that this relationship is merely a highly developed "therapeutic alliance." Some psychiatric techniques can be useful and easily adopted in developing the physician-patient relationship, or therapeutic alliance. A basic attitude or prerequisite to adopting some of these principles is a genuine interest in helping people, not just curing disease. Many originally had these attitudes. Why were they abandoned?

Young medical students, in first approaching a course in physical diagnosis, are fascinated by people as well as by their diseases. Before long, however, in our present climate, this interest in the person is squeezed his rewards come largely for utilizing highly scientific technological knowledge in handling a serious case of myocardial infarction in the coronary care unit (CCU), rather than for recognizing the depression that may follow (even though such an approach may keep the patient from achieving a successful rehabilitation after discharge). Perhaps physicians may need to be open to changing some of their own ways, even ones into which they are already comfortably settled.

When the young physician gets out into actual practice his interest in people is often rejuvenated—partly because he really always has liked patients as people. But this interest in them as people tends to get squeezed out of him again by the growing pressures of volume and time, family, regulations, insurance, malpractice, Medicare, Medicaid, the professional standards review organizations (PSROs), and hospital audits. Thus we find ourselves again focusing narrowly on the details of the symptom and the disease, rather than on the person who has them, as we struggle to meet the demands of a busy practice under the current socioeconomic constraints. Under such pressures, we can lose sight of the therapeutic alliance that has so much to do with the ultimate success of our treatment.

FACTORS INFLUENCING THE THERAPEUTIC ALLIANCE

The therapeutic alliance, or lack of it, often begins before the patient and doctor get together. It happens on the telephone when the patient makes the first appointment. The voice and attitude of the receptionist, the secretary, or the answering service make a strong impression for good or poor future relations. They may set a poor tone, and it is wise to monitor them from time to time. At the very least, it is important to pay attention to patients' complaints about telephone service, attitudes of office assistants, laboratory technicians, bookkeepers, billing agencies, or the alternate physician on call to detect whether any of them are hasty, cold, or forbidding.

It is also wise for the physician to review the physical features of his office that ensure confidentiality. Psychiatrists are especially sensitive about this, for the very good reason that patients will not tell important things about themselves if, while waiting to come in, they have heard the previous patient's secrets through the office door.

Is the office set up to provide the desired comfortable yet professional ambience? Is the light in the patient's eyes too direct or too bright? Headache patients often have intermittent yet quite uncomfortable photophobia. Is there a big block of a desk sternly separating the doctor from the patient, or are the chairs arranged so that there is a more open, informal atmosphere?

Has the secretary been cued to protect the interview from unnecessary phone calls? Patients will appreciate the doctor's answering calls that are obviously emergencies because they can picture themselves in the other patient's place; but they resent trifling interruptions during the one time they have his full attention. In general, does the office look like a friendly, personally oriented place, or like a barren, cold cubicle in an overly busy beehive of activity? What about the pictures? Do they consist only of diplomas, or are there some photos of people or beautiful objects present on the walls?

SOME PSYCHIATRIC OBSERVATIONS

From studies made while teaching "office psychiatry" to internists the author made some psychiatric observations about technique which are pertinent to this discussion. The major and probably most important one is how internists and medical doctors in general fail to make, or at least to use, certain observations that psychiatrists consider essential to diagnosis and treatment.

Psychiatrists tend to notice "physical signs" that medical physicians are not accustomed to looking for. These consist of such things as the downcast look of depression, the knitted brow of anxiety, the grimace of anger, the tapping foot of frustration, the wide-eyed stare of fright or the whitened knuckles of desperation. These signs all enter into a psychiatrist's evaluation and help him to determine the nature of a patient's illness and its treatment. Medical doctors tend to see the same signs in their patients and to consider them "interesting" but then simply "file them away." Their thinking might be: "This fellow is sick, no wonder he looks depressed," rather than, "This fellow looks depressed— perhaps that's one reason he has these symptoms."

I remember one particularly interesting case in which, as an internist, I conjointly in-terviewed a patient with a psychiatrist. I thought I was doing well, and had learned quite a lot about my patient. She was a child orphaned at an early age, who had been brought up by her grandmother and had endured a rather hectic life subsequently. I succeeded in bringing out how several of these elements related to in the history of her headache problem, and towards the end of the interview asked if the psychiatrist had any further questions. He merely asked: "Who gave you that beautiful ring?" The patient started to cry, and said, "My grandmother gave it to me on the afternoon when she died." This soon brought out many more things about the patient's relationship to her grandmother, and what it meant to have lost her. It was at this time that her headaches had begun. Later, I asked the psychiatrist what made him ask that particular question and *only* that question. The answer was suprisingly simple: "I just noticed that whenever she was talking about her grandmother she kept rubbing this ring on her finger."

The following week I had an opportunity to interview a young woman, a "hippie" type, who considered herself highly independent and able to manage her life, but was nevertheless having constant headache. There she sat in front of me, rubbing a ring. Having just learned this one little thing, I thought I'd give it a try, and finally said, "Who gave you that beautiful ring?" She broke into tears: "Elmer did, when he left me." And then we had a long talk about Elmer, who had much to do with this patient's headaches.

Let me strongly urge physicians to pay attention to these signs when dealing with headache patients, and to integrate those found into the diagnosis and into the treatment plan, just as surely as one would account for cyanosis, exophthalmos, dyspnea, or clubbed fingers.

WHEN DOCTOR AND PATIENT MEET

Having made these points, let us return to the headache patient who is meeting the physician for the first time. Even the nature of the greeting is an important source of information. Right off, the patient may be revealing what he or she wants or needs in the alliance about to be set up. I remember inviting one new patient into the office with: "Come right in, Mrs. Smith." She clutched my hand: "Please, call me Donna." One thing she clearly wanted from me in our alliance was a close friend, perhaps too close. As an alcoholic patient being presented to a conference of physicians entered the room, he immediately said, "Did any of you doctors go to McGill?" It was vital to his self-esteem that, even though he was a down-at-the-heels drunk, he had gone to McGill, and therefore had some at least one triumph to which his evaluators might relate and of which he might be proud.

In the case of many a male cluster headache patient, it is useful to note that he frequently is a large, husky, lion of a man obediently being towed in by a potent little mouse of a woman—his wife. This "Lady Macbeth" often gives the history, makes the appointments, and takes the prescriptions, while Leo sits compliantly by.

Then, there is the parent who "wishes to come in too." What kind of an alliance should the doctor make with her 17-year-old son, who is dragged in because of recurrent headaches—yet doesn't seem particularly willing to talk? Does the physician invite the mother in? Does he exclude her? Does he let her in now but make it clear that on future visits he will talk with the patient alone? The policy on this issue must be quickly but carefully considered for each patient.

I recall an irate contractor from a tradition-bound Mediterranean family who broke into my office just as I began to take a headache history from his 46-year-old son. "Whatsa matta with the kid?", he exclaimed. Perhaps the reader has the diagnosis already. What happens on the first meeting frequently sets the tone of the future relationship.

Each time a doctor and patient meet a two-way evaluation is going on. Some of these assessments are open and on the surface; others are hidden but are nevertheless very active. The physician is well aware that one important and immediate part of his job is to get exact details of symptoms and signs that will lead to diagnosis. He expects to do this, and the patient expects it of him. At the same time, if he is interested in developing a good therapeutic alliance, the physician is quietly, consciously or unconsciously, attempting to evaluate his patient's personality, his attitude toward the disease, and his attitude toward its treatment. Also, and perhaps most difficult, the physician must examine his own attitudes toward this kind of patient. If the physician's history-taking is rigid, and "strictly according to the book," the patient will soon get the feeling that *this* doctor has no empathy for him as a person, and conclude that it will be of no profit to relate personal feelings and reactions.

Thus is the crucial therapeutic alliance forged well, forged poorly, or even cast aside. It requires the physician to use the "art" of medicine; though the time it takes to master that art optimally is medical shibboleth, the time required to learn it well is within reach. This is a matter of style. Any style will be effective provided it clearly demonstrates to the patient that the physician is truly interested in him and his life as a person, as well as in the details of the medical complaint.

While taking a history and making these observations about the patient as a person, the physician may do well to ask himself, or the patient, certain questions not often found in the little books supplied in medical school. Some of these are:

Who is this patient? How does he fill his day? What family support or stress motivates and modulates his life?

Who sent him to the doctor? His wife? His boss? The Industrial Accident Board? Or is he coming of his own free will?

Why is he coming *now?* Is it because of the recent death of a friend who had similar symptoms? The social loss of a friend or family member? Or for reassurance?

What does he expect of me? Nothing? Everything? Does he expect me to be a friend? a critic? a judge? a failure (like several predecessors)? a magician?

Who are the characters in this play? The hostile wife, the alcoholic brother, the overbearing boss?

What is this symptom doing to or for him? If it is removed, what then? Is it his only means of grasping for help?

What goals should I set for myself in caring for this patient? Do I expect, as a physician, that I have to cure his disease or must fully remove his symptoms? Or can I manage to be happy with supporting the patient and keeping him out of harm's way?

Finally—Am I the best person to do it? Can I not only endure this hypochondriacal, chronic complainer with the daily headaches for more than 10 years but also wish to help him at the end of the visit more than I wish to duck him? If it's the latter answer, would it be better if I arrange for the patient to see somebody else? Am I willing to form the kind of alliance this patient seems to be seeking?

Meanwhile, the patient also has a list of questions: about the symptoms, about the underlying disease, and about the doctor. They are sometimes subconscious.

One question may well be: Am I really sure I really want to look into this problem? What is the doctor going to find?

Should I reveal everything about my troubles to this doctor, and should I do so just now? Some parts of it are rather embarassing: those coital headaches, my husband's impotence. Would he look kindly on me if he knew?

Could it be just nerves or depression? Do I sound like a neurotic? Am I?

Could my family history have something to do with it? I hope I'm not getting like mother, when she started going senile? How much will it cost? How long will it take? will I have to have a barium enema? Could it be cancer?

Should I tell him everything the other doctors said?

Other questions are not even related to the "present illness," may be partially concealed or subconscious: Would it be better if he just listened, instead of writing all the time? Will he tell me what is going to happen in a way I can understand? Will he explain why I need any tests, and if they will hurt? Can I make him interested in me? Finally, have I come to the right place?

Once the history-taking has started, there are several points worth mentioning about how to conduct it. Valuable as it is to follow up clues to emotional reactions of the patient in relation to the disease, it is nevertheless wise to be cautious as to how far and when to pursue them. If a physician is examining an abdomen for the signs of acute appendicitis, he does not palpate the right lower quadrant immediately but, rather, does so after careful exploration of the rest of the belly first, so that the patient anticipates that he is not going to be thoughtless or insensitive when he reaches the really tender spot. Clues in the history that the physician elicits as he keeps his eyes and ears open for emotion-laden phrases may reveal areas of emotional sensitivity that he should approach cautiously or later, when the patient has learned to trust him.

Surprisingly, pertinent emotional reactions may be prompted by adding two questions to each of the positive items in the standard family and past history of the patient: (a) "How did that make you feel?" and (b) "When did it happen in relation to your basic complaints?" It may not be so important that father died of a stroke as that he died a month before the patient's wedding, and that his loss precipitated an emotional crisis related to the headaches of which the patient now complains.

EMOTIONAL ASPECTS OF THE THERAPEUTIC ALLIANCE

In the course of speaking openly about emotional aspects of his illness and life, the patient may begin to cry. Most medical doctors are uncomfortable when a patient starts to cry. But such an episode can give a better insight into the patient's problems and, consequently, can strengthen the therapeutic alliance. It is wise for the physician to sit back momentarily, and to let the patient cry. After he finishes, ask if he can tell why he felt like crying and how he feels now. Patients usually feel better after crying if the physician's behavior suggests that he appreciates the needs and is sensitive to emotional factors that lie buried behind the tears.

A good therapeutic alliance usually allows the physician to ask direct questions about the patient's emotional state. What is making him so unhappy that he can't keep from crying? What are his thoughts about why he is depressed, or is even to the point of contemplating suicide?

At times, referral of a headache patient to a psychiatrist becomes necessary. There are some general principles for making this type of referral. The first visit is generally a poor time to suggest it unless a psychiatric emergency is imminent or mutual trust develops quite rapidly. Also, just as the physician needs to be thoroughly convinced that organic factors have been identified, ruled out, or otherwise accounted for, the patient also needs to be convinced on this score. It is also helpful for the doctor to have ample opportunity to observe whether the patient is in touch with his feelings and whether he has some capacity to relate those feelings to his symptoms. It may be a waste of both the psychiatrist's time and the patient's if the patient either will not or cannot discuss emotional aspects of his problem. Patients need to understand the reason for psychotherapy and have some motivation to participate in it. The recommendation that they go this route properly arises from mutual positive understanding between doctor and patient.

The majority of headache patients profit most by the supportive type of psychotherapy that is supplied by a good medical practitioner who will spend at least half of each visit discussing the patient's daily problems and habit patterns. Listening is therapy; therapy is listening. Too often the medical physician forgets this maxim and begins to think that he is "doing nothing" for a patient who "just

comes and gabs." Why is the patient continuing to do this for months and sometimes for years, his symptom unimproved by any specific therapy—but the patient nonetheless still appearing? The answer is that the *patient* is being helped, even if his symptom isn't. In the final analysis it is "how the patient is doing" that counts most.

Sometimes, the most important prescription a physician can give for the headache patient is a dose of himself. Sometimes "Tincture of Physician" needs to be taken in infrequent, large doses, at other times in frequent, small doses. At times of increased trouble this extremely important "tonic" may need to be increased in frequency and volume until the crisis is over. The patient should "report back" and be officially dismissed after such a stretch only when the coast seems clear, rather than be allowed to disappear without a trace.

The telephone is the smallest dose of "physician" that can be supplied—but it is very important as a vehicle for maintenance of support and continuity of care. Physicians should pay attention to underlying concerns in telephone calls from psychologically influenced patients, and should not restrict them unless they become pathologically frequent. Being "hard to get" or "failing to call back" can destroy the patient's confidence. Some physicians offer a daily telephone hour in which the patient can call, eliminating many annoying interruptions for other patients in the office. At other times, patients may be informed in advance that the physician does not have time (or is not in the office all the time) to personally answer all telephone calls, but that the office staff will discuss the call with him, and the physician will get back to the patient as soon as possible.

HOSPITALIZATION

At times a headache patient must be admitted to the hospital, for a more technologically sophisticated work-up, to get an intractable headache under control, and/or to learn what the patient is really like during attacks and how he reacts to the therapy or during the symptoms. It may be necessary to discuss with busy nurses and residents why such a patient has been admitted with "just headaches." There is an all-too-common attitude that headaches are somehow self-induced, not really that painful, evidence of "psychoneurosis" (in its demeaning sense), or that a willful patient is simply being "spoiled" by the physician. If the treatment team around the headache patient does not receive the physician's information and guidance, the hospital experience may do harm as well as good. For instance, nurses and housestaff sometimes wish to try sterile saline injections to determine whether the head pain is "real" or not. Such procedures not only reflect a lack of appreciation for the potent effects of placebos in normal patients but may even be dangerous, given their capacity to ravage a therapeutic alliance. Another tendency on the part of hospital personnel may be to "hold out" or even delay in responding to a patient's call for medication. It is important to inform the patient of any change in medication type or dosage, so that he might best cooperate, participate, and discuss his concerns, fears, or questions.

One should tell the patient who the residents, consultants, and social workers are, and what may be expected of them. Psychiatrists should usually be introduced with reference to their true role, rather than in the guise (true, but deceptively incomplete) of "another physician," a "headache specialist," etc.

In writing pain medication orders it is usually wise to let nurses carry out the order to the hilt, and to make it clear that the physician, may be changing the dose or frequency each day, and to keep the patient informed of these changes. It is also helpful to let the nurses know that the physician would like to be called if there are problems about orders, medicines, etc.; headache patients often have a remarkable faculty for being *right*, and are frequently expert in detecting flaws in their personal orders or management.

SUMMARY

The therapeutic alliance or physician-patient relationship is essential to the evaluation and treatment of patients with headache. Its proper incubation may take time, observing the manner and life-style of a patient, listening to his complaints, and paying added attention to factors not ordinarily considered when seeing patients. In the long run, this extra effort will frequently turn out to be a gratifying experience, and will be rewarded with warmth, friendship, and appreciation by the patients, even if they continue to experience occasional headaches. The "sacred cow" does, in fact, give good milk.

ACKNOWLEDGMENT

I am grateful to John Reichard, M.D., Chief of Psychiatry at Faulkner Hospital, for some of the ideas expressed in the text.

CHAPTER FIVE

Psychodynamics of Head Pain: An Introduction

CHARLES S. ADLER, M.D.
SHEILA MORRISSEY ADLER, Ph.D.

PSYCHODYNAMICS DEFINED

In the field of headache, many older practitioners share an important knowledge learned from two master teachers: the relationship of disquieted emotion to headache and the value of talk in relieving its pain. The teachers have been headache patients themselves and time.

Why the importance? Because in patients with severe, recurrent headaches psychological factors are prevalent, relevant, and treatable. Before elaborating on these judgments, certain concepts central to our understanding of how psychodynamics work require consensual definition, and some need a context for their use.

PSYCHODYNAMICS

A psychodynamic formulation can be either:

- the descriptive mapping out of relationships between intrapsychic forces, such as specific impulses, defenses, and perceptions of reality, or
- a developmentally oriented understanding of how experiences have shaped a person psychologically and of how current events are reawakening or being distorted by memories of those experiences.

THE UNCONSCIOUS

To understand "the unconscious" is to recognize that every person has memories, fears, and desires which remain outside of his awareness. Anyone who has watched helplessly while an important dream slips away into the shadows of the "forgotten" despite his best efforts to hold onto it, has confirmed for himself that the brain is capable of selective remembering. Information that has been repressed into the unconscious is typically inaccessible by ordinary methods of recall because of its powerful emotional charge. The underlying message in the dream comes from the unconscious, and is generally not recoverable by the dreamer alone.

THE DRIVES

To understand the basic instinctual drives is to recognize the presence in everyone of impulses toward assertion and gratification of needs. These mental constituents produce a state of tension in a person which pushes him to take some action that will reduce the excitation and alleviate the tension. Drives are biologically determined. Their aims are preservation and advancement of self and species. These inborn drives come into conflict with other forces in the psyche, such as the conscience, as a result of which they are either gratified, modified, or kept at bay—with varying degrees of success.

THE DEFENSES

Each person evolves a set—a profile if you will—of preferred mechanisms to keep unconscious information repressed and instinctual drives modulated in intensity and coordinated with reality. Their purpose is to shield the patient from potentially upsetting or disruptive inner stimuli, rather than to "defend" him against events in the external world (see Table 5.1). They work to protect the patient against anxiety, and they usually succeed. Most are automatic and unconscious.

The impulses, the forces that oppose the impulses, and the compromises that contain them may all be unconscious for a given patient. Even so, when unbalanced they can be deleterious to the patient's functioning or happiness.

PSYCHODYNAMICS: ITS ROLE IN HEADACHE

To reiterate: it is their prevalence, relevance, and treatability that makes psychological factors important in headache.

THEIR PREVALENCE

The prevalence of psychogenic contributions to headaches has long been recognized in the scientific literature. (The role professionals ascribe to psychological factors in the cause and treatment of headaches is documented in Table 24.1 of Chapter 24.) Friedman and Merritt (1), for example, reflect a common conclusion, when they assert that

. . . **an understanding of the underlying psychologic factors plays an important part in the management of migraine, for in the ability of the patient to handle emotional tension lies the most satisfactory means of preventing attacks in the majority of cases.**

THEIR RELEVANCE

The relevance of emotional factors is so well accepted that the man in the street uses the term "headache" as shorthand for any frustrating or emotion-generating situation that defies easy resolution. Webster confirms this, giving as one definition of headache, "a vexatious or baffling situation or problem".

The major symptom of headache is pain, which is highly subjective: It is a weathervane, turning with every breeze of emotion, and shuddering in its gales. That the psyche is an integral part of pain has long been known to both Shaman and charlatan.

Emotional significance also derives from the location of the pain. The head is central to the patient's sense of identity, a fact confirmed in every passport and yearbook. One study (2) located the sense of "self" immediately behind the bridge of the nose. This makes the head the most vital area of the body symbolically, as well as in actuality. In everyday language more references are made to the head than to any other body part. Only a century ago a glove in the face called for dueling pistols.

Indeed, the head is the body's command post. Receptors for all five senses are located there, and it is the site from which speech and expression emanate. Ethologists (3, 4) have shown that specific facial expressions have an innate capacity to communicate emotions in all higher animals and that this is one of their functions. The same facial muscles normally used to communicate aggression, affection, dominance, and submission are the ones implicated in tension headache. Sustained contraction of the masticatory muscles also frequently accompanies tension headaches; these muscles were anatomical foci in the crucial developmental experiences of exploring, receiving, attacking, and being gratified in the "oral stage." The vertex led the way and endured the sensations of that painful first voyage from uterus to delivery room. More than any other part of the body then, the head must be considered the central bulletin board for vulnerabilities, and pain there may accrue anxiety and meaning simply from its location.

THEIR TREATABILITY

When emotional problems are affecting headache they are usually treatable. Optimal treatment may require referral to a mental health professional, but can often be accomplished in a short period of time by the primary physician. A range of viable interventions makes the subject of more than academic interest.

In a 5- (5) and a 10-year (6) study the authors had greater success with chronic headache patients when they included a variable amount of psychotherapy in the basic treatment. For the 10-year study the added improvement was significant at the 0.01 level when psychologically treated patients were compared to those patients in whom psychological factors were not dealt with. These and other studies (7, 8) corroborate the experience of many clinicians that even seemingly resistant headache problems can usually be helped.

THOUGH RELEVANT, PSYCHOLOGIC FACTORS MAY BE ELUSIVE, AND THEIR EVALUATION FRUSTRATING

Even the physician who agrees in principle that many headaches start when the relationship between mind and body falls from harmony may find the specifics of that relationship hard to access. To the untrained eye, the signs indicating that psychogenic factors may be relevant to a given patient's headache are like those high wisps of cloud in a clear sky that the meterologist insists predict a blizzard. Like the meterologist, the psychiatrist bases his conclusions on educated observations and, in a like manner, often discerns underlying trouble that others will miss. Nevertheless, physicians—including psychiatrists—retain an understandable wish that psychodynamics could be observed like a temporal artery, pal-pated like a paracervical muscle, or auscultated like an arteriovenous malformation.

Other factors also camouflage the importance of psychological components: their roots are tangled with hereditary, metabolic, environmental, sociological, and neurological variables. When the meterologist wants to know if hail is likely, he must measure such things as temperature, wind velocity, humidity, and barometric pressure, as it is a pattern rather than a single reading which will give him his forecast. In a similar manner, the emotional factor is only one of the elements which must converge to precipitate headache. This complexity can blur the role emotion plays.

Finally, the patient cannot report psychological contributions that, due to active repression, he does not know of and cannot, by act of will, remember. This leaves the clinician with the task of listening for unconscious determinants of headache by becoming attuned to verbal associations and omissions and to behavioral signs that signal difficulties, on occasion even those difficulties the patient energetically denies.

TWO ILLUSTRATIVE STUDIES

The following two papers are offered to illustrate the type of headache investigation that probes the patient's psyche in depth, rather than to prove that their specific findings are generally applicable. Perhaps they will also whet the reader's appetite.

EISENBUD

An experimental case study reported by Eisenbud (9) in 1937 illustrates the effectiveness of unconscious conflict in inducing headaches. The patient, who entered the hospital with a chief complaint of headache, was described as follows:

Psychological investigation of the patient reveals a great deal of repressed hostility toward his father. Although his conscious

attitude was one of dutiful concern for the father's welfare, almost all of the patient's frequent dreams expressed wishes for the latter's death or injury. It was found that his headaches tended to follow such dreams with remarkable regularity, and that on days when he had headaches, the patient was irritable and seclusive. The reason he gave for his seclusiveness was his feeling on such days that if anyone were to provoke him or 'rub him the wrong way', he might become assaultive. He nevertheless suppressed these impulses . . .

At various times over a period of months the investigator would describe to the patient—after the patient had been put into a hypnotic trance—incidents designed to induce a predetermined type of emotional conflict. Before being awakened, a posthypnotic suggestion would be given to remember neither the content of the hypnotic session nor what had "happened to him" in the "incident." In this way Eisenbud implanted in the patient's unconscious specific emotional states born of conflict.

A variety of different psychodynamic situations were tried out to see what effect they had on the headaches. Circumstances in which the patient was humiliated and felt a rage that the interpersonal contingencies in the invented "situation" prohibited him from expressing always resulted in headaches later that day or the following day. Other conflicts did not have this effect. On occasion, the patient would have inadvertent contact with a person who had provoked him in one of those fabricated "incidents" and towards whom he was therefore repressing considerable anger (the anger was unconscious), and such a meeting, too, would invariably trigger a headache.

Another interesting finding was that while the memory of the fabricated event was unconscious the patient experienced headaches but no anxiety. When the amnesia was lifted through the use of hypnotic technique, the patient would become anxious, but his headaches would leave. When the amnesia was reinstated in a similar manner, the pa-

tient's anxiety would disappear, but his headaches would return.

JONCKHEERE

A different type of study, done by Jonckheere (8), also examines the relevance of the unconscious to migraine. He planned the study so that it would minimize a common but major theoretical design problem: for any investigator to accurately understand a patient psychologically, he must commit sufficient time to the evaluation. The reason for this is that material a patient relates in the first or second interview can differ significantly from that revealed later on, after sufficient trust has developed. At other times, it should be differently interpreted in light of information later disclosed. Because Jonckheere had seen each patient in the study for at least 15 hr of psychotherapy, he felt confidence that his understanding of them was reasonably accurate.

Jonckheere's first observation was that each of these patients showed signs of a similar type of conflict. Next, he tested this hypothesis further by looking for signs of such conflict both in 25 new migraine patients and in 3 headache-free control groups. This subsequent work confirmed for him the presence, in the migraine group only, of the conflicts previously observed. What were they? He found that the migraine patients had "one common characteristic": they all lived "in a state of permanent tension" with one or several key individuals. He continues:

The affective coloration of this tension can be summarized in one word: aggression—intense, sometimes ironic, often hateful. In all the cases it is repressed, cannot be expressed, and has a tendency to disappear (along with the headaches) when psychotherapy permits the patient to express it . . . The analysis of the above cases demonstrated in all the existence of an important conflict with one or both parents who are excessively severe or are felt to be dangerous, eventually becoming dominant . . . from that time the repressed aggressiveness generates the headache apparently related either directly to a current conflict or through the reactivation of an old family conflict . . . (From Jouckhecre P: The chronic headache patient. Psychother. Psychosom. 19:53–61, 1971, S. Karger, Basel, Switzerland, publisher.)

In his control cases he also occasionally saw obsessiveness and anger, but found that "it is a different type than in those suffering from headaches." He concludes that on the cornerstone of these problematic, psychologically influenced migraines were etched two words: nonexpressed aggression.

Although other studies cited throughout this book also show how important unconscious factors can be in headache, these two experiments are remarkable for the similarity of their conclusions despite the dissimilarity of their approaches.

It is because the unconscious can be shown to have such actual relevance to many cases of chronic headache that this chapter will now undertake a preliminary unscrambling of its mechanisms and motives.

THE MECHANISMS: PSYCHOPHYSIOLOGICAL VS CONVERSION

To fully appreciate how any thought or feeling can turn into physical pain or produce an illness that causes physical pain we must understand the mechanism by which it occurs.

Psychiatry has traditionally called psychological influences acting on the body through autonomic or hormonal pathways "psychophysiological reactions," and has called those acting via the voluntary nervous system (motor and sensory) "conversion reactions." In a study of 2000 patients suffering from migraine and tension headaches, Friedman et al (10) found that psychological factors could initiate headaches on either a psychophysiological or a conversion basis.

Although psychophysiological and conversion mechanisms are most commonly considered as alternatives, they can operate simultaneously in a particular patient or disease. The tension headache, for example, is thought to involve both excessive contraction of the cephalic musculature (psychophy-

siological) and centrally mediated hyperattentiveness to pain (conversion) in its pathogenesis.

Psychophysiological disorders result from the influence on the body of the physiological concomitants of excessively prolonged or intense affects or chronically held attitudes. Each "attitude" is a complex feeling state associated with a specific posture towards life, emotional tone, and with impulses towards certain types of action. Attitude has also been defined (11) as, "The way in which the person perceives his own position in a situation and the action, if any, which he wishes to take to deal with it." The attitude induces in the body those physiological preparations that will best prepare it for the actions or consequences so envisioned. Either a conscious or an unconscious attitude can affect the physiology.

Specific attitudes, each with its characteristic hopes, fears, and expectations, have been correlated with a number of medical syndromes (11–13) although, due to the complexity of the task, the conclusions are still being researched and refined.

If the affect or attitude is unconscious, the defenses employed to keep it unconscious are included in the patient's mental state. These defenses can have their own physiology, which then becomes superimposed.

Over time, the physiology accompanying these affects, attitudes, and defenses interacts with genetic vulnerabilities in the patient. When the "mixture" is right—perhaps the better word is "wrong"—the result is psychologically influenced headache made manifest. The mechanism by which the mind encourages pathophysiology is thus far more intricate than a unitary fight-or-flight response which switches on and off like a light bulb.

The conversion mechanism (see Chapter 12) involves usurpation of afferent or efferent impulses by an unconscious conflict that has been activated, producing what appears to be a physical symptom. The significance of the particular symptom "chosen" is symbolic.

Posttraumatic headaches can occasionally be triggered by the intrusion of a nonsymbolic memory. These types of percepts may fit the technical definition of illusion or hallucination, yet connote neither psychosis nor delirium. For example, an individual just returned from combat may flinch and startle if a car backfires near him. He momentarily relives the explosion of a nearby artillery round. This is a strong sensory memory, not a symbol, reawakened by the similar sound to briefly commandeer the veteran's sensory/perceptual apparatus (14). In psychiatry such reactions are most often seen in patients with posttraumatic stress disorders. In headache work they are most common following accidents.

Posttraumatic headaches resulting from a severe auto accident, for example, are sometimes revived by conditions resembling those in which the accident occurred (15). Seeing the bright headlights of a car in the oncoming lane momentarily brings the entire accident and its sensations back to mind.

THE THREE C'S: CRISIS, CONFLICT, CHARACTER

Three types of psychological problems can be related to headache: crisis, conflict, and character. A useful way to view them is in terms of whether they typically predispose to headache (character), precipitate headache (crisis), or do both (conflict). These have specific therapeutic implications as well. In general, treatment becomes increasingly long and difficult as one moves from crisis to conflict to character. Although the influence of one will usually predominate, they are not mutually exclusive. Current psychiatric terminology (16) recognizes in each patient the potential interdependence of several levels of difficulty, and attempts to account for this complexity with multifactorial diagnostic formulations. It is also a good way for the headache physician to think about his patients' emotional status.

In *crisis,* an individual is forced to cope with external pressures that border on the overwhelming: business is failing; the spouse is suing for divorce; the 14-year-old ran away from home; the house burned down. Tensions generated while trying to cope with these stressors place pressure on the physiology that causes its weakest link to snap. Sometimes that link is the substrate of headache.

When an active emotional *conflict* accentuates psychophysiological symptoms, it is because competing motivations are causing the patient to feel and act in ways both self-defeating and discomforting. Many of these reactions upset him, and he wishes he had more control over them—but he doesn't, largely because some of these motives are unconscious.

The patient with a *character* problem has suboptimal ways of dealing with the emotional contingencies of life—ways that he considers compatible with both his identity (the inner image of who he is) and with his ego ideal (the image of who he wants to be). Consequently, his maladaptive attitudes are entrenched and hard to influence. Even though friends and relatives may observe those habitual ways of handling things which repeatedly cause him difficulty, the patient believes them normal and sees no reason to change. Physical concomitants of the attitudes and affects generated by one's view of his position, role, and fate in life can influence headache, occasionally enough to give the patient cause to reconsider that view, if he can be convinced of the connection.

We will look at the relationship of these categories to the headache patient in sequence.

CRISIS

In many ways it is accurate to consider migraine, muscle contraction, mixed, and cluster headaches as disorders which can be aggravated by stress. This effect does not come from something mystical, but is the simple and direct result of an individual's physical preparation to meet the demands of demanding circumstance. Stress mobilizes biochemical and physiological changes that, in the predisposed individual, eventually lead to head pain.

One can think of stress as a catalyst and of the patient as a beaker of compounds in solution whose chemical composition represents his genetic makeup and early training. If the catalyst is a constant—the heat of a Bunsen burner, for example—certain solutions will be unaffected while others, each at its precise "boiling point," will roll with chemical activity. The situation becomes more complex when the "catalysts" are varied, as they are in life. Each chemical pulled from the laboratory shelf interacts with each solution to create its own gases, colors, and precipitates. The fact that people are more than beakers filled with chemicals only underscores the point: if even the inanimate responds with such uniqueness, we see what an extraordinarily individualized encounter stress must be when it affects a species which reacts idiosyncratically to everything from antidepressants to outfielders. Though analogy is not proof, it can remind one of overlooked conclusions. Are there any in this case?

Theoretically, at least, we can conlude that there is no "stress" independent of the person who reacts to it; a situation becomes a stress by virtue of that reaction alone. The same emergency room crises that drive one nurse to diazepam may prove a stimulating challenge to the next. Though the traumatic impact of certain events is so massive they induce a stress reaction in almost everyone— torture, war, or amputation, for example— milder situations, where individual variability plays the major role, are the ones more typically involved in the genesis of headache.

We can also conclude that before a situation can trigger the crisis physiology that leads to headache, the patient must interpret it as in some way dangerous, frightening, frustrating, infuriating, or disappointing. This assessment is in turn determined by his unique history of painful or pleasurable consequences following similar occurrences in the past.

Therefore, everyone carries forward from childhood a profile of strengths and liabilities with regard to the types of difficulties

he can handle. In one sense, then, any major change in the status quo has the potential to be experienced as stressful—to the point of triggering headaches—by someone. Even changes most people anticipate with pleasure, such as promotion or the move to a bigger house, can be stressful, and have been found (17) to increase one's chance of coming down with physical illness. (The man holding the winning lottery ticket may soon be holding his head.)

Nevertheless, the most stressful events for an individual day in and day out are usually those that in some way resemble and evoke the feeling states of troubled relationships or traumata in childhood.

CONFLICTS

The second "C", conflict, can either predispose to headache or trigger it. Conflict is a term which is often bandied about in ways that suggest mysterious or intimidating connotations known only to the few. Its meaning is actually quite direct: a person is pulled in several directions at once by strong and competing motives, some of which are unconscious. Either the impulse, or its true object, or its intensity, or the forces (such as guilt) opposing the impulse are not known to the patient. (If they were, it would simply be a choice, not a true conflict.) While the details and original sources of these struggles do involve considerable complexity, the basic concept does not.

The conflict cannot be resolved while major parts of it remain out of awareness. Therefore, one aim of treatment is to make what is unconscious, conscious, and thereby convert a conflict into a choice. Important and difficult choices can, of course, be stressful also, but their contributions to headache are through the mechanism of crisis.

Although they may first become manifest later, symptomatic conflicts usually have their origins in the struggles of childhood. During the process of socialization and maturation many of a child's wishes and impulses inevitably come into conflict with the wishes, expectations, and demands of his parents, or with the realities of society or of nature. The friction generated at this interface is anxiety. The child attempts to reduce this anxiety through a series of intrapsychic compromises between his competing motivations and the demands of reality. Many of these adaptations occur spontaneously, outside of the child's awareness.

Tenuous intrapsychic compromises predispose to conflict. The more permanent compromises collectively become part of the patient's personality or character. When a workable compromise has been incorporated into a patient's personality, that settled-upon resolution of the problem becomes part of his identity, and the books are closed. If the patient instead learns to use inefficient defenses to repress, separate off, or cope with competing demands that he only maintains a fragile peace between, the condition then represents conflict.

In conflict, a previously external struggle becomes internal; most typically, the patient takes in certain prohibitions of the parents and makes them part of his superego, while another part of him continues to react to those expectations with the original childlike feelings. Thus the originally external struggle becomes locked within a time capsule and buried in the patient's unconscious.

In patients with conflict, the ego is constantly trying to establish a cease-fire. Its ambassadors are the defenses.

Each person has a preferred set of defenses habitually relied upon since early life. Patients in whom psychological difficulty accompanies headaches are predisposed to use certain defenses, and each diagnosis tends to be associated with its characteristic (though not necessarily pathognomonic) constellation of them. Migraine patients are observed to use repression, identification with the aggressor, reaction formation, and sublimation (migraineurs also use a defense we refer to as "pseudoprogression"; see Chapter 15); patients with conversion headaches primarily use conversion and repression; patients with

muscle contraction headaches emphasize suppression and regression; patients with cluster headaches seem to favor denial (see Table 5.1).

CHARACTER

The third "C" is character, important for its potential to predispose to psychologically influenced headaches.

In psychiatry, the term "character" is a technical one. Everyone has a character. It has been defined as "the constellation of relatively fixed personality traits and attributes that govern a person's habitual modes of response" (18). Character is formed by the interaction between genetic and environmental forces, especially in the emotionally charged interpersonal environments encountered in early development.

The brain has often been compared to a computer. The personality, like the program, usually functions automatically. And just as each computer program will prove inadequate for certain tasks, each person can be overtaxed by situations his character is least equipped to handle. This can cause anxiety, often heralded by behavioral symptoms. Alternately, in some patients the anxiety is channeled into the body, with somatic or psychogenic illness appearing instead.

There is a percentage of people in whom the character is pathologically maladaptive; they have what is known as a "character disorder." This is a psychiatric diagnosis, and most headache patients do not fall into this category. The category excludes all those personality configurations normal enough to elude a formal diagnosis, yet only marginally efficient in one or several respects. It is within this latter group that one usually finds patients whose character inclines them towards attitudes which in turn make them vulnerable to headache.

Knowledge of how character develops can be used to evaluate its contribution to the transmittal of headaches within a family. This is because, in addition to genetics, headaches

TABLE 5.1
SOME PSYCHOLOGICAL DEFENSE MECHANISMS SEEN IN HEADACHE PATIENTS

Repression: The removal from consciousness of an unacceptably distressful memory, idea, impulse, or affect. This is done automatically by the ego and is outside of the patient's awareness or control. Material so removed is actively held in the unconscious. It can occur alone but is also seen to be an element in many defenses. Example: Woman unable to remember details of traumatic rape preceding headaches.

Suppression: The conscious, volitional decision to turn one's focus of attention completely away from upsetting thought content. Example: Scarlett O'Hara's, "I'll think about that tomorrow."

Denial: An external reality or some aspect of it is rejected or not fully acknowledged. Also applies to refusal to accept the presence of an obvious fact (such as illness) about one's self. Unacceptable fact may be replaced by a more comforting belief. Not volitional. Example: Daughter commits suicide by hanging, but mother insists that "she didn't mean to kill herself."

Regression: Withdrawal—partial or total—to earlier patterns of adaptation. Usually appears as more immature psychosocial and cognitive functioning. Unconscious aim: to act as one did in an earlier and seemingly more "successful" developmental level. Triggered by frustration and helplessness. Usually not intentional. Example: the ordinarily capable parent who becomes petulant and demanding when frightened by a severe headache.

Reaction Formation: Adopting in exaggerated form a socially acceptable intellectual or emotional stance that is the antithesis of strong unconscious feelings or impulses one wishes to disavow. Not a conscious decision or intended deception; the patient himself believes the exaggerated attitude to be true. Example: Solicitousness towards a person who is resented where the resentment inspires guilt.

Conversion: Resolving conflicting impulses by developing a physical reaction in the voluntary muscles or the special senses. Always entirely unconscious and symbolic; not facetious or malingering. Example: Pseudoparalysis of an arm to defend against the impulse to strike one's child.

Identification with the aggressor: Taking on the attitudes, attributes, or behaviors of a feared person or group with whom there has been a significant relationship in order to reduce the anxiety that one will become the recipient of aggression. Example: a battered child who in turn becomes abusive towards his own children.

Intellectualization: Focusing so heavily upon the cognitive and "rational" aspects of a painful situation that it precludes full awareness of the affective accompaniments. Example: Well-read patient who has endless ideas about what could be causing his headaches, but no recognition of his fears of what might be causing them.

Rationalization: The motive of an irrational behavior or infantile attitude is made to appear rational through specious reasoning. Example: Patient with dietary migraine decides that "light" beers do not count.

Sublimation: Transferring the energy originally associated with a raw or unacceptable impulse into the service of an adaptive or beneficial aim. An especially healthy defense. Example: "Bossy" impulses towards younger sister . . . lead person to later become a school principal.

Hypomanic defenses: Constantly shifting and energetically engaged activity leaves the person with no time for introspection, no time to focus on painful feelings or memories. Rarely conscious. Example: Following a sudden and potentially overwhelming loss, patient throws himself into three simultaneous projects at work, "never has time" to reflect upon or mourn the loss.

---

may run in families via identification. There are at least two mechanisms.

1. The child may simply form a primary identification with the parent who has headaches. He assumes both the self-image of "someone who gets headaches" in upsetting situations, and the propensity to act as the parent was seen to act when in pain, such as being irritable or reclusive.

2. Most people tend to raise a child as

they were raised. If the parent has emotional problems, this increases the chance of inducing similar difficulties in the child. These conflicts may be the type that aggravate headaches. This is the more common—and more important—mechanism. For example, the mother in whom the prohibition against expressing discontent was instilled early may not tolerate such expressions from her child either.

The most important way character develops is through identification. In it, the child assimilates and adopts the attitudes, rules, biases, and ideals of his parents or other significant persons in order to feel close to them. In the usual child-rearing situation, this mechanism of identification predominates. In the history of many headache patients, the balance is shifted toward identification valued for its ability to reduce discord.

As with adults, children are motivated not only by the carrot but by the stick: to please and to avoid displeasing. In this context, identification also serves to reduce the tension that would exist between parent and child when their wishes strongly conflict, and especially to avert any aggression—expressed in words, moods, or actions—which might result from that tension. Therefore, the more a parent becomes tense or angry when he does not see eye-to-eye with his child, the more valuable identification becomes to the child because it lowers the potential for confrontation. The child who adopts it has shaped his will to accord with that of the parent. In its extreme form, the process of emulation is impelled by the child's expectation that it is the only way to avoid resentment, rejection, or danger. This defines the psychological defense mechanism of "identification with the aggressor." It is, as can be seen, simply the exaggeration of a normal process.

Headache patients have also been reported to use identification to reduce guilt (2). The person in this scenario feels guilty about his hostile impulses towards someone else and tries to overcompensate by identifying with the person, thereby convincing himself that he bears no grudge. This only happens when there are strongly ambivalent feelings— not unalloyed dislike—toward the person with whom the person identifies.

Some researchers (19) believe they can discern one or several common denominators in the character structure of most patients with psychologically influenced physical illness, regardless of the specific diagnosis. Central features of this character develop before age 5. They arise from developmental struggles to gain control over the aggressive impulses that normally appear in response to the frustrations of that period. As an adult, such a patient rarely converts his hostile impulses to action; he has become, in fact, relatively unaware of their existence. The patient not only shields his relationships from anger but also shields himself from the discomfort he would feel if he confronted it. It has been theorized that the repressed impulses are instead discharged as somatic symptoms.

Another character trait frequently attributed to headache patients is masochism. The term—as used here—does not mean sexual masochism, which is a separate disorder. People are apt to think of a masochist as someone who "enjoys suffering," but so simple an explanation flies in the face of biology. It actually describes a tendency to endure mistreatment in order to reduce the anxiety that important relations will be ruptured by self-assertiveness. In contrast, the person expects—often unconsciously—his relationships will be strengthened by these submissions and sacrifices. The frequently seen difficulty in coping well with aggression reveals its presence here, too. A low self-esteem accompanies this harsh view of the contingencies of affection.

This martyr-like behavior is not engaged in for trivial needs. Monkeys have been taught to "masochistically" give themselves electric shocks to obtain food (20), and Harlow's classic studies (21) showed that, for young monkeys, the yearning to be connected to the mother transcended even that of food.

Alexithyma is theorized to be another character trait often seen in patients with psychologically influenced physical illnesses such as headache. It denotes a patient with limited ability to describe his feelings. Although the feelings are there—physiological monitoring shows that alexithymics react—these patients' awareness of feelings is short-circuited, and they only become aware of the physical concomitants of the affect. Such a patient's conversations often leave the impression that he has few feelings and no fantasies. It is as if attention is focused exclusively on outer realities: past, present, and future. For example, when asked how he felt when his sister died in a plane crash, the alexithymic patient might say, "I felt that I ought to contact my family. And then I went to my aunt's house."

It is possible to view this cognitive orientation as a defensive style. The patient may never have learned to feel comfortable with his inner world, and the alexithymia allows him to avoid it (although there are alternative explanations.) His outer world is often forced to serve functions of his inner life too, and he therefore structures it symbolically, much as a child arranges the rooms of a doll house. He often views his body as though it, too, were part of that outside world; indeed, physical sensations engendered by feelings commonly serve as a substitute for full feelings. Thus, the cognitive/emotional aspect of affect is blocked and replaced by overattention to its physiology. As he is minimally aware of his deeper mental life the patient has difficulty appreciating any connections between these sensations and emotions, or between emotions and illness. He is subject to somatic dysfunction when an adverse turn of events that most people would handle through fantasy or other emotional channels places a strain upon this adaptation. Headache is one of the conditions to which the alexithymic is prone.

TREATMENT IMPLICATIONS

What does identification of whether a patient is primarily having problems with crisis, conflict, or character suggest about how to treat him?

To the patient in **crisis** the physician should offer direct support. If he can be helped to cope with the crisis, his physiology will repair, and the headaches will take care of themselves. It is often necessary to help the person in crisis better "fit" his life-style to his profile of strengths and weaknesses so that his capacities best correspond to his obligations. Sometimes this means helping him redefine or change his role at work, at home, or in the extended family. When the square peg does not fit the round hole, it is always reasonable to search for a square hole before starting to whittle.

A patient whose headaches are aggravated by **conflict** should be helped to identify the conflict's underlying sources, to see that the struggle is probably an archaic one which did not mature along with the rest of him, and to mediate between and eventually control the unreasonable demands of his warring motivations. The means for accomplishing this is exploratory psychotherapy.

For patients whose headaches are accompanied by **character** problems the first job is to determine whether the undesirable traits are causing enough mischief to motivate the patient to change the *status quo*. If they are, the second task is to convert the character problems into conflicts. This is done by helping the patient recognize that he is both bearer and perpetrator of traits which are generating unappreciated difficulties for him and for those he loves. Once this is accomplished, the conflict is treated in the manner just mentioned. The job requires a highly trained therapist, as an overthrow of old and deep-seated characterological patterns must precede the learning of more suitable ones. During the transition the patient may experience a loss of functional stability and may temporarily have increased anxiety or other symptoms. Extensive revision of character is a task reserved for psychoanalysis, although more modest revisions can occasionally be performed by professionals with less training.

PAIN

A patient with a headache has—by definition—an *ache* (i.e., a pain) in his *head*. So, to fully understand headache, one must first understand pain, what it is, and how it is communicated (see Chapters 2, 5, and 8 also).

Pain has been described (22) as a phenomenon that at one and the same time is always **both** a sensation *and* an experience: *sensation of pain* results from stimulation of a pain receptor and propagation of the resulting impulse over afferent pathways to the thalamus and discriminative cortex.

The *experience of pain* devolves from the projection of that sensation to other areas in the neocortex, where it is interpreted. It is often more the experience of pain than the sensation which grieves the patient and brings him to the doctor. The raw pain sensation is fleshed out into the pain experience through its interaction with emotions, cognitions, memories, and anticipations; these determine both the intensity of the experience and its quality. Though the pain sensation is theoretically not subjective, the pain experience is. Many workers have acknowledged this complexity (23–26). Because of this interplay between sensation and experience, some have even gone so far as to say that "pain is always a psychosomatic problem" (22).

To understand the psychodynamics of pain, one must consider three factors:

1. The type and degree of stimulation of distal pain receptors or their proximal nerve trunks. These impulses attempt to break through the barrier which shields consciousness from extraneous or unwanted stimuli.

2. Memories of pain which, functioning as endogenous stimuli from the temporal lobe, may also attempt to capture the attention of consciousness. To do this they will often try to "ride their way in" on the back of an afferent stimulus, in the process intensifying or otherwise modifying it.

3. A highly sophisticated brain mechanism which functions as a sieve (or as the grid in an electron tube), acting to selectively enhance or filter out stimuli (in a fashion similar to that of the "attentional filter of Broadbent" (18, p 344)). Like a tough and savvy receptionist, this grid will accentuate, diminish, modify, coalesce, split, or entirely block the access to consciousness desired by each competing stimulus. The neuroanatomical substrate of this grid is probably the reticular activating substance and other subcortical structures (27). This grid has substantial power at its disposal when it needs it, as can be seen with hypnosis, which works its sleights-of-hand merely by persuading "the receptionist" to thwart or facilitate access of stimuli to consciousness. Its influence is strong enough for hypnosis to occasionally allow abdominal surgery without anesthesia (28). Conversely, patients in a deep trance have been touched with a pencil which they were told was a hot cigarette. Wincing with pain, they soon developed erythema and blistering at the site touched.

Headache patients, however, are not under the influence of posthypnotic suggestion, and it is other, primarily psychological, factors which are taken into consideration by this complex mechanism for regulating attention to painful stimuli.

Some of these factors are:

1. The real and symbolic **meanings** of the stimulus, as well as the perceived danger involved in ignoring it. Attention to discomfort in the neck will differ markedly, depending upon whether it is believed to originate from muscle tightness or bone cancer.

2. The patient's **history** of similar episodes in the past and their outcome. The influence of anxiety can be recognized here. A patient who has had only two headaches in his life, both caused by ruptured cerebral aneurysms, will find his attention drawn compellingly to any significant sensations above the neck.

3. ***Competing stimuli.*** The soldier in battle is preoccupied with stimuli which determine life or death. He will often be oblivious, not only to headache but also even to serious head injury. In contrast, the elderly woman isolated in her apartment without friends or hobbies may have too few stimuli that compete with the sensations from her cervical arthritis.

4. The expected ***duration*** of the pain. Brief tension headaches twice a year cause little attention when they come. Minor headaches that usually turn into incapacitating 3-day affairs are attended to with greater vigor.

5. ***Other needs or impulses*** which find pain useful can argue their case before "the receptionist." These include communication of emotional hurt or overload, doing penance to relieve guilt, or expressing aggression towards the family. Depression is especially prominent in this respect. Certain types of depression seem to rather generally open the floodgates of pain. It has been suggested (23) that depression can change the perception of a normal stimulus into a painful one.

Stimulation of pain receptors, memories of past pains (especially ones that occurred in the same region or were of the same type) and of their social/emotional contexts, anticipation of a pain's continuation, and the experience of sadness are but some of the forces that modify head pain and give it coloration.

To further complicate matters, the patient must *communicate* his pain experience to the doctor. Although the physician might observe the accompanying pallor, sweat, and grimace, he cannot observe the pain itself. As a result he is forced to evaluate the quality of the communication to be sure the words being used have similar connotations for both patient and doctor.

Because pain is subjective, an absolute judgment about the validity of someone's pain experience is rarely possible. When medical personnel voice doubts about the reality of a patient's pain, they are treating it,

usually unwittingly, as though it were a perception of something it is not—a hallucination. Yet, the pain rarely meets the formal criteria for a hallucination, and the patient rarely has a diagnosis, such as psychosis, in which one might expect hallucinations. With medicine's current knowledge, a physician can only determine the probably presence or absence of commonly known sources of pain. That leaves to the art of medicine the task of teaching how to accept the limits of its science and how to comfort the patient in distress who is outside those limits.

CONCLUSION

The perspective of psychosomatic medicine provides a comprehensive and balanced approach to many headache patients. This perspective rarely holds that a particular experience, emotion, or conflict "causes" a "psychosomatic disease," like the tubercle bacillus causes tuberculosis.[1] The psychosomatic approach attempts instead to recognize the many competing vectors moving the patient towards or away from a particular disease outbreak and the complex congress by which they are governed. It does not propose that illness is simply the result of overheated emotion or that it can be reversed by a determined act of will.

A tenet of psychosomatics is this: mind and body is only one way to view an illness. An alternate division, frequently more useful, is that of structure and function, and these are seen as unitary, related one to the other much like the flame and wood of a burning log are the indivisible elements of fire. Another basic assumption, therefore, is that every mental

---

[1] Even for TB, the harder one looks the more complexity that can be found. One must take into account the number and virulence of the organisms to which the patient is exposed and whether the patient's resistance is too slight or too intense (which also leads to pathology). The patient's resistance is in turn influenced by genetics, nutrition, endocrine status, concurrent illness, psychological factors, and age.

activity, greater or smaller, conscious or unconscious, is in some way reflected in the physiology and, conversely, that every event in the physiology is reflected, to some extent, in the mind (29). Can one change the shape of a violin without, however slightly, affecting its song? Or change its song without, however slightly, affecting its shape?

An anecdote told by a Canadian colleague (30) reminds us that the irreplaceable foundations of clinical medicine are empathy, perspective, and common sense:

As a young and inexperienced internist in the armed services I was forever plagued by the problems of headache which were constantly referred to me. I peered into fundi, tapped kneecaps and spinal fluids, all in a perpetual state of alarm, alerted to the ever-present possibility of a cerebral tumor. Finally, in desperation I asked the advice of an older and wiser physician. He looked out across the barren wind and rain swept plains of the air force camp where a squad of new recruits were drilling, glanced at me kindly, and said "Wouldn't you get a headache too?" (Originally published in Canodian Medical Association Journal **Volume 91, October 24, 1964.)**

The art of doctoring is helped if the physician can cultivate as empathetic an attitude towards the headache patient's foibles as towards his headaches and, also, towards his own human fallibility in diagnosing and treating them.

There is both challenge and promise in the recognition that head pain, along with the psychological distresses that orbit it, though subjective and as yet unmeasureable, have ultimately discernible physicochemical bases in the brain. This fact reassures us that they will prove to be increasingly treatable conditions within the physician's purview.

REFERENCES

1. Friedman AP, Merrit HH: Migraine. In Friedman AP, Merritt HH (eds): *Headache, Diagnosis and Treatment*. Philadelphia, Davis, 1959, p 208.
2. Kolb LC: Psychiatric and psychogenic factors in headache. In Friedman AP, Merritt HH (eds): *Headache: Diagnosis and Treatment*. Philadelphia, Davis, 1959, p 264.
3. Darwin C: *Expression of the Emotions in Man and Animals*. New York, Appleton, 1873.
4. Lorenz K: *King Solomons Ring*. New York, Thomas Y. Crowell, 1952.
5. Adler CS, Adler SM: Biofeedback—psychotherapy for the treatment of headache: a five year followup. *Headache* 16:189–191, 1976.
6. Adler SM, Adler CS: Physiologic feedback and psychotherapeutic intervention for migraine: a 10-year followup. In Pfaffenrath V, Lundberg PO, Sjaastad O (eds): *Updating in Headache*. Heidelberg, Springer-Verlag, 1985, pp 217–223.
7. Hunter RA: Psychotherapy in migraine. *Br Med J* 1:1084–1088, 1960.
8. Jonckheere P: The chronic headache patient. *Psychother. Psychosom.* 19:53–61, 1971.
9. Eisenbud J: The psychology of headache: a case studied experimentally, *Psychiatr Q* 11:592–629, 1937.
10. Friedman AP, Von Storch TJ, Merritt HH: Migraine and tension headaches: a clinical study of two thousand cases. *Neurology* 4:733–788, 1954.
11. Grace WJ, Graham DT: Relationship of specific attitudes and emotions to certain bodily diseases. *Psychosom Med* 14:243–251, 1952.
12. Dunbar F: *Emotions and Bodily Changes*, ed 3. New York, Columbia University Press, 1947.
13. Alexander FG: *Psychosomatic Medicine: Its Principles and Applications*. New York, Norton, 1950.
14. Adler CS: Discussion of: Glucksman ML: Physiologic changes and clinical events during psychotherapy. *Intergr Psychiatry* 3:168–184, 1985.
15. Adler CS, Adler SM: Psychiatric treatment of post-traumatic headache. In Solomon S, Elkind A (eds): *The Post-Head Trauma Syndrome*. New York, Spectrum Press, in press, 1987.
16. Spitzer RL (ed): *DSM III: Diagnostic and Statistical Manual of Mental Disorders*. Washington, American Psychiatric Association, 1980.
17. Rahe RH, Meyer M, Smith M, Kjaer G, Holmes TH: Social stress and illness onset. *J Psychosom Res* 8:35–44, 1964.
18. Kaplan HI, Freedman AM, Sadock BJ: *Comprehensive Textbook of Psychiatry III*. Baltimore, Williams & Wilkins, 1980, p 3315.
19. Sperling M: A further contribution to the psychoanalytic study of migraine and psychogenic headaches. *Int J Psychoanal* 45:549–557, 1964.
20. Masserman JH: The neurotic cat. *Psychol Today* 1:36–39, 1967.

21. Harlow HF: The nature of love. *Am Psychol* 13:673, 1958.

22. Langen D: Psychologic factors in the development and therapy of trigeminal neuralgia. In Hassler R, Walker EA (eds): *Trigeminal Neuralgia.* Philadelphia, Saunders, 1970, pp 149–152.

23. Dalessio DJ: Some reflections on the etiologic role of depression in head pain. *Headache* 8:28–31, 1968.

24. Frazier, SH: Complex problems of pain as seen in headache, painful phantom, and other states. In Arieti S, Reiser MF (eds): *American Handbook of Psychiatry,* ed 2. New York Basic Books, 1975, pp 838–851.

25. Friedman AP: Psychophysiological aspects of headache. In *Phenomenology and Treatment of Psychophysical Disorders.* New York, Spectrum, 1982, pp 42–50.

26. Karpman B: Psychogenic aspects of headache: a symposium. *Clin Psychopathol* 10:1–26, 1949.

27. Luthe W (ed): *Autogenic Therapy* vol 6. New York, Grune & Stratton, 1973.

28. Kroger WS: *Clinical and Experimental Hypnosis.* Philadelphia, Lippincott, 1963.

29. Green E, Green A: *Beyond Biofeedback.* New York, Delta, 1977.

30. Sloane RB: Psychological aspects of headache. *Can Med Assoc J* 91:908–911, 1964.

SECTION TWO

Assessment of the Headache Patient

CHAPTER SIX

First Things First: The Physical Workup

ROBERT S. KUNKEL, M.D.

Treatment of the patient complaining of headache commences with the first visit to the physician's office. The approach and concern shown by the physician regarding the patient's symptoms sets the stage for a successful therapeutic relationship. The physician needs to take the patient's complaints seriously even if the discomfort is primarily psychogenic. The fact that the headache sufferer seeks help is an indication he is concerned and worried. Fears cannot be allayed unless a thorough history is taken and a complete physical and neurological examination is performed. Attempts at managing the patient are less likely to be successful if it is felt that the physician is not taking complaints seriously or is not interested in listening to the patient's symptoms, even though they may be read from a list.

Although the overwhelming majority of headache complaints are not due to any structural disease or life-threatening condition, it is essential to correctly diagnose those headaches that are, so that specific surgical or medical treatment can be administered. Most patients, at least early in the course of the headache, worry that the symptoms may be from a brain tumor. A complete and detailed history followed by a thorough examination does much to reassure the patient—if the examination is normal—as to the absence of any disease.

THE HEADACHE HISTORY

The basis of the headache diagnosis rests with the history (see Table 6.1). It is unusual to turn up something on examination or testing that is not suspected from the history. A short duration of headache complaints and increasing frequency and severity of pain and/or development of new symptoms are the most important features which would make one suspect an organic cause for the complaints. It is therefore essential to find out how long the symptoms have been present. Persons may have had headaches in the past and then been free of pain, only to have a recurrence. This may happen in migraine and, of course, is typical in cluster headache. A steadily progressive course with increased pain and/or neurological dysfunction is very suggestive of an organic process.

Any headache occurring for the first time in a patient over the age of 50, no matter what the pattern of pain may be, needs to be thoroughly investigated. A nonprogressive headache pattern lasting many months or years is strongly suggestive of nonorganic headache. Migraine usually begins before the age of 30. Muscle contraction (tension) headache usually begins before the age of 50.

DIFFERENTIAL DIAGNOSIS

The type of pain described may be helpful in arriving at the diagnosis. A pulsatile, throbbing pain suggests a vascular etiology and is usually present in migraine. Interestingly enough, however, the discomfort in another vascular headache, cluster, is usually not pulsatile. The common, chronic muscle contraction headache is usually described as a

TABLE 6.1

ESSENTIAL ITEMS OF THE HEADACHE HISTORY

---

1. Number and types of headache present
2. Age and circumstances of onset
3. Family history
4. Characteristics of pain
   a. Location
   b. Frequency of attacks
   c. Duration of pain
   d. Description of pain
   e. Time of onset of attack
5. Prodromal symptoms
6. Associated symptoms
   a. Systemic
   b. Neurologic
7. Precipitating factors
   a. Environmental (external)
   b. Psychological
   c. Internal
8. Emotional factors
   a. Sleep pattern
9. Medical history
   a. Past illnesses
   b. Concurrent disease
   c. Trauma
   d. Surgery
10. Allergies
11. Medication use
    a. Over-the-counter medications
    b. Prescription
12. Response to medication
    a. Past
    b. Present

---

dull, aching pressure sensation or as a tightness or heaviness. Neuritic pains, such as occur with tic douloureux, are sharp, severe, stabbing, repetitive pains. Contary to what many think, the headache caused by a growing brain tumor is usually not intense, and visual and neurological abnormalities are often more disturbing than pain. The pain from an intracranial hemorrhage is quite severe and, of course, is very sudden in onset and is characteristically unlike any headache the patient may have experienced previously.

The family history of headache is important to obtain. Migraine is familial, and about 70% to 80% of migraineurs know of others in the family who have had migraine or "sick headaches." It is important to ask about "sick" or menstrual headache and not merely to ask about the presence of "migraine." In the past many such patients were not diagnosed as having migraine.

Patients often learn pain behavior when they are young by observing parents and other family members. An impressionable child can notice the attention, sympathy, and support a parent gets from the family when he complains of pain and, specifically, of headache. These observations can play a prominent role in fostering complaints of and disability from headache when the child becomes an adult. Many patients are unaware that their behavior reflects what they observed as children, and it may be helpful to point this out. In general, other than patients with an acute migraine attack, patients suffering the most disability and inability to perform daily tasks are very likely to have significant psychological problems.

Migraine, for the most part, occurs in paroxysmal attacks, with pain-free intervals lasting weeks or months. An individual attack may last 12–72 hr. Occasionally, a migraine will linger for many days. In the female, migraine often occurs around the menstrual period and is absent during pregnancy. If the history brings out a daily, persistent discomfort for weeks, months, or years, migraine is much less likely. Chronic muscle contraction headache or a mixed headache pattern (with both muscle contraction and vascular components) are likely diagnoses in persistent headache of long duration.

Migraine is a disorder marked by altered autonomic stability, symptoms of which include nausea and vomiting, photophobia, phonophobia, chills, and diarrhea accompanying attacks. Emotional changes such as irritability, depression, and anxiety may precede or accompany an attack. Because emotions can effect the autonomic nervous system, psychological factors can influence migraine attacks. It is therefore essential to explore the patient's psychological history, even when the diagnosis of migraine is certain. Any headache, and for that matter any medical condition, chronic or acute, is associated with some change in the psychological balance.

In discussing headaches with the patient, one can often help him identify trigger mechanisms. Specific dietary agents such as red wine, aged cheese, chocolate, and fermented foods may trigger attacks. Estrogens, as well as other drugs such as the vasodilating agents and reserpine, may also be a factor in exacerbations of migraine.

Excessive intake of caffeine has been recognized as a cause of daily headaches. Primary sources of caffeine include coffee, tea, cola, and over-the-counter analgesics. Patients awaken in a state of caffeine withdrawal in which headache is a prominent symptom. These persons take in excessive amounts of caffeine during the day. When they have no intake for several hours at night, they then awaken with withdrawal symptoms. Many such patients feel better as soon as they take analgesics containing caffeine along with their morning coffee.

Emotional stress is the most common precipitant of headaches. There is often not a direct temporal relationship between a tension headache and a stressful event, and it is wise to remember that persons with chronic tension headache may awaken with headache even though they claim to have slept well all night. Many persons feel their headache cannot be caused by tension or stress because it is present upon awakening. But muscle contraction may occur at any time.

Part of any good medical history is to note the past history of significant medical illness or trauma. Posttraumatic headaches can last for years. The severity of the discomfort is often out of proportion to the recognizable extent of injury. Seemingly minor and apparently insignificant trauma can be followed by prolonged head discomfort along with other symptoms such as lightheadedness, giddiness, weakness, fatigue, and mental dysfunction. Any previous malignancy should be noted, since headache of recent onset may represent intracranial metastatic disease. Breast carcinoma in particular may metastasize many years after the initial diagnosis was made.

EXAMINATION

After a thorough history is obtained, one should have a pretty good idea how to classify the headache. A physical examination, including a neurological examination, is mandatory on every headache patient. First, observe the patient. Note particularly any disturbance in gait. If present, it might suggest some neurological abnormality. Observe, also, the patient's mannerisms. A person with chronic muscle tension headache will often be continually rubbing or rolling his neck.

During an acute migraine or cluster attack, one will often find autonomic signs which are helpful in diagnosis. The vital signs, such as blood pressure, temperature, and pulse, are often ignored but should be recorded. Mild increases in blood pressure may aggravate migraine and, of course, significantly elevated blood pressure may be a cause of headache. Fever may be the clue to an underlying disease. Headache is a common accompaniment of any fever.

Particular attention should be paid to the head and its sensory structures, the eyes, ears, nose, and throat. Gentle palpation of the eyeballs may alert one to the possibility of glaucoma. An orbital bruit may be heard in the presence of arteriovenous malformation, aneurysm, carotid artery disease, or temporal arteritis. The fundus examination may reveal signs of increased intracranial pressure. Examination of the neck and trapezius muscles will often demonstrate tightness in these muscles in a patient with chronic muscle contraction headache. Palpation of the head and neck may reveal tender areas indicative of muscle spasm; these are often seen in people with temporomandibular joint problems. The overwhelming majority of patients who have pain related to the muscles of mastication are tense, and continually brux or grind their teeth. Only a small minority will have significant bite problems or temporomandibular joint disease.

Although attention is focused on the head, eyes, nose, ears, teeth, and neck, it is important to do a complete physical examination. Lung and heart disorders may be associated with headache, and a search for any systemic disease should be performed, especially in anyone with a recent onset of headache. Hypothyroidism can be associated with generalized aching and myalgia and may be specifically associated with chronic neck pain.

LABORATORY STUDIES

Laboratory studies are best selected after a thorough history and physical exam. They should be used to confirm a specific diagnosis or to rule out a suspected lesion (see Table 6.2). The CT scan is the best way to demonstrate structural changes within the cranium. X-rays of the neck may demonstrate degenerative changes in vertebrae and discs which may play a role in chronic muscle contraction headache. Cervical X-rays taken of patients with neck pain from chronic muscle contraction often show a straightening of the normal forward lordotic curve; they can be helpful for demonstrating to the patient how chronic muscle contraction can alter physiology. Laboratory studies may turn up anemia, electrolyte imbalance, hypoglycemia, hypothyroidism, or other abnormalities which may be clues to organic dysfunction. Although systemic problems are not a common cause of headache, they may be a factor and are worth checking at least once during the headache workup.

TREATMENT PLANNING

If serious disease is discovered, one's approach to telling the patient will vary with the patient's emotional stability. It may be better to gradually disclose the abnormality to the patient over the course of several visits, rather than to thrust a devastating diagnosis on him all at once. The physician should

TABLE 6.2

DIAGNOSTIC TESTS USEFUL IN HEADACHE EVALUATION

1. Lab: complete blood count (CBC), biochemical profile, electrolytes, sedimentation rate, endocrine function studies
2. X-rays
3. CT scan
4. Electroencephalogram
5. Angiogram
6. Lumbar puncture

never suddenly abandon the patient just because it is learned his disease is incurable.

If it is decided that psychological therapy is indicated as a part of the treatment, the primary physician should continue to follow the patient. New symptoms may develop and, of course, medical diseases may arise at any time and need to be treated. The patient with chronic headache is best treated by a team approach and should see his primary physician at regular intervals, as well as the person who is helping him with psychological problems. The initial medical evaluation should not be the end of medical care but should be the basis for an ongoing association and intermittent re-evaluation. The psychiatrist or psychologist treating the headache patient should not hesitate to get the clinician reinvolved in the care of the patient if his response to therapy does not progress. Follow-up and continuity of care is essential if one expects to help the chronic headache patient function with less disability and discomfort. If such patients are not given the time they need, they will drift from doctor to doctor, getting incomplete help (and, most likely, getting a variety of analgesics, which only compounds the problem).

The chronic headache patient habituated to numerous medications is much too prevalent today. Treatment by combined psychological and pharmacological means, using nonhabituating medications when indicated, will restore many of these people to useful, productive lives. A thorough history and physical should lead to the correct diagnosis, and the correct diagnosis is essential in directing the proper therapy, both psychological and pharmacological. The patient's confidence and faith in the treating physician play a very important role in the therapeutic program for the headache patient. This faith, trust, and confidence will only occur if the physician has convinced the patient that a thorough investigation of possible causes has been done. The history and physical examination as well as the laboratory workup is an essential part of the therapy of the headache patient.

SUGGESTED READINGS

Dalessio DJ: *Wolff's Headache and Other Head Pain,* ed 4. New York, Oxford University Press, 1980.

Diamond S, Dalessio DJ: *The Practicing Physician's Approach to Headache,* ed 4. Baltimore, Williams & Wilkins, 1986.

Lance JW: *Mechanism and Management of Headache,* ed 3. London, Butterworth's, 1978.

Packard RC (ed): *Neurologic Clinics: Symposium on Headache.* Philadelphia, WB Saunders, 1983, vol 1, no. 2.

Saper J: *Headache Disorders: Current Concepts and Treatment Strategies.* Boston, John Wright-PSG Inc, 1983.

CHAPTER SEVEN

Mythology in the Management of Headache

JOHN EDMEADS, M.D.

Headache, more than most symptoms, is invested by a fabric of false beliefs—a mythology—that may delay diagnosis and impede treatment. There are three reasons why headache is so liable to be misunderstood by those who suffer it. First, it is a very common symptom and therefore subject to ill-informed discussion by patients, relatives, and the media. Second, the more common kinds of headache, muscle contraction ("tension") headaches and migraine, are not susceptible to either confirmation or measurement by x-ray or laboratory tests. Third, physicians themselves are far from unanimous about the causes and treatment of the various types of headache, and this uncertainty is quickly apprehended by their patients and may encourage the development of misinformation.

Nor is the medical profession immune to serious misconceptions about headache. In his classic textbook of medicine, Osler (1) identified mouth breathing as a common cause of headache and recommended adenoidectomy. It may well be that our professional heirs will someday regard some of our current concepts about headache as quaint myths.

The theme to be developed in this discussion is that myths about headache abound; that they flourish because they have a grain of truth and a certain usefulness to those who nurture them; and that physicians, for reasons of their own and with varying levels of awareness of what they are doing, may support the harboring of these myths by their patients.

DIAGNOSTIC MYTHS

These take two forms. The first is a mistaken belief that the headache is due to a process that is benign, elusive, and invaribly physical. This belief usually results in the patient and, often the physician, fruitlessly searching for an underlying condition which will yield to physical treatment such as medication or surgery and has as its major consequences a waste of resources and time and delay in addressing the true cause of the headache. This may be likened to chasing a wild goose up a blind alley.

The second type of diagnostic myth is a groundless fear that the headache is due to ominous life-threatening disease. This, too, can result in needless investigation and delay in diagnosis but may also pose a risk to the patient if concern about ominous possibility impels the physician to such hazardous investigation as angiography. This may be likened for searching for a ghost in the attic.

Viewed rationally, these diagnostic chases, whether after goose or ghost, are hardly ever necessary.

COMMON GEESE:

a. "Headaches frequently are caused by *eye strain*" (2). While headaches certainly may occur in a situation of prolonged close work, these are mediated by muscle contraction accruing from prolonged maintenance of a hunched and relatively immobile posture, fatigue, and attempts at ocular convergence. Glasses are unlikely to be the whole answer, nor are tedious corrections of latent squints.

b. "Headaches frequently are due to '*sinus troubles*'" (3). Not so. Acute sinusitis, through the agencies of inflammation of pain-sensitive mucosa and suction on mucosa from impeded drainage, may cause frontal and/or cheek pain. Other sinus conditions (such as allergies, chronic sinusitis, etc.,) only rarely produce these two circumstances and thus only rarely cause headache. Criteria for acute sinusitis are fever, nasal or postnasal discharge, local tenderness over the sinuses, and abnormal sinus x-rays. A patient who does not fulfill these criteria does not have "sinus headaches." Most people who think they have "sinus headache" have either migraine or muscle contraction headaches.

c. "Headaches frequently are due to *allergies*" (4). This is an especially pernicious myth because allergies and headaches are each very common, and there are bound to be people with both. The myth is augmented by occasional instances of improvement in headache from "allergy medications" such as vasoconstrictors and antihistaminics; it is not realized that such medications may be equally efficacious in migraine. Pursuit of this particular goose leads to exhaustive skin tests with the almost inevitable occurrence of a few positive reactions, leading in turn to either assiduous avoidance of essentially harmless substances by the patient, or to inconvenient desensitization procedures, with the ultimate benefit accruing only to the practitioner who charges for them. There is no convincing evidence, either clinically or in the laboratory, that allergy is a cause of headache.

d. "Headaches are due to '*arthritis of the neck*'". (5) This, too, is a widespread myth because everybody has a neck, nearly everybody has some transient discomfort in it from time to time, and most people over the age of 40 have radiologic changes of cervical disc disease whether or not they have symptoms from it. While there seems little doubt that lesions at the craniovertebral junction (e.g., atlantoaxial dislocation, basilar invagination, etc.,) and lesions of the upper cervical spine may present with headache, there is considerable doubt that lesions lower down (most cervical disc disease is distributed from the fifth cervical interspace downwards) can produce pain referred to the head. Uncritical consideration of this possibility may lead to the unfortunately not uncommon sequence of neck x-ray, collar immobilization, "muscle relaxant" medication, chiropractic manipulation, and surgery, and may result in a patient with less money in his bank account, less confidence in his doctors, and as much headache as ever. Most patients with chronic recurrent headaches and abnormal cervical spine x-rays have common muscle contraction headaches.

e. "Headaches are due to dental malocclusion and jaw joint disease ('*temporomandibular arthritis*')" (6). Many people have malocclusion; many people have clicking jaw joints; and many people have headache. The uncritical melding of these disparate entities into a syndrome has led to a wave of enthusiasm for tooth grinding, bite plates, and even surgical assaults on the temporomandibular joint. Fortunately, this enthusiasm is subsiding, mostly because these measures frequently are not of lasting benefit. Head pain can result from dental problems or from bruxism (tooth gnashing), usually through the agency of prolonged contraction of jaw muscles, with subsequent recruitment of adjacent scalp muscles; it is more appropriately termed "the Myofascial Pain Dysfunction syndrome." Most people who consider themselves to have "temporo-mandibular arthritis" have either this MPD syndrome or simple muscle contraction headaches.

COMMON GHOSTS

Most patients, by the time their symptoms have increased to the point where they consult a physician, have had at least a momentary thought that serious disease may be present. Some carry this idea to unnatural lengths. They become excessively concerned, occasionally obsessed, by the notion that their headache may be due to brain tumor, aneurysm, or stroke, and there may be great difficulty in convincing them otherwise. The serious diseases that frighten these people are rare in comparison to the very common entities of muscle contraction headache and migraine.

a. *Brain tumors* hardly every present with headache alone; there are nearly always other neurological complaints, and some neurological deficit, however slight, is nearly always found on careful examination.
b. *Aneurysms* very seldom present with headache prior to rupture. Small leaks from an aneurysm may produce one or two episodic severe headaches, but never a lengthy history of chronic recurrent head pain. When these leaks occur, there is usually some evidence of meningeal irritation on examination, if it is looked for.
c. *Atherothrombotic strokes* (occlusive cerebrovascular disease) (7) may be preceded or accompanied by dull headaches, but patients with headaches on this basis almost always have either historical or physical evidence of atherosclerotic vascular disease.

When the physician has a legitimate suspicion that these conditions may exist, appropriate investigation will nearly always either exclude or establish the diagnosis. The best "all-purpose investigation," if available, is a contrast enhanced CT scan; this will demonstrate nearly all tumors, most arteriovenous malformations, some aneurysms, parenchymal hemorrhages, most instances of subarachnoid blood, and some infarcts. Angiography, though not without risk, will identify most of those aneurysms which might have been missed by the CT scan and will be useful in detecting some varieties of cerebrovascular disease.

WHY DIAGNOSTIC MYTHS FLOURISH

Patients' conviction that their headaches *must* be due to physical disease are prevalent, persistent, and due to a number of factors:

a. There is a natural desire in our "cause-and-effect oriented society" to have all symptoms explained on an easily understood, tangible, and mechanistic basis.
b. Diagnostic myths are reinforced and disseminated by relatives of patients, by the media, and by some practitioners, all of whom share a desire to be of help, a lack of critical faculty, and perhaps a degree of self-interest.
c. The failure of many physicians to explain their diagnosis to their patient in a confident, comprehensive, and convincing fashion may leave the patient vaguely dissatisfied, worried, and open to continuing concerns about other possibilities.
d. Possibly most important of all, some patients, reluctant to confront the possibility that their headaches may be a somatic manifestation of psychological stress, insist upon tracking down other diagnostic alternatives; they create this diversion with varying degrees of awareness of what they are doing and why. When a patient's concern about undiagnosed ominous disease tenaciously resists all reassurance, including knowledgeable explanation and exhaustive investigation, then that concern may assume the proportions of a de-

lusion and constitute a symptom of serious psychiatric disease.

Physicians also may be caught up in a diagnostic wild goose chase, again for various reasons:

a. Any physician may have a reasonable but mistaken belief that a certain physical condition underlies the headaches—that is, a simple diagnostic mistake.

b. The habitual attribution of all headaches to one specific physical condition ("Dr. Jones is a TMJ man") may signify the conquest of common sense by evangelical fervor.

c. Some physicians, knowing full well that their patients' headaches are due to migraine or muscle contraction, will perform numerous unnecessary investigations because of fear of medicolegal consequences, should a mistake in diagnosis occur.

d. Some doctors, possibly because of lack of confidence in their ability to operate along psychological lines, seem as reluctant as their patients to address the issue of emotional disturbance as a cause of headaches, and they put off the biting of the bullet by chewing with the patient as long as possible on more mutually acceptable physical possibilities.

THERAPEUTIC MYTHS

These are legion. Only three major myths will be addressed: "All headaches are psychogenic," "All headaches are biochemical," and "Any headache can be helped by medication."

"ALL HEADACHES ARE PSYCHOGENIC"

According to this myth, all headaches (excepting, of course, those due to brain tumor, subarachnoid hemorrhage, etc.,) are somatic manifestations of psychological stress and are peculiar to perfectionistic, rigid, anxious, or depressed individuals; these headaches and these individuals are always helped best by traditional, formal psychotherapy.

This is a foreshortened, formulaic version of the "migraine personality" concept. Migraine patients are viewed as invariably intelligent, compulsive, conscientious, and fastidious individuals whose headaches result from the stress imposed upon these perfectionistic people as they cope with an imperfect world. Presently, some experienced clinicians question whether the "migraine personality" might not be an artifact of self-selection; compulsive individuals are less likely than more relaxed people to accept anything less than perfect bodily function and are therefore more likely to present themselves repetitively to physicians in attempts to gain for themselves the same perfection in health and wellbeing that they demand from all other aspects of life. The observation that sufferers from migraine and tension headaches are more tense and anxious than people without frequent headaches may have some substance, but it is also difficult to verify, since it may be that anxious people are likelier to present themselves to physicians than are more relaxed individuals with headaches. It does seem, however, that headache patients in general are more anxious than patients with other conditions (e.g., epilepsy) that also present with repeated attacks; that patients with frequent headaches are more anxious than those with occasional headaches; and that of those patients with frequent headaches, anxiety levels and other indices of psychological disturbances appear on psychological testing to be higher in some headache types (e.g., muscle contraction headaches) than in others (e.g., cluster headaches) (8).

If it is true that "all headaches are psychogenic," then conventional psychotherapy might reasonably be expected to help a proportion of these patients. In fact, as practiced by many therapists, it frequently is unsuccessful. Indeed, it is not too unusual to have a "chronic headache patient" emerge from a psychiatric diagnostic interview with the Good Housekeeping seal of "no psychopathology" newly affixed despite the facts that the patient is having headaches each and every day with no evidence of physical disease and is abusing analgesic medications. This situation seems to come about for two reasons: first, these patients are very well defended, and on their best behavior can present an impression of normalcy; second, these patients often do not have conventional signs or symptoms of psychoneurosis, and "having headaches" is the only evident abnormality.

In summary, the returns are not yet in on the question of the psychogenic component of headaches, but it does appear that emotional factors probably play a role in the production of chronic headaches resistant to pharmacologic therapy and that the conventional rules of formal psychotherapy are often less effective for relieving the situation. Therefore, referral should be to psychotherapists knowledgeable about headache patients, ones chosen with as careful an eye to the appropriate matchup as is used in selecting the best medication.

"ALL HEADACHES ARE BIOCHEMICAL"

This school of thought holds that factors in the external environment (e.g., dietary amino acids, food additives, etc.,) or in the internal environment (e.g., hypoglycemia, hormonal alterations, etc.,) are largely responsible for the production of headaches and that headaches can be eliminated by adjusting these factors. This tradition, particularly as it pertains to diet and hypoglycemia, is enormously popular with patients. While it is likely that these considerations are relevant only to migraine and, indeed, to only 10–15% of migraine sufferers, much larger numbers of patients assiduously exclude certain foods from their diet, juggle their meal schedules, and consume various interesting vitamin supplements. A few physicians encourage this, sometimes because they believe, perhaps more often because they are following Vol-

taire's maxim of "amusing and diverting the patient while Nature heals." There is just enough truth in the notion that hormonal fluctuations affect headaches to encourage manipulation of these potent chemicals. Occasional successes from blind juggling are recorded; more numerous failures or adverse effects are forgotten; and the myth endures.

In summary, alteration of some environmental factors is occasionally helpful for the occasional patient with occasional headaches. For patients with frequent headaches, particularly if those headaches are of a "muscle contraction" pattern, such biochemical sleight of hand is fruitless.

"ANY HEADACHE CAN BE HELPED BY MEDICATION"

Physicians have always emphasized medication, more particularly so since advances in our understanding of the pathophysiology of headache have led to the conviction that appropriate medication should be able to normalize the disturbed physiology and abolish the patient's symptom. Thus, the vasoconstrictor ergotamine should be able to nullify the vasodilatory headache of migraine; various "muscle relaxants" should be able to break the sustained muscle contraction that underlies tension headaches; and peripherally and centrally acting analgesics should be able to block the transmission of pain. All of this, sadly, is only partly true. The pathophysiology of muscle contraction and migraine headaches is no longer as clear-cut as was once believed (9, 10). In the opinion of some workers, the distinction between muscle contraction and vascular headaches is becoming increasingly blurred (11). Medications once thought to have a very specific effect are now recognized as having many actions, any of which could be responsible for therapeutic efficacy (e.g., ergotamine not only constricts via the α-adrenergic receptor but also has a serotoninomimetic action; amitriptyline is not only an antidepressant but enhances the activity of pain-modulating systems within the brainstem). Clinicians who have stumbled through this swamp of shadowy theory and confused therapeutics have emerged with a fairly generally accepted rule of thumb:

- Patients with occasional headaches, especially if the headaches conform to a pattern of migraine or muscle contraction headaches, are in general well-adjusted individuals and obtain a good result from small amounts of appropriate medication. Patients with frequent or constant headaches, especially if the headaches are of an amorphous and ill-defined character, are almost always emotionally disturbed, hardly ever have any insight into this, practically never obtain substantial benefit from medication, but nevertheless manage to abuse medication and develop dependence upon it.

Whatever the reason for this, the moral is clear—medication is not the answer for every patient with headaches.

Patients are reluctant to discard the myth of the omnipotence of medication. Not only does this go against all their preconceptions, but—probably more important—it implies that headaches may be one situation in which the traditional patient's role of a passive recipient of therapy ("Here I am—fix me") is inapplicable. Physicians at times are even more reluctant to accept that medication is not always the answer. It goes against much of our professional upbringing; it deprives us of our most familiar therapeutic tool; and it forces us into a dialogue with our patients.

MINIMIZING THE MYTHOLOGY OF HEADACHE

To a considerable extent, patients learn the mythology of headache from society and present to physicians with misconceptions already in place. However, the kind of contact that the patient and physician make, particularly if it is early in the patient's medical experience, makes the difference between dislodging the mythology (so that a more rational diagnostic and treatment program can be pursued) and entrenching it (so that appropriate management becomes impossible, not only for that physician but also for those who inevitably will come after).

Few forces are more enduring than mythology. Extra minutes spent with the patient during the first few interviews may prevent the establishment of harmful misconceptions that hours of toil expended later cannot dislodge. In fact, one of the basic precepts for dealing with patients presenting with headache is really quite simple: "Listen to the patient," Osler said. "He is trying to tell you what's wrong."

REFERENCES

1. Osler W: *The Principles and Practice of Medicine.* New York. D Appleton, 1982, p 337.
2. Behrens MM: Headaches associated with disorders of the eye. *Med Clin North Am* 62:507–521, 1978.
3. Birt D: Headaches and head pains associated with diseases of the ear, nose, and throat. *Med Clin North Am* 62:523–531, 1978.
4. Medina JL, Diamond S: Migraine and atopy. *Headache* 16:271–274, 1976.
5. Edmeads J: Headaches and head pains associated with diseases of the cervical spine. *Med Clin North Am* 62:533–544, 1978.
6. Howell FV: The teeth and jaws as sources of headache. In Dalesion DJ (ed): *Wolff's Headache and Other Head Pain,* ed 4. New York, Oxford University Press, 1980, pp 381–387.
7. Edmeads J: The headaches of ischemic cerebrovascular disease. *Headache* 19:345–349, 1979.
8. Kudrow L, Sutkus B: MMPI pattern specificity in primary headache disorders. *Headache* 19:18–22, 1979.
9. Edmeads J: Vascular headaches and the cranial circulation—another look. *Headache* 19:127–132, 1979.
10. Olesen J, Lauritzen M, Tfelt-Hansen P, et al: Spreading cerebral oligemia in classical, and normal cerebral blood flow in common migraine. *Headache* 22:242–248, 1982.
11. Ziegler DK, Hassanein R, Hassanein K: Headache syndromes suggested by factor analysis of symptom variables in a headache prone population. *J Chron Dis* 25:353–363, 1972.

CHAPTER EIGHT

Evaluating the Psychological Factors in Headache

CHARLES S. ADLER, M.D.

SHEILA MORRISSEY ADLER, Ph.D.

PSYCHOLOGICAL EVALUATION OF THE HEADACHE PATIENT

Pain—whatever its origin—is a mental experience: not to examine the mind experiencing it would be like not listening to the heart in a patient complaining of arrythmia. In the treatment of many headache patients, a good psychological evaluation is as crucial to the therapeutic outcome as a good physical examination.[1]

The depth and nature of a fitting psychological assessment will vary with the needs of the patient and the practice of the physician. With some patients the psychological terrain can be covered quickly. In some practices it *must* be covered quickly, even though doing so is less than ideal. One point, however, is vital: even a brief psychological evaluation is better than none. The details of psychological evaluation given in this chapter will not be intimidating if one fixes in his mind its most important message: *ask a personal or psychological question of every patient, to let him know he may talk about matters of the heart.*

If one asks the patient about strains in the present and struggles in the past, it is uncanny how often his initial associations prove the headlines to his story. Even more importantly,

---

[1] As outlined in Chapter 6.

such questions also open the door to emotion, permitting its threshold to be crossed as needed later on.

It is important to learn about the patient's past in order to understand why he reacts in certain ways—including with headaches—to events in the present. We must know what sort of person is experiencing those events. The most relevant source of this knowledge is a discussion of his psychological development. Such knowledge allows the physician to appreciate whether there have been any major obstacles to that development, and aids him in gauging principal present-day reflections of the patient's successes and failures at overcoming those obstacles.

In short, it is important to learn the context of the headaches. To achieve this, the doctor constructs in his mind a rough model of who the patient is; of what—through his eyes—day-to-day experiences look and feel like; of what anticipations, frustrations, and gratifications he routinely encounters at home and work; and—because everything in medicine has its reasons—of the events which shaped him psychologically, the memories of which now color his world. One part of a headache workup is to imagine walking a mile in the patient's hat!

In addition to documenting the factual content of *what* the patient says, the evaluator needs to pay attention to *how* the patient says it, to gauge how his emotional and cognitive equipment is functioning. The formal name for this appraisal is the mental status examination. The tact required to obtain sensitive historical information is also necessary when evaluating the patient's mental status. A patient who is not in blatant psychological distress is not complimented by a request to recite serial sevens, the names of recent presidents, or the correct city and year. He often interprets such questions as a sign that the doctor is not sure whether the patient is "losing his mind." The best—and kindest—mental status examination is therefore one that the patient does not know has been performed. As the need to organize and communicate one's history—and to further evaluate which aspects of it may have contributed to physical problems—is a significant mental challenge requiring both good memory and an ability to abstract, a patient's mental status can usually be inferred from a comprehensive initial interview.

Thus, evaluation of the patient's present can disclose stressors which might be acting as precipitants of headache; evaluation of the past reveals his potential predisposition to headache and to specific present-day strains. This knowledge allows the physician to visualize the sources contributing both to head pain and to the patient's overall distress. The reward for this effort is a more effective treatment plan.

RATIONALE FOR THE PSYCHOLOGICAL EVALUATION OF THE HEADACHE PATIENT

The ability to fully evaluate psychiatric aspects of a headache complaint is important for several reasons:

1. Headaches are mankind's most frequent source of recurrent pain. Patients who have them are lifelong companions of a medical career.

2. The doctor must determine when a patient coming for headache really has another chief complaint in mind that he is either too anxious about, or ashamed of, to bring forward directly. In these cases the headaches merely serve as a ticket of admission into the doctor's chambers. The patient may only mention his recent chest pain, insomnia, or impotence offhandedly, and just as he is leaving. Therefore, especially if headaches have been present for years, it is useful to learn early on what motivates the patient to seek help for them now. Even if headaches remain the primary problem, such information helps the interviewer to discover which aspect of them most distresses the patient.

3. Besides being part of the evaluation, taking a good psychiatric history is often the start of treatment itself. The initial session is the single most important opportunity to establish rapport with the patient, as it may be the first time he has been asked to reconstruct his perceptions of the most significant emotional and physical events in his life. Many chronic headache patients have pilgrimaged to renowned specialists and clinics, yet have never felt they were given a chance to tell their own story fully, without having to race the clock to do so.

4. When psychological problems complicate the headache picture, taking a complete psychiatric history is also a way to begin learning how likely it is that the patient will be able to involve himself in productive psychotherapy. The job of resurrecting potentially disturbing memories and organizing them in the presence of a physician is a difficult one. The patient unable or unwilling to do this is less liable to benefit from subsequent exploratory therapy. Insight-oriented therapy may have little to offer the patient who describes his childhood in a stereotyped and innocuous fashion, or who recalls the factual details of his past but becomes confused when asked to also relate how he felt about them. On the other hand, the patient who

has shared his life's story may consider this contact with the doctor as an emotional investment, one he would not want to feel had been squandered. He is therefore likely to be openminded if psychotherapy is recommended.

In contrast, the patient who felt the initial interview was tense, or intimidating, or too brief, or too narrowly focused on physical symptoms, may assume a passive attitude in which he expects his role in treatment will be to answer questions and receive medications, much as he does when he visits his doctor for a chest cold. The physician has thus incurred a liability: it will be harder to expect the patient to view his headaches as related to the gestalt of who he is and how he reacts to situations, or to have him actively participate in treatment, or share responsibility for its outcome.

5. If psychotherapy is seen to be indicated, a final aim of the evaluative session is to enumerate, as far as possible, specific and reasonable goals for treatment based on the patient's age, character, level of disability, and financial constraints (see Chapter 24.)

Thus, although the usual emphasis in the diagnostic interview is on what the examiner can learn from the patient, it is equally important that he be aware of what effects his words or actions have on the patient. The doctor must win the patient's confidence by demonstrating thoroughness, respectfulness, sensitivity, and compassionate curiosity if he is to set the stage for the evaluation to be the first step in a helpful treatment relationship.

TAKING THE PSYCHIATRIC HISTORY IN HEADACHE: TECHNIQUES

We have found that certain techniques ease the task of obtaining a more accurate and informational history from headache patients. These involve:

1. *A neutral beginning.* Do the first evaluation before reading discharge summaries, psychological test reports, or other doctors' impressions. If such records are reviewed only after the patient has been seen, one has the benefit of these opinions without the liability of being swayed by them towards a particular diagnostic conclusion.

2. *Allow adequate time.* The physician should not feel pressured into completing his diagnostic evaluation in a single session unless the history seems unusually clear-cut. Techniques that save time often forfeit opportunities. In history-taking, patience with interest is as important as skill—there are no shortcuts.

3. *Nonverbal behavior.* If the patient were an actor in a silent film, what would be the impression made by his posture, gestures, dress, and mannerisms? If one did not understand the language he was speaking, what would be deduced about how he was feeling from the tone, rhythm, and rate of his voice? Most important: Do these impressions amplify or contradict the patient's verbal messages?

4. *Learn from the patient.* Patients, like physicians, often have their own unspoken differential diagnosis. A great many subliminal cues may have gone into its formulation. One should inquire, therefore, about the patient's unshared thoughts about what may be wrong, even with the patient who worries that his suspicions may be "just silly." It is surprising how often such "silly" thoughts turn out to be important diagnostic clues to physical problems, important worries to be relieved, or valuable metaphors for psychological conflicts related to headaches.

5. *Juxtaposition of ideas.* Be attentive to the timing and sequence of a patient's statements. If a patient follows statement A with statement D, statement D may

bear some important relationship to statement A, even if it appears the patient is just slipping off the subject.

6. *Phrases and colloquial expressions.* Pay attention to the particular phases and colloquial expressions the patient uses. This is especially important for the ones he employs to describe his headaches, his family, or himself. The patient who says, "these headaches are killers, they really do a guy in," is not only using figures of speech—he might be indicating concern that what is causing his headaches could kill him. Consider what the patient's figures of speech would mean if one took the words literally, especially if he seems to use certain expressions over and over.

7. *The physician's emotional reactions.* One of the physician's most accurate and underused tools for psychological assessment is an awareness of his own emotional reaction to the patient, and he should make full use of it. A vast amount of subliminal data has been absorbed by the interviewer's five senses at the end of the session, and his intuitive mind has integrated this material with a sophistication yet to be matched by computers. To tap this resource it is only necessary to ask oneself certain questions after the interview has ended: "If I were in her place, how would I feel inside? What feelings would I have to push from my mind to act as she does? How would I feel if I were her husband? Does talking to her leave me unexplainably annoyed? Depressed? Weary of politely returning those excessive smiles?" Many masked depressions can be recognized this way. Still trying to imagine yourself in her place: "What might motivate me to enter psychotherapy, or to cut back on analgesics?" The more the physician uses this tool, the more he will discover which questions yield him useful information. Not only does the ability to use empathy as a diagnostic tool increase

with practice, but the physician may find those moments of contact one of the most satisfying rewards of clinical practice.

8. *Recurring patterns.* Listen for recurring patterns, whether emotional, cognitive, or behavioral. This is done in much the same way one attempts to characterize pathognomonic patterns when investigating any chronic disease. The psychological evaluation, however, involves documenting more than just the situations to which the patient is exposed, as it must include his interpretation of them, the fantasies and memories triggered by them, and his emotional reaction to them. What is harder—or, depending upon one's perspective, more challenging—is to remain aware throughout the interview that some of this information the patient may be reluctant to reveal because it is embarrassing, and some of it he will be unable to reveal because it has been repressed and is unconscious.

9. *Don't lead the witness.* To obtain the most important information, the patient needs leeway in setting the pace and direction of the conversation. In particular, true-false questions trace a path largely determined by the interviewer. Open-ended questions allow the interviewer to be guided towards the patient's most significant areas of concern.

10. *Specific vignettes and examples.* Always ask for specific vignettes and examples. These are invariably more revealing than generalizations and unelaborated conclusions.

11. *Ask questions that require the patient to evaluate himself.* Certain questions help the physician judge the patient's ability to see himself from a more objective, external perspective. Does he feel that there are particular types of situations in which he overreacts? Can the patient relate how a family member would describe his behavior during a headache,

or how that family member would characterize his personality?

12. *Respect resistances.* Respect the patient's resistances and emotional limits. Confrontation has limited usefulness in the psychotherapy of headache patients, and only rare usefulness in their evaluation (and then only by those highly skilled in its use). Provocative confrontations have no place. Tact is needed to reduce the patient's shame when he reveals troublesome areas, and empathy is required to determine when the limits of the patient's emotional tolerance have been reached in a particular area or for a particular day.

13. *An incremental approach.* Approach difficult material in a stepwise manner. When palpating an acute abdomen, one invokes a soothing mannerism and only arrives at the painful spot last. The same method helps when interviewing. The doctor's words should be as circumspect as the surgeon's fingers.

14. *Don't catalogue.* Allow the line of inquiry to flow naturally in response to the patient's priorities and emotional reactions rather than attempting to catalogue all potentially relevant information. It is more important to make empathic contact than to conduct an emotional review of symptoms. Although any theme which elicits feelings from the patient deserves further inquiry, if a correct rapport is established, any specific area of content can be returned to on a later date. Thus, the interview is tempered to avoid a traumatic impact upon the patient.

15. *Repeat phrases the patient uses.* Use the same phrases the patient does to describe what he is feeling or his rationale for feeling it. If, for example, from what has been said the interviewer expects that the patient gets furious at his stepson, but he prefers to describe it as only being "cross," one should honor the patient's choice of words. "And can you describe a little more the sort of things

you say when you are cross?" In a similar manner, if a depressed patient insists that his depression is only due to the headaches, he can be asked whether the head pain was ever so severe that it made him feel it just was not worth going on.

16. *Relevant analogies.* Use analogies from a patient's cultural or occupational background. These can help to clarify concepts that the patient might otherwise have a hard time getting a handle on. Only assume a patient will understand scientific terms as complicated as those used to describe medical breakthroughs in the magazines he reads. (It also helps, when evaluating a patient's communications, to remember the significance in different cultures of acknowledging pain, or of visiting a doctor.)

17. *Acknowledge the patient's strengths.* Show interest in the patient's strengths as well as in his difficulties. The typical patient is apprehensive when first seen by a doctor and may be unreasonably ashamed of his inability to have mastered his symptoms. These feelings are accentuated by the need to relate in unbroken sequence only the troubled parts of his history. If also asked to share his achievements, he becomes more at ease in the interview and has less trepidation about the next one. A knowledge of the patient's emotional resources will also prove useful if he later enters treatment. Finally, this approach conveys from the start that the physician does not view the patient in the overly critical manner in which a headache patient is often liable to view himself.

18. *Family history and psychodynamics.* Use the family history as a source of psychodynamic as well as genetic information. The patient may be less guarded in revealing perceptions and fantasies related to headache when talking about his father's migraines than when talking about his own. Observations about or

associations to a family member's headache problem may also be relevant for the current patient, and a mental note should be made of this for later exploration.

19. *Appraise all important relationships.* Since disordered interpersonal relationships are so often critical to the headache patient's emotional difficulties, he should feel free to describe all relationships—in addition to those within the nuclear family—that he thinks were important influences in his development, or are important to his current equilibrium. Lovers, grandparents, pets, teachers, aunts, employers, and coaches may all have had special relevance.

TAKING THE PSYCHIATRIC HISTORY IN HEADACHE: CONTENTS

We have found that certain topics are more likely to be problematic for the psychologically influenced headache patient. While all of these topics need not be covered, even in a comprehensive evaluation, we present them all here for the physician's discretional use.

1. *Why now?* Are there any new symptoms (physical, psychological, or social) impelling the patient to seek help now? What changes would he envision if he became headache free?

2. *The first headache.* The first headache the patient can recall, along with his initial reaction to it, can be important. Circumstances surrounding this headache often give clues to a specific conflict or stress which remains relevant to the headaches. Can he remember what had been on his mind? Sometimes the patient has repressed these details by the time he is first seen, and it is only in later visits that decreased resistance permits more illuminating specifics to come to light.

3. *Dates and times.* The specific date or time of year when the headaches began can be psychologically important, especially if the headaches started abruptly or recur at the same season each year. Some headaches are tied to the anniversary of a trauma, most often the death of a close relative. It is the regular timing of exacerbations that is the key to diagnosing such an anniversary reaction. One should be especially alerted if the relative died of a head injury or had headache as a symptom of his final illness. Such a patient's headaches may result from pathological identification with the deceased relative.

4. *Friends and relatives.* Is there a recurrent difficulty in the patient's relationships with relatives, friends, or doctors? For example, does he always wind up feeling used by people or forced to carry a disproportionate share of every burden? Is such a pattern apparent to the examiner in relationships that the patient views as normal?

5. *Response to frustration of effort.* Does the intensity of the patient's reactions to frustration or failure generally reflect its realistic importance, or can they be equally intense to a failure which is objectively minor?

6. *Expectations of himself.* What does the patient expect of himself, and how does he feel he has lived up to those expectations? This is part of evaluation of the superego, and in some measure may need to be deduced from circumstantial evidence the patient presents, rather than be asked about directly. Does he expect the same of others? If not, how did he learn to treat himself differently?

7. *Expectations of him by others.* Attempts to gain information about expectations of himself will often lead the interview in the direction of what was expected of the patient as a child, how these expectations were enforced, and by whom. What were the patient's earliest reac-

tions to these expectations? Did he think them fair? Was physical punishment used or threatened? Was he ever struck in anger about the face or neck?

8. *Anger.* What clues signalled that his parents were angry or moody? Did the parents ever fight? If so, how did the patient feel when he heard or saw it? Did his parents tolerate anger in their children? If they did not, what techniques did they use to suppress it? Was there an unusual intensity of brother-sister animosity?

9. *Hypersensitivity and criticism.* Is the patient unusually sensitive to what he expects others will think of him? To their overt criticism? To their anger? How does he react if he feels their anger is unjustified? How well does he assert himself if his self-assertion threatens to displease people?

10. *His own story.* If the patient were writing his own story for a candid autobiography to be published posthumously, what would he describe as the most important influences on his development? Why?

11. *Good times and safe havens.* What were the best times the patient can remember? How did his family function then? What gave him the most solace when he felt hurt, attacked, or misunderstood? With whom did he feel most secure? In whom did he confide?

12. *Illness in childhood.* Because serious illness in childhood will often set the emotional tone for relating to illness in later life, one wants to know the patient's earliest experiences with illness. Did he have any protracted hospitalizations during childhood? Was anyone else in the immediate family seriously ill? If so, how—as a child—did he try to make sense out of what was wrong, what was happening, and what might happen?

13. *Loss, grief, and mourning.* Details about important losses should be obtained as far back as the patient can remember, as unresolved grief is frequent in headache and other psychologically influenced dis-

orders. It is important to get a picture of how the patient reacted to each major loss and, in particular, whether he allowed himself sufficient time to cry, remember, and grieve. Did he feel he had to be strong, set an example, or not upset the children (or the parents, or the husband or wife), and did he therefore stifle these normal feelings? Besides the death of friends and relatives, other significant losses can include the death of a pet or the loss of a goal or dream, a religious faith, a beloved home or community, a physical attribute or prowess, or one's native country through emigration. Sometimes the loss is a purely internal one, such as when the realization crystallizes that an important relationship is based on misconception, self-deception, or fantasy; such an existential moment can herald an enduring despair.

14. *Medication issues.* Psychodynamic information can be garnered while reviewing the patient's medications. Does his attitude towards medication use suggest that he feels an angry entitlement to complete and immediate pain relief? Does his habit of taking medication in anticipation of pain indicate excess anxiety? Does he use anticipatory medication in fear that a headache might interfere with a frenetic life-style, or cause him to let people down? One also wishes to know if drugs are taken for the anxiety or depression that can masquerade as pain or accompany it. Although the wishes of the patient who emphatically states during the first session that he dislikes medications and would prefer to get along without them should be respected, what else does this request reveal? Unusual strength and autonomy? Undue mistrust? Specific aversive experiences with drugs? A struggle to deny strong dependency wishes? Paranoia? It might be any of these. What can one conclude about the psychology of the patient who reports troubling side effects

from a long series of chemically unrelated drugs?

15. *Health care history.* What was the patient's prior experience with medical care and with the physicians who provided it? If past doctors were perceived as less than competent or as hurtful, the patient must be treated with particular care. Do the actual details he relates bear out these perceptions? Does the patient have a history of misinterpreting doctors' motives? If so, it is important to learn from these other doctors' experiences and plan a therapeutic approach to take if, due to transference, one finds himself repeating them.

16. *Sequences, stressors, and diaries.* Most patients realize that they must pay careful attention to those events immediately before or during a headache, if they hope to correlate emotions with headaches. As a result, these overt stressors or emotional blowups are usually identified. There is, however, more complexity to the question of timing than meets the eye. Some patients will bring to their first appointment a diary, in which they have diligently recorded stresses and headaches; they have wracked their brains, but insist that they find no connection between the two. Some problems with this approach are:

   a. Since emotional triggers may precede migraine by considerable space (a mean of 2–3 days in several recent studies, (1, 2) the patient may not have thought back far enough. To his mind, the events of yesterday bear no relationship to the headaches of today.

   b. The patient may have taken copious notes on the external stressors, but not recorded feelings engendered in response to them. As that feeling state is the common denominator of these triggers, his notes will only reveal a confusing sequence of dissimilar situations.

   c. Sometimes it is the symbolic meaning of an event, as determined by repressed memories and unconscious attitudes, which ignites the headache tinder. Because the patient is unaware of these memories and attitudes, he cannot see how the event has any relevance for him and discounts its emotional importance.

   d. Stress, conscious or unconscious, is specific and selective. The patient may argue that his migraines were relieved when he was hospitalized for a cholecystectomy, and may be puzzled as to why, if his headaches are really triggered by emotions, they did not become worse at that time. This patient is not aware that the most important stress for him, and for his headaches, may be the responsibility he feels in his job as a weather forecaster, and that this particular stress is relieved by the enforced hospitalization.

   e. Besides the immediate triggers of individual headache episodes, there are longer, more gradual shifts in the patient's level of psychological adaptation, with corresponding periods of increased vulnerability to headache. The accountant with tension headaches, for example, may need to separate his increased vulnerability to headaches during the tax season from his specific vulnerability when old Mr. Smith arrives on April 14th carrying two shopping bags of tax receipts.

At the end of an evaluation, if it is decided that the patient needs therapy, it is helpful to answer any questions that he has about the therapist's background or about the nature of the proposed treatment. This acknowledges that the assessment has been a bilateral one, in which the patient has also been deciding whether therapy and therapist are right for him. If he makes a deliberate choice that they are, it bolsters his commitment to stick with treatment if difficult moments are later encountered. Furthermore, because this approach reflects the doctor's respect for the patient, it augments the patient's respect for the doctor.

A sincerely conducted interview is rarely experienced as a waste of time by the patient, even if it does not turn up material relevant to the headaches or requiring further elaboration. It allows the patient to step back and gain a better perspective on the course of his life and on the role of the headaches in it. Sharing these perceptions often confirms for the patient the doctor's interest in his experience as an individual. Even single evaluative sessions seem to have a salutary effect upon a surprisingly large number of patients.

PSYCHOMETRIC TESTING

As an adjunct to the clinical interview, psychometric tests can sometimes alert the physician to problems that he may have missed. These tests are easier to justify to the patient as part of the routine initial workup than they are further along in treatment. As with other tests, their function is advisory, and does not replace clinical judgment.

The most commonly employed psychometric test is the MMPI (Minnesota Multiphasic Personality Inventory). It is important to point out that one cannot rely on its findings for a comprehensive understanding of the patient, or consider it as a substitute for a psychosocial interview. The MMPI can assist as a screening tool to alert the physician to gross psychiatric disturbances and to suggest the appropriate diagnosis. Such overt psychopathology is not commonly encountered with headache sufferers, however, and the MMPI has not been found useful for eliciting the subdiagnostic nuances of psychological dysfunction that often exacerbate headache (3).

In skilled hands, the projective tests, such as the Rorschach and Thermatic Apperception Tests, in which the patient is required to create a picture or a story from minimal cues, are more subtle and more useful. Like a test with essay questions, these can reveal things a multiple choice test misses. Psychological test results are occasionally reviewed with a patient to stimulate his curiosity and motivation.

Neuropsychological instruments for evaluating headache are best chosen by the clinical neuropsychologist after conversing with the physician about the case. If, for example, the primary question is whether part of the patient's mental picture is the result of subtle organic impairment, the neuropsychologist can tailor a suitable test profile which will sometimes localize as well as detect lesions.

PUTTING FINDINGS IN PERSPECTIVE: DO THEY MATTER?

If the psychiatric history and mental status exam do reveal psychological problems, there is still the difficult task of determining how they bear on the headaches. Basically they may be related in one of four ways:

1. *Contributory*—Psychological factors can contribute to the physiological changes that precipitate headache, intensify the patient's perception of pain, or alter the significance he ascribes to it. They may, in other words, be contributory.

2. *Resultant*—Psychological problems may result from the strain of coping with chronic pain and its anticipation.

3. *Symptomatic*—Both headaches and psychiatric manifestations may be symptoms of a primary illness, such as an endocrine disease, cerebral neoplasm, cerebrovascular anomaly, etc.

4. *Independent*—the patient's psychopathological symptoms may be entirely unrelated to his headaches.

We will survey these four types of interaction in sequence, giving examples of the types of problem seen in each.

CONTRIBUTORY

Psychodynamic factors that accentuate a patient's liability to headache are covered in the chapters specifically devoted to that headache category (Chapters 11–15, 17, 18, and 20). If we approach this interaction from the opposite direction, however, we see that some psychiatric diagnoses are more likely to be associated with headache complaints or to significantly color any clinical headache picture; these include: depression, somatization disorder, marital or family conflict, psychogenic pain disorder, and schizophrenia.

DEPRESSION

There is consensus among headache specialists that depression is a frequent cause of headaches and a still more frequent participant (see Chapter 29). The question to be decided invariably becomes whether the depression is a natural, indeed inevitable, result of chronic pain. A patient's attribution of serious depression to pain is usually incorrect (4). More often, the depression comes first. Freeing such a patient from his depression will usually help his headaches.

The presence of depression is sometimes obvious; yet, there is also the patient who sighs and looks sad but becomes evasive if the doctor suggests depression. He only wishes to discuss his head pain. Such a patient is generally not trying to deceive the doctor; rather, he has deceived himself, as he has truly pushed from awareness or simply takes for granted the dejected state in which he passes his days.

SOMATIZATION DISORDER

The somatizing patient can present with a complaint of headache, the true nature of which is identified by the company it keeps: ubiquitously malfunctioning organ systems. Headache is but one symptom in the lineup.

Such a patient may demonstrate ruminating self-involvement, scanty relationships, and a stream of talk which is superficial and unappreciative. Although he comes for appointments obligingly, the visits are not motivated by the pain relief he obtains; indeed, he may insist that "nothing has ever helped my headache." His tale will often encompass many doctors, many surgeries, many rejections, and will be related in a vocabulary which includes many medical terms related to his illness.[2] Such a patient may unconsciously use his symptoms to maintain contact with people in an otherwise isolated life. His real illness is not defined by symptoms, as the doctor who tries to stamp out these brushfires soon finds out, but by the hopeless withdrawal of attention into his own body which generates them. This, rather than the headache, is what needs treatment.

MARITAL OR FAMILY CONFLICT

These can also cause or contribute to headache. Featherstone and Beitman (5) found that most intractable migraines are an enduring monument to insoluble marital disharmony and that the identified patient need not be the one with greatest psychopathology. In evaluating these situations, the physician should consider not only whether family stress coincided with the onset or exacerbation of headaches but also what adaptive function—if any—the headaches might serve in the family equilibrium. What roles, in other words, do the headaches require different family members to play? For example: Do the headaches serve to prevent a family breakup, or to modulate its propensity to fight? Is it the only way 11-year-old Tommy can pass the word that his family needs help without feel-

---

[2] This patient is not to be confused with the intelligent layman who has been exposed to a great deal of personal family illness, as a consequence of which he has tried to educate himself about his problems.

ing disloyal? Are little Julia's headaches her only way of saying that her parents scream at each other all night, or that she is the victim of physical or sexual abuse? Even in less dramatic cases, the patient's family is always a vector influencing his liability to illness and the threshold at which help may be sought for it. Families can either help patients cope with headaches or can covertly demand that the headaches continue. The physician should be alert to the possibility that family pathology is a source of difficulty when:

1. Headache is stubbornly entrenched in a way that is baffling from a strictly organic viewpoint.
2. The patient is reticent to talk about the most superficial matters related to family relationships.
3. A family member, like a bailiff, always accompanies the patient to the office.
4. Appointments are routinely made and cancelled by a family member other than the patient himself.

PSYCHOGENIC PAIN DISORDER

A close relative of the conversion reaction, psychogenic pain disorder may make its appearance in the head as atypical facial neuralgia. As in conversion reactions, the pain distribution is symbolic rather than anatomic. Kolb (6) notes that the pain in this syndrome is frequently initiated by an emotionally significant event, such as being struck in the face in a humiliating context. Alternately, the patient gives a history of a painful facial lesion present at the time of a psychologically disturbing experience; when later events reactivate the original psychological troubles, the facial pain is also revived. The character structure in these patients has been portrayed as masochistic.

SCHIZOPHRENIA

Schizophrenic patients are frequently reported to show a diminished capacity for physical pain which may be more than just a byproduct of their impaired ability to communicate it. When they do report pain, however, it can be difficult to assess: even description of a typical tension headache might become obscured by the patient's ideosyncratic language, inappropriate affect, and loose associations. On the other hand, the schizophrenic patient might hallucinate headache or develop a delusion that he has headache.[3] Delusions are hallmarked by their bizarre and unvarying description, which takes on the quality of recitation rather than communication. One patient, for example, regularly described headaches caused by "small devils who crawl onto my scalp and drill holes in it with square and triangular bits." Such delusions may have symbolic or communicative meanings for the schizophrenic that are unrelated to pain *per se*. A frequent delusion in schizophrenia is that of transmitting or receiving thoughts or of being controlled by an "influencing machine" implanted in the brain. Awkward attempts to convey these perceptions could be miscommunicated as headache.

RESULTANT

Psychological problems which result from head pain can be considered secondary factors, because they are consequences of the headache's pain, its chronicity, unpredictability, and treatment. The best tool to determine whether a symptom is secondary is an accurate history of the patient's premorbid functioning, of when the headaches began, and of when the psychological symptoms began. To be considered a result of headache, depression—for example—must not only follow the onset of headaches but also must follow it by enough time for disability and social impair-

---

[3] Raising the serious philosophical question of whether a patient with a delusion or hallucination of headache actually experiences pain or only *thinks* that he has experienced pain—it would seem a rather metaphysical difference.

ment to have set in. Generally, though not inevitably, the longer a patient has had headaches, the more important secondary psychological factors are. The patient often needs help to differentiate cause from consequence. To complicate matters, secondary factors may themselves ultimately contribute to initiation and maintenance of headache and may even remain after the headaches have been relieved.

"Headache-maintaining factors" can be defined as apparent benefits that incidentally accrue to the patient for having headaches. For example, the children may stop whooping it up, the husband may leave work early and act attentive, and the patient may have an excuse to take pills that ease anxiety as well as headache.

Although these headache-maintaining factors are often referred to as secondary gain, this term is not preferred, first, because it has acquired a pejorative rather than a descriptive connotation and, second, because it is inaccurate: these short-term benefits ultimately cause the patient more trouble than gain.

One example of a headache-maintaining factor seen in some patients is a tenuous family equilibrium that requires one member to continue in the sick role to prevent the family's breakup in divorce. Another example is the patient who feels he will have to take on responsibilities beyond his ability at work or in school if he gets better. The husband who finds that he is able, through nightly headache, to avoid the demands for intimacy required during sex is in a similar position, although this situation is seen more frequently by script writers than by doctors. A rationalization for using narcotics (or barbiturates or benzodiazepines) which can numb the tension and depression of a nonfulfilling life along with the head pain is a frequent secondary problem afflicting headache patients.

When pain is present for years, it becomes an abandoned cave which some ragged psychological or interpersonal need will eventually crawl into and put to its own use. Initially unrelated psychological problems find shelter there, and in time the pain becomes a bureaucratic institution in the mind's economy—many needs acquire a vested interest in maintaining it. Therefore, even when a headache does not have its origin in emotional dysfunction, it can be parasitized by emotional difficulties later on. This is particularly likely if headache is present in childhood, while the patient's adaptive strategies are still forming.

These "secondary headache-maintaining factors" must be differentiated from what is known as "primary gain." A primary gain is an internal psychodynamic benefit, the need for which antedates the onset of a symptom and directly contributes to its causation. A conversion reaction is motivated by primary gain. The mechanism here is always unconscious.

It is also important to distinguish headache-maintaining factors from malingering. Although the former can increase the patient's reluctance to give up the sick role, this influence is usually not conscious. The malingerer, on the other hand, will be likely to show other attributes of an antisocial personality and will be conscious of his intent to create the symptoms for a specific purpose. Kolb (7) makes this important point:

The physician must be extremely careful in arriving at a conclusion that the patient is malingering. The accusation of the patient's conscious willfulness in presenting a complaint usually terminates the physician's therapeutic value.

"Secondary dysphoria-enhancing factors" can be defined as disagreeable consequences of the headaches that compound the problem of pain. They are occasionally more detrimental to the patient's overall adjustment than the head pain itself, and thereby add to the patient's motivation to get well. Examples include:

1. A debilitating combination of loss of self-esteem, helplessness, social withdrawal, and depression in the face of inevitably recurring pain is a major contributor to the

disability associated with frequent headaches.

2. Anxiety, which comes from not being able to predict when a headache will start, how long it will last, how severe it will be, or what plans it will sabotage, is common. The feeling of being at the mercy of the headaches may result in anticipatory use of analgesic or ergot preparations as the patient becomes increasingly less tolerant of vague premonitory symptoms.

3. This in turn may lead to habituation or addiction, shame about being dependent upon medications, and feeling resentful about the need to rely on a physician's sometimes unpredictable attitude and availability for such vital relief.

4. As noted previously, disabling headaches routinely disrupt family funcitoning.

These factors show that the total impact of chronic headache upon a patient's life far exceeds his enduring the sensations of pain.

SYMPTOMATIC

One reason a patient with a long-standing headache history may be motivated to consult a doctor late in life is the onset of a different type of headache superimposed upon the original. The new headache may be an important indicator of a new disease. Just as the cerebral neoplasm may be presaged by a not very troublesome headache of recent onset, it may also be heralded by apparently minor changes in psychological functioning, such as increased forgetfulness or personality deterioration. The list of causal agents for this type of headache is long (see Chapter 6).

The primary condition may be toxic (mercury), metabolic (hypokalemia), endocrine (hypothyroidism, hypoglycemia), infectious (tuberculous meningitis), allergic, autoimmune, cerebrovascular (microemboli), traumatic (subdural hematoma), or neoplastic (metastatic breast cancer.) Either systemic or strictly intracranial disorders may be responsible. The differentiation from other relationships between psychological problems and headache is made by relevant physical and laboratory findings, and often includes signs of organicity in the mental status examination, along with a parallel progression of both physical and mental symptoms over time.

INDEPENDENT

The patient whose psychopathology is unrelated to his headache complaint is potentially the most misleading. If mental difficulties are florid, it is tempting to presume them guilty of causing the headaches, even in the absence of specific evidence that this is so. The problem is compounded if the psychiatric condition makes a crisp communication of symptoms difficult. Ideally, one would like to see in each patient specific stressors, personality characteristics, and past experiences which would give an intelligible psychodynamic reason for head pain, but this ideal can rarely by actualized. As in all areas of medicine, one usually winds up working with the best assumptions he can bring to bear on a clinical picture, and these fall considerably short of perfection. The physician must not only make peace with this state of affairs, but also should extract gratification from his efforts to approximate that ideal.

CONCLUSION

Although the examiner will initially wish to fix in his mind an aerial map of the patient's psychological terrain, few evaluations need ever, in fact, exhaustively cover all areas presented in this chapter. Time will allow each clinician to find the most effective techniques in his hands, and the patient's subconscious, appreciative of the physician's open-minded interest, will generally respond by providing the clues that will guide the physician's inquiries to the most important questions and to the general source of the problem.

In the challenging job of evaluating the psychosomatic status of the headache patient, it helps to pay fastidious attention to the mind struggling to balance its competing emotions, as best it can, within that vault of inflamed or traction-sensitive structures.

REFERENCES

1. Dalkvist J, Ekbom K, Waldenlind E: Headache and mood: a time series analysis of self-ratings. *Cephalalgia* 4:45–52, 1984.
2. Levor RM, Cohen MJ, Nabiloff BD, McArthur D, Heuser G: Psychological precursors of migraine and related personality factors. *Headache* 24:174, 1984.
3. Adler CS, Adler SM: Pitfalls in the interpretation of psychometric testing of headache patients. *Cephalalgia* 5 (Suppl 3):212–213, 1985.
4. Arena JG, Andrasik F, Blanchard EB: The role of personality in the etiology of chronic headache. *Headache* 25:296–301, 1985.
5. Featherstone HV, Beitman BD: Marital migraine: a refractory daily headache. *Psychosomatics* 25:30–38, 1984.
6. Kolb LC: Psychiatric and psychogenic factors in headache. In Friedman AP, Merritt H (eds): *Headache: Diagnosis and Treatment*. Philadelphia, F. A. Davis, 1959, pp 259–298.

CHAPTER NINE

The Psychiatric Aspects of Headache in Children

R. SCOTT BENSON, M.D.

Headache pain, like all pain, is an intangible symptom with multiple and diverse etiologies. The absence of other signs and symptoms leaves us to ponder the mysteries of the unknown in search of a rational explanation which will lead to a rational intervention aimed at giving relief. In this process, the direction taken is determined by the physician's program of diagnostic thinking. Often, the search for a physiological explanation is unrewarding. One tendency is to end up assigning the patient to a global diagnostic grouping, "psychogenic." Since psychiatry is part of medicine it is subject to its demands for rigorous scientific thought, and this is the spirit in which one should pursue symptom evaluation in psychiatry. Such a program should lead to a psychiatric diagnosis, with its attendant treatment alternatives and prognostic implications. The purpose of this paper is to suggest such a program by describing cases of headache in children and comparing them to present psychiatric diagnostic categories (1).

Headaches are a frequent complaint in children. Studies by Sillanpää in Finland demonstrated the ubiquitous nature of this symptom (2). Eighty-two per cent of the children questioned reported having a headache in the year of the survey. Forty-seven per cent had headaches on a monthly basis. Over 10% described headaches characteristic of migraine.

In spite of their widespread occurrence, childhood headaches are rarely the subject of psychiatric study. Headaches are found in the normal development section of the *Basic Handbook of Child Psychiatry* (3). They are also referred to in the psychosomatic medicine section, but the discussion is limited to a classification of patients with tension, migraine, and conversion headaches (4). This style of descriptive diagnosis is similar to that presented in the neurological literature (5).

In his review of headaches in children, Rothner (5) identifies several types of psychopathology contributing to psychogenic headaches. The patient may have simple anxiety and tension, severe depression, or conversion hysteria. He also identifies stress as a major precipitant of migraine headaches. This association of migraine with emotional stress is repeated throughout the migraine literature (6–8). Among other things, this close association of migraine attacks with life stresses led to the development of a migraine personality profile by Krupp and Friedman. The validity of this type of formulation has been debated (4, 7).

The American Psychiatric Association's Diagnostic and Statistical Manual III (DSM-III) recommends specific diagnostic criteria for psychiatric illness. Application of these criteria to the information generated in an adequate diagnostic evaluation should lead to a diagnosis. The publication suggests the use of a multiaxial diagnosis, which allows one to utilize a larger segment of the information gathered in a clinical interview.

In children, an adequate psychiatric evaluation consists of interviews with the child and with the child's parents or guardians; information from the school, preferably gathered from an interview with the child's teacher; and an educational evaluation, which includes testing for intelligence and achievement. Additionally, psychological testing to determine personality characteristics may be indicated. Integration and synthesis of this data should provide the most likely diagnostic possibility, an assessment which is confirmed or modified by observing the child and his response to treatment.

To determine whether grouping children with headaches by diagnosis is the most useful division, a representative sample of children with headache would need to be evaluated. The best source of such patients would be pediatric clinics where children with headaches are treated. The limitation of this paper, and of all other papers from neurology clinics, is that the selection of cases referred by primary physicians may bias the sample. Therefore this chapter will primarily consider children who were first seen because of psychiatric difficulties and who were then found to have frequent headaches as part of their symptom complex.

Evaluation of these cases suggests that the children met the specific diagnostic criteria for four distinct psychiatric diagnoses. They are: Pathologic Separation Anxiety, Borderline Personality Disorder, Major Depression, and Psychological Factors Affecting Physical Condition.

PATHOLOGIC SEPARATION ANXIETY

The essential feature of this diagnostic category is excessive anxiety on separation from major attachment figures. Headaches and other somatic complaints are a frequent finding.

Tom, age 9, was seen in consultation with his pediatrician following hospitalization to evaluate a change in personality. He had been physically well, with adequate school performance, family, and peer relationships, until 4 months prior to his hospital admission. This occurred 1 week after his Christmas vacation from school. At that time he began to complain of vague stomachaches and headaches. These symptoms would frequently interfere with going to school, and at times would interrupt his school day. Tom's prior adjustment in school had been outstanding. He functioned at his level of ability and was well liked by his peers. His teacher was perplexed by his recent difficulties, and had wondered if he was angry with her.

At home, he insisted on prolonging his bedtime rituals and asked his parents to stay in the room until he could get to sleep. During these nighttime "visits" his conversations would focus on his concerns about illness and death, and he frequently brought up memories of his grandfather's death 2 years earlier.

Outpatient evaluation and symptomatic treatments had been unsuccessful in finding the cause of his problems or in providing consistent relief. Evaluation in the hospital setting, including EEG, CAT scan, and radiological studies of gastrointestinal function, failed to demonstrate physical illness.

Interviews with Tom's parents, both together and separately, showed them to be stable in marriage, work, and health. There had been no significant changes in the family since Tom's younger brother was born 5 years before.

The grandfather had been an important figure in Tom's earliest years, but he moved away when Tom was 6. They had only visited intermittently since that time. His death from a heart attack was unexpected. Tom attended the funeral without apparent incident. To all appearances, the grieving process had been managed well by both parents and children.

During his interview Tom seemed relaxed, and talked easily about his illness. He felt worried much of the time and constantly anticipated that "something bad" was going to happen. Although he worried about his parents' health, he could give no clear reason for the worries. His dreams centered on the theme of being alone, or of his parents' becoming ill or getting injured. Aside from missing his friends from school, he did not feel sad. He said his headaches occurred when he would think about having to go to school or to bed. They usually were associated with an uneasy feeling in his stomach. The headaches were relieved by aspirin.

A diagnosis of Pathologic Separation Anxiety was made. Treatment for Tom was a combination of medication (imipramine) to control his overwhelming death anxiety and dread, and brief psychotherapy to help him overcome the anticipatory anxiety which interfered with his return to school. Informative sessions were held with his parents and his teacher. He had prompt relief of the somatic symptoms, and in 2 weeks was attending school without difficulty.

BORDERLINE PERSONALITY DISORDER

The characteristic feature of these children is instability in almost all areas of functioning—home, school, and with peers. This lack of stability in their dealings with the world reflects an internal state of turmoil which can be demonstrated by a careful psychiatric examination.

The specificity of this diagnosis as well as the use of personality diagnoses in children is heavily debated (1,9,10). This diagnostic category can also be used to identify the child's level of personality organization, rather than to define a specific personality disorder, and it is this usage which is preferred. An alternative diagnosis for patients under 18 years of age, Identity Disorder, has many similarities to the "borderline" diagnosis. However, patients who fit this category have strong and specific concerns or confusion about their identity, but do not show the intensity of mood disturbance seen in borderline patients.

Lucy was 13 when she was taken to the emergency room following an overdose of Fiorinal and Elavil; these had been prescribed for complaints of headaches and depression. After being stabilized on the pediatric wing she was transferred to a psychiatric unit for evaluation and treatment planning.

She was the oldest of three children living with her mother and stepfather. This was her mother's fourth marriage. Lucy's father had been part of the family until her 5th year, when he moved from the area. Visits were for 3 weeks in the summer, and were described as pleasant. She had tried living with her father when she was 11, but it ended after 4 months because of inadequate school performance and a poor relationship with her stepmother.

After her return home, Lucy's school performance continued to deteriorate. Educational evaluation and intelligence testing provided no evidence that she had a learning disability. At age 12 she began being truant from school; when she did show up, she was frequently tardy. Staff at her school expressed some concern that her current group of friends was exerting a bad influence. Lucy resisted her school counselor's efforts to intervene in those relationships. Conflicts at home continued to increase. She refused to do household chores, or to come home after school, preferring to visit at her friend's houses. In the meantime, she developed an intense attachment to a 17-year-old dropout who was suspected of being a drug dealer.

Her parent's responded to this behavior by threatening her with severe restrictions and other punishments, but they were usually unavailable to monitor the restrictions which they had set.

In addition, Lucy's younger siblings became afraid of her rages. The extent of those rages was discovered only after her hospitalization. She had beaten her brother on one occasion following a minor provocation and had chased her sister through the house with a butcher knife after they had argued about an afternoon snack.

She had been to her physician before the start of 7nth grade. A review of systems uncovered daily headaches, described as a generalized, dull, "bad" feeling over the cranium. She described her mood as one of constant boredom; her only enjoyment came from being with friends. Thoughts of committing suicide were denied.

A variety of medications were tried for the headaches, but all proved ineffective. This included Elavil, which was increased to 75 mg per day but continued to be ineffective nonetheless.

On the afternoon of admission she had discovered her boyfriend talking with his old girlfriend. After a screaming outburst with him she left school and, on arriving home, emptied her bottles of Elavil and Fiorinal. She was found by her mother, who arrived home from work shortly after the ingestion.

Further history from Lucy revealed two prior episodes of suicidal behavior. In one, she had swallowed 15–20 aspirin when she was just 11 years old; in the other, she had taken some antibiotics given for a bladder infection at age 13. The patient also discussed recurring dreams in which she vividly saw her parents being decapitated. Members of the nursing staff said that she had shared information with them about her sporadic episodes of drug abuse and sexual activity.

In the initial stages of treatment she suddenly appeared to become healthy and participate actively in individual and group therapy. She eagerly sought contact with her therapist and praised his insightfulness. When her spurious "flight into health" was not rewarded with special treatment or privileges, she then began to pit the hospital staff against her parents. Ultimately, her father began to complain about the cost of treatment, allied himself with Lucy against the hospital staff, and helped her to escape to his house. Efforts to have Lucy return to the hospital or to again involve her in outpatient treatment were unsuccessful. (It should be noted that there are also elements suggestive of an antisocial personality disorder in this young woman's case history.)

MAJOR DEPRESSION

The use of DSM-III criteria for diagnosing major depression in children has recently been widely recommended (11, 12). Previous concerns that it would not be possible to detect associated symptoms of depression in children have not been borne out by experience.

John was referred by his school counselor because of a sharp decline in school performance. His teacher and parents had been frustrated in their attempts to maintain him academically. An evaluation by his pediatrician failed to demonstrate any physical pathology which would account for this decline.

An interview with his parents revealed additional information. John's best friend had recently changed schools, and since then John complained of having no friends. He no longer played with children in the neighborhood, but spent most of his time alone in his room. Although he assured his parents he was doing schoolwork, assignments were never finished. It was difficult to arouse him in the morning, even though his parents thought he was sleeping more hours than usual. He had become finicky in his eating habits, but his parents attributed that to his age. They in turn attributed his complaints of dull, bifrontal headaches to the poor eating. These had been coming increasingly often over the course of the illness. Headaches could begin at any time, but were most frequent in the morning. Although they typically improved with aspirin, some discomfort would continue throughout the day.

At 12, John was the middle of three boys. The family had lived in the same area since John was 2. His mother was hospitalized for depression following the birth of their youngest child, when John was 5. She had been successfully treated with antidepressants at the time, and had had not depressive symptoms since then. She was concerned about the possible effect of her hospitalization on John's present difficulties.

The school counselor was concerned about John's attitude and irritability. Although he had displayed difficulties in the classroom and with teachers, the referral was only made after he was in a fight in the lunchroom. Testing had previously demonstrated "high normal" intelligence.

On examination John was sullen, responding to questions with one-word answers, and after considerable delay. When asked about his best friend he became tearful. He agreed that his life had become difficult and, in response to a direct question, indicated he had thought of suicide, but would not act on it because of religious teachings. Psychological testing showed him to be preoccupied with death, guilt, and feelings of worthlessness.

John's case fits the diagnostic criteria of major depression. As is not uncommon, it was associated with a family history of major depression. He was treated with imipramine and outpatient therapy. There was a dramatic improvement in his symptoms after taking the medication for 5 days.

After 1 month his parents called to report that he was showing less energy, and to express their concern that he was getting ill again. When this was discussed with John, he admitted that he had stopped taking his medication; since he felt well, he had seen no need to continue it. Medication was restarted, and this was again followed by relief of symptoms. After 8 months his medication was discontinued with no recurrence of the depression.

PSYCHOLOGICAL FACTORS AFFECTING PHYSICAL CONDITION

This diagnostic category refers to a physical condition which is initiated or exacerbated by psychological factors. The physical condition must have demonstrable organic pathology or a known pathophysiological mechanism. Tension headache and migraine are specifically included.

Identification of the relevant psychological factors in this disorder requires a careful evaluation. To meet the criteria for this diagnosis, environmental stimuli must be shown to have both psychological significance for and a temporal relationship to the onset of the physical condition.

Kristin was 11 when she began to complain of frequent occipital headaches. Following its onset, the pain of a typical one increased steadily, unaccompanied by aura, throbbing, or vomiting. Headaches usually started after school let out. They interfered with her homework and other afterschool activities. For several years she had been actively involved in dance and music, and had recently begun swimming competitively. She was the oldest of three children and the only girl. Her father worked for an insurance company; her mother was planning to begin work in his office. They described their marriage as stable. The mother's cousin had died of a brain tumor.

In school Kristin was popular, with many friends. Her schoolwork reflected high intellectual ability, and she was enrolled in a program for the academically gifted.

Kristin was seen by her pediatrician for the persistent headaches. The lack of findings on physical examination along with the above history lead to the diagnosis of tension headaches.

In discussions with the patient and her mother, they were reassured about the unlikelihood of malignancy and were encouraged to review Kristin's overly crowded schedule. There was some concern expressed at the father's uninvolvement in Kristin's problems.

After 1 month, in spite of significant decreases in afterschool activities, her symptoms remained unchanged. A neurological consultation confirmed the diagnosis of tension headache. The parents then requested a psychiatric referral due to the continued impact of the head pain on Kristin's activities and school performance. On examination Kristin was anxious but able to actively discuss her headaches and their impact on her life. She described no unusual thoughts, sadness, irritability, change in sleep patterns, or change in appetite. She recalled a dream about caring for a kitten. When it was suggested that her headaches might be related to worries, she reported that she did worry about becoming pregnant. This was explored over subsequent sessions and was found to be connected to some sexual activity she had engaged in with an older male cousin during a visit the previous summer (when the headaches began.) Kristin had been frightened that she would become pregnant, but was afraid to say anything for fear that she and her cousin would be in trouble.

Kristin was helped to discuss what had happened with her parents. Several more sessions were required to clarify sexual and other concerns that came to light as a result of these discussions. On follow-up 6 months later, she was headache free and enjoying her previous level of outstanding functioning.

DIAGNOSTIC CRITERIA AND TREATMENT CONSIDERATIONS

The DSM-III criteria for diagnosis of Separation Anxiety Disorder requires excessive anxiety about separation from major attachment figures, manifested by three of nine possible symptoms. Tom's illness fits the criteria by having: (a) complaints of physical symptoms on school days; (b) unrealistic worry about harm befalling his parents; (c) persistent reluctance to go to school; and (d) reluctance to go to sleep without being next to his parents. Additional symptoms which would support this diagnosis are (e) unrealistic worry that a calamitous event will cause separation; (f) avoidance of being at home alone; (g) repeated nightmares involving separation; (h) signs of excessive distress upon separation; and (i) withdrawal, apathy, or sadness when not with a major attachment figure.

Treatment must address two issues: the inability to participate in usual activities and the subjective distress. The superiority of a combined approach using imipramine and behavioral techniques has been demonstrated. Although medication may be necessary for relief of subjective distress, it is ineffective for the anticipatory anxiety which accompanies this condition. Anticipatory anxiety can be managed with the combined efforts of patient, physician, parents, and school personnel.

Borderline personality disorder is considered when there is a pattern of current and long-term dysfunction with significant impairment in social or occupational functioning or subjective distress. To make the diagnosis, five of the following must be found: (a) impulsivity in two areas that are potentially self-damaging; (b) unstable and intense interpersonal relationships; (c) intense anger; (d) identity disturbance; (e) affective instability; (f) intolerance of being alone; (g) physically self-damaging acts; and (h) chronic feelings of emptiness or boredom. This symptom cluster is under continued study and comparison with other diagnostic categories (9). Clarification of this diagnosis allows a greater precision in identifying etiologic agents (10).

It has not yet been clearly determined what treatments will be most effective for this condition. Usually a combination of hospitalization, environmental control, psychotherapy (individual, group, or family), and medication is necessary. Antidepressants may help the dysphoria; major tranquilizers sometimes modulate the intense anger and impulsivity. It is typically a difficult condition to treat, and most cases end up with only partially successful outcomes.

Although headaches and other somatic complaints are frequently seen in Major Depression, other signs and symptoms are used to make the diagnosis (13, 14). The first criteria is dysphoric mood, loss of interest, or lack of pleasure in all or most of the patient's usual activities. Four of the following must be present for at least 2 weeks: (a) appetite change; (b) sleep disturbance; (c) psychomotor agitation or retardation; (d) loss of interest or pleasure; (e) loss of energy; (f) feelings of self-reproach or guilt; (g) subjective difficulty thinking or concentrating; and (h) recurrent thoughts of death or suicide. Organic illness causing depression (such as pancreatic cancer) and normal bereavement must be ruled out.

The use of medication for treating depression in children has only recently been evaluated (12, 15). A variety of medications are available with no clear advantages among them. Imipramine has been the most widely studied. Medication is recommended as one element of a comprehensive treatment program. Significant suicidal preoccupation may necessitate hospitalization. A combination of individual and family therapy may be required. Intervention with the schools is often necessary.

When a demonstrable physical illness— including migraine or tension headaches— accounts for the headache, the diagnosis "psychological factors affecting physical condition" is considered. The judgment that psychological factors are involved requires evidence of a temporal relationship between the stimuli and the initiation or exacerbation of the headaches. Uncovering meaningful and relevant psychological factors in children often requires extensive evaluation, as such factors may be obscure. Frequently these include poor school performance, the need to maintain a family secret or to appease an alcoholic or mentally ill parent, or the wish to sustain a faltering marriage.

Treatment for this condition requires identification of the most etiologically central fears, fantasies, and experiences. This process will in turn be helped or limited by the family's psychological mindedness and by their willingness to enter into a therapeutic relationship. Family therapy may be a useful setting in which to identify and resolve such aggravants to health (16). Errors can occur when the patient's refusal to accept the physician's judgment is interpreted as always representing resistance. Medication is not indicated in this condition, except as needed for management of the physical condition.

EVIDENCE FROM STUDIES

Some recent controlled studies suggest a frequent association of predisposing personality or psychological factors in many pediatric patients with headache, even though specific DSM-III criteria were not used. However much it is preferable to establish and plan treatment based upon a specific psychiatric diagnosis, the implications of these and similar general studies cannot be overlooked in children with chronic headaches in whom no firm diagnosis can be made.

In a study by Guidetti et al (17), 35 children (mean age 10) with idiopathic headache underwent clinical examinations and psychological tests; similar study was done on a normal, age-matched control group for comparison. Patients in the headache group had significantly more feelings of being excluded from the family group, insecurity, and repressed hostility towards important school or family figures.

A study by Lanzi et al (18), using psychometric testing and parental interviews, studied 20 pediatric migraine subjects. Eighty-five per cent demonstrated repressed anger preceding the attack. In 40% of the subjects, events such as a death in the family, an important separation, a sharp quarrel between the parents, or scholastic problems were seen just before the onset of childhood migraine. The authors hypothesized that certain unconscious emotions may modify brainstem neurotransmitters, inducing the neurohumoral and vascular changes that underlie a migraine attack in biologically predisposed subjects.

Maratos and Wilkinson (19) examined 47 migrainous children medically, neurologically, and psychiatrically, and compared them to matched controls drawn from a dental clinic. An "emotional upset" was the most frequently reported (86%) precipitating factor in migraine attacks. A significantly higher proportion of migrainous children also showed signs of neurotic disorder (mainly, anxiety or depression), and they evidenced a greater prevalence of neurotic disorder during the previous year as well. This increased prevalence was found to be associated with a disturbed parental relationship and especially with certain factors related to their mothers (who were older than the median and had higher "malaise scores"). The proportion of parents whose marital relationships were less than "close and positive" was four times as great among the parents of disturbed migrainous children than among those of the nondisturbed children or among those not subject to headaches.

In a classic study by Bille (20), 99.3% of all school children between the ages of 7 and 15 in Uppsala Sweden (pop. 70,000) were studied for migraine. This amounted to a large (9059) and complete population, thereby eliminating potential sampling errors. They were also followed up over the subsequent 30 years (21). A battery of psychometric tests showed the migraine children to be "more sensitive, less physically enduring, more tidy, and more vulnerable to frustration than the control children. According to their own descriptions and those of their parents, the migraine children were more anxious, tense, and nervous, and exhibited a more perfectionistic attitude than the control children" (21).

SUMMARY

In 1881, a British pediatrician, William Henry Day (22), in a textbook of pediatrics, devoted an entire chapter to headaches in children.

Many of his comments, such as, "Headaches in the young are for the most part due to bad arrangements in the lives of children" are equally applicable today. Yet few controlled studies have explored the association between the elusive symptom of headache and psychological factors (similarly elusive).

It is apprent that headaches are frequent in children and are often unaccompanied by physical findings. When emotional factors are probable, a comprehensive evaluation of the child and of his interactions at home, at school, and with his peers should produce a psychiatric diagnosis. This evaluation will require a considerable amount of time and physician involvement, and it is one in which participation of the child and parents is necessary.

The DSM-III diagnoses most frequently associated with headache in children seem to be the following: Separation Anxiety Disorder, Borderline Personality Disorder, Major Depression, and Psychological Factors Affecting Physical Condition. Other conditions can also be associated with headaches. Delineation of these conditions as distinct has promoted the development of effective treatments and encouraged research when no effective treatment has "been available." Application of appropriate psychiatric evaluation and treatment can often produce relief of the psychiatric symptoms and of the associated headaches.

REFERENCES

1. *Diagnostic and Statistical Manual of Mental Disorders,* ed 3. Washington, D.C., American Psychiatric Association, 1980.
2. Sillanpää M: Prevalence of headache in prepuberty. *Headache* 23:10–14, 1983.
3. Goldings HJ: Development from ten to thirteen years. In Noshpitz JD (ed): *Basic Handbook of Child Psychiatry.* New York, Basic Books, 1979.
4. Prugh DG, Eckhardt LO: Psychophysiological disorders. In Hoshpitz JD (ed): *Basic Handbook of Child Psychiatry.* New York, Basic Books, 1979.
5. Rothner AD: Headaches in children: A review. *Headache* 19:156–162, 1979.
6. Krupp GR, Friedman AP: Migraine in children: A report of fifty children. *Am J Dis Child* 85:146–150, 1953.
7. Prensky AL: Migraine and migrainous variants in pediatric patients. *Pediatr Clin North Am* 23:461–471, 1976.
8. Shinnar S, D'Souza BJ: The diagnosis and management of headaches in childhood. *Pediatr Clin North Am* 29:79–94, 1981.
9. Perry JC, Klerman GL: Clinical features of the borderline personality disorder. *Am J Psychiatry* 137:165–173, 1980.
10. Shapiro ER: The psychodynamics and developmental psychology of the borderline patient: A review of the literature. *Am J Psychiatry* 135:1305–1315, 1978.
11. Carlson GA, Cantwell DP: Diagnosis of childhood depression: a comparison of the Weinberg and DSM-III criteria. *J Am Acad Child Psychiatry* 21:247–250, 1982.
12. Kashani JH, Husain A, Shekim WO, Hodges KK, Cytryn L, McKnew DH: Current perspectives on childhood depression: an overview. *Am J Psychiatry* 138:143–153, 1981.
13. Kashani JH, Barbero GJ, Bolander FJ: Depression in hospitalized pediatric patients. *J Am Acad Child Psychiatry* 20:123–134.
14. Ling W, Oftedal G, Weinberg W: Depressive illness in childhood presenting as severe headache. *Am J Dis Child* 120:122–124, 1970.
15. Petti TA, Bornstein M, Delameter A, Conners CK: Evaluation and multimodality treatment of a depressed prepubertal girl. *J Am Acad Child Psychiatry* 19:690–702, 1980.
16. Minuchin S, Fishman HC: The psychosomatic family in child psychiatry. *J Am Acad Child Psychiatry* 18:76–90, 1979.
17. Guidetti V, et al: Psychological perculiarities in children with recurrent primary headache. *Cephalalgia* 3 (Suppl 1):215–217, 1983.
18. Lanzi G, et al: Psychological aspects of migraine in childhood. *Cephalalgia* 3 (Suppl 1):218–220, 1983.
19. Maratos J, Wilkinson M: Migraine in children: a medical and psychiatric study. *Cephalalgia* 2:179–187, 1982.
20. Bille B: Migraine in school children. *Acta Paediatr Scand (Suppl)* 51:1–151, 1962.
21. Bille B: Migraine in childhood and its prognosis. *Cephalalgia* 1:71–75, 1981.
22. Day WH: *Diseases of Children.* Philadelphia, Blakiston, 1881.

Symptom Formation and the Meaning of Diagnostic and Therapeutic Procedures to the Patient

CHAPTER
TEN

CHASE PATTERSON KIMBALL, M.D.
FRED OVSIEW, M.D.

THE ASSESSMENT OF PAIN

Pain and pleasure are two polarities along a continuum of feeling, a continuum which can be observed, to varying degrees, extending down the phyla of animals and even of plants. Pain may be viewed as an overwhelming, pervading, emotional state. Similarly, pleasure is often a phenomenon totally encompassing body and mind, at least for brief periods. Pain, whatever its source, is usually characterized by certain behaviors; their nature and complexity are dependent upon the discriminatory and sensate capacities of the species. These behaviors are rooted in the organism's capacity for arousal. Withdrawal is viewed as the most fundamental response to pain (as in Kandel's aplysia studies) (1). Attack may be a secondary response, less common than withdrawal. Both depend on a total body behavior consolidating emotion and action into a single, simultaneous response.

Pain may be experienced at various levels of the nervous system. It will be a more specific sensate experience at the periphery of the stimulus pathways, but may, further up,

be experienced as emotion, or even as an all-consuming feeling state. For a greater or lesser period of time, depending upon their intensity, either pain or pleasure may be so powerful as to blot out all other feeling states.

The field of medicine could be viewed as primarily existing to relieve a patient's experience of pain. Headache is one of the more common painful experiences which practitioners of medicine are called upon to relieve. Unfortunately, headache pain is sometimes thought of as an entity in itself and is therefore treated without establishing a diagnosis first. Even today, many of the oldest and most commonly used drugs for headache are analgesics and sedatives, the specific effects and mechanisms of which are still awaiting definition.

Pain is clearly an individual experience. One person's pain is never identical to the pain of any other. We are only in the early stages of shaping words that might effectively relate the pain of one to the pain of another.

A fundamental question is: "How does one know what is painful?" In the earliest years of development, the infant may express pain by a cry and/or a withdrawal. The concerned attendant to the situation—mother, father, caretaker, physician—will have some perceptual threshold above which they will sense that the child is signaling his discomfort. The caretaker will try to respond to the infant's distress, relying on intuition and empathy to interpret what the child feels, wishes, or needs, on the basis of his overt behavior. The mother might assume that the cry reflects hunger, and thereby might seek to stifle the cry by thrusting her breast or a bottle into the child's mouth. This usually succeeds; but when it does not, the attendant looks for another explanation. Perhaps the child is cold, or has a fever, or a rash. She may search for the undone diaper pin. She may tentatively suggest colic. Or, should all this fail, she may become more and more frustrated, may even panic. Her actions and expressions are communicative, perhaps even contagious. The infant now has an aura of pain which is, in a sense, more tangible than the sense of hunger, the diaper pin, or the colic.

A number of discreet stimuli are eventually incorporated into a sense of pain. These extrapolations from the pain may be partial or complete. They may act as omens of pain—or more than omens. Thus, having associated a needle with pain, the mere sight of pin or needle is frequently stimulus enough for the individual to "feel" pain, and the child begins to cry in anticipation of the prick. In a sense, he cries not only in apprehension of the prick but also because the very sensation of the prick is already induced in him by the sight of the needle. Other symbols associated with needles, even in the absence of an actual needle, may induce a state of apprehension; they cause him to anticipate and fear "the unseen needle."

Thus, the doctor's office or emergency room, the physician's white laboratory coat, the smell of anesthetic and medicinal compounds, or other reminders of hurtful past procedures might all forebode harm for the child. As an antidote to this, clinics, emergency centers, and hospitals attempt to remove common symbols that have been found to precipitate such reactions.

The reactions of parents, staff, and others will augment or ameliorate the reactions of the patient to these symbols. Therefore, birthing rooms, for example, are frequently made to appear similar to one's bedroom. Such maneuvers attempt to provide the serenity and familiarity of home, and thereby to reduce the anxiety—and the pain—surrounding parturition. The presence of a significant other person, maybe the unruffled husband or mother, may further serve to diminish pain. On the other hand, the despairing spouse or beside-herself mother-in-law may create histrionics that turn the birthing environment into a nightmare of fears, fantasies, jealousies, and conflict.

The typical physician tries to act in an objective and concerned manner with the patient. He has learned a limited number of meanings for pain, e.g., Where is the pain; What is it like? In a sense, the physician is thus more limited in his interrogation and therapy than is the naive mother, as the latter is also probing the situation with something other than words. She is cuddling and infantilizing the child against her warm breast, rocking him back and forth. She is reviving, in the midst of pain, a pleasurable, symbiotic experience. She speaks in a placating way, assures by her behavior that things will be alright—unless or until she is unsure, concerned, or becomes frustrated, angry, tired, or hungry.

Thus, many experiences and meanings may be superimposed on the meaning of a painful experience. (For example, one of the authors (CPK) can never be sick without visually recalling the 16-year-old farmgirl with the peach-colored blouse, who fed him floating island pudding in his crib when he was three. The remembered image is a placating one.) With each new pain experience, both negative and positive associations to pain may be reinforced or added to, objective ones as well as subjective.

In medicine it might be said that we never get close to really understanding pain without knowing and even feeling some of the misery of the patient. The child who eventually becomes a patient has learned, perhaps (as in the example) from his mother initially, and from his physician subsequently, the language of pain. The problem is: in our analysis and treatment of patients, can we adequately address pain in our patients without experiencing something of the empathy of the mother, however inexperienced she might be?

Pain or hurt, physical or symbolic, can also be viewed as punishment. Punishment is sometimes bewildering: What did I do?—the patient wonders inside. What have I done to deserve this? In addition to bewilderment, there may be a sense of anguish, loss, abandonment, uncertainty, alienation, or separation from others, especially from the well. These feelings are further augmented if the patient is isolated in a hospital or nursing home, away from relatives and friends. External bureaucratic controls erode the patient's autonomy, resulting in a lessened sense of self. To a large extent, the confined patient is held captive, usually without access to clothing and with limited cash. The hospital's schedule of tests, appointments, examinations, meals (or lack of meals) is enforced for the convenience of physicians, nurses, and technicians. Restricted visiting hours diminish the availability of support from family and friends. Hence, many aspects of illness, at least as it is investigated and treated within the hospital setting, add to fantasies of punishment, restrict freedom, threaten unknown and painful procedures, and diminish self-worth. Each of these in their own right may increase the patient's expanding perception and conception of pain, not only in the present but also when faced with subsequent, potentially painful processes.

In the above, the authors have addressed some of the concerns that Thomas Szasz outlined in his book *Pain and Pleasure* (2). He identified the physician's approach to pain as being one most concerned with pain's "public signature," that is, with its tangible somatic vectors; he identified the individual and idiosyncratic experience of pain as its "private signature." It is in the area of the private signature that we must address the patient with headache. However, training has imbedded in physicians a desire to rule in or to rule out; to weigh each objective factor; to make a definitive diagnosis and to then confirm our impression with an ever-increasing number of diagnostic tests and one-by-one trials of therapeutic procedures.

Many of these pain concepts are especially applicable to organ systems which are viewed as most vital to the individual. Head pain, especially, is seen as menacing because of the fears and fantasies to which it gives rise. This is made significantly worse if the pain is accompanied by an altered state of consciousness. Such an alteration greatly exaggerates the fantasy of having had a stroke or brain tumor, as does the presence of seizures, stupor, excitability, or paresis. Such symptoms, alarming enough for the medical staff, are more so for the patient and his family. For most, despite the increasingly sophisticated techniques utilized to assess and surgically intervene to correct intracranial pathophysiologic processes, the trephining or opening of the skull is held to be the ultimate violation, an act almost reserved for the gods.

When, as physicians, we turn our attention to head pain, our demeanor towards the patient commonly takes on an increased gravity. The head towers above the body; it has displaced the soul upwards from the heart, and in our present cathexis of brain as the end-all and be-all of human existence (3), has captured it. This is a far cry from the Greeks' concept of bile for explaining the various afflictions and mood states experienced by Hellenic citizens (4). For so many centuries, the mysteries of the brain lay unexplored. Both lay-persons and physicians are in awe of the brain and what affects it, as it seems the very key to our will and our existence. Those who would approach it venture into a still largely unexplored and quasispiritual territory. This is despite the rapid accumulation of knowledge and technique, neuroendocrine transmitters, neuropeptides, receptor sites, genetic and epigenetic enzyme deficits, tumors, and trauma aside. Not the least of these advances have been more moderate strides in elucidating aging processes, Alzheimer's disease, and other affective, cognitive, and conative deficits and disabilities (5).

LANGUAGE AND THE INTERPRETATION OF HEAD PAIN

As was already discussed, pain has both objective and subjective components (6). The expression given to pain is influenced by many things: individual, intrafamilial, and cultural factors (local and general); the type of medicine practiced regionally; and the availability of physicians or other healers (7, 8).

Of foremost importance are the words and actions patients use to identify pain. These should be carefully attended to and recorded. Graham et al (9) and Grace and Graham (10), in several articles, identify verbal samples characteristic of different segments of the United States population in which the expression of somatically localized pain is metaphorical. Individuals subject to headaches frequently use such expressions as: "She is a pain in the neck" (if not elsewhere). Mothers of two-year-olds frequently tell the latter that they "give their mother a headache." The latter statement may be quickly, if only transiently, adopted by the precocious 2 or 3 year old who begins to have "headaches just like Mommy." (This does not mean that headaches are not also picked up from Daddies.) More often, Daddies cannot concentrate at home because the noise junior makes causes him to "have a headache." In these situations, the headache is likely to be related to increased tension in muscles of the forehead, temple, and neck. These so-called "tension headaches" may be viewed partly as "modelled" ones, or as based upon conversion mechanisms adopted from significant models: parents, teachers, friends.

In another sense, they are learned. Individuals who are puzzled, frustrated, worried, or in conflict develop the habit of wrinkling their brow, gritting their teeth, grimacing to express concern, annoyance, ambivalence, or anger. On the other hand, expression of pleasurable affects, such as by smiling or grinning, may be relaxing, despite the fact—or maybe because of it—that different muscles are tensed.

Some headaches can only be described as "angry headaches." They are often attributed to persons who make the patient angry. Their mechanisms may be vested in tension of muscles such as frowns or clenched teeth—causing facial pain. This is sometimes accompanied by aggressive stances which can cause tension or pain elsewhere in the body. Facial pain or tension may be manifested by taut or tight-lipped smiles, sometimes betraying ambivalence or half-amusement.

Thus far we have paid special attention to words patients use to describe their symptoms. We try to approximate an understanding of what a patient's words mean by drawing upon our own experiences with other patients in pain. At the same time, the physician may be unintentionally suggesting, conveying, persuading, or shaping a definition of pain, one which may or may not correspond to the patient's actual feeling or to his intended meaning. At the same time, the physician might mentally discard other statements by the patient, such as "It (the head) feels like garbage" (which probably means "I feel like garbage"). On the one hand, the physician gropes for closer approximation to his patient's meaning, however inarticulate, garbled, or vague the words used to communicate it. On the other hand, however, he may have quietly and to his satisfaction settled on his own definition of what he thinks the patient means by "pain." Note that there is a reciprocal interaction between the patient and the physician which defines the pain. Such reciprocal processes result in a definition which is at best a compromise between the patient's and the physician's points of view. Generally, the more rushed the circumstances, the greater the polarization. One should not underestimate the importance of these "semantics," especially if the language becomes overly florid. The patient who expresses his symptoms in terms such as, "It feels as if a herd of elephants are galloping through my head," may have this vivid experience based on mental illness, histrionic posturing, or merely poetic license. But the physician may dismiss such a statement peremptorily, without bothering to find out which of those it is.

GRIEVING STATES

States of grief are frequently associated with pain or other physical symptoms, especially those symptoms that the deceased had in life or during the terminal illness. Especially during early phases of grief, a similar pain may be experienced by the bereft (11). This is usually transient, but in delayed or unresolved grief there may be an inappropriate and pathological holding on to the deceased through the unconscious adoption of one or more of his terminal symptoms. This is especially true if there had been a symbiotic relationship between the patient and the deceased. These symptoms may become relatively fixed for a period of time, causing friends and physicians to show concern for the survivor.

Delayed grief responses may merge with or become indistinguishable from pathological grief states, that is, they may take on characteristics of frank depression. The expression of grief states has been well portrayed by artists throughout history: people suffering from it are pictured as having vacuous, dry, staring eyes; a mask of melancholia, with furrowed brows, hollowed cheeks, and tensed mouth; a bent head, hunched shoulders, with the arms frequently cradling the withdrawn self; or, hands may be passively outstretched, as if in supplication of alms. The general demeanor is one of despair, emptiness, and limpidity.

Far from being a passive state, grief, despite its appearance, is a cauldron of emotions—emotions that are mixed, bittersweet, ambivalent, hostile, self-placating, antagonistic, protagonistic, self-pitying, attacking, and

withdrawing. They may be viewed as a withdrawing of emotional investments from the external environment and back into a preoccupation with the self. There is in this narcissistic posture a regression in which the individual is engrossed only by his own wounds which, while they may be seen as symbolic, are given substance through somatic expression. One of those expressions may be headache.

A SCIENTIFIC AND PROCEDURAL WAY OF EVALUATING HEADACHES AND THEIR TREATMENT

The origin of most headaches is not easy to determine. As we have considered above, much has to do with the learning of language and the individual's definition of pain, aches, and feelings. Are there times when a headache is not a headache? Objective classification is not especially difficult. One goes through the common diagnoses in his head, then the more esoteric ones and, finally, perhaps the idiosyncratic ones based on his own experience. This process begins even before the patient is first seen. What is important here is that, whether or not one is consciously aware of it, the interview communicates, as well as obtains, information. Thus our interview may implant symptoms, signs, and possible diagnoses in the patient's mind. These may induce iatrogenic confusion or problems, ultimately causing unnecessary anxiety and apprehension. Therefore, the interview is not a benign procedure.

Nor is the physical examination. It is even more intrusive. For many patients, both fear and trembling accompany interrogation or examination. Hearts skip beats; pulse rates are elevated or sometimes slowed; blood pressure rises; sweat glands perspire harder; reflexes become exaggerated; pupils dilate; mouths dry up; peristalsis increases; and headaches are precipitated. The physiology the patient has in the office is not representative of most situations in his day to day life. For full evaluation, some patients need to be placed in a quiet and darkened environment prior to, before, and occasionally after, the examination.

The examination comes before the really invasive procedures, procedures that from our objective perspectives we tend to view as ordinary and benign. For physicians, routine x-rays give rise to only casual thoughts about irradiation and cancer. Isotope studies may cause more concern. But have you ever put your head in a CT scanner? Do you know what it is like to lie absolutely still for 20 minutes for a CT scan? Have you imagined the "science fiction" fantasies that a patient might have during a positron emission tomography (PET) scan?

Except for anecdotes, we have comparatively little data concerning these "ordinary" techniques. And we have not yet even considered intravenous arteriograms, or the theatres in which these take place, or the partly-overheard, parsimoniously cryptic dialogues of the investigators performing these procedures. What half-information is conveyed during this process? Which fears are allayed? Which are augmented? To what extent and how often does the individual with something wrong with his head fear he is losing his mind, becoming insane, losing control, suffering from a relentless and invasive deterioration of the brain and cognitive processes—and ascribing to every casual comment of a nearby house officer clues or answers to his dreaded questions?

HOW PATIENTS GET REASSURED

Having completed an appropriate psychological and neurological diagnostic inquiry, the physician will have arrived at a diagnosis and be ready to decide on treatment. If the diagnosis is a benign one, he will wish to communicate this in the most reassuring way, so as to set the patient's mind at rest, thereby reducing as well the patient's subsequent use of medical resources. The more chronic the patient's disorder, the more important it will be to set the stage for an empathic, long-term

relationship. If he has diagnosed a psychiatric disorder, the primary physician will wish to institute proper treatment himself or, when indicated, to make a referral.

Reassurance or, more broadly, the therapeutic use of the relationship between doctor and patient, has been an element of treatment as long as there have been doctors. Through much of medical history it has been the only effective element of treatment, with specific remedies being unknown. It remains today the bedrock of medical treatment, whether or not specific remedies are put to use, are unknown, or are unnecessary. Certainly physicians are taught to "reassure the patient" if possible. Oddly enough, then, they are not taught *how*. Only a few papers we know of comment on this aspect of medical care (12, 13). Like other forms of medical intervention, reassurance can be done well or badly; the patient does better if the doctor does it well.

This part of treatment is often referred to, sometimes in a derogatory way, as the "placebo effect." But clinical experience and some systematic research have shown that it is a potent element of the physician's total treatment. Fitzpatrick and Hopkins (14) studied patients seen in British neurological clinics for headaches not due to structural lesions. At follow-up 1 year after the consultation, most patients had experienced considerable improvement. The factor measured at the time of consultation that proved to be most strongly associated with improvement was satisfaction with the consultation; initiation of, or changes in drug treatment had an independent and more modest association. Several interpretations of this finding are possible, but the authors conclude that patients who felt the consultation personally valuable in relation to their concerns experienced improvement due to nonspecific "placebo mechanisms." This conclusion is consistent with our clinical experience.

Other work by the same authors (15) and by Grove et al (16) points toward a similar conclusion. Both studies found that after a neurological consultation, patients visit their general practitioners for headache less often. Unfortunately, Fitzpatrick and Hopkins did not find that this necessarily meant a reduction in headache; many patients simply reduced their visits despite continuation of their symptoms. Further, Grove et al found no fall in total visits, that is, apparently new complaints arose to bring the patients back to their doctors. Nevertheless, the conclusion seems reasonable that the consultation as a psychological fact is potent, regardless of the specific treatment offered. It should, however, be noted that these studies from Great Britain and Australia may not reflect accurately the situation in the United States, where neurological referral is more common and general practice less so.

It must also be made clear that these psychological effects are not limited to the patient with a psychiatric disorder. Psychiatric symptoms, distressingly common in the general population, can be expected to be at least as common in the general headache population. Thus, in a careful study by Fitzpatrick and Hopkins' (14), 18 of 95 patients could be rated as "extensively psychiatrically impaired." (We have simplified their more complex tabulation.) But 65 of 95 patients were rated as having fears of serious illness, and the majority of those did not have psychiatric symptoms. These data reinforce our clinical impression that even the psychologically healthy headache patient should be assumed to be worried and to require proper reassurance.

How then should this reassurance be delivered? We offer the following suggestions.

(a) The patient cannot be reassured unless the doctor knows what he is worried about; there is no such thing as "reassurance in general." Thus, part of the history-taking must explore the patient's concerns in the way discussed above. Only then will the doctor be able to reassure specifically that, for example, "You don't have a tumor" or "This is different from what your father died of." Much of the time, the single, simple question "What do you think is the matter?" will reveal much of what the doctor needs to know.

(b) The patient is less likely to be reassured by negatives. "The CT-scan doesn't show anything wrong" may mean to the physician that the possibility of tumor is effectively excluded. To the patient unfamiliar with the diagnostic power of the history, the examination, and the various investigations—and perhaps too worried to think rationally in any case—this statement means only that the physician has not yet figured out what the matter is. In the worst case, he takes it to mean that he had better find a smarter doctor, one who *will* find something—for, after all, he knows perfectly well that *something* is wrong, or else he would not have such a bad headache.

We believe it more helpful to say to the patient something like, "We have learned from the history and examination and tests that this is the kind of headache that results from muscle contraction," or "from spine disease," or even "from worry and depression"—adding, as suggested above, whatever specific reassurance is indicated, for example, "and the scan shows that you don't have a tumor." One of us has found it useful to say, when consulting on a worried headache patient who has already seen several doctors who "couldn't find anything wrong," that doctors are very good at finding dangerous problems, but that figuring out what exactly is causing less dangerous ones, like the common cold, is sometimes harder.

(c) The consulting psychiatrist is not the ideal agent of reassurance. It is best for the patient to be reassured by the primary physician. Many patients will consider the mere facts of psychiatric consultation or referral to be a dismissal, unless or sometimes even if it is properly handled by the primary physician. The difficult patient who has not been responsive to proper reassurance, or who has not been reassured in a competent manner, may not be amenable to psychiatric evaluation either.

We have found that the most useful approach is to involve the psychiatrist early. As soon as the physician concludes that psychiatric factors are of significance, he can approach the patient with the idea of consultation. "This is the kind of headache that can come from several different causes: a problem inside the skull, or an abnormal blood vessel, or excessive worry or depression. I want to look into all these possibilities."

Obviously, not every patient can have a psychiatric consultation. But it is not unusual for a neurologist to arrange an extensive workup—CT scan, lumbar puncture, even hospital admission—firmly expecting in advance that the only pathology to be found is psychological. Yet, a psychological workup is not arranged. From the point of view of most consulting psychiatrists, they would rather see an occasional patient "unnecessarily," one in whom structural pathology is ultimately found, than to recurrently face patients angry because psychiatric referral was discussed with them only after "everything else had been ruled out." Patients who feel "dismissed" are less likely to cooperate in a psychological evaluation (and perhaps more likely to seek a second neurological opinion).

(d) The opposite of dismissal is invitation—first, invitation to tell the whole psychological story, but also an invitation to return. An additional visit, even if only a brief one, may allow the patient to reveal concerns he hid the first time around, especially if the invitation to return is done in a way that indicates the doctor is interested. Even in so limited and often impersonal a setting as a neurological clinic, the offer to "Come back in so I can see how things are going" may prove a powerful therapeutic agent.

(e) Opinion is divided on whether patients find procedures reassuring per se. On the one hand, Fitzpatrick and Hopkins (15) did not find that the ordering of procedures was associated with satisfaction or, thence, with symptom-reduction. On the other hand, the issue is unsettled, and probably cannot be settled in general. It is only by understanding his particular patient's concerns and expectations that the physician can decide wisely about psychological interventions. Here again, the simple question "What do you think should be done?" may provide a wealth of data. The patient may reveal, for example, that he will be unsatisfied unless he has an utterly unnecessary investigation, seeming important to him only because of an identification with a relative or friend who had the study, unsatisfied, that is, unless the physician can expose this concern to the light of day and set the patient's mind to rest. As stressed in other sections, the management of chronic headache patients requires periodic follow-up visits, regardless of the presence or absence of new symptoms. This assures the patient of the physician's availability and caring concern. Many of these visits will be spent talking over family situations, financial problems, and even transportation difficulties. While the physician may feel frequently overwhelmed by his inability to "do something" for the patient, this attention often provides help that is impossible to justify in a pathology laboratory. A major part of the periodic evaluation will be to ensure that there has not been an onset of new symptoms such as depression, cognitive dysfunction, or intercurrent somatic disease. These will be most easily investigated by questions identifying changes in work schedules, sleep habits, appetite, sexual behavior, and patterns of socialization.

REFERENCES

1. Kandel ER, Kriegstein A, Schacher S: Development of the central nervous system of Aplysia in terms of the differentiation of its specific identifiable cells. *Neuroscience* 5(12):2033–2063, 1980.

2. Szasz T: *Pain and Pleasure*. New York, Basic Books, 1957.

3. Eckstein G: *The Body Has a Head*. New York, Harper & Row, 1969.

4. Taylor HO: *Greek Biology and Medicine*. Boston, Marshall Jones, 1922.

5. Wolff HG: *Headache*. New York, Oxford University Press, 1963.

6. Engel GL: "Psychogenic" pain and the pain-prone patient. *Am J Med* 26:899–918, 1959.

7. Melzack R: Gate control theory. In *The Puzzle of Pain*. New York, Basic Books, 1973.

8. Ramsay RA: The understanding and teaching of reaction to pain. In Kimball CP, Krakowski AJ

(eds): *The Teaching of Psychosomatic Medicine and Consultation-Liaison Psychiatry. Bibliotheca Psychiatri* 159:114–140, Basel, S. Karger, 1979.

9. Graham DT, Stern JA, Winokur G: Experimental investigation of the specificity of attitude hypothesis in psychosomatic disease. *Psychosom Med* 20:446–457, 1958.

10. Grace WJ, Graham DT: Relationship of specific attitudes and emotions to certain bodily diseases. *Psychosom Med* 14:243–251, 1952.

11. Westberg G: *Good Grief.* Philadelphia, Fortress, 1962.

12. Kessel N: Reassurance. *The Lancet:*1(8126):1128–1133, 1979.

13. Wehlage DF: The art of doing "nothing." *Chicago Med* 85:175–176, 1982.

14. Fitzpatrick RM, Hopkins AP: Referrals to neurologists for headache not due to structural disease. *J Neurol Neurosurg Psychiatry* 44:1061–1067, 1981.

15. Fitzpatrick RM, Hopkins AP: Effects of referral to a specialist for headache. *J Roy Soc Med* 76:112–115, 1983.

16. Grove JL, Butler P, Millac PAH: The effect of a visit to a neurological clinic upon patients with tension headache. *Practitioner* 224:195–196, 1980.

CHAPTER ELEVEN

Multiple Headaches in Cases of Multiple Personality Disorder

RUSSELL C. PACKARD, M.D.
FRANK BROWN, PH.D.

Jesus asked him "What is your name?" "Legion," he said. "There is a host of us." **(Mark 5:9)**

Multiple personality disorder (MPD) is a dissociative disorder that has been somewhat poorly characterized and at times has been quite controversial. According to Bliss (1), MPD has actually been described through case reports for centuries, Paracelsus perhaps giving the first clinical description of a case in 1646. Ellenberger (2) credited Rile with first recognizing the existence of separate or multiple personalities in 1803. Since then, several criteria for diagnosis have been offered in the literature, the organizing principle for most definitions being the degree to which the alternate personalities can be distinguished as separately conscious entities capable of independent behavior.

Although the purpose of this chapter is not to discuss MPD per se, it should be pointed out that the disorder is frequently either unsuspected or misdiagnosed as schizophrenia, manic-depressive illness, temporal lobe epilepsy, sociopathy, or borderline personality disorder (3). The diagnostic criteria for MPD listed in the 3rd edition of *The Diagnostic and Statistical Manual of Mental Disorders* (4) are:

a. Within the individual exist two or more distinct personalities, each of which is dominant at a particular time.

b. The personality that is dominant at any particular time determines the individual's behavior.

c. Each individual personality is complex and integrated, with its own unique behavior patterns and social relationships.

More recent articles on MPD have strongly stressed the importance of amnesia, either partial or complete, as a clinical characteristic of the syndrome (5). The diagnosis of MPD is confirmed when the therapist is confronted with a distinct and separate personality. In approximately two-thirds of reviewed cases, it was not until an alternate personality spontaneously revealed itself to a surprised and unsuspecting clinician that the diagnosis was made (3).

In two separate reviews of MPD cases, headache has been described as the most frequent somatic complaint, with a frequency of 53% in one series of 38 cases (3) and 91% in another series of 11 cases (1). The description of the headaches, however, has usually either been in general terms such as "headache," or by a patient's own description, such as "a violent headache'' (6). In the few accounts where the headaches have been described in more detail, they are often characterized as extremely painful, "migraine-like head-aches," which commonly occur with the switching of personalities (5, 7, 8). Even these cases, however, did not elaborate on how the diagnosis of migraine was derived.

One of the more complete descriptions is noted in a paper by Ludwig et al (7), in which a male patient presented with a history of memory lapses preceded by severe head-aches. The headaches were described as a band-like pressure around his head that would progress to the vertex in a skull cap distribution. When he would regain aware-ness of himself, the headache would be gone, and he would feel relaxed. It is worth noting that in this case the initial diagnosis was psy-chomotor epilepsy, which changed when

TABLE 11.1

SUMMARY OF PERSONALITIES AND HEADACHE DESCRIPTIONS: CASE 1

PERSONALITY NUMBER	AGE	PERSONALITY FEATURES	HEADACHE DESCRIPTION
1	24	The patient; main personality. Smokes, wears hair brushed out long. Somewhat blunt in speech and manner. Denied knowledge of other personalities. Worked as a secretary.	Two types: (1) Several years of intermittent bitemporal throbbing associated with nausea and vomiting. Come out of the blue. (2) Dull constant daily headache on top and sides of head. This type often brought on by stress at work.
2	13	Ponytail—initially shy but talkative. "I don't have a name." Nicknamed, "Sweet girl." Doesn't like smoking.	Dull, frontal, constant headache between eyes. Points to a place between her eyes. Relieved when playing cards.
3	18	Lived in a different state with an older man. Irritable. Smokes. Forms unstable relationships. Frequently beaten. Threatened suicide.	Chronic daily headache in the back of her head, radiating to the temples. Sometimes "feels sick."
4	10	Nickname: "Pink Pajamas." Afraid of physical abuse by her mother. History of abuse? "Hates smoking."	Constant frontal headaches in forehead. Never goes away.
5	6	No name. Little detail other than "absolutely hates smoking." Constantly tries to talk husband out of smoking.	No headache but complains frequently of her "mouth hurting."
6	? (18–25)	Second most dominant personality. "Pretty girl." Seductive. Likes nightgowns. Husband finds her "hard to resist." Smokes.	Intermittent, dull frontal headache. Has days without.
7	? (20's)	No name. Only present once for 20 min. Seemed at ease with herself. Calm and understanding.	? No headache according to personality no. 2.

hospital personnel observed the emergence of differing personalities during memory lapses.

This chapter describes three cases of multiple personality disorder in which specific attention is paid to the reported headaches.

CASE 1

A 24-year-old housewife was referred for evaluation of headaches. She had been recently diagnosed as having multiple personalities; a total of seven different personalities had been identified. For simplicity of presentation, these differing personalities will be noted by number (see Table 11.1). The patient's dominant identity was personality no. 1, also referred to as "the patient" or "the husband's wife."

The patient first came into the office accompanied by her husband, who introduced her as personality no. 2, a 13-year-old. She had a shy, somewhat youthful smile and a ponytail held back with a rubber band. She seemed to have a considerable knowledge of the other personalities, and said that four others besides herself had headaches. Most of the history with regard to the other personalities and their headache types was obtained from this "no. 2" and from the husband. Fortunately, the examiner also had the opportunity to interview personality no. 1, after the husband was able to talk "no. 2" into taking a nap on the examining table. (The husband remarked that a nap frequently served as a way for a new personality to appear.) The 13 year old, prior to settling down for the nap, complained of a constant dull frontal headache centered between her eyes.

After about 2 min of sleep in semidarkness, personality no. 1, the wife, suddenly bolted upright on the examining table, held her head, and stated she did not know where she was. She immediately reach up, pulled the rubber band out of her hair, and began fluffing out her hair. The patient then asked for a cigarette and, while holding her head, began to complain of a terrible, pounding, bitemporal headache, accompanied by mild nausea. She went on to describe her headaches in detail (see Table 11.1), to which the husband added some further pertinent observations (see Table 11.2).

An EEG performed on personality no. 1 was normal, and a diagnosis of multiple headaches in a case of multiple personality disorder was established. Devising a comprehensive treatment plan for six different headache situations and seven different personalities was like trying to work out an arrangement for seven families in one house to share the bathroom. Because of the difficulties inherent to such an approach, it was elected to try and treat one headache and one personality at a time, while the patient continued in psychotherapy to resolve her MPD problem.

A trial of Bellergal Spacetabs was prescribed for the vascular headache symptoms of personality no. 1. Only a small supply was given since personality no. 3 (the 18 year old) had recently threatened suicide because personality no. 1 had changed her hairstyle. (The husband also felt somewhat exasperated because none of the other personalities liked the new hairstyle either, and he felt obligated to try and explain to each one why the change had been made.)

Another difficulty arose when the patient did not return for follow-up the next week to either her neurologist or psychologist. The husband said his wife had just disappeared. After a few days he officially reported her missing. Three weeks later the psychologist received a telephone call from personality no. 3, who was in southern California. She was crying, and said she had just been beaten up by her boyfriend again. This was followed by a call from personality no. 2 a week later, who was by then at a telephone booth in Texas, saying she was scared and had run away. She was advised to wait there for her husband,

TABLE 11.2
OBSERVATIONS BY HUSBAND ON
PERSONALITIES WITH HEADACHE: CASE 1

1. Increased headache intensity noted immediately before and briefly after a switch.
2. About 2 min after a switch, headache was less intense. (Confirmed by examiner when Personality no. 2 switched to no. 1).
3. All would feel sleepy or "blah" before a switch.
4. Personalities no. 5 and no. 7 did not experience headaches at times of switch—did feel sleepy or listless.

who went to meet her, but by the time he arrived she was gone. Neither patient nor husband was heard from again.

Maintaining outpatient contact with an MPD patient is often so difficult that it may be one indication for hospitalization.

CASE 2

A 19-year-old woman presented with chief complaints of amnesic spells and headaches over the past 2 years. In addition, she had recently been apprehended for writing bad checks, a situation for which she claimed no memory.

Two years before being evaluated, the patient experienced several "bad headaches" associated with nausea and vomiting. She was hospitalized by a neurologist and had a normal neurologic examination, EEG, CT head scan, and spinal fluid studies. Pain medication containing aspirin, butalbital, and caffeine provided only fair relief of symptoms. Six months later she saw a psychologist about three times for difficulty sleeping.

Her headaches continued on and off until 2 months prior to evaluation, at which time she started having "small lapses of memory." These memory lapses would usually be preceded by a brief period of dizzy, lightheaded feeling and were typically followed by a bad headache. The amnesic spells would often last several hours, during which she would apparently carry out unplanned activities, i.e., shopping at the department store instead of the grocery store, looking at new cars, etc. Most often, the patient would simply be unable to account for the lost time. The first thing she would become aware of was usually a severe, bitemporal, throbbing headache and loss of the sense of time. The headache often lasted 3 hr and was distinctly worse during the first 20 min. She described her headaches as "typical migraines" which were often accompanied by nausea and vomiting. Pain was usually unilateral, but could be bitemporal, and was pounding in nature. As these episodes continued she started to discover different clothes in her closet, rearranged furniture in her house, and a new perfume which tended to set off migraine attacks. At first she was concerned, and believed that her husband was responsible

for these new events. She confided that his behavior was beginning to worry her!

Additional history was obtained from the husband. He first noted a change in his wife's behavior at a homeowners association meeting. His wife, who was generally reserved, started talking rather loudly, and sounded like "a completely different person . . . uninhibited." When they arrived home she told him that she was not his wife, and refused to give her name. He naturally thought she was kidding. But his concern mounted when she then separated her jewelry into two piles, saying one was for Anne (his wife, the patient), the other for herself. Later, she identified herself as Paula, age 21. Paula knew all about Anne, but Anne knew nothing about her. The husband spontaneously stated that Paula was "another individual, another identity."

Neurologic examination, repeat CT head scan, and EEG were all normal. The patient appeared quiet, a bit withdrawn, and backward. She used makeup sparingly, and seemed apprehensive and nervous, with little facial expression.

The differential diagnosis was between complex partial seizures, a dissociative disorder, or MPD. Complex partial seizures were excluded because of the long periods of amnesia during which goal-directed behavior occurred, as well as the normal EEG.

The possibility of MPD was discussed with the patient and her husband. She was taught to relax with the help of self-regulatory techniques, and the suggestion was made that during a countdown from 10 to 1, she would reach a state in which Paula would emerge, or at least would have an opportunity to. Although the patient was initially reluctant to do this, she ultimately agreed. During the countdown, the patient appeared to doze briefly. Suddenly, Paula emerged, feeling slightly tired but smiling.

Paula was bubbly and restless to the point that she did not want to remain seated. She squirmed in the chair and soon stood up, asking if she could "get out of here and go for a drive." She described herself as a "free spirit," and admitted that Anne did not know about her. "I come and go whenever I want." This was followed by the statement, "I don't really care about her husband either." Paula had apparently been "present" for years, but

TABLE 11.3
SUMMARY OF PERSONALITIES AND HEADACHE DESCRIPTIONS:
CASE 2

PERSONALITY NAME	HEADACHE DESCRIPTION
1. "Anne," 19 year old presenting personality with memory lapses. Generally reserved, quiet to withdrawn, little facial expression and sparse use of makeup.	Intermittent, unilateral or bitemporal, pounding. Accompanied by nausea, vomiting, and photophobia lasting about 3 hr. Precipitated by certain types of perfume.
2. "Paula," 21 year old alternate personality. Bubbly, restless; impulsive, socially friendly but immature, suspicious, friendly but distinct and self-centered. A "free spirit."	No headaches. Wore perfume that would precipitate a headache in Anne.

first came out when Anne was in grade school learning to talk on the telephone. "I wanted to do that too." No other childhood memories could be recalled. She liked bright colors and expensive things, "all the things Anne never gets for herself." Curiously, Paula had never experienced a headache, even after the personality switch. It was explained by her that "Anne gets headaches because she is too inhibited." Paula also seemed to take delight in the fact that her perfume would set off headaches in Anne. After the interview, Paula started reading a magazine. Anne then re-emerged with a throbbing headache, nausea, and photophobia. Her last memory was relaxing while listening to the biofeedback tape. The patient is currently in psychotherapy (see Table 11.3).

CASE 3

Personality no. 1 (Rose) was a 33-year-old woman who came for a headache evaluation. She had a known multiple personality disorder, and had been in treatment for it for approximately 8 years. Rose apparently grew up simultaneously with personality no. 2 (Glenda). They were both 33 years old.

Rose had constant, daily headaches. They were aggravated by stress. She described a dull pressure all over and in her eyes. Sometimes the muscles in her neck felt tense. She had not experienced visual change,

dizziness, nausea, or vomiting with these headaches.

For the past month she thought, "I might be the only personality left." This was creating a good deal of stress, since "I used to spend a lot of my time in bars, and now I have to learn to be a mother." (Glenda was a single parent of an 8-year-old boy and now Rose was having to change her ways in order to care for "Glenda's child.") She tended to let her feelings out and talk about them, whereas Glenda tended to keep hers inside because "she doesn't want to hurt people and doesn't stand up well."

Rose described Glenda as a "mother-type" who had headaches that were periodic, pulsating, severe, and disabling. They were accompanied by nausea and vomiting, and she often had to go to bed for 3 days at a time. Afterwards, Glenda would feel totally drained. Rose thought Glenda had headaches like this because she "holds things in."

Personality no. 3 (Angie) was a 19-year-old female who had intermittent, mild, dull headaches. She was "a peacekeeper" who also tended to suffer from intermittent "deep depressions." Her headaches were always very brief, and usually only occurred when she became upset. They never lasted an entire day.

Personality no. 4 (Lynne) was 4 years old "and never gets any older." She had never been sick and never had a headache.

TABLE 11.4
SUMMARY OF PERSONALITIES AND HEADACHE DESCRIPTIONS:
CASE 3

PERSONALITY NAME	HEADACHE DESCRIPTION
1. "Rose," 33 year old presenting personality but had been a former alter personality. Mildly depressed. Probably alcoholic. Independent. Stressed by responsibility of having to "become a mother."	Dull pressure type of constant daily headache. All over, behind eyes. Neck tense. Worse with stress.
2. "Glenda," 33 year old former main personality. A "mother type" but unmarried. Kept feelings inside. Didn't want to hurt people. Didn't stand up well.	Periodic, pulsating severe and disabling headaches. Associated nausea and vomiting. Lasted 1–3 days.
3. "Angie," 19 year old. A peacekeeper. Often depressed.	Brief, intermittent, mild, dull headaches, lasting less than a day. Stress related.
4. "Lynne," 4 year old. Never gets any older. Never been sick.	Never had a headache.

Rose reported that the headaches of each personality (except no. 4) would intensify or be precipitated after a switch in identity and that the new person would be "drained," especially if the previous one had been quite upset. However personality no. 4 usually felt tired or drained, but never had a headache.

Rose also reported that when a personality emerged it often tended to suffer problems incurred by the previous one, i.e., if Rose had been out drinking in a bar, Glenda would sometimes wake up with a hangover. Also, if Glenda had been down for 3 days with a terrible headache, Rose would often feel "totally drained" (see Table 11.4).

DISCUSSION

These patients seemed to confirm reports in the literature that headaches associated with MPD appeared to build in intensity or be precipitated immediately prior to and/or after a personality shift (7). Although one of the authors observed that personality no. 1 in Case 1, and Anne in Case 2, emerged from a switch with a vascular type headache, this was not true in every case. The headaches often varied considerably, and many switches occurred without evident headaches (e.g., Paula in Case 2, as observed directly by the examiner). The husbands were also aware of switches occurring without headache, as were "alternate personalities." At a minimum, though, patients tended to feel drained, blah, or tired after a switch.

Several other factors were intriguing. One was that in all three cases, each personality with headache clearly described a different type of headache, with variations in quality, location, frequency, or severity. In Case 1, only one personality reported a vascular-type headache (no. 1); the others usually suffered from chronic muscle contraction headaches (with a possible combined headache in personality no. 3.) Some headaches might have been diagnosed as psychogenic, but further information would have been needed to do so with certainty. In Case 1, at least one personality (no. 7), and possibly two, did not seem to have headaches at all. In the two remaining patients, personalities were also identified who were without headaches.

These cases raise some interesting questions about the mechanisms of headache and about the interplay between characterological and physiological factors. Although the list of such potential questions is nearly endless, one purpose of this chapter is merely to stimulate the reader to raise questions of his own. Clearly the most intriguing paradox is how just one individual could experience vascular headache symptoms, as we would currently interpret them, while sharing the very same body with as many as six other personalities, each of whom was free of vascular headache symptoms. And how do we explain, physiologically, a chronic, daily headache, possibly sustained muscle contraction or combined in nature, which leaves no trace of itself after just 2 or 3 minutes of a transition into another personality state? This type of chronic daily headache patient is often a vexing problem in clinical practice, one that proves stubbornly resistant to analgesics, muscle relaxation exercises, antiinflammatories, muscle relaxants, and antidepressants. The explanation that all daily headaches noted in these cases are merely "psychogenic" or "hysterical" is unlikely to be correct.

Taken individually, each personality seemed to have a unique headache problem, as unique and distinctive as its sense of self. If we were to diagnose Anne in Case 2, or Rose in Case 3, as a "typical migraineur" with all the inherited or biochemical or neurological factors that "cause" migraine, we must assume they are still present when the other personalities expropriate that same body. Migraine researchers who would prefer to divorce personality considerations from the study of physiologic processes must account for why this pool of migraine precursors and chemicals does not continue to cause attacks during the reigns of alternate personality states or, turning the question around: What are the personality factors involved in "allowing" a vascular headache of the migraine type

to emerge? Why does the perfume act in only one?

Other studies of MPD cases have found that some psychological testing results are often significantly different among the different personalities (7–9). Physiological differences in EEG (7, 10), galvanic skin response (7, 8), and visual evoked responses (3, 8) have also been noted. This growing body of psychological, physiological, and neurophysiological data suggests that profound bodily as well as mental changes may accompany the shift into different personality states.

Could these changes be similar to phenomena found in some headache situations? Might similar mechanisms be operative when a migraine patient experiences a mood disturbance before the onset of headache? We might even wonder: Do patients develop headache instead of dissociating into a different personality state? Are headache and dissociation related? The present study at the least suggests a clear and definite relationship between personality and bodily functioning. It is certainly remarkable that one body has the capacity to react in so many ways.

Although MPD is a common disorder, it should be emphasized that many cases seem to be overlooked, unsuspected, or misdiagnosed. This point was stressed repeatedly in a recent symposium on MPD (11). (The material from this conference provides a wealth of further information on diagnosis, etiology, and treatment of MPD.) Severe headaches have been cited as a sign suggestive of MPD, especially if they are associated with other factors, such as time distortion, time lapses, being told of disremembered behavior, observers' reports of noteworthy personality changes, or the discovery of productions (such as writing or art) or of objects among one's possession which can neither be recognized nor accounted for (12).

The "alternate" personalities may also give clues to underlying psychodynamics that are "unconscious" in the primary personality. In the second and third cases, observations were made about the primary (migrainous) personalities "holding things in" or not expressing anger or feelings. This type of observation has been made in many previous studies of personality factors in migraine, although currently there is no consensus about a "typical migraine personality."

Treatment of the headaches in MPD may be considered on an individual personality basis, but cannot be divorced from the complex task of treating the underlying disorder itself. Decisions about headache treatment are based on criteria similar to those used with other patients. Pharmacologic treatment is obviously limited, however, if some of the personalities are unstable, suicidal, or uncooperative. Treatment of MPD itself is discussed elsewhere (13, 14).

It is suggested that patients with MPD and headache might be ideal for studying, in a more sophisticated fashion, the blood flow differences, electrophysiologic, and biochemical changes known to be associated with different headache types. These studies might suggest answers to the most elusive question of all: How does headache involve the entire person—body, mind, and personality?

REFERENCES

1. Bliss EL: Multiple personalities: a report of 14 cases with implications for schizophrenia and hysteria. *Arch Gen Psychiatry* 37:1388–1400, 1980.

2. Ellenberger HF: *The Discovery of the Unconscious.* New York, Basic Books, 1970, pp 126–141.

3. Putnam FW, Post RM: Multiple personality disorder: An analysis and review of the syndrome. National Institute of Mental Health, Section on Biological Psychiatry, personal communication, 1983.

4. *Diagnostic and Statistical Manual of Mental Disorders,* ed 3. Washington, D.C., American Psychiatric Association, 1980.

5. Coons PM: Multiple personality: Diagnostic considerations. *J Clin Psychiatry* 41:330–336, 1980.

6. Franz SI: *Persons One and Three: A Study of Multiple Personality.* New York, McGraw-Hill, 1933, p 176.

7. Ludwig A, Brandsma J, Wilbur C, et al: The objective study of a multiple personality. *Arch Gen Psychiatry* 26:298–310, 1972.

8. Larmore K, Ludwig AM, Cain RL: Multiple personality: an objective case study. *Arch Gen Psychiatry* 31:35–40, 1977.

9. Brandsma JM, Ludwig AM: A case of multiple personality: Diagnosis and therapy. *Int J Clin Exp Hypn* 22:216–233, 1974.

10. Thigpen CH, Cleckley H: A case of multiple personality. *J Abnorm Soc Psychol* 49:135–151, 1950.

11. Kluft RP: An introduction to multiple personality disorder. *Psychiatr Ann* 14:19–24, 1984.

12. Greaves G: Multiple personality: 165 years after Mary Reynolds. *J Nerv Ment Dis* 168:577–596, 1980.

13. Kluft RP: Aspects of the treatment of multiple personality disorder. *Psychiatr Ann* 14:51–55, 1984.

14. Wilbur CB: Treatment of multiple personality. *Psychiatr Ann* 14:27–31, 1984.

SECTION THREE ☐

Psychiatric Aspects of Specific Headache Syndromes

Clinical and Psychodynamic Aspects of Tension Headache

CHARLES S. ADLER, M.D.
SHEILA MORRISSEY ADLER, Ph.D.

DEFINITION

On this there is agreement: the image of tension headache conveyed to the public in television advertisements little resembles the chronic tension headache seen by the medical specialist. In the televised version, a tired and irritable (but still beautiful) woman in a noisy social gathering presses her brow with the back of her hand and announces her headache to a kindly friend. The kindly friend gives her two extra-strength relief pills. In the next scene it is dawn, and on the deck of her sailboat is our lady, refreshed and smiling.

From the headache clinics of the world come different allegories, such as the one Lance quotes (1) from Shakespeare's *King Henry V*:

In peace there is nothing so becomes a man
As modest stillness and humility;
But when the blast of war blows in our ears,
Then imitate the action of a tiger;
Stiffen the sinews, summon up the blood,
Disguise fair nature with hard-favour'd rage;
Then lend the eye a terrible aspect . . .
Let the brow o'erwhelm it . . .
Now set the teeth and stretch the wide
nostril . . .

For such patients the extra-strength, over-the-counter pain relievers no longer work. Or work only in prohibitive quantities, or result in all manner of side effects, or actually wind up perpetuating the headaches.

These examples illustrate how much the chronic tension headache—the type this chapter will address—differs from the occasional tension headache. Its causes may be different as well as its solutions.

Few medical syndromes are as wedded to the emotions as tension headache or are as riddled with debate. Much of that debate revolves around the fundamental question: What is tension headache? Is the condition primarily mental or physical? Is the "tension" in the emotions or in the muscles?

Unfortunately, this common headache, like the common cold, routinely slips through the fingers of science. When, as a starting point, one looks for a definition of the chronic tension headache, he is immediately confronted by ambiguity. Sjaastad (2) points out that even headache specialists have not unified their thinking about this syndrome. Diagnostic criteria are variable enough to allow an assortment of poorly defined headaches to gather under this label.

One reason the diagnosis lends itself to overinclusiveness is because it is often partly correct. In most people, head pain of any origin will result in reactive muscle contraction that can, if sufficiently prolonged, turn into tension headache. The cause of a tension headache is, in other words, sometimes another headache, such as migraine, or another source of pain, such as cervical arthritis.

Another source of diagnostic confusion is self-generated. It arises from attempts to give tension headaches with different trigger mechanisms separate names. Friedman et al (3) proposed to separate "muscular headache" from tension headache, with the former term to be applied if the triggering event was physical rather than psychological. Other authors (4) segregate tension headaches caused by depression into a category of depressive headaches. When an important element in a tension headache's causation is centrally mediated hyper-attention to pain, many clinicians loosely refer to it as a conversion headache, even when the hyper-attentiveness is just one contributor to the clinical picture. Although these different perspectives often add to our understanding of etiological factors in this syndrome, the habit of renaming the headache merely adds to our uncertainty.

The minimally illuminating phrase "psychogenic headache" is also heard in hallway consultations. Does it mean tension headache with important psychological contributions? A true conversion headache? Or is it to be understood as some additional headache category? Only the person using the term knows for certain.

It is the authors' position that there is a distinct chronic tension headache syndrome, which can be defined as follows: the painful, final stage of a chain of events involving prolonged spasm of the cervical and/or cephalic musculature, centrally mediated hyper-attentiveness to pain, and probable intramuscular vascular restriction. It can be initiated by a variety of somatic or psychological triggers in an individual who habitually reacts to tension with his muscles, and who is largely out of touch with his somatic sensations. When an emotional problem triggers tension headaches, the patient is usually only partially aware of its source.

CLINICAL FINDINGS

DEMOGRAPHICS AND PREVALENCE

Most people have had at least one acute tension headache in their life, perhaps following a drive through foul weather and piled-up traffic, or after a tense day on the planning committee. Its prevalence tells us that the mechanism of tension headache is not exotic. Problem tension headaches are about as common as problem migraines. Like migraines, they are significantly more frequent in women, especially married housewives or semiskilled workers (5). Fifteen percent of tension headache patients started having symptoms before age 10 (1). The syndrome is most common in the 3rd and 4th decades (3) but may be lifelong.

SIGNS

There are a few signs, and none is pathognomonic. They basically consist of evidence of excessive contraction of the voluntary musculature accompanied by a diminished awareness of that contraction. Shoulders may be hiked up and, when asked to relax them, the patient at first looks surprised, then lowers them, but only halfway. The forehead often betrays a scowl, and wrinkles may seem like permanent features. The neck may be hyperextended and limited in spontaneous motion. The patient may sit on the edge of the chair, or think he is relaxed when in fact his toe remains pointed at the ceiling from tension. If the examiner tries to move the patient's jaw freely with his hand it often seems to fight back, almost involuntarily. Diffuse tenderness of the scalp and, in particular, wincing tenderness of nodules known as trigger points, may be observed. The trapezius and paraspinal muscles of the neck are often contracted, tender, and sore, although it may not be easy to reliably assess the spasm by palpation alone. The teeth are occasionally worn down by constant nighttime grinding, colorfully described as "fang sharpening" (1).

SYMPTOMS

The pain is steady and nonpulsatile, and has been described as dull, heavy, drawing, tight, or pressing in nature. Its intensity and even its location may vary slowly over time. Common locations are the brow, occiput, and neck, although it may, especially when advanced, be all over. It rarely awakens the patient, emphasizing the importance of centrally modified perception in this disorder. In sharp contrast to migraine, it is occasionally made better by alcohol or amyl nitrite, and made worse by ergotamine. Head pain typically begins or is exacerbated at a time of overt stress (or during its anticipation), rather than afterward as occurs in migraine. When mild, stiffness and aching may be reduced by a gentle rolling movement, but when acute, the head may be cradled in the hands like a fragile egg, as unsupported movement brings too much pain to be attempted. In contrast to migraine, the patient may report that the pain has continued nonstop for weeks, months, or years.

In published accounts of tension headache, many psychological symptoms have been reported. They are usually recounted along with the description of the pain. This makes it harder to determine which invariably accompany tension headache and which rather accompany a psychological disorder that can cause tension headache.

Psychological symptoms obtained from self-descriptions by tension headache patients portray them as often irritable, tense, depressed, prone to episodes of weeping, overconcerned about the opinions of others (6), easily embarrassed, worried, unduly fearful of making mistakes, overly conscientious, ambitious, restless, afraid of going insane, moody, dependent, prone to self-doubt and feelings of inadequacy (7), perfectionistic (8) and, occasionally, compulsive. A panicky anxiety is sometimes seen, especially during exacerbation, and the patient may show signs of significant regression. Many of these symptoms are explained most economically by the concepts of chronic anxiety and masked depression.

The specific life experiences and predominant emotions generated by each patient's psychopathology do, however, clearly affect the clinical picture. Where the psychodynamics reflect an unconscious biting anger that harkens back to the oral stage of development, muscles of mastication, such as the temporalis, may become preferentially involved. When depressive elements are more prominent, the clinical picture may be that of frontal pain. One patient could not free herself from ruminating about her mother's constant warning, "I'm going to break your neck!"—and naturally her neck, invariably protected by a neck collar, was the site of her pain.

TESTING

Minnesota Multiphasic Personality Inventory (MMPI) studies of tension headache have repeatedly shown elevated depression, hysteria, and hypochondriasis scales (9). Kudrow and Sutkus (10) found this elevation greater than in migraine, yet less than in conversion headache. A study by the authors (11) questions the validity of the MMPI for understanding psychological aspects of headache, however, and found the test's emphasis on diagnosis caused it to miss the more subtle psychological problems typically aggravating headache.

Many reports have found elevated levels of resting electromyographic potential from recording leads placed over the cephalic region (9). One may not always get such a reading, however, and some workers have questioned the replicability of this finding. At least one study (12) points out the need for stringent diagnostic criteria in experiments that would contest this long-established doctrine. It is also important to remember that, like a charley horse elsewhere in the body, an overcontracted, fatigued, head or neck muscle may ache long after the contraction has ended (13), a fact which may partially account for these seemingly contradictory findings.

ADDITIONAL FINDINGS

Numerous studies, such as that by Friedman and his colleagues (14), are cited in the text. A few representative additional ones include the following.

Dalessio (15) finds that the great majority of such patients are depressed, and considers their pain a symptomatic manifestation of that depression. He notes an atypical symptom of depression frequently seen in these patients: polysurgery.

Martin (8) evaluated 50 patients with tension headache, and found that 20 of them met the criteria for psychoneurotic depression (frequently the result of a prolonged grief reaction). In addition, 41 showed grossly evident tension, and the remainder handled emotional conflicts by using denial. They usually welcomed the opportunity to discuss possible sources of their tension, and were typically aware that it was relevant to the headaches. He documented the following as common problems: difficulty leaving home, passive submission to a domineering spouse, broken marriages, impotence, frigidity, poor work records, and specific emotional problems. He concluded that symptoms centered around three themes: dependency, sexuality, and control of anger. In his view the perfectionism, rigidity, and hypochondriasis represent the patient's unsuccessful attempts to gain control over his intolerable feelings.

Howarth (16) evaluated 72 tension headache patients referred to a neurological clinic, and appraised the effects of supportive psychotherapy on 67 of them approximately one year after it had concluded. The initial visit was an hour or less, and subsequent sessions were shorter. In the interviews he encouraged patients to discuss ways to minimize present problems and prevent similar future ones. Sixty-eight percent of these patients had anxious and obsessional traits and were diagnosed as "insecure personalities." The 21% whose headaches coincided with a significant environmental stress had a much better prognosis than did those in whom personality disorder predominated. Howarth saw less evidence than other authors for the central role of anger in the etiology of tension headaches.

PATHOGENESIS

Both psychological and somatic factors can either predispose to, or trigger, tension headaches. We will consider each combination in turn. It is important to keep in mind that these factors only result in headache if and when they elicit the necessary physiological reaction: sustained contraction of head and neck muscles over time, accompanied by a lowered pain threshold and intramuscular vascular restriction.

The pathogenesis starts with a problem, the burr under the saddle. Although physical triggers and commonplace stresses may play this role, the trigger is usually some psychosocial aggravant which derives its importance from factors in the patient's unconscious. (These three are not, of course, mutually exclusive.) Heightened emotional tension evokes and sustains physical preparation for fight-or-flight. Since both fight and flight involve action, the body automatically prepares for this by tensing its muscles.

Friedman (5) points out another important fact: scalp muscles react to stress as skin does. Since scalp muscles are less essential than others in war or panic, their blood supply is rerouted to muscles actually used for fighting. This deprives the scalp muscles of nutrients. Yet, most modern stressors are social, and require the person to use those very same scalp muscles for smiling, talking expressively, etc., during periods of tension. If at such times he is also experiencing veiled fear or anger, it will cause him to tense up, and his blood supply will be diverted to his "fighting muscles" in preparation for releasing anger or defending himself against the anger of others. Unfortunately for his headache, the day at the office slips into the night at the cocktail party without denouement. And the fight-or-flight preparations—undischarged—remain.

But because no one wants to go around feeling as though he is constantly *en garde,* psychological defenses automatically come into play to keep the patient from recognizing the nature and intensity of his emotions. These defenses make him partially unaware of his state of physiological preparedness— such as muscle tension—and of its implications.

This capacity of the mind to remove motor behavior from awareness is vividly seen in demonstrations of arm levitation during hypnosis. Following a suggestion to that effect, a person in a hypnotic trance can hold his arm out from his body in a position that would normally soon cause discomfort—but the subject is not only oblivious to discomfort, he may even be unaware that he has raised his arm. It is perhaps in a similar manner that the tension headache patient loses awareness of the extent to which muscles are tightened, and instead only recognizes, in time, the consequences of that contraction: pain.

Whether the tension headache actually begins with spasm of scalp and neck muscles, or with constriction of arteries supplying those muscles, or with both simultaneously, is unclear. In any event, it is hypothesized that the vasoconstriction leads to both muscle ischemia and a buildup of metabolic waste. Because muscles in spasm do not perfuse as well, the spasm accentuates the effects of vasoconstriction. The vasoconstriction, in turn, seems to make the spastic muscles more sensitive to pain (17). At this point in pathogenesis, the pain often generalizes to the entire region, and even if the patient can stop contracting his muscles, he will not immediately become pain-free. The constant pain and spasm chase one another like a dog and his tail. The headache now has a life of its own, independent of the factors that initiated it.

An additional factor suggested as having a role in perpetuating this cycle is interference by the spasm with intermittent, alternating movements of neck and face muscles, that is, with the head's normal rhythm of nodding and bobbing. Because this rigidity further impedes vascular flow, it disallows the muscles time for recuperation, and interferes with replenishment of blood-borne nutrients (17).

SOMATIC PREDISPOSITIONS

Patients who tend to react to both intrapsychic and environmental sources of stress somatically and, in particular those who characteristically react with their musculature, are at greater risk. This is also true of patients with poorly exercised muscles or stooped postures, in the first case because the muscles cannot take as much strain, and in the second because more strain is placed on them. It is also not clear whether some people have a genetic tendency to vasoconstrict their external cranial circulation during stress. If genetics do play this role, it has not impressed researchers with as forcefully as have genetic contributions to migraine.

Certain unique attributes of cranial muscles make them particularly vulnerable to being targeted by emotional tension. Many of these muscles have a limited excursion, and the aches that prolonged isometric use can inflict upon a muscle are like those the assistant holding a retractor experiences during a long operation. Also, throughout the higher species, these muscles are used for displays of challenge, aggression, threat, and submission, as described by Darwin (18) and by ethologists such as Lorenz (19). One can imagine, for example, the menacing expression of the alerted guard dog or, more to the point, the grimace of distress that comes over the face of an angry, wailing, infant. In short, the muscles of the head and face are primary effector organs for emotional communication, and it is not surprising that they suffer when the emotions to be expressed are unremitting, brutal, or desperate.

SOMATIC TRIGGERS

As discussed earlier, pain in the head from any source can stimulate a reactive spasm in muscles serving that region. Because of this, some have suggested that muscle contraction in tension headache may be the result, rather than the cause, of pain. Because prolonged muscle tension in many areas of the body leads to an aching pain that ebbs when muscles relax, this theory seems unlikely. Nevertheless, local pathology (or even an extrinsic irritant, such as tight eyeglasses) can be the stimulus that initiates a cycle of true tension headache in a predisposed individual. Some commonplace triggers of this nature are: certical spondylosis, neck trauma, latent strabismus, improper bite, cracked or infected teeth, infected sinuses, and a series of mechanically disadvantageous positions in which people habitually hold their necks (the Sistine Chapel syndrome.) Certain occupations are particularly hazardous: these include draftsman, computer operator, and microbiologist.

Still, psychiatric difficulties are so prevalent in the chronic form of this disorder that even when a somatic trigger is found, one will occasionally still find a concomitant emotional disturbance. The elderly gentleman with cervical arthritis may also be depressed. His headaches may clear up when the depression is treated, even though his arthritis remains.

PSYCHOLOGICAL PREDISPOSITIONS

The preeminent relevance of psychodynamic factors to tension headaches is recognized by most researchers. Although it could be argued that by excluding muscular headaches they changed the odds, Friedman and his coworkers (14) found that of the several thousand tension headache patients interviewed, 72% acknowledged being anxious, and the primary treating physicians considered all of them to have important, and generally longstanding, psychopathology. They point out that the frequency with which the tension headache patient is aware of emotional distress and connects it, to some extent, with his headaches, contrasts sharply with the typical story from the patient with conversion head-

aches. Equally important is their observation that, although most tension headache patients were aware of the presence of emotional distress, "in the majority of our cases the fundamental psychological factors were largely unconscious."

They assert: "The most frequently observed conflicts . . . were those over hostile impulses" (3). Much of that hostility was directed against family members or their substitutes. Guilt about aggression was also prominent. Finally, tension headache patients often had conflicts about identity, and struggled with unconscious wishes to remain dependent.

Childhood History

The tension headache patient often describes a rigid family background in which he was the recipient of insistent nagging, belittlement, or overt or covert cruelty from his caretakers (8). His attempts to be assertive as a child were often squelched. As a result of this background, when interpersonal difficulties arise in adulthood he is prone to excessive anger and fear, and may encounter marked difficulty when dealing with frustrating, competitive, or potentially hostile encounters with people. Indeed, prolonged exposure to such encounters frequently results in headache.

It has been reported (8) that most tension headache patients had been closely associated with someone with a head or neck injury, usually a parent or sibling. There may be partial identification with this person by means of the symptom.

Anger

We have observed that the most problematic emotion for the tension headache patient is usually anger that he attempts to stifle. It is often a primitive anger, and it is often countered by primitive attempts at suppression. Epigenetically, it may best correspond to the type of anger experienced during oral phases of development. Other emotions are also strong; a situation that incites someone to chronic anger generally gives him reason to feel anxious and depressed as well. In addition, people who go around angry often fear the consequences of that anger getting out of hand, both in terms of what might happen to others and in terms of the retaliation it might provoke. Anger that, for whatever reason, cannot be effectively acted upon yet cannot be forgotten, in time leads to feelings of powerlessness and depression. If one had to accord primacy to a single emotion in tension headache though, it would be anger.

In some cases it is possible to view chronic tension headache as a simultaneous expression of aggressive impulses and the defenses against them. While the scowl automatically expresses aggression—recall, for a moment, the image from Shakespeare—the patient simultaneously braces the muscles to disguise that aggression even, to a degree, from himself. Out of fear and out of civilization, adult *homo sapiens* struggles against those automatic expressions of anger that the house pet uses to show his displeasure: snarling, bristling, and hunching its shoulders. When the picture involves such attempts to muzzle anger, the patient's features often look strained, or his face seems frozen into a mask of tension.

We have observed that the tension headache patient tends to regress to an earlier developmental level when threatened. His emotions generally seem to be more raw and unrefined than those of the migraineur. He frequently appears to be hanging on to his emotional equilibrium in spite of a bunched-up rage which he is trying—unsuccessfully as a result of the headaches—to just go on about his business and ignore. He often wishes to impose his will on relationships, but lacking the diplomacy frequently seen in the migraineur, is more likely instead to engage in passive-aggressive and dependent behaviors to force others to come around to his way of having things. In the long run this is not satisfying and usually not even successful.

Aggression in the Family

If aggressive impulses build to intolerable levels, the need to discharge anger may blind the patient to the point of striking out at the nearest target. The most frequent objects of this anger are family members. This may take many forms.

The patient may have unsuspectingly recreated in his home life the same problems he thought he left behind in his family of origin. At one level this is motivated by the hope of finally overcoming them, but more often than not he finds he cannot transcend these problems with his family of marriage either.

Alternatively, transference distortions may cause him to misperceive a realistically different current situation and see it as though it were a replay of an upsetting past relationship. The metaphor does not really apply, yet he cannot help reacting as though it did. These distortions may be active when a patient ends up feeling bullied or cowed by his family. If the patient has unconscious vengeful impulses for hurtful events from his past, these can also partake in the family drama.

Despite popular opinion, minor suburban chores such as negotiating with the architect or getting the kids to the orthodontist do not, of themselves, cause chronic tension headache. Feelings about what they represent, might.

Anxiety

Anxiety is so prominent in tension headache patients that some investigators (8, 20) consider the disorder primarily an epiphenomenon of anxiety. Nevertheless, even if one accepts that the muscles are tense because the patient is anxious, the question "Why is he anxious?" follows. Often it appears to be because he sees the world as a place where he can rarely feel secure enough that someone will not attempt to compete with, bully, or belittle him, if not physically, then emotionally. The fact that he, too, is sometimes filled with bitter or brooding anger only reinforces the impression that survival of the fittest is the golden rule of human relationships.

Dependency

The universal need to occasionally feel relaxed and looked after in the presence of others must fight an uphill battle if people are seen as potentially demanding, cruel, or hurtful. Emotional struggles of the type the migraineur seems to have overtly accepted or at least compromised on long ago are still in tumultuous engagement within the tension headache patient. The contingencies of his childhood environment prevented many such a patient from forming an identity comforting and stable enough for him to feel secure. His difficulty maintaining a firm sense of identity inevitably sabotages his confidence and self-esteem. As a result, he is more liable to feel disenfranchised from people and in search of safe haven for as long as it lasts, that is, until the expected outbreak of aggression or rejection disrupts it. Such a patient may wish to be noticed and seen as hurting, but be fearful that if he calls attention to himself it might only provoke annoyance or anger. His attachments formed in adulthood are often seen to involve a hostile dependency in which dependent strivings are entwined with aggressive dynamics. These transference aspects of his relationships can cause him to both hate and fear the very people he loves.

PSYCHOLOGICAL TRIGGERS

The concept that a certain orientation towards people and events can predispose to tension headache needs to be integrated with the more familiar concept that a stressful life event or interpersonal situation can initiate a tension headache. Such an integration can come from recognizing that it is the individualized perception of and reaction to an external event—largely determined by one's prior orientation—that usually determines whether it will prove stressful for a given patient and in

what way. "An assessment of the problem of stress is inevitably bound up to some degree with an estimate of personality" (16).

The frequency with which emotional situations precipitate tension headaches is high (16). Emotions or situations especially liable to aggravate conflicts that trigger the physiology of tension headache include frustration, anger, competition, loss of a loved one, blows to the self-esteem, a sense of being inadequate to the task at hand, threat of injury, and threat of loss of control. These start the ball rolling.

Some life events are upsetting enough to produce a tension headache even in people without a predisposition to this disorder. Frazier (21) believes that severe situations can cause tension headache in patients who are otherwise emotionally healthy.

In general, however, the magnitude of a stressor, its power, duration, and specificity required to trigger a tension headache, decreases proportionately the more the patient resembles the tension headache-prone individual. In some people these traits are so pervasive that any number of external precipitants can flip the headache switch. For others, personality factors are so minimal that only extraordinary events or trauma can have this effect.

Nevertheless, even the patient in whom predisposing characteristics are strong usually develops a headache in response to a specific situation, and the more that external pressures have contributed to the onset of tension headaches, the better the prognosis. Prognosis is worse when headaches seem to be a reflection of chronic bitterness or a malignant attitude towards life. Yet, even in the latter case, removal of the stressful situation was invariably found to reduce pain (16).

COMBINED HEADACHES, CONTRASTED DYNAMICS

Psychological similarities are often noted between patients prone to tension and those prone to migraine headaches. Because these two types account for over 90% of the headaches seen in clinical practice, their differentiation is a frequent diagnostic dilemma for the headache practitioner. The exercise of trying to contrast psychological factors accompanying migraine with those accompanying tension headache patients will sharpen the reader's appreciation of psychodynamic elements often seen in each disorder. Although knowledge in this area is still partial, questions about this distinction are asked frequently enough to warrant consideration, however tentative the conclusions or subject to later modification.

If the physician develops sufficient feel for them, psychodynamic attributes can be entered into the diagnostic equation, a suggestion first tendered by Alvarez (22). Many seasoned headache specialists find that certain patients display psychological characteristics which, while not in and of themselves pathognomonic, feel right for migraine, while others strike the examiner as more compatible with tension headache or with cluster. Although based on clinical observation, this application currently best fits into the art of medicine, and supplements more basic means of arriving at a diagnosis.[1]

For the sake of clarity, this discussion may at times appear overly simplified or inclusive. It should be kept in mind that this is a description of patients with problematic and treatment-resistant headaches in whom the psychological contributions are strong.

Certain differences between migraine and tension headache attacks are quite apparent. For example, more tension than migraine headaches have a psychological trigger

---

[1] One day medicine may understand the relevant details well enough to construct a formal psychological profile and structured interview test based on them similar to the one developed by Friedman and Rosenmann (23) for assessing the type A (or coronary-prone) individual. Questions in such a test are specific to behavioral observations in the disorder, and in that way differ from more general psychometric tests, which are as limited in testing for susceptibility to migraine as they are for predicting patients who will one day develop coronary disease.

(5). Also, once a migraine has settled in, it is more likely to end only after having run its course. This goes with the observation that while 55% of tension headache patients responded to a placebo, only 25% of migraine patients did (3), although we stress that this is not to recommend placebos.

The patients themselves also differ on superficial analysis: while even during an attack a migraineur's behavior is often "considerate of others, controlled, and outwardly calm," the acutely symptomatic tension headache patient is more likely to display "transient depression and dejection, withdrawn social behavior, irritability and irascibility, a sulking unwillingness to assume responsibilities, and poor judgment with open expression of impulsivity, hostility, and destructiveness" (7).

Psychologically influenced patients with both types of headache have a developmental history in which they were often exposed to situations that accentuated normal childhood conflicts. From these histories it appears that the future tension headache patient often tries to manage the resulting tension through psychological and physical regression to earlier modes of functioning, while the future migraineur often tries to handle it through a precocious pseudoprogression in the direction of adulthood and responsibility. To help him accomplish this, the young migraineur often identifies strongly with his parent or early caretaker. His tension headache counterpart's reactions are liable to lead in the opposite direction, that of greater self-involvement and isolation.

Therapy with many migraine patients reveals that their motivational emphasis is on reducing anxiety about possible disenfranchisement from others, especially from parenting figures. As a child, the migraine patient often attempted to shield himself from that possibility by developing attitudes designed to please others and to deflect or reduce their potential resentment. Efforts to revise his wishes to make them compatible with the parents usually led to a strong identification with that parent. While the identification reduced the risk of loneliness, painful feelings and resentment at being caught in this situation may have had to be repressed and may not have been sufficiently dealt with. If a similar relationship later in life reactivates these feelings, they may press for release from the unconscious. It is often when this release is denied them that psychologically influenced migraine headaches are triggered or exacerbated.

The patient with tension headaches is frequently caught up in trying to cope with more consciously accessible anger, anxiety, and resentment about some currently aggravating situation. He may hide these feelings from others, but typically has been unwilling to fully relinquish his anger and is unable to fully shake his own awareness of it. (A subgroup does, however, totally deny emotional problems.) As a result, he must direct more of his conscious mental energies towards its containment. Anxiety often comes from fantasies of verbal bullying or physical aggression or from fear that his own anger will erupt into action.

A tension headache patient in whom these dynamics are operative responds to the stress by retreating to an earlier level of psychological functioning (perhaps to the oral-aggressive stage), and his physiology manifests the counterparts of that regressed state.

In contrast, the patient whose dynamics are liable to ignite the genetics of migraine learned at an early age that, with effort, he could mold himself in the direction his caretakers (or their substitutes later on) wished, and that that type of sacrifice was more compatible with his character style. Yet it is generally accepted in psychiatry that when someone makes such wholesale accommodations he still, at some level, feels his acceptability is contingent. Of particular importance is this: by late childhood such a patient often finds he is truly acceptable, even to himself, only if he does things flawlessly. As a result he may not know how to stop cleaning house or volunteering for committees. Only the pressure to keep volunteering may be conscious, however.

The tension headache patient is more likely to report having been motivated as a child by the wish to avoid punishment. Sometimes he will recall obedience being fostered through threats or spankings. Sometimes the punishment depended as much upon the parent's momentary mood as it did upon the child's behavior. The story commonly reported by the migraineur is that, although he might have contended with both a certain type of distance from his caretakers combined with firm behavioral expectations by them, he could earn a stable—even a moderately comfortable—reprieve through conformity.

Thus, although the tension headache patient typically continues to feel the smart of injustice and to wrestle with the resentment of authority it engenders in him, the psychologically destabilized migraine patient more typically faces his problems by repressing any resentment, by trying to mature too rapidly, and by prematurely identifying with the dominant parent so as to become that authority. In the process, the migraineur may lose much of the carefree and naive spontaneity that most adults remember as one of the bonuses of childhood, its place taken by a constricted, precocious mastery of duties and attitudes appropriate to a later age. He frequently recruits the psychological defenses of repression, reaction formation, identification with the aggressor, sublimation, and pseudo-progression to achieve these ends. The tension headache patient, on the other hand, often prefers to engage such defenses as suppression, regression, and the resort to action.

To assist his defenses, the migraine-prone child often incorporates a superego that resembles the expectations of the parent, scorns his more childlike impulses and feelings, and gives definite but minimal credit for hard work. The tension headache patient is more likely to develop a rougher, more action-prone superego that closely approximates his frequently reported view of authority: it threatens and belittles him, invokes guilt, and warns of retribution.

Some patients prone to tension headache anticipate a potential for humiliation in close relationships. Where this is the case, they often feel the safest route to a relationship will involve disguising resentment and then manipulating, or behaving passive-aggressively, to pressure others to come around to their way of having things. This modus operandi may also be the product of identification with insensitive or hurtful parents. In short, it may be the only way they know, and if it does not work, they feel helpless and alienated.

Because problems in past relationships are often relived in present ones, one explanation of anxiety and depression in tension headache patients may be their frequent proneness to feelings of futility stemming from a conviction that there is no behavior they can predictably count on to retain affection or to parry distressful exchanges.

This is in sharp contrast to the paradigmatic migraineur, who initially reacts to similar interpersonal threats with energetic attempts to do the things that will gain others approbation, even if at times these actions are based more on what the patient thinks is right than on empathy. While the migraineur frequently capitulates to behavioral expectations of the outside world (as interpreted by his superego) to maximize rapprochment with it, the tension headache patient tends to capitulate to his own intense feelings. Sometimes, when the tension headache patient appears submissive, it is found to be because he feels defeated by other people's perceived power and latent aggression; underneath, he often expresses the wish to escape, or even to turn the tables.

Each of these views of human interaction leads to a different cognitive/emotional state, which in turn puts pressure on a different segment of the physiology. Different symptoms, tension versus migraine headache, arise from the specific pathogenic potentials of these physiologies. Patients with tension headache are more likely to see the world in terms of action, and to unconsciously tense their muscles to prepare for it. Patients with migraine are more likely to prepare themselves to think things through.

Since the combined migraine/tension headache is a well-known syndrome, these disorders cannot be psychologically incompatible. There are at least two ways to explain this coexistence. Both stem from the observation that combined headaches almost invariably start with migraine, onto which the tension headache component is slowly grafted.

1. A patient predisposed to migraine can also develop an acute, situationally triggered regression, along with the feelings, behavior, and physiology that accompany that regression. This is especially likely following a long period in which his migraine coping style has proven unsuccessful. The regression-related feelings predispose to the addition of a tension headache.

2. Because head pain from any source, including from frequent migraines, can cause a reactive, spreading spasm in the cranial musculature, frequent migraine may act as a physical trigger of the tension headache component. Overly frequent use of analgesics to treat the migraines may exacerbate this progression.

To repeat: these are summations and condensations based upon the detailed reporting of many headache patients. They will not capture the spirit or essence of every patient with psychological problems affecting these diagnoses, and even the question of whether the process itself—summation and condensation—is a valid undertaking remains an open one for the authors. Hopefully, time and utility will someday answer it.

TREATMENT

Tension headaches can be treated with medication, psychotherapy, self-regulatory therapies, and physical therapy. These treatments compliment one another and can be used together, with the particular mix determined by the needs of the individual (24). Indeed, for the patient unable for years to break free of constant headache, a combined push is mandatory to break through the layers of hopelessness, habit, and pessimism that encumber his motivation.

MEDICATIONS

Antidepressant medications are currently drugs of choice (for specifics, see Chapters 13 and 24). Although anxiety is an important contributor to tension headache, many patients can be effectively treated with nonsedating antidepressants such as imipramine. Sjaastad (2) has described a type of headache with many similarities to tension headache, but which is specifically responsive to doxepin.

Ataraxic drugs, especially those with a muscle relaxant capacity, can help the patient through relapses associated with life crisis. Though useful while the patient is learning to relax or to solve his problems by other means, they are rarely indicated for therapy *ad infinitum.*

Narcotics are often necessary during acute exacerbations of tension headache. The patient in acute pain should be given an analgesic strong enough to provide relief. In light of the background from which many of them come, these patients may interpret the withholding of analgesics on moralistic or other grounds, even rational ones, as a sign of cruelty. For the same reason, if one must halt long-term analgesic use, major or minor, because it is blocking a remission, extra effort may be required to convince the patient that this difficult step is not taken in disregard for his comfort—that, on the contrary, it should help him eventually have less pain. In this way one anticipates and tries to avoid specific transference problems in the doctor-patient relationship.

SELF-REGULATORY TECHNIQUES

Both electromyographic feedback and generalized relaxation techniques, such as autogenic training or progressive relaxation, are frequently used to good effect with the tension headache patient. These are covered in Chapter 32.

PHYSICAL THERAPY

A variety of physical therapy techniques can help tension headache patients, including hot hydrocollator packs, massage, strengthening exercises for the neck, and ultrasound for the neck and shoulders. Patients who find local application of hydrocollator packs helpful should purchase some for home use. Physical therapy works best if it is done by a sympathetic and knowledgeable physical therapist with whom the physician remains in communication.

PSYCHOTHERAPY

This is discussed in Chapters 28–31.

CONCLUSION

It is important to remember that the tension headache patient often arrives at the doctor's office both disabled and discouraged. His life is often in crisis or chronic diarrary, and the words "tension headache" are only the headline to that story. One is usually pleasantly surprised that it is the rare patient who does not want to get well, and the still rarer one who cannot surprise the physician with initially unrecognized strengths which he can rally to use in his own recovery.

REFERENCES

1. Lance JW: *Mechanism and Management of Headache,* ed 3. London, Butterworths, 1978.
2. Sjaastad O: So called tension headache: a term in need of revision. *Curr Med Res Opin* 6 (Suppl 9):41, 1980.
3. Friedman A, de Sola Pool N, Von Storch T: Tension headache. *JAMA:*151, 1953.

4. Diamond S: Depressive headaches. *Headache* 4:255–259, 1964.

5. Friedman AP: Characteristics of tension headache: a profile of 1,420 cases. *Psychosomatics* 20(7):451–461, 1979.

6. Frazier SH: Complex problems of pain as seen in headache, painful phantom and other states. In Arieti S, Reiser MF (eds): *American Handbook of Psychiatry, ed 2.* New York, Basic Books, 1975, pp 838–851.

7. Kolb LC: Psychiatric and psychogenic factors in headache. In Friedman AP, Merritt HH (eds): *Headache, Diagnosis and Treatment.* Philadelphia, F.A. Davis, 1959, pp 259–298.

8. Martin MJ: Tension headache: a psychiatric study. *Headache* 6:48–55, 1966.

9. Budzynski T, Stoyva J, Adler CS, Mullaney D: EMG feedback applied to tension headache: a controlled outcome study. *Psychosom Med* 25(6):484–496, 1973.

10. Kudrow L, Sutkus BJ: MMPI pattern specificity in primary headache disorders. *Headache* 19:18–24, 1979.

11. Adler CS, Adler SM: Pitfalls in the interpretation of psychometric testing of headache patients. *Cephalalgia* 5 (Suppl 3):224–225, 1985.

12. Haber JD, Kuczmierczyk AR, Adams HE: Tension headaches: muscle overactivity or psychogenic pain. *Headache* 25:23–29, 1985.

13. Speed WG: Muscle contraction headaches. In Saper JR (ed): *Headache Disorders.* Boston, John Wright-PSG, Inc., 1983, p 115.

14. Friedman A, Von Storch TJC, Merritt HH: Migraine and tension headache: a clinical study of two thousand cases. *Neurology* (NY) 4:773–787, 1954.

15. Dalessio DJ: Some reflections on the etiologic role of depression in head pain. *Headache* 8:28–31, 1968.

16. Howarth E: Personality and stress. *Br J Psychiatry* 3:1193–1197, 1965.

17. Robinson CA: Cervical spondylosis and muscle contraction headache. In Dalessio D (ed): *Wolff's Headache and Other Head Pain, ed 4.* New York, Oxford Press, 1980, pp 362–380.

18. Darwin C: *Expression of the Emotions in Man and Animals.* New York, D. Appleton, 1873.

19. Lorenz K: *King Solomon's Ring.* New York, Thomas Y. Crowell, 1952.

20. Kolb LC: Psychiatric aspects of the treatment of headache. *Neurology* 13:34–37, 1963.

21. Frazier SH: The psychotherapeutic approach to patients with headache. *Mod Treatment* 1:1412–1424, 1964.

22. Alvarez WC: The migrainous personality and constitution; the essential features of the disease: a study of 500 cases. *Am J Med Sci* 213(1):1–8, 1947.

23. Friedman M, Rosenmann RH: *Type A Behavior and Your Heart.* New York, Alfred A. Knopf, 1974.

24. Adler CS, Adler SM: Psychiatric treatment of the headache patient. *Panminerva Med* 24:167–172, 1982.

Chronic Headaches and the Dysthymic Pain Disorder: Profile and Treatment of a Variant of Depressive Disease

CHAPTER THIRTEEN

DIETRICH BLUMER, M.D.
MARY HEILBRONN, Ph.D.

Since the early papers of Diamond (1) and Lance and Curran (2) in 1964, the significance of depressive traits in chronic headache sufferers has been generally well accepted, and antidepressant drugs have been widely used for their treatment. The role of a depressive disorder has been particularly associated with the so-called tension or muscle contraction headaches (3).

In 1960 Paoli and colleagues (4) first reported the effectiveness of an antidepressant (imipramine) in the treatment of various pain conditions. Although many isolated reports followed over the years, all attesting to the success of this type of therapy, antidepressants until recently were not systematically used in the treatment of the many poorly defined, nonspecific or atypical pain syndromes (5) of unclear etiology, such as low back pain (6). Surgical "rescue attempts" persisted for a long time as a primary treatment approach. With the advent of behavioral treatment for

chronic pain (7), it became more recognized that chronic pain tends to persist if it is treated as due to a local lesion, or treated according to the model of acute pain (8). The goal of behavioral treatment for chronic pain is to deemphasize the pain complaint while reactivating the patients and guiding them to a better life in spite of their pain. Behavioral treatment for chronic pain is generally carried out on specialized inpatient units. Treatment of chronic pain with antidepressant drugs, on the other hand, can be carried out on an outpatient basis and can result, if carried out systematically, in freedom from pain in a substantial portion of the patients (9–11).

We have identified chronic atypical or "nonspecific" pain as a depressive disorder with characteristic clinical, premorbid, psychodynamic, genetic, and other biologic features. While certain traits of classic melancholia tend to be absent (notably the episodicity and the psychotic features), the relationship to the spectrum of depressive disorders can be well demonstrated. With George Engel (12), in earlier work, we have termed this variant of depressive disease the Pain-Prone Disorder (13), in lieu of somewhat stigmatizing terms such as psychogenic pain (DSM-III) or pain-neurosis (14), and in preference over less specific terms such as chronic pain syndrome (15), chronic benign pain (16), or abnormal illness behavior (17). More recently we (18) proposed the term dysthymic pain disorder as a substitute for the term pain-prone disorder to convey our concept of the disorder as a variant of depressive disease.

The dysthymic pain disorder manifests itself with pain of highly variable location. Patients with dysthymic pain disorder who complain of chronic headache have not, in our experience, proven to be different from patients with pain located elsewhere (19). Invariably, and by definition, the pain is not caused by a specific somatic disorder, although it may be preceded by or associated with such a disorder. Low back pain, for example, is frequently triggered by a banal injury, and chronic headache is frequently associated with muscle contraction.

Identification of the dysthymic pain disorder allows for a positive diagnosis, rather than a diagnosis by exclusion, and would thus allow for prompt recognition and early appropriate treatment. Furthermore, knowledge of the dysthymic pain disorder as a variant of depressive disease provides a rational basis for the hitherto largely empirical use of antidepressants for chronic pain syndromes and for the psychological management of these patients.

THE DYSTHYMIC PAIN DISORDER

Our view of chronic pain as a relatively homogeneous disorder, termed the dysthymic pain disorder with its characteristic clinical, biographic, biologic, and psychodynamic features, is based on the evaluation of over 2000 patients with chronic pain carried out over the past 20 years. An increasingly comprehensive standardized evaluation protocol was developed for these patients (20) Since 1978, at the Henry Ford Hospital, we have carried out treatment for chronic pain with antidepressants on an outpatient basis. Our pain clinic would accept for evaluation and treatment any patient with the chief complaint of persistent pain in the absence of related somatic findings, regardless of motivation for treatment, involvement with litigation, dependence on drugs, or presence of overt psychiatric disturbance.

The clinical features of the dysthymic pain disorder are listed in Table 13.1. The patients present with chronic pain of obscure origin, which in the great majority is continuous in nature. In spite of repeated negative examinations, they display a pronounced pre-

TABLE 13.1
CLINICAL FEATURES OF THE DYSTHYMIC PAIN DISORDER

Somatic complaint
  Continuous pain of obscure origin
  Somatic preoccupation
  Desire for surgery
"Solid Citizen"
  Denial of conflicts
  Idealization of self and of family relations
  Ergomania (prepain): "Workaholism," relentless activity
Depression
  Anergia (postpain): lack of initiative, inactivity, fatigue
  Anhedonia: inability to enjoy social life, leisure, and sex
  Insomnia
  Depressive mood and despair
History
  Family (and personal) history of depression and alcoholism
  Past abuse by spouse
  Crippled relative
  Relative with chronic pain
Syndrome
  Inability to appreciate and verbalize feelings (alexithymia)
  Relentless activity (ergomania)
    ⟶ Inactivity (depression with anergia)

occupation with the painful body part(s). The persistent desire for a surgical solution is marked in many.

Even after years of disabling pain and dependence on others, most patients maintain an image of themselves as "solid citizens." They deny difficulties in their interpersonal relationships, often describe family members in idealized terms, and often perceive themselves as highly independent types. Their dislike of any scrutiny of their personal life is very strong. They usually have a history of generally relentless activity prior to the pain onset. The original industriousness ("workaholism"), overactivity, and trend to overachieve of these patients may have been manifest since childhood and is highly characteristic. We have chosen the term *ergomania* for these premorbid traits. The excessive self-sacrifice for the benefit of the family suggests a masochistic trend as well as a marked need to please in order to be accepted.

With onset of the chronic pain, these patients lose their initiative and zeal for work. The contrast of their excessive premorbid activity with their present fatigue and helplessness is striking. This anergia becomes associated with anhedonia, an increasing inability to enjoy social life, leisure time, and sexual relations. While the appetite is usually maintained, insomnia often develops. Almost invariably, the patient attributes his depressive symptoms—the anergia, anhedonia, and the sleep disorder—to the pain. The depression is viewed as a natural consequence of the chronic pain, and this is the prime reason the depression remains *masked*. The pain itself, for which there is no somatic cause, must rather be viewed as the somatized expression of a painful affective state of concealed inner agony.

Beyond their self-sacrifice in relentless work, the patients often have a history of overt masochism, in the form of marked submissiveness and the suffering of abuse. Their proneness to choose a spouse who turns out to be alcoholic, promiscuous, brutal, or otherwise abusive had earlier brought on prolonged suffering as they tended to remain the victims of their masochistic bond. Chronic pain paradoxically begins, as a rule, when there is relief from the abuse. They tend to be intolerant of success.

The psychodynamic factors behind the anxiously maintained image of the "solid citizen" can be evidenced by sensitive psychologic tests and by the study of the few patients who lend themselves to intensive psychotherapy, or may be evident by scrutinizing the clinical findings.

Table 13.2 summarizes the psychodynamic features of the dysthymic pain disorder. The patients tend to show all the characteristics of alexithymia (21, 22). Alexithymia is the inability to recognize and verbalize one's feelings and is a common finding in psychosomatic disorders. Little emotionality is displayed, although many are close to tears, with steady efforts to remain in control. The stiff upper lip is maintained. Tragic life events may be cited in merely factual manner while all concern focuses on the body parts in pain. Underneath a detached attitude there is a different set of core issues. Strong needs to be accepted and to depend on others, as well as marked needs to receive affection and to be cared for, are present. These basic "infantile" needs have never been acknowledged by the patient, who had assumed early the precocious role of an active, independent, and caring individual. Passive-submissive and masochistic trends are in evidence, and combined with a marked eagerness to be accepted by others, manifest themselves in subservient industriousness for the sake of the family.

By relentless activity and work performance the inner insecurity and guilt had

TABLE 13.2
PSYCHODYNAMIC FEATURES OF THE DYSTHYMIC PAIN DISORDER

EGO-IDEAL (RIGIDLY MAINTAINED)	CORE NEEDS
To be independent	To depend
To be active	To be passive
To care for others	To be cared for

been soothed and a certain acceptance gained, but the dilemma sooner or later becomes too painful. After a significant loss or disappointment, with or without advent of a painful injury or ailment, pain occurs, and a drastic shift takes place. It transforms the "solid citizen" into an invalid and heightens the same painful dilemma. The needs to depend, to be passive, and to be catered to, which had not asserted themselves, are still unacceptable, and the urge to be viewed as a strong and independent individual persists. This explains the enormous need to maintain a physical problem as the culprit. Notable is the overcontrol of anger and aggression, which instead become turned against oneself (masochism).

Of extraordinary importance is the finding of alcoholism or of unipolar depression requiring psychiatric treatment and hospitalization, not only in several of the patients themselves (preceding or alternating with the chronic pain) but also frequently among their relatives (5). This suggests that the disorder belongs to Winokur's depression spectrum disease (23). Many relatives also suffered from chronic pain. We had earlier documented a high incidence of biologic markers for depression in a consecutive series of 20 patients with dysthymic pain disorder: 40% were nonsuppressors on the dexamethasone suppression test (DST), and 40% had an abnormally short REM latency (24). There was a highly significant correlation between DST cortisol levels and REM latencies. Later data suggest that the incidence of these biologic markers for major depression (melancholia) is not as high from larger populations of patients with dysthymic pain disorder (18, 25).

COMPARISON OF PATIENTS WITH TENSION HEADACHES AND CHRONIC NONCEPHALIC PAIN

In a series of comparisons, we were unable to detect any significant differences among patients with dysthymic pain disorder grouped according to body parts affected, laterality, or peripheral versus central location of their chronic pain. We compared, then, the psychobiologic profiles of patients whose pain was localized to the head with those of patients whose pain was localized to single and multiple areas elsewhere (18). Of the initial 627 consecutive chronic pain patients referred to the Henry Ford Hospital Pain Clinic after no physical cause for their pain could be substantiated, there were 32 patients who complained of headache only. A total of 53 patients sampled complained of a single pain located elsewhere, and this group served as a control group. A second control group of 53 patients with chronic pain of multiple (excluding cephalic) location was randomly selected.

All of these 138 pain patients had undergone our standardized psychiatric-psychologic evaluation for pain, and all met our diagnostic criteria for the dysthymic pain disorder. Comparison of the two control groups indicated the groups could be collapsed, averaged, and treated as a single control group.

Demographically, the headache patients did not differ significantly from the combined control group of noncephalic chronic pain with the exception that the headache patients were younger in age (37.2 versus 45.3 years). No significant differences appeared between the headache group and the control group with respect to premorbid traits, family histories, or other biographic features. Importantly, no significant differences emerged between the groups in response to antidepressant treatment. Of the patients who were cooperative in treatment, 23% of the headache and 19% of the control patients became totally pain free; 69% of the headache and 58% of the control patients showed improvement.

The headache patients differed significantly from the control patients on only three features: (a) fewer of the headache patients reported that their pain was continuous in nature (63% versus 88%); (b) a greater number of headache patients denied having any emotional problems (59% versus 30%); and (c) a significantly higher number of headache patients reported suicidal attempts or gestures (22% versus 8%). The depressive traits characteristic for the pain-prone disorder are otherwise present in almost identical fashion among the headache and other pain patients. Of interest was a trend in our data for manual laborers to develop pain in their bodies and limbs, while patients who chiefly use their head at work were more vulnerable to suffer headaches.

On the basis of these data we conclude that chronic headache generally referred to as tension or muscle contraction headache can be understood as the chief symptom of "masked depression" or, more specifically, of a variant of depressive disease which we term the dysthymic pain disorder. Accordingly, it should be viewed as a psychobiologic disorder and treated systematically with antidepressant medication.

TREATMENT

Treatment with antidepressants is aimed at the biologic basis of the disorder in an attempt to eliminate chronic pain and the other symptoms of depression. Other treatment efforts aim at pain control and are often listed under the heading of pain management.

Behavioral modification consisting of persistent deemphasis of the pain and gradual reactivation is carried out by many pain clinics, usually on an inpatient basis, and can be very effective with well-selected patients. The principles of this operant conditioning aimed at the "unlearning" of pain behavior have been well established by Fordyce (7, 8). Lake (26) reports that many patients can learn to control both autonomic and musculoskeletal responses associated with various types of pain and may control their pain through their own self-regulatory efforts. Several different types of biofeedback and relaxation techniques have proven effective in pain management, but may be most useful when combined with appropriate pharmacotherapy.

Treatment of the chronic pain patient is more effective if it is carried out with an understanding of his psychologic difficulties. It has been emphasized that the patient with

dysthymic pain typically has an enormous need to view himself as a solid and mentally sound individual who is victimized by a physical pain. In the course of fruitless pursuits to find and eliminate a physical cause of pain, the patient has become increasingly sensitive to any implication that the pain may be imaginary, at best something obscure, and at worst feigned or a sign of madness. While some patients are able to verbalize their fears ("Do you think I'm crazy?"), many choose to go untreated for fear of becoming "a psychiatric case." Their bias against anything psychiatric represents a difficult challenge to the treating psychiatrist. Indeed, we have found that our patients with dysthymic pain tend not to be suitable candidates for exploratory psychotherapy, but are best treated psychopharmacologically in a supportive yet firm manner, in the setting of a pain clinic.

The patient should be told that there is no mechanical cause for the pain, that the pain nevertheless is very real and must be chemically treated, and that so-called antidepressants are the drugs of choice. A more open-minded patient can be told that he suffers from a form of depression which has a physical expression. It can be helpful to point out to the previously overachieving patient that he tends to expect too much from himself.

Two points must be made clear to the patient at the beginning of treatment. First, while insomnia tends to improve promptly, the pain responds slowly, and much patience may be required before the most effective type and dose of medication is established. Second, the side effects may require a slower introduction or a replacement of the drug; the side effects need to be promptly reported so that proper adjustments can be carried out. The physician needs to be available by phone, reassuring and supportive. Explaining the treatment to the spouse or next-of-kin may be very helpful.

The dysthymic pain disorder is a serious and disabling disease. Antidepressant medication must be prescribed *lege artis,* as for major depression. We generally use a sedative-type antidepressant for patients with insomnia (e.g., amitriptyline or doxepin), and imipramine for those without sleep disorder, in daily increases of 25 mg, from 25 mg b.i.d. to 50 mg, t.i.d. Further increases are only prescribed if necessary, after at least 3 or 4 weeks have passed, in stepwise increments to a maximum of 300 mg daily. If particular concern over side effects is warranted, one may use the secondary amines Norpramin or nortriptyline instead of the tertiary amine tricyclics. The doses, of course, are less (by at least one-third) in patients past the age of 60, and are only cautiously increased. The very elderly may be best started with a tricyclic dose of as little as 10 mg. Preference for serotonergic antidepressants is not justified; in point of fact, we have recently been impressed with the effectiveness of the noradrenergic antidepressants desipramine and maprotiline, which tend to have less side effects.

Changes from one antidepressant drug to another are usually mandated by the presence of side effects. Antidepressants other than those cited may be just as effective. Once the maximum dose of an antidepressant is achieved and is judged ineffective after prolonged administration, we implement a combination therapy of the antidepressant, at a lesser dose, with lithium carbonate (brought to a low therapeutic level), or with small doses of a neuroleptic (we use a ratio of 30 mg of amitriptyline to 1 mg of trifluoperazine, or their equivalents, i.e., 90–100 mg of amitriptyline and 3 mg of trifluoperazine, up to 150 mg of amitriptyline and 5 mg of trifluoperazine). With the exception of lithium carbonate, which should be prescribed in two or three daily doses, all medication can be given as a once daily (h.s.) prescription. However, it helps many anxious patients if they can take some medication distributed over the day. The MAO inhibitors, phenelzine and tranylcypromine, are also effective for chronic pain.

Most effective, in our experience, is the combination of (a) antidepressant medication prescribed competently and systematically, as for a major depressive disorder; (b) a steady, supportive, and positive guidance on the part of the physician; and (c) a firm approach insisting on more activity while ignoring the pain as much as possible. The patient, however, must be repeatedly advised to pace himself and not to maintain superhuman expectations of himself. He must not relapse in his premorbid pattern of ergomania. Practical counseling about problems present at home or at work should be carried out.

Results of our systematic treatment of chronic pain with antidepressants, obtained over the past 5 years, justify a hopeful attitude. We have reported 1-year and 2-year follow-up studies of an initial group of 129 pain-prone patients treated with antidepressants (9, 10). The success of our treatment was further supported by a recent survey of the treatment response of 391 patients who complied with treatment in our Pain Clinic (11). The sample was randomly selected, and mean duration of the pain complaint was 6 years. Of these 391 patients, 37% showed very significant improvement, with 20% becoming nearly or completely pain free. Only 11% showed no improvement at all. Compliance was the major problem among our pain-prone patients. Approximately 35% of the patients referred to our Pain Clinic dropped out of treatment very early, with two or less follow-up visits. The high dropout rate may reflect those patient's distaste for a psychiatric approach, suggesting the need for primary physicians to recognize and appropriately treat patients with dysthymic pain.

Patients with chronic pain generally require prolonged use of antidepressants. The main problem tends to be the weight gain which occurs with tricyclic drugs. In general, antidepressants can gradually be phased out and finally stopped completely once the patient has achieved a meaningful and active life style.

We conclude that treatment with antidepressant drugs, enhanced if necessary by lithium or a neuroleptic, can be highly effective, regardless of chronicity or location of pain, in the cooperative patient. The psychopharmacologic antidepressant treatment, prescribed *lege artis* as for major depressive disorders, should be carried out with an understanding of the pain-prone patient and with the appropriate psychologic approach.

REFERENCES

1. Diamond S: Depressive headaches. *Headache* 4:255–259, 1964.

2. Lance JW, Curran DA: Treatment of chronic tension headache. *Lancet* 1:1236–1239, 1964.

3. Speed WG: Muscle contraction headaches. In Saper JR (ed): *Headache Disorders: Current Concepts and Treatment Strategies.* Boston, John Wright-PSG, 1983, pp 115–124.

4. Paoli F, Darcourt G, Cossa P: Preliminary note on the action of imipramine in painful states. *Rev Neurol* (Paris) 102:503–504, 1960.

5. Blumer D, Heilbronn M: Chronic pain as a variant of depressive disease: the pain-prone disorder. *J Nerv Ment Dis* 170(7):381–406, 1982.

6. Nachemson AL: Pathophysiology and treatment of back pain: A critical look at the different types of treatment. In Buerger AA, Tobis JS (eds): *Approaches to the Validation of Manipulation Therapy.* Springfield, IL, Charles C Thomas, 1977, pp 42–57.

7. Fordyce WE: *Behavioral Methods for Chronic Pain and Illness.* St. Louis, Mosby, 1976.

8. Fordyce WE: Learning processes in pain. In Sternbach RA (ed): *The Psychology of Pain.* New York, Raven Press, 1978, pp 49–72.

9. Blumer D, Heilbronn M, Pedraza E, et al: Systematic treatment of chronic pain with antidepressants. *Henry Ford Hosp Med J* 28(1):15–21, 1980.

10. Blumer D, Heilbronn M: Second year follow-up study on systematic treatment of chronic pain with antidepressants. *Henry Ford Hosp Med J* 29(2):67–68, 1981.

11. Blumer D, Heilbronn M: Antidepressant treatment for chronic pain: Outcome study of 1000 patients with the pain-prone disorder. *Psychiatr Anna* 14(11):796–800, 1984.

12. Engel G: "Psychogenic" pain and the pain-prone patient. *Am J Med* 26:899–918, 1959.

13. Blumer D, Heilbronn M: The pain-prone disorder: A clinical and psychological profile. *Psychosomatics* 22(5):395–402, 1981.

14. Blumer D: Psychiatric considerations in pain. In Rothman RH, Simeone FA (eds): *The Spine, Vol II.* Philadelphia, Saunders, 1975, pp 871–906.

15. Black RG: The chronic pain syndrome. *Surg Clin North Am* 55:999–1011, 1975.

16. Crue BL (ed): *Chronic Pain: Further Observations from City of Hope National Medical Center.* New York, Spectrum, 1979.

17. Pilowsky I, Spence ND: Illness behavior syndromes associated with intractable pain. *Pain* 2:61–71, 1976.

18. Blumer D, Heilbronn M: Depression and chronic pain. In Cameron O (ed.): *Presentations of Depression: Depressive Symptoms in Medical and Other Psychiatric Disorders. New York, John Wiley & Sons, in press, 1987.*

19. Blumer D, Heilbronn M: Chronic muscle contraction headache and the pain-prone disorder. *Headache* 22(4):180–183, 1982.

20. Blumer D: Psychiatric aspects of chronic pain: Nature, identification and treatment of the pain-prone disorder. In Rothman RH, Simeone FA (eds): *The Spine, Second Edition.* Philadelphia, Saunders, 1982, pp 1090–1117.

21. Krystal H: Alexithymia and psychotherapy. *Am J Psychother* 33(1):17–31, 1979.

22. Sifneos PE: Clinical observations on some patients suffering from a variety of psychosomatic diseases. *Proceedings of the Seventh European Conference on Psychosomatic Research,* Basel, Karger, 1967.

23. Winokur G, Behar D, VanValkenburg MD, et al: Is a familial definition of depression both feasible and valid? *J Nerv Ment Dis* 166:764–768, 1978.

24. Blumer D, Zorick F, Heilbronn M, et al: Biological markers for depression in chronic pain. *J Nerv Ment Dis* 170(7):425–428, 1982.

25. Blumer D, Heilbronn M, Rosenbaum A: Antidepressant treatment of the pain-prone disorder. *Psychopharmacol Bull* 20(3):531–535, 1984.

26. Lake AE: Biofeedback and headache management. In Saper JR (ed): *Headache Disorders: Current Concepts and Treatment Strategies.* Boston, John Wright-PSG, 1983, pp 191–231.

CHAPTER FOURTEEN

The Migraine Patient: Descriptive Studies

CHARLES S. ADLER, M.D.
SHEILA MORRISSEY ADLER, PH.D.

Since Hippocrates, the medical community has increasingly recognized the importance of psychological factors in migraine. In the last century alone, medical investigators have illuminated many details of the association between migraine and contributing psychodynamic factors. Nevertheless, even physicians interested in headache who accept the importance of psychological factors approach this subject reluctantly. Several things contribute to this paradox.

First, only a percentage of migraine patients have noteworthy psychological contributions to their illness. Even then, these are often obscured by healthy or adaptive functioning in other contexts. The physician has probably observed most of his migraine patients to be compliant, hard working, and successful; they often have devoted a greater than average portion of their mental activities to developing character through cultivation of society's traditional values and adherence to its expectations. Specific strengths of character most admired in medical circles, such as self-discipline, are the very ones physicians share with many migraineurs.

Such a patient does not look "psychological." In particular, he contrasts sharply with the common, but usually false, stereotype of the psychologically influenced pain patient: angry, depressed, and somatizing, a person who finds in pain a way to avoid responsibilities or to give in to self-pity or irascibility. The physician will instantly recognize that to characterize his migraine patients this way would be inaccurate and unfair.

Yet psychological factors can insert themselves into the headache picture in other, more subtle ways, and these too must be considered. These presentations may even be diametrically opposed to the unappealing stereotype just described. Such forces operate in patients who carry on *despite* the handicap of migraine, with its genetics, its discrete physiological changes, and its often prostrating pain. Because these influences say "keep pushing," rather than "give in," they may derail the diagnostician who anticipates psychological factors to come dressed in bolder garb.

A second factor that commonly constrains the physician from broaching psychological issues with migraineurs is his understandable concern over his relationship with his patient. Might the patient believe the doctor to be questioning the reality of his pain, and thereby offending his pride? Imagine the physician to be impugning the just-mentioned pejorative description to *him*? Will he think the doctor is suggesting that his frequent efforts to keep going are to be rewarded only with a psychiatric label, making him hurt or angry? Or might the referring physician react with dismay when he later hears that a psychological tack had been taken?

Each of these possibilities is a real risk. Discussion between the physician and the patient, however, is usually part of the preferable approach despite them. For example, consider this: many patients are too hard on themselves, an attitude which often fuels behaviors which ultimately trigger migraine. They sometimes anticipate that the physician's attitude towards them will resemble their own self-critical feelings. One way to correct this critical self-concept is to encourage the patient to express feelings about himself, and to find that the doctor has a different, and more favorable opinion. Thus, by broaching emotional topics in treatment, a physician can begin to convince the patient that talk can repair, not diminish, self-esteem. The authors would caution, however, that such an approach is generally effective only if the physician is convinced of the value of talk himself.

A third source of reticence to broach the issue of psychodynamics of migraine may be found in discouraging past experiences with psychiatric consultation. For example, the physician may remember a consult that offered psychodynamic explanations which were impossible to translate into practical interventions of direct assistance to his patient. (If this is the roadblock, for the good of the patient, please persevere.)

Finally, the thought will recur that many less complicated and time-consuming ways to treat migraine are in common use. The physician knows that well-selected medications and infrequent follow-ups provide a satisfactory protocol for the typical patient with occasional migraine. Most migraineurs will—and should—be treated this way. Why add complexity?

For those patients in whom psychological pressures significantly accentuate the migraine predisposition, however, the standard treatment is an incomplete solution. Touraine´ and Draper (1) tell us why:

Migraine is an essential quality of the sufferer. It belongs in the fabric of his personality like the bony structure of his skull. . . .

Thus, although the physician can usually select medications that reduce or largely eliminate migraine attacks, there is one group of patients for whom this simpler approach will not suffice, and another for whom it leaves unsolved problems even more distressing than head pain, problems that now and in the future will seriously impede love and work. An analogy might be made to treating the angina pectoris patient with nitroglycerin to reduce his chest pain, but ignoring his diet, lack of exercise, 2-pack-a-day cigarette habit, and frenetic, coronary-prone life style.

HOW THESE CHAPTERS ARE ORGANIZED

Chapters 14, 15, and 16 form a unit addressing the current level of understanding of the psychodynamics of migraine. Our aim is to present this material in a manner that does not burden the reader. Nevertheless, three chapters are devoted to this subject because we did not want to oversimplify a complex field by prematurely dismissing valid dissenting viewpoints. While we wish to impart the concept of common psychodynamics in a coherent and usable fashion, it would be disappointing if these ideas were taken as doctrine. Preferably, the reader will finish these chapters educated to appreciate some common nuances in the emotional lives of a complex and far from homogenous group of patients. The reader will undoubtedly find his own best applications for this knowledge. It is our hope that one of these will be an increased sensitization to factors that trigger, amplify, or maintain migraine's chronicity in his patients.

This information in these 3 chapters can be divided into six sections. Section 1 looks at migraines' demographics and gives a brief overview of how the physiology reacts with the person. Section 2 confronts the controversial topic of personality and migraine by presenting characteristics migrainologists have observed repeatedly in several thousand patients with the disorder. (In this and other sections we let the authors "speak for themselves" whenever possible.) These Section 2 portrayals are more like snapshots than motion pictures. In Chapter 14, we begin Section 3 with a discussion of two methods of study, "statistical" and "observational," and of the different types of knowledge that can be best acquired from each. Findings from some representative psychometric studies on migraine are also presented.

The second part of Chapter 15 begins the fourth section, and takes a chronological look at the major "observational studies" of the past century, and at the contributions each researcher makes, or attempts to make, to understanding the psychodynamics of both the migraine patient and the migraine attack.

Chapter 16 begins with Section 5, which deals with a theoretical construct: the modal "psychologically influenced migraineur." This device is employed for convenience and for clarity. In the first half of the chapter, the life history of this apocryphal figure is reviewed, highlighting common experiences, reactions, defenses, strengths, trouble spots, and so forth. A developmental approach is continued in the sixth, and final, section, which synthesizes the accumulated information with the author's observations and conclusions gained from an in-depth treatment of several hundred psychologically influenced migraineurs.

DEMOGRAPHIC STUDIES

The demographic evaluation of migraine is complicated because many migraine sufferers are reluctant to acknowledge their disorder: approximately half never consult a physician about it. They are also loathe to admit headaches when applying for health insurance, employment, or the armed services (2). An additional problem for determining incidence may relate to the frequency with which physicians in different countries recognize and report the disorder: countries in which migraine seems most prevalent are also those in which physicians are at the forefront of headache treatment.

Nevertheless, it is estimated that 5–10% of the overall population has migraine, and that an even larger percentage of patients seen in medical practice do (2). Migraine is reported more frequently in urban areas, ei-

ther because of the greater strain of city life or because of urban dwellers' more frequent consultation with specialists. Although not restricted to any social or economic groups, there is controversy about whether migraine is (2) or is not (3) more frequent in individuals whose work is chiefly mental, such as professionals and executives. Women are nearly three times more likely to have this disorder than men; that this is not true before pubescence emphasizes the important role of endocrine factors.[1]

Migraine has a hereditary component. Some authors (1, 4, 5) suggest that observation and imitation of a migrainous parent or sibling could also play a role in transmitting the disorder within families. This seems unlikely, as migraine manifests itself in autonomic dysfunctions that are consistent between patients and not under voluntary nervous system control. A more probable interpersonal contributor is when the future patient incorporates into his identity attitudes and expectations of the afflicted family member that eventually pressure a genetic migraine trait into becoming manifest.

PHYSIOLOGY AND MIGRAINE

One thing is clear: whatever its causes, each migraine episode unfolds as a well-defined clinical syndrome whose common symptoms bespeak a common physiological sequence (see Chapter 22). Both common and classical forms are exacerbated by increased responsibility, stress, or change. However, classical

---

[1] From a developmental perspective, it is also possible that something about the responsibilities of the female role or about the relationship between a mother and a daughter could increase the female child's risk of developing migraine. The female child, for example, usually develops a stronger identification with the mother than does her brother. The significance attached to the menarche, a psychological as well as a physiological event, might also play a role in the delayed onset of sex differences. These factors would be in *addition* to the established hormonal ones.

migraine is more likely to appear unexpectedly than is common migraine, which usually
has at least some buildup (6); and recent
work by Olesen et al (7) suggests fundamental differences between the pathophysiology
of these subtypes.

In clinical practice the more prevalent
common migraine seems somewhat more
susceptible to psychological influences than
does its classical counterpart. For purposes of
this chapter, however, these psychological
differences are too slight to justify separating
the disorders.

Although the lion's share of clinical research has been directed towards the aura
and headache phases of migraine, a well-documented prodromal period precedes them.
Researchers (8–12) also describe a prolonged cycle of shifting mood, activity levels,
and minor somatic symptomatology between
headaches. The letdown into headache is often in decided contrast to an energetic mental
state which the migraineur strives to maintain
in the interval period, and which he seeks to
recapture as soon as the headache is over.[2]

Although the postheadache phase may
be marked by exhaustion, it is sometimes described in terms of rejuvenation. Patients may
make comments such as it being "the one
time when I feel like the person I really want
to be . . . refreshed and renewed" (1).

---

[2] One way in which this cycle may be related
to the interaction between psychiatric triggers and
migraine is the following: many migraineurs prefer
to cope with important problems or anxiety-provoking tasks by using their intellectual and cognitive capacities, rather than by resorting to action.
Intellectual activity is known to be associated with
dilation of cerebral vessels (13). Perhaps when this
state of anxious attentiveness is no longer needed,
when either "the performance" is over or the attempt to cope with the problem intellectually
seems doomed, there is a shift in the physiology
that is so abrupt that the sudden contrast—like a
stuck door that is being pushed on and unexpectedly breaks free—precipitates an attack of psychophysiologically triggered migraine (see Chapter
22).

PERSONALITY AND MIGRAINE

In the search for correlations between psychological functioning and headache, it is
doubtful that anything has been pursued
more doggedly than has the attempt to document personality traits shared by patients with
migraine (Table 14.1). This quest caught the
interest of many early pioneers in psychosomatic medicine. Their studies led them to describe a constellation of character traits later
nicknamed "the migraine personality."

Many physicians react negatively when
"personality" is broached in the headache
context, almost as though the term referred to
a concept so rigid that its employment should
be considered not only outmoded but also
offensive. Used badly, it is, and the authors
bear no sentiment for or against its retention.
The *flexible concepts* underlying its *correct*
use do deserve some discussion, however.
Thus, we will let the concepts speak for themselves; afterwards, any suitable term can be
applied to those worth retaining.

In psychiatry and psychology, "personality" and "character" are technical terms with
similar meanings. They can be defined as the
way a person habitually perceives, approaches, and acts in new situations. Everyone has a personality, comprised of various
"personality traits." Our personalities largely
reflect the strategies we developed to adapt to
emotional contingencies that prevailed during
childhood. Personality style evolves from
each person's reliance upon that preferred
behavioral/emotional repertoire which he believes will offer his best chance to feel well and
to act correctly in life. It is based on his experiences, convictions, and inner conclusions
(conscious or not) about the dangers, rewards, and imperatives of interpersonal relationships.

Each personality style allows its owner to
handle some of life's problems better than
others; it may also lead the owner to repeatedly feel caught in specific types of conflict.
The nature of someone's personality determines which attitudinal states he is likely to
continuously or repetitively experience. An

TABLE 14.1
PERSONALITY ATTRIBUTES COMMONLY DESCRIBED IN CONJUNCTION WITH MIGRAINE

AUTHOR	OBSERVATIONS
Friedman (4)	Intense, orderly, striving, overly conscientious, meticulous in performance. Conditioned to use his wits to the exclusion of his feelings.
Karpman (5)	Compliant, anxious to please; chief goal is to be accepted by virtue of overconscientious efforts to do perfect work.
Selinsky (16)	Excessive sense of responsibility which makes its appearance early in life; inclined to act as main support for younger siblings or aging parents, or to voluntarily contribute to the support of indigent relatives.
Frazier (17)	Bright, perfectionistic, knowledgeable; highly developed intellectual techniques for dealing with stresses; overly sustained states of emotional restraint; overly rigid controls and techniques for dealing with stress; controls manifested by such characteristics as perfectionism, neatness, ambitiousness, efficiency, rigidity, and stoicism. React with anxiety when a stressful situation invades their supercontrolled environment. Difficulty dealing with incessant, intense stimuli such as occur at puberty, menstruation, and maturation. Build lives for themselves with too much environmental demand, yet, at the same time are hypersensitive to this overload; thus, situational as well as psychodynamically caused anxieties ensue.
Jonckheere (18)	Obsessional, ambitious, compulsive. Repressed aggressiveness and an absence of imaginary life forces them to discharge their needs into somatic life.
Touraine and Draper (1)	Appear always to be turning backward into themselves; create first impression of detachment or partial self-absorption. Certain warmth of personality is lacking; deliberate, hesitant, insecure; do not make easy social contacts, yet force themselves to do so in compensation; extremely sensitive to criticism, seek cause of problems within self; assume unnecessary burdens, responsibilities; anxious, anticipate catastrophe; quickly discouraged; do not lose themselves in the art of living; detailed, perfectionist checking and rechecking of work; emotions are deep but expression of them appears to be frustrated; often found to use daily laxatives or frequent enemas just to keep self cleaned out.
Wolff (19)[a]	Always on the go. Sometimes, particularly in men, quality of studied poise, with tense facial expressions, quick moving eyes, uneasy laughter. Refer to themselves as quick-tempered, temperamental. *Troubled attitude towards bodily inadequacy:* blatant disregard for loss of sleep and common sense limits of work or pursuit of goals between attacks; stoical in waiving reasonable restrictions; unduly sensitive at being reminded of headaches; disregard for body as long as it functions well, but react with resentment when it interferes with attainment of their ends; unwilling to adapt themselves to limitations of organism. *Troubled relations to parents:* marked attachment, excessive dependence on mother in over one-third of patients; poor emancipation; incomplete development of self-reliance. *Social relations:* cautious, circumscribed; courteous, gracious manners enable them to conduct social relations at arm's length; protect themselves from intimacy that might engender friendly criticism; give impression of being aloof, detached, even cold, despite demonstrated desire to be thought well of; although critical themselves, seldom allowed themselves to be in a position that might provoke criticism; self-righteous, satisfaction of being right led to impression of lacking humility at times; free expres-

Table 14.1 Continues

TABLE 14.1 Continued

AUTHOR	OBSERVATIONS
	sion of enthusiasm or deep affection curtailed; inherently conservative and cautious; opposed elements representing change in community; disliked expediency as administrative policy.

Ambition and drive to success: prominent in nine of ten subjects; attempt to dominate their environment; conscientious, perfectionistic, persistent, exacting; attempt to bring order wherever possible; meticulous, fastidious, well dressed even when not well heeled; neatness rather than attractiveness or fashion is prevailing effect of dress.

Orderliness: Keeps lists and index card systems; stamp collecting popular, likes classification of things; free expression of fantasy or philosophy not related to data is rare; sometimes marked exceptions, such as disorderly household; love of formalism, nicety of detail in aesthetics; in music prefers Bach, Haydn, and Mozart.

Perfectionism and efficiency: extremely hard working, great deal of energy, push, and striving; frequently become secretaries of social or professional organizations; expend endless effort to obtain perfect result, flawless data; allocate responsibility poorly, preferring to do tasks themselves for fear they might be done wrong; single-minded persistence at tasks makes interruptions extremely distressing; tendency not to stop task until completed, leading to long, irregular hours of intense application; not always pleased with their own achievements, even when these are objectively high.

Doubts and repetitions: found frequently, and often related to fear of being found wrong and criticized; lead to related difficulty, that of trouble making decisions; also lead to procrastination, delay, and avoidance in taking a stand; sometimes engage in ritualistic behavior, such as with personal toilet; difficulty throwing things out and, as a result, drawers and cupboards in disarray.

Caution and economy: getting a "good bargain" important even if it involves sacrifice of time and energy; seeks out goods of full and lasting value; finds waste, extravagance extremely distasteful; in contrast, sometimes generous with larger sums; shows efficiency, impatience, dislike of wasting time as well as money.

Inflexibility: Impatient with character qualities opposite to theirs; although they themselves frequently create schemes, systems, arrangements, etc., for others, they show great difficulty in complying with or adapting themselves to similar systems imposed on them by others; resistance to change manifested by strong-headedness, stubbornness, "nonpushability," and difficulty with compromise or readjustment; at times prefer defeat to modification; often the type who need to be convinced by work associates that proposed changes were really their original idea.

Resentments: present and strong in two-thirds of subjects; harbor deep resentments, feelings of being injured; would not talk this out with the person they resented but instead remain ostensibly friendly; unable to forgive others and often also unable to forgive themselves; develop and sustain pernicious emotional reactions such as tension, dissatisfaction, and resentment in reaction to the experience that other human beings and environmental conditions are not just so. Emotions commonly seen include anxiety and short-lived, intense rage reactions associated with revengeful and spiteful feelings; also, long sustained superficial, pervasive uneasiness or anticipation of untoward events; usually fail to correlate these mental states with migraines; sometimes obtain pleasure from the feelings of being alert and striving.

TABLE 14.1 Continued

AUTHOR	OBSERVATIONS
	Genuine relaxation seldom attained: goal in work more important than the process of attaining goal; accomplishment seldom brought more than transient pause; one task quickly followed the next until migraine interrupted.
Kolb (20)	Have trouble with personality structure that is apparent between, as well as during headaches, and this is one of the factors predisposing to chronicity; may have trouble with childbirth, nursing of children, strenuous hours of work, poor living habits. Subject to inferiority feelings, fear of making a mistake. Scrupulous, ambitious, overconscientious. Problems with insomnia, irritability, restlessness. Fantasies of rejection by significant persons. Leads to retaliatory fantasies. Unconscious hostility beneath agreeable, considerate exterior.
Alvarez (21)	Above average intelligence, with a distinctive personality and sometimes a distinctive appearance; sometimes so distinctive that one can suspect the nature of the trouble the minute the individual walks into the office . . . her eyes are bright and expressive, her face is intelligent, and her responses and movements are quick. Few mention . . . headaches, and some even conceal the fact; a few are so resentful of their handicap and the fact that it causes them to break engagements at the last minute that they will even deny its existence.
Alexander (22)	Repressed dependency needs which patient tries to overcome by overcompensatory striving. Attempts to repress aggressive thought as well as to block aggressive actions.
Fromm-Reichmann (23)	Tend to repress hostility, especially in close relationships. Fear affective exclusion if they do not meet family standards. Ambitious, competitive; delicate sensibilities.
Dalsgaard-Nielsen (24)	Sensitive, perfectionistic, and tending to bottle up emotions. "Migraine can be precipitated by emotional stress in 68%, but in no patient was this the only known precipitant."
Selby and Lance (25)	In review of 500 cases found 67% liable to migraine attacks precipitated by emotional factors; 42% described as having "normal personalities."
Khouri-Haddad (26)	Inability to cope with stress threatening self-esteem. Tendency to relapse into periods of deflated self-esteem accompanied by anger, depression, increased headaches.
Graham (27)	Overtax congenitally vulnerable nervous system by pushing beyond its limits, denying it sufficient repose and pacing.

[a] It might be pointed out that Wolff saw no conflict in placing these observations side by side with more measurable data about migraineurs' carotid pulse variations, obtained in conjunction with Graham (28).

attitudinal state includes a bias towards certain perceptions, and towards the characteristic emotions generated by those perceptions. The pattern of physiological response that characterizes this complex can, if prolonged, induce or accentuate specific psychophysiological diseases. This is why personality in migraine has been studied so intensively: it is because personality can influence vulnerability to headaches, even when within the normal range. This effect is similar to the way someone with an inherited propensity towards coronary disease can influence that propensity by dietary preferences he learns in childhood and later perpetuates.

Sometimes a person's personality is sufficiently pathological to be considered a "personality disorder." The reactions of a patient in this category are usually aberrant enough to grossly interfere with his functioning. Co-workers and neighbors may think the person "troubled" or "difficult," even if they cannot always put into words exactly what makes him so. Of course, just as in any group, some migraineurs have personality disorders. With most migraineurs, however, the degree of dysfunction, if present, is subdiagnostic. Thus, the difficulties experienced by him, though real, do not announce themselves to the casual observer. Returning to our analogy, one has to eat an unusually strange or deficient diet to garner a medical diagnosis, but can eat in a way sufficient to compromise his cardiovascular status merely by habitually positioning himself in a fast-food line. If one excludes these "personality disorders" from consideration, a range of "personality traits" remain that do not lead to a diagnosis but are, nevertheless, more or less efficient, productive, or compatible with the genetics of migraine; they can, therefore, cause trouble and warrant our attention.

Researchers who have written about "the migraine personality" refer to a theoretical construct. It is their image of the quintessential migraine collage constructed from attitudes and behaviors they have repeatedly observed in patients with this illness. No individual fits this stereotype exactly, and statistically many will be expected to situate themselves several standard deviations away.

Psychological factors are only one vector among many contributing to the appearance of migraine. A plethora of combinations can sum up to migraine or its absence. If the picture includes a strong genetic tendency, combined with increased susceptibility to biological (hormonal, dietary) triggers, migraine may result in the absence of personality traits often associated with migraine. If personality features are present, but the genetics are not, one may see the traits, but no migraine. That so many combinations are possible keeps things confusing for those trying to theorize about cause and effect. For example, a patient with psychological characteristics often attributed to migraineurs may have a genetic vulnerability to both migraine and ulcers; his job takes him to Indonesia, where the food is unfamiliar and he must struggle not to feel homesick; and he develops an ulcer instead of headaches.

In short, personality traits often found in migraineurs can sometimes be seen not only in patients with other illnesses, but also even in the asymptomatic man in the street. The diversity is accounted for by genetic makeup, the nature of the personality, and types of environmental stressors. Differences in *genetic makeup* may cause particular organs to be more susceptible to overactivation in response to a variety of stresses, or more likely to break down in response to prolonged general autonomic activation. Subtle qualitative differences in the *nature of the personality* result from childhood experiences which emphasized one or another aspect of basically similar developmental conflicts; this can include differences in defensive maneuvers that the patient enlists to cope with threatening inner and outer realities and their symbolic equivalents. (Like individual affects, each defense is marked by distinctive somatic preparations.) Finally, chance throws different *types of environmental stressors* into one's path.

These factors—genetics, personality, and life events—can set the stage for migraine headaches, tension headaches, or other specific diseases, determine the patient's overall susceptibility to psychological influences on illness, and predict what types of stress in adult life will be most likely to revive early difficulties in a way that can aggravate illness. If adulthood's inevitable strains can be managed without resorting to earlier coping methods, the potentially vulnerable individual may remain asymptomatic. Because of this complexity, the concept of the migraine personality has generated its full measure of controversy.

Among the criticisms of the migraine personality theory is the concern that, as only half the people who get such headaches seek medical attention, the ones who do may have more psychopathology. Because perfectionistic character traits are attributed to this "migraine personality," another argument goes, perfectionistic migraineurs are naturally more discontented by occasional migraines than are nonperfectionistic ones. As a result, it is this first group which typically comes for treatment, thereby biasing the population studied to include the perfectionistic character trait. Yet another criticism is that the number of migraine patients studied psychologically is not vast.

Undoubtedly, there is some self-selection among patients, especially those who see psychiatrists or psychologists; yet, each of these criticisms also has fallacies. Consider that:

(**a**) Perfectionism would logically drive a patient to the doctor for any significant problems, not just migraine. Patients with most illnesses are not considered perfectionistic.

(**b**) In the United States alone, over 10 million migraine patients come for treatment, and a good percentage of them have been seen by physicians interested in psychosomatics. Though these observers and their approaches are different, their observations, while not identical, are routinely similar.

(**c**) Those migraineurs who do not visit doctors have been found (14) to have less frequent headaches. Yet, because there is effective treatment for migraine, one must wonder what other than a psychological reason would keep quite so many of these patients away.

On a practical level, it is less important to determine the psychological status of migraine patients who avoid doctors, because the physician will only be called upon to treat patients who do seek help.

Perhaps a more important question— and definitely one that is more taboo—is: To what extent have compulsive characteristics often seen in neurologists and other physicians unwittingly influenced patient selection, patient retention, or an investigator's perceptions of the personalities of patients? About this, we have, as yet, no answers.

Unfortunately, the idea of frequently shared personality traits in migraine—what- ever its validity, if used well—can be, and frequently is, oversimplified and used incorrectly, as if it were a magic formula. In this context its use will most certainly prove disappointing to the clinician or insulting to the patient. The presence of migraine headaches should never permit one to presume personality characteristics in a patient unless these are also observed in him independently. The concepts to be elaborated can be helpful if they are used to guide an evaluator's line of questioning, but neither to replace nor inhibit his curiosity about the individual before him. Understood this way, knowledge of frequently noted personality features in migraine may save the physician time by directing his inquiries towards fruitful topics.

All personality traits, functional or dysfunctional, have a reason for their existence. That reason is occasionally revealed by the patient's history. The logic accounting for their existence may be flawed, but it is a type of logic nonetheless. The logic may be childlike, primitive, and based on incorrect or anachronistic assumptions. It is always important to understand, insofar as is possible, however, what functions those traits were intended to serve when they were first incorporated into the personality. By uncovering those intended functions and the imperfect logic that sponsors them, the patient may eventually choose to relinquish them.

Many adjectives have been enlisted in the attempts to delineate personality characteristics of the migraineur. The words chosen by different authors, though sometimes repetitious or overlapping, are often insightful by virtue of a novel emphasis.

The information offered in this chapter is primarily descriptive rather than analytical. These are the psychological signs and symptoms of migraine, presented from a phenomenological, rather than an etiological, perspective. Some of these attributes are conceptual constructs extrapolated from the patient's behaviors and statements. Perfectionism, ambition, sensitivity, and poor self-confidence cannot be observed directly, but must be concluded on the basis of other observations.

Similarities have been noted between these traditional descriptions of the migraineur and adjectives applied to the Compulsive Personality Disorder.[3] Despite resemblances, the two are different. The patient with a compulsive personality disorder usually lacks the migraineur's self-sacrifice and striving for acceptance. Technically speaking, less character features can be traced to the oral stages of development in the compulsive. Also important, few migraineurs reach a diagnosable level of psychological impairment. The so-called "migraine personality" is merely a suggested constellation of frequently seen attributes. The authors stress that, although migraineurs frequently show compulsive attributes, it is a mistake to think of the psychologically influenced migraineur as a watered-down compulsive.

Before leaving this topic it is important to point out that the compulsive *personality* is different from the obsessive-compulsive *neurosis* (obsessive-compulsive *disorder* in DSM-III), the latter being an anxiety disorder marked by clearly defined obsessions and compulsions. The frequent search for "neuroticism" in migraine patients, particularly through the use of psychometric tests, suggests that this distinction may have been a source of confusion in the past.

Most investigators have remarked upon the relatively stable adaptations of migraineurs and on their penchant for success. The migraine patient has frequently achieved

social or professional advancement, due to a high degree of drive. This is sometimes combined with a marshalling of organizational capacities to use intelligence more efficiently to achieve goals.

From the descriptions in Table 14.1 a picture emerges of that theoretical being whose personality quirks so agitate the genetics of migraine: he is hard working, hard driving, ambitious, precise to the point of perfectionism, yet intolerant of imperfections in himself or others; unsympathetic to the needs of his body; preoccupied with order and arrangement; thrifty, cautious; sometimes given to stubbornness; subject to self-doubt and to the attempts to overcome it; affectually rigid, with difficulty in letting down his guard in relationships; socially polite but rather formal, conscientious, punctual, dutiful, habit bound, and accomplished or successful in his professional life, if not always entirely creative. He is largely out of touch with his own needs and feelings, but is highly attuned to his own expectations and those of others. At times he seems driven to control his environment and have the people in it march to his drumbeat; at other times there is a contrasting and even masochistic willingness to subvert his own best interests in deference to the wishes and expectations (or presumed expectations) of others.[4] Because he views needs which might conflict with what he believes is expected of him as a potential source of anxiety he is frequently out of touch with those needs, whether they be for sleep, relaxation, or physical affection. Both the needs themselves and the anger at subjugating them must therefore often make their appearance in disguised fashion, typically—though not necessarily—disguised to the patient as well as to others. When a full awareness of the needs and of the anger at their frustration threatens to erupt

---

[3] The American Psychiatric Association's *Diagnostic and Statistical Manual III* (29) states that the patient with a compulsive personality shows: ". . . restricted ability to express warm and tender emotions; perfectionism that interferes with the ability to grasp the big picture . . . excessive devotion to work, and productivity to the exclusion of pleasure; and indecisiveness . . . preoccupation with rules, efficiency, trivial details, procedures, or form . . . always mindful of their relative status in dominance/submission relationships . . . decision making is avoided, postponed, or protracted, perhaps because of an inordinate fear of making a mistake . . . a depressed mood is common . . . they tend to be excessively conscientious, moralistic, scrupulous, and judgemental of self and others. . . ."

[4] It is as if the migraineur will on occasion even submit to unreasonable demands, but only if he first internalizes and makes them *his own* unreasonable demands, i.e., demands of himself via his superego. This would explain the seeming paradox between the tendency to control and the tendency to submit.

into consciousness, a migraine attack often intervenes and aborts the process. In some patients, these reactions are conscious, yet the feelings are strong enough to trigger the physiology anyway.

"Real patients," of course, do not come neatly packaged like eggs in a box. There are dramatic variations on this theme; every practicing physician will be able to think of many.

Throughout these chapters it is hoped that the interested reader will also give himself, on occasion, the opportunity to refer back to these original reference works. Many have both eloquent and readable expositions of findings.

REFERENCES

1. Touraine GA, Draper G: The migrainous patient: a constitutional study. *J Nerv Ment Dis* 80:1–204, 1934.

2. Friedman AP, Merritt HH: Migraine. In Friedman AP, Merritt HH (eds): *Headache, Diagnosis and Treatment*. Philadelphia, F.A. Davis, 1959, pp 201–249.

3. Knopf O: Preliminary report on personality studies in thirty migraine patients. *J Nerv Ment Dis* 82:270–285, 400–414, 1935.

4. Friedman AP, von Storch TJC, Merritt HH: Migraine and tension headaches: a clinical study of two thousand cases. *Neurology* 4:773–788, 1954.

5. Hunter RA: Psychotherapy in migraine. *Br Med J* 1:1084–1088, 1980.

6. Graham JR: Migraine: clinical aspects. In Vinken PF, Bruyn GW (eds): *Handbook of Clinical Neurology*. Amsterdam, North-Holland, 1968, pp 45–58.

7. Olesen J, Lauritzen M, Tfelt-Hansen P, et al: Spreading cerebral oligemia in classical, and normal cerebral blood flow in common migraine. *Headache* 22:242–248, 1982.

8. Blau JN: Migraine prodromes separated from the aura: complete migraine. *Br Med J* 281:658–660, 1980.

9. Blau JN: Resolution of migraine attacks: sleep and the recovery phase. *J Neurol Neurosurg Psychiatry* 45:223–228, 1982.

10. Rafaelli E, Menon AD: Migraine and the limbic system. *Headache* 15:69–78, 1975.

11. Dalkvist J, Ekbom K, Waldenlind E: Headache and mood: a time-series analysis of self-ratings. *Cephalalgia* 4:45–52, 1984.

12. Levor RM, Cohen MJ, Naliboff BD, McArthur D, Heuser G: Psychological precursors' of migraine and related personality factors. *Headache* 24:174, 1984.

13. Grinker RR, Robbins FP: The head and the special senses. In Grinker RR, Robbins FP: *Psychosomatic Case Book*. New York, Blakiston, 1954, pp 109–142.

14. Henryk-Gutt R, Rees WL: Psychological aspects of migraine. *J Psychosom Res* 17:141–153, 1973.

15. Karpman B: Psychogenic aspects of headache. A symposium. *Clin Psychopathol* 10:1–26, 1949.

16. Selinsky H: Psychological study of the migrainous syndrome. *NY Acad Med Bull* 15:757–763, 1939.

17. Frazier SH: The psychotherapeutic approach to patients with headache. *Mod Treatment* 1:1412–1424, 1964.

18. Jonckheere P: The chronic headache patient. *Psychother Psychosom* 19:53–81, 1971.

19. Wolff HG: Personality features and reactions of subjects with migraine. *Arch Neurol* 37:895–921, 1937.

20. Kolb LC: Psychiatric and psychogenic factors in headache. In Friedman AP, Merritt HH (eds): *Headache, Diagnosis and Treatment*. Philadelphia, F.A. Davis, 1959, pp 259–298.

21. Alvarez WC: The migrainous personality and constitution, the essential features of the disease; a study of 500 cases. *Am J Med Sci* 213:1–8, 1947.

22. Alexander F: *Psychosomatic Medicine; Its Principles and Applications*. New York, W.W. Norton, 1950, pp 155–163.

23. Fromm-Reichmann F: Contribution to the psychogenesis of migraine. *Psychoanal Rev* 24:26–33, 1937.

24. Dalsgaard-Nielsen T: Migraine and heredity. *Acta Neurol Scand* 41:287–300, 1965.

25. Selby G, Lance JW: Observations on 500 cases of migraine and allied vascular headache. *J Neurol Neurosurg Psychiatry* 23:23–32, 1960.

26. Khouri-Haddad SE: Psychiatric consultation in a headache unit. *Headache* 24:322–328, 1984.

27. Graham JR: *Treatment of Migraine*. Boston, Little, Brown, 1955.

28. Graham JR, Wolff HG: Mechanism of migraine headache and action of ergotamine tartrate. *Arch Neurol Psychiatry* 39:737, 1938.

29. American Psychiatric Association; *Diagnostic and Statistical Manual of Mental Disorders, Third Edition*. Washington DC, American Psychiatric Association, 1980.

CHAPTER FIFTEEN

The Migraine Patient and the Migraine Attack: Clinical Studies

CHARLES S. ADLER, M.D.

SHEILA MORRISSEY ADLER, PH.D.

The psychological characteristics commonly observed in migraine patients, as outlined in Chapter 14, are fairly static observations. Though helpful, they fail to clarify the relationship between those characteristics and the triggering of headache. This chapter will present these dynamic views of the interchange between mind and body in migraine. We will review chronologically the thoughts of the major theoreticians who have addressed this problem. But first, because most recent studies emphasize psychological testing, it will be useful to consider briefly the relationship of psychometric data to clinical observation.

TWO ROUTES TO KNOWLEDGE

One way to acquire information about a medical syndrome is through statistical or actuarial methods. With this approach, one "looks where the light is." To do this, he tries to obtain numbers, preferably large ones, on which he can shine the familiar light of mathematical and statistical analysis. Once the data are collected in numerical form, there is little uncertainty about what one must do to arrive at a clear yes, no, or maybe. The logic and precision with which numbers can be used to reach conclusions is satisfying to investigators

and is theoretically the ideal way to process clinical information.

There are two prerequisites for using this approach: First, the information to be statistically processed must be *accurate*. Second, the information must be *relevant*. Accuracy and relevance are easier to certify when the system being studied is a simple one, or when tightly limited variables within that system can be isolated and studied alone.[1]

Human beings in pain are not simple systems. They function on many levels, some of the most important of which are consciously inaccessible. If it is to be useful, the level a test measures needs to correspond to the level the physician is trying to investigate in the patient. If these are in accord the test saves time and adds standardization. But this is not always the case. Therefore, for example, the accuracy of data obtained from a paper and pencil questionnaire, even one conducted with integrity and forethought, and the accuracy of the conclusions reached on the basis of this

---

[1] Hine et al (1) have written a thought-provoking article about similar concerns currently being debated among philosophers of science regarding inherent limits in the application of experimental techniques to psychological phenomena.

data, may be inherently low because of its method of collection.[2] Such a questionnaire might ask "Do you often feel anger?" and the patient might answer, without conscious deception, "No, in fact I never get angry," an answer akin to "Actually doctor, my pulse never varies." Thus, such questions may either answer how much a group of patients gets angry or how much they *are aware* of getting angry or, more likely, some mixture of these two.

The other requirement is that data be relevant to the important issue in the study, and to the question the investigator thinks he is answering. All data mean something. The difficult question to answer is what, really, any given set of data means. If an investigator collects information using the Minnesota Multiphasic Personality Inventory (MMPI), for example, he still needs to know whether the test posed the right questions for evaluation of headache patients, or whether, instead, it took a very accurate look at not quite the right thing. The answer to this question partially depends on the intended use of the information obtained. The MMPI may ask questions excellent for screening out patients with overt psychopathology, yet less useful for studying the subclinical nuances of headache dynamics. Of course, these same standards apply to any psychometric instrument, not just the MMPI.

It should be noted that biopsy reports, blood chemistries, x-rays, etc., refer to a different and theoretically more "objective" order of information than that obtained by the clinical examination. In contrast, the analyses from psychometric testing are ultimately based on diagnostic impressions obtained in a clinical interview, and therefore do not tap an inherently "higher"—or at least alternate—order of information. Put differently, there is no pathology laboratory for personality; there are no biopsy specimens that might contradict the patient's statements. Thus, despite their convenience, the clinician must be on guard against viewing psychometric results as a court of higher appeal to a well-run clinical interview. A recent study by the authors (2) reviewed their experience with 53 chronic, psychologically influenced migraine patients who had been given an MMPI during their intake. All received psychotherapy and a 10-year follow-up (3). In only three cases did the intial MMPI reveal problems, and in none did it give the investigators clues to the specific, clinically relevant psychological themes that were actually aggravating the patients' headaches.

The other approach, or route to knowledge, is that of analyzing small numbers of individuals with such thoroughness that one is sure of both the accuracy and the relevance of the data; this method also has its drawbacks. First among them is the limited number of patients that can be seen. This is because relatively few individuals are qualified by training to make sophisticated psychodynamic assessments, and is also due in part to the time and expense involved in making such an assessment. The limited sample size gives undue weight to chance, and findings may prove anecdotal rather than replicable. Second, there is a tendency for patients with more obvious psychopathology to be referred to such specialists; this predisposes to greater psychopathology among migraine patients who come to their attention. Finally, because more complex questions are typically asked, there is less consensus on the interpretation of data collected this way.

Because systems being studied can usually be sufficiently isolated in traditional biomedical research, the statistical approach to problems has gained favor over the in-depth observational one in recent years. As can be seen from the foregoing discussion, however, each technique has inherent strengths and weaknesses. Progress in understanding psychological influences on headache can best be made if these are factored in when planning new studies and acknowledged when interpreting their findings.

---

[2] Just as information gained about astronomy before the telescope allowed observers to probe beneath the superficial appearance of the skies could only yield inherently limited conclusions.

THE PSYCHOMETRIC APPROACH

The findings of some representative, statistically oriented studies on migraine may be summarized as follows.

Phillips (4), in a review article, concluded that several psychometric studies failed to support the view that migraineurs had increased neuroticism. This was also the finding of his own study, which relied on the Eysenck Personality Questionnaire. It surveyed 39 randomly selected medical patients who had migraine, but were not coming to the clinic for that reason.

Lucas (5) evaluated 1300 identical twins to study genetic factors in migraine. He found concordance rates of 26% in identical, and 13% in fraternal, twins. This finding is of interest because, whatever it reveals about the role of "nature" in transmission of migraine, it clearly demonstrates the effect of "nurture." Lucas found that if two individuals have an identical genetic makeup and one has migraine, only 1 time in 4 will the other develop migraine. His study thereby suggests that the dominant factor in the appearance of actual migraine symptoms is experience, which in 74% of the cases can deny access to the migraine genotype.

Passchier, van der Helm-Hylkema, and Orlebeke (6) studied both migraine and tension headache patients with a variety of psychometric instruments. Migraineurs were found to have elevated achievement motivation when compared with controls, as well as more rigidity (though less than tension headache patients), greater fear of failure, and reduced impulsiveness. Duration of attacks positively correlated with the amount of rigidity and achievement motivation.

Rorschach studies by Cooper and Friedman (7) and by Kaldegg (8) failed to show uniform personality patterns in migraineurs. The Kaldegg study did find evidence, however, that migraine patients strove to remain in command of a situation. If they were unable to, or if something "interfered with their rhythm," a state of tension resulted that might be resolved by a migraine attack.

Specific findings in the Rorschach evaluations of 50 patients in a carefully controlled study by Ross and McNaughton (9) yielded the following formal interpretation: "persistence towards success, difficulty in sexual adjustment, perfectionism, inflexibility, conventionality, and intolerance." Neither instability nor disability ratings were abnormal in the migraine group. They recommended that future Rorschach studies compare patients at different stages of the life cycle.

Timsit (10) studied 120 migraineurs with the Rorschach examination. He notes that formal interpretation of movement responses in the inkblots are like dreams, "closely related to deep and unconscious processes." With migraineurs, these were found to be of a "psychosomatic" pattern, "mainly characterized by '. . . static perception,' repressiveness or repression of movement, with 'kinesthetic' shock and petrified or devitalized contents, such as 'puppets,' 'sculptures,' 'statues,' and 'cartoons'." There were also signs of hypersensitivity, strict rational control, and somatic concerns focused on the head. This sign, the lack of sufficient movement responses, was seen to be due to a blocking of unconscious aggressive fantasies. Aggression in relationship to the head itself was also seen; many patients saw in the inkblots the "Winged (and headless) Victory of Samothrace."

The Comprehensive Textbook of Psychiatry (11) notes that "The Rorschach excels all other tests as an aid in making neuropsychiatric diagnoses . . ." Therefore, its comparatively limited utilization to date for evaluating migraineurs is unfortunate, and the ambiguous conclusions of the studies that have been performed suggest a need for continuing replication by examiners well trained in its interpretation. Use of other projective tests, such as the Thematic Apperception Test (TAT) might be helpful also in detecting common psychodynamic themes in migraine patients.

Arena, Andrasik, and Blanchard (12) administered a battery of psychometric tests to chronic headache patients (migraine, tension and combined). Patients were separated into groups based on the percentage of their life that had been spent with headaches. When personality traits of the groups were compared, the differences were insignificant, ". . . indicating that the percentage of life one spends with head pain has no differential effect on a number of psychological test measures. One interpretation of the above results is that the characterological personality traits so often found in headache sufferers are not a result of the pain experience, but in fact were present before the pain problem started."

The MMPI has been extensively administered to headache patients of all diagnostic categories. In a review article, Harrison (13) pointed out that a common MMPI profile for migraine and many other headache patients includes what has been termed the "Conversion V": elevated scores on hypochondriasis, hysteria, and depression scales. It often implies that anxiety is incorporated into physical complaints and that the patient is using compulsive defenses. Although the conversion V is regularly seen in the MMPIs of both migraine and tension headache patients, its full significance—if any—is uncertain.

Kudrow and Sutkus (14) found essentially normal MMPI profiles for migraineurs, which was in contrast to what they found for several other headache diagnoses.

Rogado, Harrison, and Graham (15) compared MMPI findings in 150 migraine, cluster, and control patients. Both headache types showed somewhat more psychopathology than did the control group; most evident were obsessive-compulsive traits.

For their large study of migraine patients, Henryk-Gutt and Rees (16) used three psychometric tests, a psychiatric history, and an observation period. They compared migraineurs who were not currently in treatment to a control group. Subjects filled out an abbreviated MMPI (in which female patients showed elevated anxiety and somatization scores), a BUSS scale (higher hostility scores), and an Eysenck Personality Inventory (higher neuroticism scores.) Over the 2-month observation period, subjects recorded headache attacks and consciously recognized sources of stress. The authors concluded that psychological influences were important precipitants of migraine, as over half of the 120 recorded attacks were related to emotionally stressful events. In addition, more than half of the subjects reported that they had their first migraine during a period of stress. Migraine subjects chosen at random from the civil service register only recorded one-fourth as many attacks as did migraine patients at a headache clinic.

These investigators were unable to confirm excessive ambition or obsessional tendencies in the nonpatient migraine population. They further found that neither the quantity nor the intensity of the stressors to which migraine subjects were exposed during the 2-month monitoring period differed, objectively, from stressors to which the controls were exposed; yet, the migraineurs had significantly more subjective distress in comparison. They concluded that migraineurs must be constitutionally predisposed to experience a greater than average reaction to a given quantity of stress.[3]

THE OBSERVATIONAL APPROACH

EARLY STUDIES: GLIMPSES OF THE WHOLE

It has been said that there is nothing new under the sun, and certainly the observation of

---

[3] A difficulty with this conclusion—and it may be only a semantic one—is this: "stress" cannot be objectively measured because it is a subjective experience. The experience of stress is based on the cognitive and emotional significance ascribed to a given situation, which is in turn based upon the memories, conscious and unconscious, that the patient has of similar encounters in the past. If by "constitutional" Henryk-Gutt and Rees mean all things learned and genetic that shaped the person prior to the onset of the disease (which we suspect they do) their conclusion is warranted, but if the term only refers to chromosomal factors, it is not.

Junkerius (17) in 1734 confirms this view, reading, as it does, like the coat of arms of the psychologically determined migraine sufferer: "ira, in primis tacita et suppressa" (initially anger, unspoken and suppressed). When he advanced this as the prime psychological contributor to migraine, he sounded a note that has echoed from study to study down to the present day.

In 1873 Liveing (18) published *On Megrim, Sick Headache, and Some Allied Disorders,* a work considered by some to be the first comprehensive exposition of migraine and which was still cited as a standard reference 50 years later (19). He believed that emotional disturbance was one of three "exciting causes" of migraine. "Accessory causes" included "marriage with childbearing, nursing and caring, working late at night, mental exertion, competitive work like examinations, worries and competition in business, and poor hygiene of living as is common among professional men."

Tilney (20) concurred with Liveing's view that emotional strain and competitive spirit, if not the causes of migraine, as least influence the course of it.

Ulrich (19), in 1912, published a study of 500 migraineurs which reinforced this view still further. She noted that such things as "lasting strain, mental trouble, and want" may not create migraine, but will drive it from a background condition to the foreground of experience.

In 1926 Crookshank (21) observed that migraineurs were "thinkers rather than doers." He considered their self-contained and reserved outward attitude to be deceptive, as the personality underneath was actually in an unstable equilibrium.

Weber (22), using observations from classical psychoanalysis in 1932, described sharply conflicting feelings in migraine, such as repressed guilt arising from hostility towards people with whom there were close affective ties. Attacks were seen to be triggered in particular by events which wounded the vanity.

GRACE TOURAINE AND GEORGE DRAPER: AMBIVALENT EMANCIPATION

In 1935 Touraine and Draper (23) published thorough case portraits of 50 patients with migraine. Their study was undertaken to see whether migraineurs "represent a special design of total personality . . . a migraineous constitutional type." It concluded—with vigor—that they did.

The central theme around which problems typically developed was thought to be the patient's incomplete emancipation from his mother. This was manifested by extreme alternations in the impulse to wrest an individual personality from the common substrate of the mother-child relationship. It was a relationship which the mother was invariably found to dominate. Touraine and Draper reported that their patients' earliest memories were of insecurity in interactions with the parent. Patients overcompensated for this insecurity by striving to become unusually close to the mother—by, indeed, becoming, in the process, very much like her.

An impulse to "complete the self," of which the mother was felt to be part and parcel, was seen in the patient's recurrent attempts to return home and, by so doing, to ameliorate a pervasive sense of insecurity. These "returnings" routinely failed, however, and before long the impulse to leave again reasserted itself.

A central insight into the genesis of this struggle is then offered:

Thus it would appear that the mothers of the migrainous have withheld recognition of their offspring's individuality. The effect of this neglect is to encourage identification with the mother in the case of the daughters; and in the case of sons to retard or prevent the usual masculine escape. In short, unconsciously the migrainous person is unable to view herself as an individual apart from the mother, and the idea of separation is apparently insupportable (23).

In other words, men and women react differently. The woman frequently assumes a more active role, taking over the mother's responsibilities and contributing to her financial support, yet all the while feeling bitter resentment at her inability to escape the mother's influence. By means of the repetition compulsion the migrainous woman was then seen to reenact similar troubles with her own child and,

inevitably passes on the pattern for safety which lies in perpetual identification with the mother. . . . A sense of unreality pervades her relationship to her own family and one observes a wearying attempt to attend to the technique of maternal duties without in any way giving of herself . . . the tragedy . . . is that she has little of herself which can be called herself to give (23).

The male migraineur, in contrast, adopts a more passive attitude towards the mother and assumes fewer responsibilities for her, "preferring instead to continue to live within the maternal protection." Though not necessarily living at home, at some level he seems unwilling or unable to challenge her authority.

What triggers specific attacks? The delicate equilibrium between independence and union can be ruptured either by intensified conflict with the mother, making the status quo intolerable, or by something that implies a rift is about to take place. These influences can be either conscious or unconscious. Thus ambivalence about separation is revived from childhood, with one part of the personality trying to stay with the mother at all costs, the other part trying equally hard to individuate and break away.

They conclude that although migraine results from the triggering of disordered physiology in patients with a particular constitution, that disordered physiology is secondary to (and precipitated by) the emotional discharge.

OLGA KNOPF: OVERPROTECTED AND OVERSENSITIVE

In a study reported in 1935, Knopf (19) evaluated 30 migraineurs at New York's Bellevue City Hospital to see if they had character traits in common. She primarily saw patients from the lower socioeconomic strata, many of them Eastern European immigrants.

In the families of her patients she found the oldest or youngest children most likely to develop migraine, and attributed this to role expectations accompanying those positions in the family order.

Overall, she was struck by the similarities in the personalities of her patients, particularly in what she concluded were the underlying psychic structures. Her study recognized that, as years go by, a given illness may evoke similar somatopsychic personality changes in initially dissimilar patients and, thereby, blur the distinction between cause and effect. She therefore tried to get a picture of the patient's mental/emotional makeup before onset of headaches. However, she found most patients reluctant to admit to "bad" qualities, preferring to present themselves as having been model children.

Of the attributes observed, some are familiar: ambitious, reserved, repressed, dignified, sensitive, domineering, resentful, and with a constricted sense of humor. But, the term that conveys her overall impression is new: the "goody-goody."

What is a "goody-goody"?

The *Thorndike-Barnhart Dictionary* offers the following, perhaps somewhat ancient, definition of goody: "an old woman of humble station." (This image of acting old, even older than one's age, comes up again in Chapter 16.) The *Oxford Dictionary*, choosing to define "goody-goody" by example, cites the following quote from Goethe: "Oh! If they had but the heart to commit an absurdity!"

Perhaps one can remember from school years that the "goody-goody" was apt to be fussy, oversensitive, and wanting things just so; sometimes they also showed a stuffy or bossy righteousness which set them apart.

In the overwhelming majority of cases she found both the start of the illness and its exacerbation to be immediately preceded by psychologically traumatic events "similar to those preceding other types of personal maladjustment." She especially noted the importance of menarche and pregnancy, and found incomplete genital stage adjustment in all women in the study.

She concluded that her patients

. . . were to a large extent, overprotected children, who had grown up with an increased feeling of inadequacy due to their particular constitution as well as to their particular situation and their personal interpretation of their circumstances (19).

Knopf believed that the increased sensitivity, submissiveness, and isolation that she saw in these patients were their means of trying to both compensate for and protect themselves from feelings of inadequacy.

Some of her observations may have been skewed by psychosocial influences prevailing in the immigrant cultural and social milieu of New York's ghettos.

FREIDA FROMM-REICHMANN: RESENTMENT REPRESSED

In 1937 Fromm-Reichmann (24), a scholarly psychoanalyst working at the Chestnut Lodge, published a frequently quoted paper containing her observations about migraine based on the psychoanalysis of eight patients with this disorder. As Chestnut Lodge is a private facility devoted to long-term, residential treatment, she was able to understand these patients in great depth, and she found them all to be struggling with severe, unresolved ambivalence. "They could not stand to be aware of their hostility against beloved persons; therefore they unconsciously tried to keep this hostility repressed, and finally expressed it by the physical symptoms of migraine." One patient, for example, recognized that she felt "guilty of treason" and developed a headache each time she did not totally agree with one of her mother's ideas or resented one of her mother's decisions. (This patient was eventually able to use this insight to abort migraine attacks during the analytical hour.)

Fromm-Reichmann asks, and then tries to answer, two questions: "Why is the ambivalence so intense?" and "Why is it expressed through the head?"

With regard to the first question, she found that her migraine patients

came from very cultured and somewhat conventional old families with a particularly strong solidarity within the family and a highly developed family pride. Within groups like these aggression against each other is, as we know, extremely taboo. If one member of these families should dare to express hostility against another he would be punished by exclusion, that is to say by losing the protection of his family background, which means being abandoned in the struggle of life. This fear of punishment by being deprived of the family's protection was rather decidedly the fundamental reason for repressing hostility in all my migraine patients (From Fromm-Reichmann F: Contribution to the psychogenesis of migraine. *Psychoanal Rev* 24(1):26–33, 1937, © 1937, Human Sciences Press, New York.)

In contrast to the temporary, suppressed, or only superficially repressed aggressiveness she saw in other patients, she states: "I have the impression that migraine always seems to be one specific expression of deeply repressed, continuous hostility against beloved persons. . . ."

Fromm-Reichmann concluded that it was the intensity of the vengeful feelings and of their destructive unconscious aims which strongly motivated the migraine patient to repress his hostility, as its recognition might disable the wished for relationship. In addition, she observed her migraineurs to be "refined above the average," and therefore, decided that they also repressed anger because "their sensitive conscience could not bear to realize it."

One of her patients illustrates these themes with the following verbatim account:

We were raised with the law: 'we family members belong together and love each other' as if that was the eleventh commandment, and when a child, unconsciously obeyed this law very strictly. However, as I note today, I secretly hated my mother with all my heart because of her enormous family pride and especially because of one fundamental proof of it she gave me: she would not take care of me when I was ill because her family vanity made her imagine that no family member ought to be ill at any time. But she heartily enjoyed taking care of invalid persons who were not family members. We children had to help her at that job. Consciously I admired mother's procedure very much; however, I became secretly furious whenever I had to pay a visit to one of her proteges, and I regularly came home with a migraine attack (Fromm-Reichmann F: Contribution to the psychogenesis of migraine. *Psychoanal Rev* 24(1):26–33, © 1937, Human Sciences Press, New York)

The conservatism and power of many of these patients' families may have been greater than usual due to the costs of being treated at Chestnut Lodge. Yet her basic observation, that aggression was taboo and punished by exclusion, has been replicated by other investigators in other populations.

Her second question, "Why the use of the head?", runs into problems which can be anticipated from its very phrasing. Such a question is appropriate for a conversion reaction, where the target organ or function is "chosen" for unconscious and symbolic reasons; the question should not even be asked about a psychologically influenced physical disorder like migraine, where any symbolism is apt to have only been tagged on later.

Her patients were competitive, and valued intellect. She hypothesized that in their fantasies they wished to destroy their competitor's intellect, along with its concrete symbol, the head. Guilt about this impulse and expectation of "an eye for an eye" (talion law) retribution, made them instead turn this aggression towards themselves. The ensuing headache punished the forbidden impulse with a cruel but specific justice.

We should view this last hypothesis critically. Although such fantasies may be more common in migraineurs, it is probably due to their understandably added attention to the symptomatic head and to their frequently competitive natures. The relationship of the fantasy to the headache is unlikely to be causal. Still, these mistakes do not obviate Fromm-Reichmann's more accurate insights.

HAROLD G. WOLFF: DISRUPTED DUTY

In the same year that Fromm-Reichmann publisher her findings, Wolff published the now classic article "Personality Features and Reactions of Subjects with Migraine" (25). Chapter 13 has already described his observations on personality features common to the migraineur. This section, in contrast, will cover his observations of what triggers individual attacks. He saw two overall patterns. In the first, the patient lives in a state of unremitting tension which, without the impingement of obvious incidents, gets punctuated by headache. In the second, and far more common pattern, this same tension exists as a backdrop against which headaches are initiated by sudden intensifications of mood in the direction of excitement, anticipation, joy, anger, resentment, disappointment, surprise, horror, or even by severe or prolonged effort.

Wolff sidesteps hypothesizing a sequence of psychodynamic events leading up to a migraine attack. Yet his detailed description of events that might precede one gives clues to how he viewed that progression.

These are what he observed to be specific migraine triggers.

Relations to Parents. Tension and other negative emotions in the context of contact with the parents often triggered headache. One married woman experienced severe homesickness each time she wrote to her mother, and afterwards would develop headaches. Another would develop attacks shortly after she answered the scolding letters of an overbearing and disgruntled father whom she had been supporting for years. She described herself as answering his letters with a mixture of strong resentment and loyalty.

Social Relations. The mere anticipation of social intercourse frequently triggered anxiety related to the thought of meeting new and perhaps unsympathetic persons. Some patients tried to cope with this common precursor by only arranging social contacts on the "home field," where they felt more secure.

Reaction to Bodily Inadequacies. Failure to adjust to real or perceived physical inadequacy increased the frequency and intensity of attacks. The most characteristic attitude towards these inadequacies was intolerance.

Time Bound Factors. Most people accommodate to days when they are not up to their usual self, lack energy, motivation, and "oomph," by expecting less of themselves; the migraineur does not, and his refusal often triggers a headache. They showed an unwillingness to bow to these low points in their energy cycles. The patient who was invariably less efficient on Mondays would drive himself to the same standard of performance that applied on Thursday—and predictably spent Monday evening in a bed in a darkened room.

Fear of Failure to Excel. The fear, not just of failure but of failure to excel, precipitated some attacks.

Ambition and Frustration in Work. Ambitiousness often made work a centerpiece in his subjects' life styles. Frustrations related to the work place, especially situations that interfered with the satisfaction of fulfilling responsibilities, were particularly difficult.

Added Responsibility. In contrast, it was sometimes added rather than reduced responsibility that increased the frequency and severity of attacks. The increased responsibility could come from external sources, but equally often came from self-imposed, perfectionistic standards. One conscientious military officer regularly experienced headaches when it was his turn to be "officer of the day."

Hurry. Apprehension that it might be impossible to finish a project in time, or that time pressures would force a job to be done incompletely, was a precipitant.

Any Sudden Letup in Pace. Any change of program leading to a slacking off of tension, release from discipline or restraint, or "letdown" could initiate a headache. The first days of vacation, for example, especially when preceded by the strain of preparation and packing, would frequently be disrupted by migraine.

Criticism. Criticism—and even just the anticipation of criticism—commonly provoked attacks.

Resentment. Sustained resentment predisposed to episodes of migraine.

Apprehension and Despair. Either state might start or worsen attacks in certain subjects.

By mentally telescoping these triggers that Wolff identified, a pattern—even, perhaps, a meaningful sequence—emerges. This process paints the picture of a person insecure with parents and peers, trying to overcome this state by extreme self-discipline and hard work; he is intolerant of the roadblocks to such a performance imposed by his body's limitations, and attempts to overcome those limitations by not honoring them. This adaptation can be derailed by circumstance (job gets finished, job becomes too difficult to do perfectly, time off interrupts completion of job), or by interpersonal factors such as criticism. The failure of these defenses again brings him face to face with his original resentment, insecurity, and sadness, and culminates in a migraine.

HERMAN SELINSKY: FAULTY BIOLOGY

Two years after Wolff's publication, Selinsky (26) synthesized his own evaluations of 200 migraine patients, and portrayed attacks from a biological perspective. The theoretical position he espouses, though common to thinking of the time, today might be considered on the border between the bold and the exotic. He noted that organisms constantly seek to strike a balance between the push of their inner desires and the restraints of their environments. He calls up the image of an amoeba attempting to master an object in its path, first by engulfing and incorporating it but, should the object prove noxious, by ejecting it.

The following explanation is then proffered: "As a psychobiological phenomenon the migrainous attack represents an attempt to eject, reject, and withdraw . . ." Migraine symptoms "express dramatically the fearful helplessness and frantic effort to reject something offensive and insufferable to the ego of the subject. . . ." He considers migraine a physiological expression of the "riddance urge." Vomiting and the forced retreat from light and people are examples of phenomena he cites as evidence.

But what is the patient trying to rid himself of? Selinsky states that migraine represents "an inhibitory reaction to an aggressive impulse which permits the suffering subject to withdraw from the situation." Is it the provocative situation or the aggressive impulse that the patient is trying to reject? On this point, the theory is unclear.

In short, Selinsky views migraine as a faulty homeostatic protective device, neither desirable nor adequate, as is true of many biological mechanisms intended to protect, but the best the individual can muster given his physical limitations and psychological inhibitions. He admits that while one can be certain these biological principles are valid, one cannot have similar confidence about their relevance to migraine. To the extent that he is conceptualizing the rejection as symbolic rather than reflexive, we can instead be confident—for the same reasons that applied to some views of Fromm-Reichmann—that they are not.

WALTER ALVAREZ: THE LITTLE ENGINE THAT COULDN'T

Alvarez (27) studied 500 patients with migraine. In a style combining keen observation with Edwardian gentility, he reported that, despite an inherent delicacy of constitution, migraineurs always kept their engines at the strain, and because they overworked their delicate machinery it would frequently break down in headache. His basic thesis is that migraineurs have a definite, often instantly recognizable, physical constitution and characterlogical temperament. These two factors are typically at odds, leading to exacerbation. He describes migraine patients as alert, quick, and conscientious, yet also as overresponsive to strains that do not affect others and subject to becoming overtired. They nevertheless do not yield their "overcommitments to worthy enterprises." An excessive inner pressure to please others and to be liked, and a wish to "keep the peace at any price," are behind their inability to say no to unreasonable obligation, whether expected of them by the chairman of the Junior League or by their own conscience.

ARNOLD FRIEDMAN: AGGRESSIVE ENERGY MISMANAGED, ENERGY RESERVES DEPLETED

Many soldiers who returned from the Second World War suffering from headaches were seen at the Montefiore Hospital Headache Clinic, newly started at that time by Friedman. Soon thereafter (with von Storch and Merritt), he published an article (28) detailing physical and psychological observations of 2000 (subsequently expanded to 5000) migraine and tension headache sufferers. He found psychological factors were relevant to 90% of chronic headache patients. In ensuing decades, extensive publications have linked his name to both the physical and psychological aspects of headache. What did he observe about migraine? He states (29):

For a brief psychological characterization of a person with migraine, I would say that he has not successfully learned to handle aggressive energy, either his own or that of others, and that during his early years he was conditioned to value the approval of others more than his own.

Although he does not believe in a "migraine personality," he describes in migraine patients many characteristics ascribed to it by other authors. He finds, for example, that "a patient with migraine is generally intense, striving, orderly, overly conscientious, meticulous in performance, exacting in his requirements of others and himself, and tends to become immersed in a morass of detail" (29).

In his experience, the onset of migraine corresponds to times such as adolescence when, "with increasing responsibility and decreasing energy reserve a difficult way of life becomes harder to maintain." The individual attack usually "erupts in a setting of unconscious anger associated with sustained resentment, anxiety, and frustration in what may be thought of as a state of energy depletion" (29). "Clinically, the most frequently observed conflicts were those concerned with hostile and aggressive impulses of an intense and destructive nature. Some subjects developed the headache because they reached the limit of their capacities to tolerate their repressed or suppressed anger" (30).

In addition to hostile impulses, Friedman observed signs of unconscious guilt in migraineurs. He reminds his reader that pain can also function as self-punishment, and reflects upon the fact that in many rituals both primitive and modern, suffering and guilt are bedfellows.

Some characteristics of patients refractory to standard treatments are also delineated (30). First, more have a family history of migraine. Second, they show significantly less tolerance for emotional trauma, perhaps, he hypothesizes, due to unstable autonomic nervous systems. Third, they often display nonspecific personality disturbances, manifested by rigidity, heightened aggression, or sexual difficulties. Finally, "the most significant difference . . . is that in the refractory cases there is a pronounced deficiency in the mechanism whereby patients handle their aggression."

FRANZ ALEXANDER: BRAIN AS OVERLOADED SYMPATHETIC CAPACITOR

Alexander (31) was a pioneer of psychosomatics. He espoused the position that differing mental conflicts evoke correspondingly different physiological reactions; they thereby each potentiate different, yet specific, psychophysiological diseases. With migraine, Alexander believed the problematic conflict involved aggression that the patient not only needed to keep from reaching the stage of action, but also even from reaching the theater of consciousness. He detected analogous conflicts over aggression in hypertension and rheumatoid arthritis, and hypothesized that the level of physiological preparation for aggression at which the impulse is blocked differs in the three disorders.

Alexander reasoned that the migraine patient attempts to simply deny strong yearnings to be dependent and instead pushes to just get on with his life. To achieve this goal he strives to maintain an ongoing alertness. The continuous pressure to remain keen overstimulates his sympathetic nervous system. However, unconscious ambivalence over hostility interferes with adequate discharge of aggressive tensions that have built up in sympathetic nervous system channels. In a constitutionally predisposed individual, a migraine headache might result when a case-specific trigger opens the gates to this dammed up sympathetic energy.

JOHN R. GRAHAM: MIGRAINE AS RELUCTANT POLICEMAN

For over 50 years Graham has been gently encouraging medical practitioners to accept the notion that migraine cannot be understood or treated if taken out of the context of the patient's emotional, work, and family life. He sees the migraineur as having a characteristic temperament, one which only makes a good "fit" with certain life styles. Patients who get into serious trouble with migraine have usually not respected these constitutional liabilities. Everyone knows that if the shoe doesn't fit, yet one insists on wearing it, pain will ensue. The same is true for the limitations circumscribed by the genetics of migraine, actual attacks of which he has referred to as "the ticket which is given by nature's policeman for speeding" (32). In other words, "the biological meaning of the migraine attack is that this congenitally poorly equipped neurovascular system has been pushed beyond its limits of adaptation and needs a chance to recuperate." If this requirement for more compatible "pacing" is disregarded by the physician or "fixed" by his medicines, the "patient may not be learning to drive properly and to treat his machine with respect" (32). Though medications are useful, especially over the short term, they do not replace an insistence on proper reorganization of the way of life.

Graham suggests that a starting point for the consideration of migraine is its genetic underpinnings: "Since migraine may pursue an individual from the cradle to the grave, many features that have in the past been considered its etiology must be limited to consideration as trigger mechanisms only," the female hormonal cycle being one such example.

His position is captured in the following quote (32):

This is the anchor to which all other theories should be tied—namely, that the migrainous individual is genetically ill-equipped to deal with a number of stimuli from the external or internal environment, with the result that symptoms develop when proper adaptation cannot be made. This inadequacy may be great or little depending on inheritance, and will be revealed to greater or lesser extent according to the demands placed upon this inadequate system by life's varied exigencies which call for its action and find it more or less wanting. Some individuals, by virtue of a particularly driving or perfectionistic personality may place frequent and severe demands upon this deficient system, and thus create more frequent and severe illness. Here again, their personality is not the fundamental cause or specifically related to the disease but merely an attribute which serves to accentuate the underlying genetic defect (From Graham JR: Migraine: clinical aspects. In Vinken PJ, Bruyn GW (eds): *Handbook of Clinical Neurology.* Amsterdam, North-Holland Publishing Co., Elsevier Science Publishing Co., Inc., Biomedical Division, 1968, pp. 45–58.)

However far one's theoretical wanderings in the field of migraine lead, it is always reassuring to have as a fall back position the common sense perspectives of John Graham.

RICHARD HUNTER: SIMPLE PSYCHOTHERAPY FOR THE RECALCITRANT PATIENT

In 1960, Hunter (33) published his psychological observations of 35 medically recalcitrant migraine patients treated in psychotherapy. He stated that they all, "gave the impression of having some disturbance or unhappiness in their lives," and that this was found to be due to something other than the headaches. Psychological disturbances were seen to relate to migraine in one of three ways: (*a*) The very first migraine attack followed an emotional trauma. (*b*) Acute psychological factors precipitated a series of headaches. (*c*) Chronic emotional difficulties persistently aggravated existing migraine.

Most of these patients were helped to have significantly fewer headaches, psychiatric symptoms, and medication usage when he treated them with a straightforward and largely supportive psychotherapy. Interestingly, he found that

Improvement was not related to new or additional drugs since none were given; indeed, the best results were obtained in those who finally took minimal or no drugs at all, even during attacks.

MELITTA SPERLING: PREGENITAL REGRESSION, OMNIPOTENT RAGE, NARCISSISTIC GRATIFICATION

The somewhat convoluted theoretical position taken by Sperling (34) places great emphasis on the role of unconscious fantasies in the genesis of migraine. She considered that all 24 migraineurs she analyzed possessed "pregenital character structures" (which is to say, formed before the oedipal stage at age 5). Indeed, she viewed all "psychosomatic diseases" as representing "the expression and fulfillment of specific fantasies and impulses of a pregenital nature." The specific fantasy that accompanies each illness varies, however; with migraine she envisions the following sequence in the unfolding of an attack:

In migraine the basic similarity in them [the fantasies] is that they deal in various ways with attacks on the head. The situation which precipitates a migraine attack represents to the patient a situation of complete helplessness. In the psychosomatic patient, such a situation leads to an instant, transitory regression to the level of primary narcissism. On this regressed level he deals with the (traumatic) situation omnipotently. The psychosomatic patient establishes omnipotent control by mobilizing the somatic channels for instant wish fulfillment and for the discharge of rage . . .

In other words, a migraine represents an acute attempt to reinforce the repression of a dangerous aggressive impulse which, by means of the head pain, is at the same time partly discharged and gratified in unconscious fantasy.

While some of her insights are valuable, one has the feeling that it is constantly necessary to separate the wheat of insight from the chaff of overinterpretation, as they are both presented to the reader quite definitively.

PAUL JONCKHEERE: THE COCOONS OF FURY

Jonckheere (17) found that migraineurs lived their lives "in a state of permanent tension" with one or several key individuals. The basic cause of the tension was repressed anger. These relationships echoed ones in childhood between the patient and a domineering parent. Eleven of sixteen migraine patients were both obsessional and aggressive. Their headaches were helped when the aggression could be ventilated in psychotherapy. His work is described in greater detail in Chapter 5.

LAWRENCE KOLB: THE CONSEQUENCES OF "SHUNNING"

Kolb (35, 36) reports that migraineurs typically come from achievement-oriented fami-

lies in which direct expression of anger is punished by temporary exclusion from the family's affections. He notes that with careful questioning one will obtain accounts of actual, as well as fantasized, rejection or attack by significant people in the patient's life. These are situations to which the migraineur sometimes reacts with fantasies of destructive retaliation.

He further states that:

If one looks at the repetitive situations in which these headaches occur and their psychological, emotional significance to the particular individual, it is usually apparent that they are always related to the arousal of hostility (35).

In addition, Kolb describes the critical import of an overdeveloped superego to the character of many migraine-prone individuals. It is only with difficulty that the moral dictums of that superego can be modified by later experience. Given this family background and the strong impulses that need to be checked from within, it is easy to see how such a tyrannical superego might flourish.

When the developmental process is such that gratification is provided only upon conformity to the wishes of others or when it comes only with the suppression of such feelings as those of fear, anger, rage, love, or sexuality, the basis is laid for a rigid, self-demanding personality in adulthood—they [migraine patients] are generally incapable of expressing their feelings as a means of obtaining the respect and affection of others. Therefore they tend to repress all emotional expressions and desires (36).

Kolb also points out that early developmental influences cause the future migraineur to develop a particular attitude towards his body—an attitude of shame and inadequacy, as though he had an "inherent defect." This has unfortunate implications for his ability to later adapt to physical illness.

A.R. FURMANSKI: PROJECTED AMBIVALENCES; SUBLIMATED IMPULSES

A surprisingly comprehensive and underreported study was published by Furmanski (37) in 1952. The study is based on his evaluation of 100 migraineurs—an uncommon number, considering that he is a psychoanalyst. He presents a dynamic view of the psychological and developmental issues involved in migraine, focusing on how and why specific impulses and defenses are synthesized into a character structure typical for migraine.

Psychologically influenced migraineurs are seen to have areas of difficulty throughout the spectrum of pregenital issues. His study sorts these out in a way that shows which attributes can be traced to which stages, needs, and defenses.

Most of what he describes has been mentioned before: repressed resentments, yearning for closeness, sublimations, reaction formations, and compulsivity, for example. Also this: guilt over the aggressive impulse is allayed by excessive work, a desire to serve others, to give to others, and to be altruistic. Also noted: the search to acquire sumbolic substitutes for love. Also: in superego formation the following must be considered:

Hostile feelings of the child are projected onto the parents. Even a lenient parent may be considered severe by an ambivalent child. It is these distorted impressions of the parents that the child incorporates into his superego. This process makes the superego of an ambivalent person a forbidding, ultra-moral force, which has a powerful control of the ego's self-esteem (From Furmanski AR: Dynamic concepts of migraine. A character study of one hundred patients. *Arch Neurol Psychiatry* 67:23–31, Copyright 1952, American Medical Association.)

Thus it is more than just the parent, even more than just the child that must be considered. One must factor in the compatibility of child with parent, as a needy and sensitive child may be frustrated by a normal—but reserved or impatient—parent.

All in all, it is the only partially successful attempt by the migraineur to overcome a strong aggressive instinct with a strong impulse to find acceptance and love—and to be loving—that most lingers in Furmansky's mind when the words have fallen away.

SHERVERT FRAZIER: A TREATABLE DISORDER

Frazier published numerous articles on psychiatric features of migraine (38). His image of the migraine patient is similar in many respects to previous authors' views of the patients' developmental experiences and of their dynamic reactions to them. He emphasizes that when the flint of situational complexity is struck against the rock of characterological rigidity, the spark produced is that of anxiety—and it is not difficult to name the tinder or the fire of migraine!

Most importantly, though, is the strength with which he affirms that psychological contributions to migraine are often correctable through psychotherapy. He accomplishes this less by assertion than by example: he outlines a full and traditional psychodynamic treatment for migraineurs (39). And isn't that, after all, what we have all hoped to see at the end of this long theoretical journey?

CONCLUSION

We are now facing a challenge not unfamiliar to physicians or other scientists. It is to combine these many, partly overlapping ideas into a construct of migraine unified enough that it is useable, yet not so comfortably homogenized that it is formulaic. This is what we hope to stimulate in the next chapter.

REFERENCES

1. Hine FR, Werman DS, Simpson DM: Effectiveness of psychotherapy: problems of research on complex phenomena. *Am J Psychiatry* 139:204–208, 1982.

2. Adler CS, Adler SM: Pitfalls in the interpretation of psychometric testing of headache patients. *Cephalalgia* 5 (suppl 3):212–213, 1985.

3. Adler CS, Adler SM: Physiological feedback and psychotherapeutic intervention for migraine: a ten year followup. In Sjastaad O, Pfaffenrath V, Lundberg PO (eds): *Updating in Headache.* Heidelberg, Springer-Verlag, 1985.

4. Phillips C: Headache and personality. *J Psychosom Res* 20:535–542, 1976.

5. Lucas RN: Migraine in twins. *J Psychosom Res* 20:147–156, 1977.

6. Passchier J, van der Helm-Hylkema H, Orlebeke JF: Personality and headache type: a controlled study. *Headache* 24:140–146, 1984.

7. Cooper M, Friedman AP: An evaluation of Rorschach patterns in patients with headache symptoms. *NY State J Med* 54:3088, 1954.

8. Kaldegg A: Migraine patients: a discussion of some test results. *J Ment Sci Lond* 413:672, 1952.

9. Ross WD, McNaughton FL: Objective personality studies in migraine by means of the Rorschach method. *Psychosom Med* 7:73–79, 1945.

10. Timsit M: Rorschach movement responses, distortions and chronic headache. *Cephalalgia* 5 (suppl 3):240–241, 1985.

11. Kaplan HI, Freedman AM, Sadock BJ (eds): *Comprehensive Textbook of Psychiatry III.* Baltimore, Williams & Wilkins, 1980.

12. Arena JG, Andrasik F, Blanchard EB: The role of personality in the etiology of chronic headache. *Headache* 25:296–301, 1985.

13. Harrison RH: Psychological testing in headaches. A review. *Headache* 13:177, 1975.

14. Kudrow L, Sutkus BJ: MMPI pattern specificity in primary headache disorders. *Headache* 19:18–24, 1979.

15. Rogado AZ, Harrison RH, Graham JR: Personality profiles in cluster headache, migraine, and normal controls. *Arch Neurobiol (Madr.)* 37 (suppl):227–241, 1974.

16. Henryk-Gutt R, Rees WL: Psychological aspects of migraine. *J Psychosom Res* 17:141–153, 1973.

17. Jonckheere P: The chronic headache patient. A psychodynamic study of 30 cases compared with cardiovascular patients. *Psychother Psychosom* 19:53–61, 1971.

18. Liveing E: *On Megrim, Sick Headache, and Some Allied Disorders.* London, J. & A. Churchill, 1873.

19. Knopf O: Preliminary report on personality studies in thirty migraine patients. *J Nerv Ment Dis* 82:270–285, 400–414, 1935.

20. Tilney F: Headache and migraine. *Bull NY Acad Med* 6:69–88, 1930.

21. Crookshank FG: *Migraine and Other Common Neuroses.* London, Kegan Paul, 1926.

22. Weber H: The psychological factor in migraine. *Br J Med Psychol* 12:151, 1932.

23. Touraine GA, Draper G: The migrainous patient: a constitutional study. *J Nerv Ment Dis* 80:1–204, 1934.

24. Fromm-Reichmann F: Contribution to the psychogenesis of migraine. *Psychoanal Rev* 24:26–33, 1937.

25. Wolff HG: Personality features and reactions of subjects with migraine. *Arch Neurol* 37:895–921, 1937.

26. Selinsky H: Psychological study of the migrainous syndrome. *NY Acad Med Bull* 15:757–763, 1939.

27. Alvarez WC: The migrainous personality and constitution, the essential features of the disease: a study of 500 cases. *Am J Med Sc* 213:1–8, 1947.

28. Friedman AP, von Storch TJC, Merritt HH: Migraine and tension headaches: a clinical study of two thousand cases. *Neurology* 4:773–788, 1954.

29. Friedman AP: Psychophysiological aspects of headache. In *Phenomenology and Treatments of Psychophysical Disorders.* New York, Spectrum, 1982, pp 42–50.

30. Friedman AP, Merritt HH: Migraine. In Friedman AP, Merritt HH (eds): *Headache, Diagnosis and Treatment.* Philadelphia, F.A. Davis, 1959, pp 201–249.

31. Alexander F: *Psychosomatic Medicine: its Principles and Applications.* New York, W.W. Norton, 1950, pp 155–163.

32. Graham JR: Migraine: clinical aspects. In Vinken PJ, Bruyn GW (eds): *Handbook of Clinical Neurology.* Amsterdam, North-Holland, 1968, pp 45–58.

33. Hunter RA: Psychotherapy in migraine. *Br Med J* 1:1084–1088, 1960.

34. Sperling M: A further contribution to the psychoanalytic study of migraine and psychogenic headaches. *Int J Psychoanal* 45:549–557, 1964.

35. Kolb LC: Psychiatric and psychogenic factors in headache. In Friedman AP, Merritt HH (eds): *Headache, Diagnosis and Treatment.* Philadelphia, F.A. Davis, 1959, pp 259–298.

36. Kolb LC: Psychiatric aspects of treatment of headache. *Neurology* 13:34–37, 1963.

37. Furmanski AR: Dynamic concepts of migraine. A character study of one hundred patients. *Arch Neurol Psychiatry* 67:23–31, 1952.

38. Frazier SH: Complex problems of pain as seen in headache, painful phantom, and other states. In Arieti S, Reiser MR (eds): *The American Handbook of Psychiatry, Second Edition Volume 4.* New York, Basic Books, 1975, pp 838–851.

39. Frazier SH: The psychotherapeutic approach to patients with headache. *Mod Treatment* 1:1412–1424, 1964.

CHAPTER SIXTEEN

Psychodynamics of Migraine: A Developmental Perspective

CHARLES S. ADLER, M.D.
SHEILA MORRISSEY ADLER, Ph.D.

AN APPROACH TO THE PSYCHOLOGICALLY INFLUENCED MIGRAINE PATIENT

The naivete of overgeneralizing about psychological problems that spur migraine has been documented by many authors (1). They have described the psychological circumstances attendant to headache exacerbations, and have observed that these differ from person to person. Indeed, each migraineur is as unique as his thumbprint. They each are seen to have differing histories, differing life circumstances, and differing levels of successful functioning in love and in work. Any attempt to understand psychological influences on migraine is, of course, made difficult by this great variability in the individuals who have the disorder. In this, however, migraine does not differ from other illnesses in which psychological factors sometimes are important, and psychodynamic analysis of patients will still reveal certain common themes which apply to the diagnosis with greater than chance frequency.

When the physician can view the psychologically influenced migraineur from a developmental perspective, he is also enabled to consider the patient's way of life, including the parts that sometimes give him trouble, from the vantage point of adaptations laid down during the patient's upbringing. This allows the physician to consider the patient's way of life empathically, as a coping style forged to meet the stresses of our common world in as healthy and productive a manner as possible. It is from this empathic perspective that we have found the best treatment plans arise, gratifying to the physician, respectful of the patient, not evasive of the emotional aspects to the disorder and, most importantly, successful in helping the patient with both his headaches and with his overall satisfaction in life. Thus, the physician is able to see what it is that the migraine patient is trying to do, what about his ways of doing things are or are not successful to that end, and how some of these attempts lead to headaches.

There is in migraine what can seem, at first glance, to be a paradox: the contrast between the number of "psychological" adjectives which have been compiled and pondered about migraineurs, and their apparent successfulness despite such problematic psychiatric traits. These are often, after all, the very individuals we would select as our attorney, physician, accountant, or neighbor; indeed, a recent survey showed 21% of the British parliament are migraineurs. When we come around to seeing many of the problems these patients create for themselves as strengths gone awry, however, we can begin to appreciate this fact: the same characteristics which commonly account for the migraineur's successes may also account for his liabilities.

The migraineur is often high-strung and performance oriented. This is due in part to the genetics of an alert and sensitive nervous system; in many, it is also a consequence of the extremes to which the migraineur subjects that nervous system. He has likely cultivated an approach to living which pushes him to take on more than the average person. Often, he has tried to augment his behavioral and intellectual performance to earn praise from others and from his own superego. However, this pressured life style necessarily requires him to make compensatory cutbacks in areas of his life others would take for granted—for example, providing himself with sufficient sleep, or recreation, or release of emotion. Such needs have often been pushed aside so effectively for the sake of performance that even the migraineur may be unaware of their strength.

If, when pushing in one direction and cutting back in another, the migraineur feels pressured into ignoring the warning signals of his body and exceeds appropriate limits, his physiology typically gets set up for trouble. At this point he often encounters a backlash from these previously neglected needs, which now reassert themselves. When this occurs, the feelings are often strong from neglect, uncomfortable from unfamiliarity, or awkward and alternating from his lack of practice in dealing with them. One goal in helping the psychologically influenced migraineur is to allow him to become aware of both his striving motives and his neglected ones, of the two competing sides of this split in motivation, to claim ownership of both, and to feel pleasure from both. Yet, he must also learn to integrate them. It is when these alternate, or reach for their extremes, that the patient is

in greatest danger of exacerbating headaches.

The medical world should not be deceived into thinking that inapparent feelings are absent feelings, just as the patient himself needs to learn this. Eruption of the patient's feelings may trigger an attack of headache, but it is more commonly their acute suppression which elicits one.

In treatment, the physician must ally himself with the patient's pride in his real life accomplishments and with his wishes to have more of these. Yet, at the same time he must cautiously tread the line between empathy for the patient's pride and an uncritical acceptance of the demands of the patient's strident superego. Thus, in treatment the goal is not to remove the ways he has used to adapt, but to teach him how to supplement these. We wish to add things, not remove them—with the possible exception of a critical edge to the superego.

To truly appreciate the liabilities of the migraineur, therefore, one must also focus on his strengths, as they are part and parcel of the same thing. It is a corollary, and our experience, that to best treat his liabilities, one must do so from a base relationship which acknowledges and even utilizes his strengths.

As we have seen, frequently noted strengths include:

> high energy
> organizational capacities
> committment to thinking and planning things through
> active investment in activities and organizations
> committment to accomplishment
> alacrity
> responsibility

Yet, to treat the migraineur in a psychologically influenced headache exacerbation it is evident that we must also look squarely at the liabilities of his coping style, as it is these which have eventuated in problems. In so doing certain repetitive themes have been observed[1]: Anger or ambivalence towards loved ones; poor emancipation from home; the experience of self-sacrifice in close relationships; resentment which is unconscious; feeling burdened by responsibility in certain situations; overly strict superego; perfectionism; insecurity; rigidity; anxiety; lack of kindliness towards the needs of his body and intolerance of the restrictions imposed by its limitations; and an ambition to accomplish things. To this list we will add a theme frequently seen in our clinical practice, which we refer to as "pseudoprogression."

It has been our experience that the most common stressor for the psychologically influenced migraineur is this: *he is often unsure that he will be up to the task before him.* Despite the constant striving, at his back he ever anticipates the potential to not meet criteria, his own or those he expects from others. This feeling is intensified if the job has inherent ambiguity or must, by its nature, remain only partially solved. In turn, he often employs defenses and overcompensations which sometimes help, but which occasionally make matters worse. The key affect is anxiety, though it is generally inapparent.

A self-description (2) of the type of doubts routinely suffered by such a migraineur is found in the words of Russell Elkinton, M.D., who served as Professor of Medicine at the University of Pennsylvania and editor of the *Annals of Internal Medicine:*

Throughout my adult life, a major psychological stress stemmed, I believe, from my desire as a compulsive perfectionist to do well professionally while endowed with relatively modest abilities, i.e., I was playing under tension in the big league of academic medicine. Such tension must have contributed to lowering the threshold for my genetically determined migraine headaches.[2]

Thus, to fashion an effective treatment plan, one of the most important things to discover is why, in these generally competent and successful people, there exists beneath the surface this paradoxical anxiety. This leads to a discussion of the theme of pseudoprogression. In those patients who have used this defense and/or coping style, its recognition also helped us to make sense out of the riddle of anxiety.

Pseudoprogression basically refers to the behavioral, emotional, or cognitive consequences in the adult of his attempts as a child to mature too rapidly, either to escape certain pressures of his early environment, or to reap certain benefits which accompany precocity.[3] While it is easier to learn form than substance, to learn words than to learn their implications, doing so is not conducive to underlying feelings of confidence or security. It is the adult's remembered experience of facing tasks prematurely in childhood along with expectations of high performance which sets the tone for anxiety when facing similar situations in adulthood, even if the reality of the patient's capacity to do a more than adequate job is now no longer an issue.

To better appreciate the major psychological influences on migraine, we need to see how these are understandable within the context of certain aspects of the patient's developmental history, just as the embryologist must at times clarify the origin of an otherwise inexplicable medical condition. That is the purpose of what follows. It will be followed by a discussion of common psychodynamic

---

[1] These themes usually relate to, and sometimes amplify, each other. Many of these terms also need subtle refinements to catch accurately the flavor of how what is seen in the migraineur differs from what is seen in other patients to whom these same terms might be applied.

[2] At this point in the paper, its coauthor, John R. Graham, M.D., added this: "(In the second author's opinion, the patient's view of himself and his accomplishments is an unduly modest one. It is important to record, however, since it reveals his own opinion and concerns.)"

[3] Similar observations have been made in other conditions, such as with victims of child battering. However, the concept has not been previously applied to migraine, and it further appears that the tone of this adaptation differs considerably in the different disorders in which it may be manifested. Clarifying exactly how it differs will not be attempted in this chapter.

themes seen in the psychologically influenced migraineur.

The reader should keep in mind that while our theorizing in this section is based on careful observation, it is only a current gathering point of knowledge. We invite the reader to add his own observations to what will surely bear revising by, in Heberden's (3) words, "a more enlightened posterity."

THE MIGRAINE PATIENT AND THE LIFE CYCLE

Although this section refers to dynamics frequently seen in the psychologically influenced migraineur, we are not implying that these are universal in migraineurs or necessary for migraine. Rather, they are psychodynamic constellations which, as Graham (1) has pointed out, wreak particular havoc on the migraine constitution, and so are seen more often in problematic or intractable patients.

CONSTITUTION

"Constitution" is the starting point for considering migraine. The home environment of the migraine patient is alone insufficient to fully account for his developing this disorder. A genetic predisposition is a necessary condition for psychodynamic factors—or any other factors—to trigger migraine.

The findings of Ottaviano and Guidetti (4) dramatically underscore this point. In an interesting prospective study, these researchers tested 1184 neonates for reactivity to standard stimuli of various types: light, heat, hunger, pain, noise, etc., and selected out 95 who scored in the highest, or "hyper-sensitive," range. Such an infant might react with a Moro response and crying to the same pinprick which caused most neonates to only retract their legs. These infants were then neurologically reevaluated several times a year for at least 10 years, and were compared to a control group ($N = 85$) selected from the normally reactive children. At the end of the

study, certain illnesses and symptoms were found in the hyper-reactive children to a significantly greater extent than in the controls, but none was more unequivocal than idiopathic headache and unexplained bouts of stomach pain (as seen in childhood migraine): 56% of the hyper-reactive subjects developed such headaches, compared to 2.5% of the controls. Although it remains an open question whether a genetic predisposition is a sufficient as well as a necessary condition for migraine, this study seems to affirm that a physiological predisposition is critical to migraine. Our attention should now focus on determining which things make it symptomatically manifest and which things keep it dormant—as was the case in 44% of the temperamentally "hyper-reactive" children.

One way to discover when problematic traits frequently described in adult migraineurs first appear is to review psychological traits seen in children with migraine.

With these observations in mind we will now direct our attention to the home environment of the child.

HOME AND CHILDHOOD

EARLY ENVIRONMENT

Several psychiatrists with extensive experience treating migraineurs have described their impressions of the home environment of the child who eventually develops migraine. Kolb (5) stated that:

Parents are remembered as undemonstrative in their feelings towards the child with firm and demanding discipline.

Frazier (6) notes that these children:

Come from families who take great pride in attainment, follow rigid forms of behavior, and deny the expression of direct or verbal aggression. Because such families punish those who defy these standards by excluding them from the family group any feelings of resentment or hostility towards the parent or another close person tend therefore to be deeply rejected or

TABLE 16.1

SOME REPRESENTATIVE DESCRIPTIONS OF PERSONALITY TRAITS OBSERVED IN CHILDREN WITH MIGRAINE

AUTHORS	OBSERVATIONS
Bille (24)	Migraine children exhibited a more restrained, deliberate, and perfectionistic attitude . . . the children . . . admitted more symptoms indicating manifest anxiety, tension, and nervousness than the control children . . . The migraine children were rated by their parents as more anxious and apprehensive than the control children but also more sensitive, less physically enduring, more tidy, and more vulnerable to frustration . . . temper tantrum . . . was found to be more common . . . Conflicts at school or home, anxiety, disappointment, or other mental stress were given by every third child as some of the most common attack-provoking factors. . . . tests [were] one of the five most common attack-provoking causes.
Wolff (12)	Delicate, shy, withdrawn, obedient to desires of parents; sober, polite, well-mannered; did school work conscientiously; in contrast, displayed unusual stubbornness or inflexibility in certain situations; sometimes even obstinate, argumentative, or disobedient; occasionally had temper tantrums when frustrated or pushed; not pugnacious as children, not "hoodlums" as adolescents; preferred to set their own pace; trustworthy, energetic, respected, admired; given special responsibilities and special privileges at an early age. Exceptional attachment to mother sometimes, but not universally noted; took good or even excessive care of toys; lockers were kept in order; neat and clean all day; difficult for them to part with toys of the past.
Graham (1)	Feeding problems and colic in infancy; motion sickness as a small child; recurrent bouts of abdominal pain and vomiting in the school years related to highly stimulating experiences of either a pleasant or an unpleasant sort.
Knopf (10)	Sensitive; shy, unable to make friends easily; ambitious, resentful, jealous; worried and cried easily; unusually high marks in school; ambition noted in other areas as well (such as pride in never missing school or being independent of men); same ambition also appeared among less educated patients; frequently heard the statement "I was always held up as an example to the other children."
Friedman and Merritt (21)	Psychodynamic mechanisms noted to play an important role even in migraine of young children. Above average in intelligence, sensitive to emotional and physical stress, numerous neurotic traits.

repressed, producing conflict with the associated anxiety.

He expands upon this theme in another publication (7):

As children (and this is especially true of first children) they are pushed to perform and produce beyond their capacity. This naturally heightens their feelings of inadequacy and frustration. Many migrainous patients seem to continually relive these early failures.

In a similar vein, Friedman (8) stated that:

The majority of our patients come from families with rigidly adhered to norms of behavior who place high value on achievement. Family members who defy or express conflict over behavioral standards are punished in subtle ways, and the rigidity of the family structure denies the patient a normal outlet for aggression and emotion. Thus conflict, with its associated anxiety over the inevitably emerging hostility, along with the pressure to conform to family standards so that the desired relationships may continue, triggers the headache.

Furmansky (9) found that 89% of 100 migraineurs considered one or both parents "strict in training and discipline." Eighty percent of these same patients saw one or both parents as undemonstrative of affection, and all but one patient had parents with one attitude or the other. Similar observations by other psychiatrists and neurologists are cited in Chapter 15.

These statements reflect what is commonly heard in practice: that the migraine-prone child often comes from an achievement-oriented family where his infractions of rules or direct expressions of anger are little tolerated, and cause him to be held in tacit disaffection and rebuke.

The earliest years of a child's life are in many ways the most demanding of a parent. Surely they are the most disruptive of schedules and the least flexible. During infancy, despite the pleasures of raising a child, there is the reality that one parent must be in constant attendance, and must subordinate other routines to feedings. In the "terrible twos," willful surges towards autonomy and stubborn battles for control are characteristic.[4] Between the ages of 2 and 4 the child first learns to accommodate frustrations and becomes acquainted with himself as an autonomous individual. He discovers that there are times when he can "be in charge of himself." However, he also needs to maintain good relationships with mother and dad, and so begins the process of learning when and how to internalize anger. This is the time when he first experiments with expressions of anger to discover just how far he can go. If he is punished harshly, erratically, or unjustly he may learn that it doesn't pay to show these feelings, and that it might be even better if he could learn not to have them. This is also the stage at which the child becomes aware of his emerging capacities. If he experiences too much pushing and urging to accomplish developmental steps, there is a risk that the foundations of self-doubt and shame may be laid down.

This is the description of a standard developmental struggle between parent and child. At a certain age, the child's desire for unfettered autonomy and control of relationships is normal. These desires eventually conflict with his competing needs for guidance, security, and approval. The frustration and doubt he feels as a result of this inner clash is a natural part of growing up. He must make choices.

Usually, the child overcomes this impasse by compromise: he yields many of his behaviors in the face of his parents' wisdom and authority, and in turn is allowed to express his true feelings. He is comforted by the recognition that his choices will expand as he grows. Yet this image of healthy childhood and normal development can go awry in many ways, and in the psychologically influenced migraineur it frequently does.

In the history of many patients who get into trouble with migraine, the "price" of a stable adaptation to parental expectations is that the child must make premature and unduly rigid compromises to maintain it. Migraine patients typically describe that children were not the central purpose around which their nuclear family was organized. Parents often had professional interests or active engagements elsewhere. When these patients describe their upbringing, there is frequently a sense that children were viewed as part of a team (the family) which was working towards some goal (or several), even if that goal is not

---

[4] Epigenetically, between ages of 2 and 4 a child's attention is typically directed to enteroceptive stimuli in an attempt to learn bowel and bladder control. This is a specific point of contact between interpersonal psychosocial factors and control of the autonomic nervous system's physiology, one of only a few such points in development. As such, it may be an important focus for development of psychologically influenced physical illnesses. Research in physiological feedback and self-regulatory techniques has shown that people can routinely learn to change the diameter of blood vessels by attention to enteroceptive stimuli. Because the developing migraineur primarily maneuvers through his world of expectations by using his intellect, he might also learn to dilate his cranial vasculature to that end. Thus he would get into a "thinking mode" to prepare himself to face interpersonal situations, with the physiology accompanying this mode including cerebral vasodilation. When he switches back out of the thinking mode due to frustration, to a surge of emotion replacing thought, to fatigue, or simply because the job he set out to do is now done, the rebound—and the headache—ensue. The formulation of this psychophysiologic mechanism is naturally speculative.

easily apparent: the children's enjoyment of childhood was usually not that goal, or at least not one of the primary ones. They were expected to pitch in and take responsibility at an early age, in a task-oriented fashion. Maximizing a talent of the child (e.g., tennis, piano) might have been one of those family goals. It need not have been the child's. While this philosophy typically will instill initiative and self-discipline in the child, it also has liabilities. Yet, the immediate difficulties are rarely high enough to preclude maintaining some sort of an equilibrium within the family structure.

For many of the parents described by migraineurs, some common child rearing situations are poorly tolerated. Case histories reveal the following picture: one or both parents of the future migraineur frequently has a domineering personality, yet secretly does not feel "up to" or even resents certain limitations and sacrifices involved in the raising of children. Especially burdensome are those requirements that oblige him to tolerate strongly differing opinions, heated emotion, delay, or ambiguity. The parent's impatience is intensified by those demands of parenthood that deplete his life style of some of its rhythm and order. In an attempt to quell these feelings, the parent may expect the children, especially the older ones, to assume chores and duties which are at times excessive.

Indeed, one or both parents frequently have a definite image of what a "good child" should be, and may possess little flexibility to modify that image in light of the actual youngster at hand. Many a future migraineur picks up this message from cues both overt and covert. One of the consequences of this is a pervasive feeling of insecurity. If the primary parenting figure is also a migraineur, as is common statistically, the child's insecurity may be generated by that parent's limited comfort with the vicissitudes of children's behavior and feelings, and by the child's long-term adaptations to this situation. In such a home atmosphere the migraine-prone child's normal wishes to be childlike conflict with his similarly normal strivings for security and praise; he channels his mental resources into reconciling these competing primary needs.

The resulting intrafamilial tension pressures the migraineur to internalize his parent's expectations of obedience and smooth functioning conformity. More than most, he winds up feeling sufficient security and self-esteem only if he tows the line. Thus he tries, usually with considerable success, to become serious, responsible, hard working, and dependable. To a degree, this effort has its desired effect, as it reduces the parent's impatience and may even cause him to be pleased or proud. The child may initially do this simply because it is expected of him and because it reduces tension; in time, however, he may conclude, though not necessarily consciously, that life will be easier if he can act "more grown up," as he feels he has to anyhow. And, as time continues, his motivation to be this way increasingly comes from the pleasure of mastery itself, and from the rewarding feedback of accomplishment.

The mechanism by which the child adapts to parental expectations includes his automatic repression of resentment about having to modify himself so much. If the parents also exert pressure to perform, both his frustration and resentment may be accentuated. He learns that to ensure feeling approved of, or even, at times, to simply claim sufficient positive attention, it is essential to embrace "the program" of being helpful and not being underfoot. Retaining his place in the family's favor is felt to be contingent upon his making these concessions to "the program" without apparent resentment and without much discussion about his yearning to play softball instead of Schubert.

These future migraineurs often expect punishment to include impatience, intolerance, or chilly criticisms, that lead to a feeling of condemnation or emotional isolation. They can especially anticipate this reaction to the type of childlike antics and stubborn behaviors that a rigid parent might consider "willful." The margin of safety before the parent's evident resentment is reached often seems narrow.

SIBLINGS

Some migraineurs relate that when a sister or brother was born, the older child was expected to help with many routine childcare responsibilities. This gave further impetus to identify with parental attitudes. On occasion, sibling rivalry (10) resulted from competition for positive parental attention which was in short supply relative to the children's needs or wishes for it. Competition appears to increase when the amount of attention available is experienced as too meager to be shared. This is one factor which can contribute to a child's striving "to be the best" in later life.

Knopf (10) observed that migraine is more frequent in the oldest or youngest child of a family. She noted that the eldest daughter in the family is typically expected to assume a high level of responsibility for household chores, which may include escorting and monitoring the younger children. Knopf believed that this stimulates pleasure at wielding authority, and a desire for similar authority and "prestige" later in life. Nevertheless, the role of "deputy mother" may itself cause "greater mental strain." Conversely, the youngest child often has a prolonged childhood, which also exacts submissiveness and eventual resentment. Having a sister as a "second mother," with her childlike bossiness, jealousies, and pretensions, as well as her inevitable ambivalence about the role, can contribute to these resentments. Accordingly, in therapy it is often beneficial to review the relationship between the older siblings, and the migraineur.

ADOLESCENCE

It should be remembered that adolescence is the time in anyone's life when one is faced with the anxieties of puberty and all that it engenders—decision making about one's education, and career choices—which will significantly affect one's future. Adolescence and early adulthood are difficult times for many migraineurs, which perhaps contributes to the frequent inception of headaches at this time.

Touraine and Draper (11) remind us that it is at this age that the patient must first leave home and stand alone as a responsible adult. Flexibility, compromise, and even intimacy are suddenly expected by many, and in a range of situations. The tacitly accepted compromises that united and stabilized the family now must be renegotiated with new individuals. This is a task everyone must undertake. If, however, the compromises that bound the adolescent's immediate family were rigid, as is typical for the migraineur, he will often be distressed if he finds outsiders are unwilling to interact on the basis of them. Wolff (12) observed adolescents with migraine to be unusually preoccupied with moral and ethical problems, and likely to be disappointed if their peers did not share in these preoccupations.

Many of the compromises to be negotiated at this and subsequent stages—with the new boss, the new mate, the new baby—are important and cannot be avoided or absolutely determined in black-and-white terms. Emotions must be shared, and to do so meaningfully, old authoritarian protocols rarely suffice.

ADULTHOOD

Major transitions throughout the life cycle, even expected ones, can disrupt equilibria and trigger periods of increased headache activity. These include leaving for college, starting work, changing jobs, getting married, moving, becoming a parent, and retiring. Not surprisingly, *unexpected* life crises, such as the death of a relative or being fired, can also precipitate a string of headaches.

PARENTING

As one might glean from the discussion of childhood, for many migraineurs the responsibilities of childrearing often have greater potential to cause distress than they do for others. This is particularly true if the child is "difficult," delinquent, contentious, or for some other reason stimulates in the patient increased anxiety and resentment about the parenting role. This is sometimes covered over with a reaction formation, in which the patient appears energetically devoted to his children and too concerned with their welfare. Though they want to be good parents, and in many ways are excellent ones, it is common to find deep resentments and anxieties about the task surfacing intermittently.

WORK

As mentioned earlier, work is one setting where the insecurities engendered by not feeling "up to the task" are often stimulated. On the job, patients are constantly being challenged with new projects which they are trying to meet under the watchful eyes of peers and superiors. Anxiety is accentuated when the patient's level of ambition is high. Often, the better the patient's performance, the more he is asked to perform—sometimes setting up a vicious cycle, especially if he finds requests difficult to refuse. Occasionally, the migraineur will unconsciously avoid promotion, and in this way set up things to protect himself from still greater insecurity. Many jobs, especially ones at the executive level, are not amenable to arranging in the types of routines and time schedules that can be set up for home and leisure activities.

Russell Elkinton, M.D., in collaboration with John R. Graham, M.D., recently published a study (2) outlining the variations in his own migraine symptomatology over 45 years. During this period he not only practiced academic medicine as a university department chairman, but also served many years as chief editor of the *Annals of Internal Medicine*. He was "dubious, indeed indignant" when it was first suggested to him that emotional and mental tensions might be relevant to his attacks of migraine. Therefore, he decided to score his days of tension per week to compare it with a daily "headache score." He ascertained that 89% of all headaches oc-

curred on a day of tension or on the succeeding one. He also observed that a changing threshold for initiation of migraine allowed some days of tension to be unaccompanied by headaches (see Fig. 16.1).

SATISFACTION IN MARRIAGE

Problems of childhood that remain unsolved are often recapitulated in marriage; the migraine patient's life is no exception to this phenomenon.

Psychologically influenced migraineurs caught in unsatisfactory marriages often strive to maintain them nevertheless. They frequently construct rather formal marriages, ones in which an ambivalent preoccupation with obligations interferes with intimacy, even if the general tenor of the relationship is loving.

Knopf (10) states that "the same overweening ambition may be seen when we look at the basic martial difficulties." Touraine and Draper (11) observed that female migraineurs usually choose a somewhat passive mate, frequently an old acquaintance, and that marriage itself is commonly viewed as a matter of expediency. Wolff (12) saw marital and sexual problems as further expressions of migraineurs' frequent inability to adapt. In particular, he reported that they were often resentful when the marriage partner couldn't be forced into desired attitudes, manners, and customs, or when life situations impinging on the marriage would not bend to arbitrary standards.

Featherstone and Beitman (13) concluded that "daily common migraine appears to be a marker of marital dysfunction" after finding that only 17% of 40 married patients with "daily common migraine" (in which one would suspect a tension headache component) responded to prophylactic medications, while fully 71% of the unmarried ones were helped by this same treatment.

When headaches can be traced to marital problems, we have often seen female patients marry domineering husbands by whom they then feel trapped and intimidated, re-

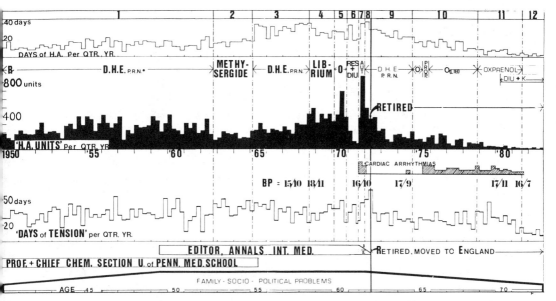

Figure 16.1. *Thirty-three years of headache data recorded over 12 periods of treatment during the years 1950–1982. DHE p.r.n., dihydroergotamine, as necessary; Res & Diu, resperpine 0.1 mg daily, hydrochlorthiazide 25 mg daily; O, no drug treatment; Aut, autogenic exercises; Prop, propranolol; Lib, librium; Oxprenol, oxprenolol; DIU + K, diuretic + potassium (taken for mild hypertension). (From Elkinton JR, Graham JR: Forty-five years of migraine—observations and reflections "from the inside" by a physician-patient. Cephalalgia, 5:187–195, 1985.)*

sponsible for, and furious at. Such a patient may speak of her husband in hushed tones with a mixture of awe, fear, and disdain. The husband's behavior often resembles that which the patient remembers in a dominant parent. Headaches sometimes follow the husband losing his temper or threatening to do so. Although she may be frightened by her husband's irritability and defer to him outwardly, she rarely bends to understand or compromise with him. Sometimes when the patient feels trapped and victimized a talk with husband and children yields another impression: a strong willed and controlling wife—the family turnkey.

Another frequently seen pattern is this one: the patient grows increasingly disappointed in her partner's lack of ambition, withdraws respect, disdains affection, and becomes resigned to either resentful endurance or divorce. The marriage partner has not lived up to expectations which, though similar to those by which the patient judges herself, are excessive.

Although there seem to have been fewer studies about male migraineurs in marriage, Wolff (12) reported that they often anticipated being catered to by their wives, although this wish may be hidden under a superficial bossiness. For example, he noted that the male migraineur, in spite of outwardly aloof behavior, would frequently insist that his wife "fuss over him" when he was indisposed with headache. Wives of these men sometimes reported feeling like they had "another dependent child."

Marriage can also provide the migraineur with an environment which facilitates his neutralizing negative childhood experiences and, in the comfort of his new family, allows him to stretch and grow. Such a marriage is conducive to a healthy maturation which mitigates the headache predisposition.

SEX ROLES, GENDER ROLES

It is not hard to imagine that if one lives with repressed anger, or habitually tries to shelter himself from intense feelings, a sudden openness to tender emotions in the bedroom would be difficult if not threatening. The needs and satisfactions of the heart have been too long blocked, and the migraineur is unlikely to tinker with the lid of Pandora's Box for the sake of a transitory pleasure.

As with romance, sex is an appetitive behavior which entails a certain messy uncertainty and, when in force, insists that desire be in control, not reason. Such unpredictability can put the patient in a position where he risks coming under the spell of the sensate passions, or being rejected and falling prey to the dominance of other emotions, and these are circumstances which make many migraineurs apprehensive. Therefore, a common finding is that sexual adjustment is rarely trouble free. Sexual activity may also provoke reproach or the anticipation of reproach from a tradition-oriented family. Finally, by their very nature sexual needs put one in a position of depending on someone else for full gratification.

A different pattern emerges for men and for women. Wolff (12) sees the sexual difficulties as subordinate to migraineurs' generally inflexible standards and reduced spontaneity. He reported sexual dissatisfaction in four of every five women, found them to hold "inelastic" notions about sex, and to have infrequent sexual contact. Sexual relations were typically viewed as a "reasonable marital duty." Because the wives did not attach great importance to sex, problems here did not seem to interfere with an ostensible devotion to their mates.

Knopf (10) found that married women made a somewhat better sexual role adjustment than unmarried ones, but "not one became fully reconciled to it." Touraine and Draper (11) put it more bluntly: "A satisfactory adjustment in the sexual sphere is not found." Yet an alternate view is that of Furmansky (9), who found that "the majority of the migraine persons in the study were able to reach a mature sexual adjustment."

Wolff questioned whether, for a patient with a rigid personality, the female sex role

might not be harder to carry out than the male role. This difference could explain why sexual frequency among men is reported (12) to be more typical of societal norms. With men, excessive committment to work sometimes led to a reduced interest in sex.

Neither perversions nor overt homosexual behavior are common (9). Considering the traditional values, strong superegos, and diminished emphasis on libidinal sensations typically encountered in the patient with migraine, this finding is not surprising.

MENSTRUATION, PARTURITION, AND NONEROTIC SEX-ROLE ACTIVITIES

Patients commonly say that their parents showed closeness and approval in other than physical ways. Touching and signs of physical affection from the parents are reported to be diminished in the histories of migraineurs—male and female—compared to those of other patients.

Patients are often inadequately prepared for menarche as well as for dating and sexual decisions. Wolff (12) found that migraineurs frequently overreacted to the discomfort associated with menstruation. He noted that sexual information was generally acquired late "partly because of lack of interest and partly because of too great an embarrassment." Practically all of Knopfs' (10) patients had a distorted or inadequate concept of the female role; some had not been prepared for menstruation at all. In Selinsky's (14) study, women "almost uniformly resented being female and suffered a great deal during the menses."

Kolb (5) believed that the same threat of arousing hostility which triggers migraine in other circumstances also instigates attacks accompanying menstruation. He found that women whose migraine intensified during pregnancy or menopause showed rivalry towards men and an unwillingness to accept the feminine role.

One could speculate that menstrual migraine might be accentuated by an unwillingness to yield to the typically reduced capacity to accomplish things at this time. None of this should be taken to minimize the effect of hormonal shifts on the underlying threshold for an attack.

Wolff (12) describes fear of pregnancy among his patients, citing their reluctance to meet the limitations imposed by caring for a child. He also reports that these women are frequently unwilling to accept the loss of body form induced by pregnancy and "to make cutbacks in social and industrial life." Knopf (10), too, found this disinclination to have children.

MIDDLE AND OLDER AGE

There are existential considerations which can interfere with a patient being relieved of migraines after a certain point in midlife. He may have particular ambivalence about relinquishing them if crucial life choices have been based upon the disability of the chronic and unpredictable head pain—not having children, for example (15). If the clinician is alert to this theme its effect can often be mitigated through discussion.

It has been suggested (16) that when migraine diminishes with advancing years it may be because beneficial life experiences have modified the patient's personality or have reduced his repressed hostility. In addition, the responsibilities of parenthood decrease with age, and activities at work either become more predictable, or retirement intervenes. By middle age people also grow more competent at and familiar with work routines, while in older age there is a tendency for others to assume more "responsibilities." The role of grandparent is more casual than the role of parent. Finally, there is a reduction, biologically, of sexual and aggressive drive levels.

One problem for the older migraineur is this: he must deal with the problem of not having the same reservoir of energy with which to keep up fast-paced behavior patterns he has often established for himself, and which others now expect of him. Normal loss of energy in old age is a specific stressor affecting what many migraineurs rely on heavily to maintain their psychosocial equilibrium. Chronic illnesses that sap energies can have the same affect.

COMMON PSYCHODYNAMIC THEMES

These, then, are some of the salient areas of development in the life of the psychologically influenced migraineur to which the clinician should be alert. Perhaps one can observe that many developmental areas that prove troublesome are not obvious to anyone but the migraineur himself. He is often putting forth a diligent effort to be a stalwart citizen of the community, and is fulfilling many responsibilities.

In this section, we will look at various themes that appear with greater than chance frequency when, in the safety of the physician's office, the psychologically influenced migraineur describes his difficulties and begins to put his life in perspective.

In looking at a vast number of migraineurs (2000), Friedman et al (17) found that patients left childhood with "considerable insecurity with resulting tensions which are manifested in inflexibility, overconscientiousness, meticulousness, perfectionism, and resentment." As for refractory migraine, Friedman (8) found a pronounced deficiency in the mechanisms whereby patients handled their aggression. Although we have heard this particular theme echoed again and again, we would suggest that anger or aggression in the migraine patient is best understood when viewed in the context of other problem areas, such as lack of kindliness to the self, pseudo-progression, and insecurity, areas to which we will next direct our attention, both as to their manifestations and their clinical roots.

ANGER AND RESENTMENT

Anger is perhaps the most widely accepted influence on migraine. Nearly all theorists agree that trouble in managing it plays at least some role in many exacerbations. The anger is typically described as repressed. Situations that intensify anger frequently lead to headache periods; events in the patient's life which acutely threaten to release anger from the unconscious often trigger an individual attack.

To more fully understand the relationship between anger and migraine, several things should be pointed out:

The type of anger-producing situation which exacerbates migraine is specific: it is one in which the patient feels caught or trapped in a position from which he can neither extract himself nor adequately solve. Australians, in fact, have nicknamed migraine "trap headache" (16). This is further aggravated if the patient believes that even the feeling of anger is forbidden, and that he must not only suppress it but repress it. The circumstance in which these two factors are most likely to come together and lead to the sense of being "caught" is when anger is elicited in intimate or long-term relationships.

Emotions in long-term relationships are characteristically complex, and chronic resentment may thwart all of the patient's attempts to either solve or escape them. Such a feeling state is typically not an unfamiliar one for the migraineur. He commonly perceives that he had to repress anger "just to get along" in his family of origin. Thus, when an analogous circumstance arises in adulthood, the migraineur may be especially vulnerable. He may have thought that the trapped and angry state was left behind following the emancipation of reaching adulthood. But in certain situations it again reasserts itself, dredging up all too familiar resentments and defenses. Thus the anger-inducing conflict in adulthood reawakens memories of old resentments and feelings of helplessness; the anger is intensified by its resonance with those

memories; and old means of trying to cope with the situation are also revived.

Migraineurs are often portrayed as being secretly angry all the time. This image may be deceptive. Because migraine can be specifically triggered when the patient has significant repressed hostility towards a loved one, this is also the time that the headaches get worse and when the patient comes for treatment; but he may not harbor such anger at other times. Nevertheless, *there is a subgroup of recalcitrant migraineurs who are constantly angry,* who bear an abiding grudge. They may re-experience these feelings with a sequence of acquaintances, friends, and relatives, all of whom have become targets for negative transference.

Finally, the anger need not be unconscious to work its effect upon the extracerebral circulation. If the resentments are strong enough, and come on fast enough, headache may be initiated even if the anger is consciously accessible. This can be seen most clearly with those patients in psychotherapy who learn when and why they are feeling resentful, yet still can't, in all situations, calm themselves down enough to prevent an attack. In the long run, however, such insights characteristically do mitigate the migraine diathesis.

How does this anger usually get started?

As we have noted, anger is one part of the ambivalence that everyone occasionally has in response to the limits and frustrations inherent in growing up. Ideally, a child has some permission to express this anger appropriately, but then must also learn, over time, to understand its sources and to control it. In the future psychologically influenced migraineur, this normal anger is often blocked by his fear that expressing it will cause a palpable discomfort for the parents and elicit strict countermeasures. These measures may include the withholding of interest, approval, or respect—sometimes even interpreted as the withholding of love. More importantly, a child may fear exposing thinly defended anger in the parent if he becomes angry or disobedient. In the parents, the flexibility required to comfortably negotiate a child's anger may be lacking, and this is what makes disciplining a child so difficult for them. Thus, the future migraineur is less likely to develop an appropriate level of comfort with anger.

Ultimately, these contingencies in the home environment square off against the child's impulses and needs. He must learn to gratify his needs "within house rules." This means reducing or eliminating those irregularities, unpredictabilities, emotional outpourings, and defiant stances to which children are heir, while at the same time maximizing the image of family harmony, obedience, loyalty, helpfulness, successfulness, self-reliance, and maturity. Such "good behavior" also serves to draw mother (or father) back if they are in a hassled, disinterested, or critical mood—at least temporarily. It may even draw them closer—temporarily. Repeatedly making these concessions molds the youngster's personality in ways that allow his yearnings for acceptance to avoid clashing with more defiant elements in his nature.

If feelings of resentment the patient experienced as a child follow him into adulthood, they are likely to be repressed or, if too strong, taken over by his superego and redirected back toward the self. When this happens, the patient commonly experiences his anger disguised as guilt or depression. This dynamic is motivated by his fear of disrupting important relationships. A guilty depression may therefore arise partly from the psychological defense against aggressive impulses. Classical theory would explain this dynamic as being those same aggressive impulses turned against the self. If this defense breaks down, and the resentments threaten to emerge, a migraine may be in the works.[5]

---

[5] A useful insight in psychotherapy comes when the patient recognizes when and how often he feels anger, but also sees that now, as an adult, he can call upon powerful interpersonal "tools" to manage it. These tools were not present at the time the anger was originally banished.

By the time of adulthood anger is often still a problem. The patient has several reasons for overcontrolling it. First, it has been so long repressed, that he may find its strength difficult to gauge, which is disconcerting to him. Also, recognition of anger throws off the very equilibrium the patient relies upon to keep things going and, in particular, precipitates the interpersonal disharmony he is constantly trying to ward off.

Resentment, then, is the most typical form of anger, and the potential for poorly managed resentment is more typical than its omnipresence. Trouble handling anger may be more problematic than its quantity. Finally, it is usually the underlying situation which is causing the anger, rather than the angry emotion *per se*, which needs to be focused on in treatment.

AMBIVALENT ATTITUDE TOWARD THE SELF—LACK OF KINDLINESS AND TOLERANCE

Another common observation of psychologically influenced migraine patients is: they do not always treat themselves well by traditional standards. Sometimes the patient will express this directly, perhaps with some bitterness, and blame it upon an unalterable crush of responsibilities. At other times it is simply evident to the physician as the patient describes his day-to-day activities: the lack of leisure time, the bowing to the needs and expectations of others, the skipped meals and late nights at the office, all of which puts him at risk for a migraine attack. Good work may be accomplished by this frenetic pace, yet the benefits often seem to be for others, and frequently at a cost to the patient, ranging from irritation to headache.

The physician may be slightly perplexed by the intransigence of this pace; even those patients who acknowledge how distressing it is rarely heed the physician's reasonable advice to slow down, to cut back, to delegate responsibilities, or to say "no." In these commitments, the patient seems to allow his own desires and the welfare of his body to be put last. In part this is a conscious tradeoff for accomplishment. But a portion of what appears "voluntary choice" may be less so than the patient believes, as it is primarily driven by anxiety and superego. Even when he agrees that he should make cutbacks, an anxiety intrudes which prevents its actualization, and he instead finds some eminently plausible "reason" to keep pushing.

There are many reasons for this life style, some sounder than others. And to understand why someone would choose this *modus vivendi* we must look at identification, superego, and self-sacrifice.

Many a future migraineur, discomfited by feelings that push him towards behavior he expects will displease, controls these feelings by identifying with a parent. The child incorporates parental expectations as he sees and interprets them, not always correctly, and sometimes in the midst of fear. By the time he is an adult he is still unlikely to have reappraised these expectations in a less pressured atmosphere, or to have selected characteristics sympathetic to his own wishes and reflecting a reasonably clear perspective on the outside world. As a result, the patient's superego may become as rigid and demanding as his inner image of a parent seen through a child's eyes. In many ways this resolution works hummingly: if the child is like his parents, he can do what he wants and not displease them, because what he wants is what they want. However, the premature timing of this identification results in an inappropriately rigid superego and an excessively intense identification. As a result, his adult behavior is impelled by a strident superego, completed too young, a situation which has some serious long-term liabilities.

One of these liabilities is that a normal and loving rapprochement with the inner self is compromised or squelched when the patient too fully makes his perception of the family's expectations his own. He may feel it

means renouncing permission to be sufficiently assertive in pursuing such needs as sufficient sleep, relaxation, and sexual gratification. When the migraineur has this type of superego, it frequently expects even the wish for such self-expression to be denied.[6]

Other liabilities are incurred if the migraineur projects the expectations he has of himself onto neighbors, bridge partners, doctors, employers, and spouses. When this occurs, the patient becomes liable to react to these "parent substitutes" as he did to his early caretakers, reenacting with them the same initiatives he used in the early years of his life to win praise and placate resentments.[7]

Our discussion of identification leads naturally to a more specific discussion of superego, as superego is largely formed through this process. It then becomes the repository of the contents of identification, actively transmuting these into the attitudes and behaviors of the adult. In the words of Anna Freud (20): "When a child constantly repeats this process of internalization and introjects the qualities of

_____

[6] This willingness of an organism to sacrifice important aspects of "self" for security can be seen in animal experiments, and is thus more than theoretical. Harlow (18) showed that infant monkeys would choose the anxiety reduction provided by clinging to a rocking, terrycloth manikin even in preference to food, and Pavlov (19) could get dogs to shock themselves to obtain food. Although shocks and food deprivation have nothing to do with migraine, the wish for security often does. However, such sacrifice is less obvious if, as a result of identification, it is disguised as ego-syntonic, or "voluntary" behavior.

[7] The authors have observed that female migraineurs tend to view their father's life style as more meaningful and even significant than that of their mothers. They would more frequently wish to emulate and identify with him. This was observed even when the father had a temper, or was frequently away and emotionally unavailable, causing anger at him. His life was still admired as the one filled with vitality; to win his respect and approval was prized. The mothers, in contrast, even when empathized with, were often viewed as consigned by fate to a more dreary role.

those responsible for their upbringing, making their characteristics and opinions his own, he is all the time providing material from which the superego may take shape.''

Because it was "set" too early, the superego of a theoretical problem migraineur usually functions with a stern countenance. For the patient to obtain this inner image's permission for time off is no easy matter—it will sometimes not relent even in the face of a migraine. Even when he feels justifiably proud when maintaining the pace and actualizing the accomplishments which his superego desires, this migraineur can never quite shake free of his underlying insecurity. There may still be uncertainty about whether he will yet fail to live up to his own expectations and risk criticism, anxiety, or shame.

Adult perfectionism[8] is a direct carryover from the way a child imagines that grownups do things. Certain "formulae for adulthood" have been internalized during childhood; and, as the jobs of adulthood loom large in the eyes of a child, these seem to carry with them the requirement of extra hours, extra work, and extra capability. There is anxiety that without these ingredients—and without, perhaps, some good luck—the job of being a productive adult will not be managed well. Both the pressured life style and the insecurity are inevitable consequences of these perceptions.

As most adults are usually less concerned than this about having an occasional failure, such a migraineur will typically—barring bad luck—get more done. Yet, success fails to convince him that the next project will not again require the same all-out effort, at the end of which, though he may be relieved and gratified, he may also be energy depleted and headache prone.

---

[8] It might be noted that this "perfectionism" frequently emphasizes doing enough and "not doing things wrong," rather than doing them extraordinarily "right" in some novel way; thus the term may be a slight misnomer.

INSECURITY AND RESPONSIBILITY

A sense of underlying insecurity is also frequently encountered in psychologically influenced migraineurs, even though its presence may be inapparent to the outside observer (21). The patient may have learned to compensate for the resulting discomfort for so long that he almost takes it for granted. Because he is rarely given to complaining or to showing the familiar social signs of insecurity, it frequently goes unnoticed. The consequence of this is that he is often not seen to need, and usually does not receive, the normal amount of social support.

Also sometimes observed in these patients is a certain subtle sense of loneliness, usually referred to by other terms: for example, the patient is thought to be "just reserved." The loneliness is typically not clearly reflected in his behavior, and must be deduced by other methods.

More than any other factor, feelings of responsibility interact poorly with this insecurity on a regular basis. Sometimes, what is usually stressful for one reason, such as the anxiety associated with surgery, is less stressful from the standpoint of migraine headaches as the hospitalization releases the patient from his usual responsibilities. Other events which stress the migraineur may do so, to a greater extent than is usually assumed, because they require him to be accountable. An excellent vignette illustrating the role of relief from responsibility in ameliorating migraine is that of the self-report of Dr. Elkinton (2):

We have tried to indicate the many stresses and tensions associated with the frequent and severe attacks over more than a quarter century in the professional and personal life of this patient—a man with a compulsive perfectionist temperament . . . But the striking diminution and disappearance of his migraine over the ensuing decade when the patient at the age of 62 retired from his professional responsibilities and exchanged his hectic urban-suburban life in America for a quiet un-

pressured village life in rural England (the home territory of his English wife) strongly suggest that psychic factors play a major role in his disease.

PSEUDOPROGRESSION

All people require defense mechanisms to get by in life, to be their shield against the proverbial arrows of fortune. The psychologically influenced migraine patient typically uses a profile of what are termed "high level" defenses, that is, those which are more complex, sophisticated, and adaptive: reaction formation, identification with the aggressor, repression, intellectualization, sublimation and, occasionally, suppression (see Chapter 10). These are in the repertoire of many a migraineur, and are used to cope with the responsibilities he has taken on or has been handed. Another defense we have observed the troubled migraineur to frequently give a history of having used is the one we refer to as pseudoprogression.

Pseudoprogression occurs when a child shortcuts emotional or behavioral stages of development in the adaptational attempt to grow up so fast that he can deflect problems and gain emotional closeness, praise, or autonomy. In the process of shortcutting epigenetic maturation, however, he also shortchanges it and, sadly, himself. A child using this defense quickly learns the ways of adulthood, because the ways of childhood are simply not looked upon favorably by his family or by himself; he becomes a "90-month wonder."

Pseudoprogression is a defense in many ways the opposite of regression. In regression one slips back into past ways of functioning in the hope of again finding the successes of a happier time. In pseudoprogession, it is time future where the grass looks greener. The child using this defense attempts to skip ahead to become the "little adult" that authority figures in his life seem to want in the

belief that this offers his best chance for happiness. Pseudoprogression may either operate in several areas of a child's life or in only one. Though it may be cognitive, behavioral, or emotional, it is most commonly seen to be a mixture of all of these.

In addition to being a means for smoothing out relationships with parents and other adults, getting their attention, garnering their praise, tempering any intolerance, and avoiding their displeasure, other motives can initiate and maintain pseudoprogression. One of these motives is, in curious fact, the opposite of getting closer to the parent: that is getting along, to a greater extent, without him. If the parent is often moody or unavailable for advice, the child may feel a sense of security in learning the "how to's" of taking care of his needs alone. Then he is not as dependent upon the parent's availability or fluctuating state of emotions. He feels greater control over his life. For many children this desire for independence is the dominant motive behind pseudoprogression. Both the wish to be close and the wish to be independent may be operative simultaneously. The desire to gain more control over an erratic physiology may also play a role here. In addition to environmental determinants, many internal factors—one might even say "choices"—influence which children will take this route, to what degree they will take it, and with what level of success.

Some actual advantages accrue to the child using this defense which, despite their defensive functions, will serve the child well throughout life. These include: (a) Rarely given to "childish behavior," he harmonizes well with the expectations of many adults, parents, and teachers. (b) He can be more independent than his childhood peers. (c) He is diligent and self-disciplined.

Because the child matures too rapidly, however, not allowing the slow, epigenetic building blocks of development to be carefully laid and fitted to each other, not allowing the integrated resolutions which occur in unhurried maturation to form and set, this maturation may be gerry-rigged and brittle. The reasons are: first, it is built on too little experience and, second, it is constructed at an age when the cognitive abilities available to the child for use in its construction are less developed. [Piaget (22) has found that, even for intellectually gifted children, certain capacities cannot develop before the necessary age is reached.] This premature enrollment in adulthood is only partially successful at achieving the child's aims: simply put, some things can't be rushed. Therefore, the adult migraineur who has taken this route still shoulders his burden of unsolved childhood problems and conflicts, though now they are out of sight if not truly out of mind. However, it is important to realize that under specific types of stressful provocation these hidden liabilities can resurface.

An example of how these early childhood adaptations set the patient up for later insecurity is the following. One woman recalled how, as a 7 year old in a private convent school, she had wished to achieve the state of spirituality that the nuns praised so highly in their favorite students. To this end she carefully learned, through imitation, to assume the hand, head, eye, and knee postures she observed them using at prayer, and which she believed were the keys to piety—which she was indeed convinced was its identity. To shore up her efforts, the Latin prayers heard at Mass were also—untranslated—committed to memory. Although the nuns praised her for such behaviors, before long she developed doubts about herself because the expected state of mind did not follow.

The psychic structure that results from pseudoprogression may work well in most situations, but when confronted by atypical or ambiguous ones the patient may lack the flexibility to consider complex variables with openmindedness, compassion, creativity, or wisdom. Instead, he is overcommitted to memorized "rules and formulae of adulthood." Thought and action tend toward the highly focused, with all the benefits and limitations of that orientation. The patient's perceptions and decisions are too much driven by his superego, wherein these formulae reside; and every superego is a bureaucracy.

Although the more mechanical problems of life may be frustrating or insoluble, the most complex, ambiguous, and multitiered situations in life are usually close interpersonal relationships. They are also the situations where success or failure may mean the most to the person. As a result, these are typically the ones which place greatest strain upon this adaptation.

Some of the inherent liabilities of this adaptation are accentuated when adolescence or adulthood arrives, perhaps as signalled by the menarche, leaving home, getting married, starting work—events typically associated with the onset of migraine. By now, one's peers have caught up and are not hampered by the rigid image of adulthood to which the pseudoprogressed individual has become accustomed. The person who has not pseudoprogressed has had the luxury of more trial-and-error learning, and has grown into adulthood with greater flexibility in his view of the rules of the game of life, and with more empathy towards his own desires. In contrast, the person who has pseudoprogressed is in many ways still burdened by a mode of coping with adult tasks which retains the striving and anxious energies he brought to challenges when he was young. Nevertheless, this individual's behavior continues to satisfy his conscience while earning the respect of authority figures in the home and work place. While he may learn greater flexibility, he is also, by this point, often simply a prisoner of habit, as his past adaptations remain successful in many areas where his colleagues' coping styles are not. The early advantages of pseudoprogression often become increasingly combined with liabilities unless the patient outgrows or supplements this style through corrective experiences (perhaps in college or in marriage) which allow him to "fill in" learning which was bypassed or foreshortened, or is aided in doing so in psychotherapy.[9]

Pseudoprogression is not a tactic whose relevance ends when childhood does. It leaves the residual effects referred to earlier, and can also be taken off of the shelf by the adult patient when facing any novel or anxiety-inducing situation. This may manifest itself by his getting the superficial hang of things quickly, but stopping before a deeper appreciation can be obtained.

Thus pseudoprogression is both a means of coping with anxiety-provoking stressful situations and, at the same time, is itself a source of anxiety and stress. In the short run it helps a person to overcome obstacles; in the long run it may, in part, create them. The advantages and disadvantages of this coping style are reflected in the dichotomy seen in adult migraineurs mentioned in the introduction.

As a result of pseudoprogression, these patients often have learned how to take charge of their own lives early on, for better or worse, and at the time they are seen for treatment years later almost don't know how to let other people help them out with the problems in their lives. This is why the approach to treatment must be careful, cautious, and considered.

---

[9] "Identification with the aggressor" may be accentuated by pseudoprogression. This defense, though described more fully in Chapter 10, can be summarized in the words of Anna Freud, who first defined it: "By impersonating the aggressor, assuming his attributes or imitating his aggression, the child transforms himself from the person threatened into the person who makes the threat" (20). When identification with the aggressor and pseudoprogression are both present, the child needs to learn early from role models the "hows" and "whats" of acting in an adult fashion, even though the "whys" may be scrimped on. This throws him into an earlier identification with his primary caretaker, usually the one who is strict or domineering, as it is this parent whom the patient wishes to placate or avoid. In essence, the identification with him becomes more rigid and more rote through its acceleration.

MOURNING

We can see that the wish to maintain stability in important personal relationships is a major contributor to the psychologically influenced migraine diathesis; so, too, is a need to shield oneself from focusing on the resentment which inevitably accompanies the perception of paying too dearly for security and esteem. During development these needs are both satisfied and defended against through the use of various high level defenses presented previously. The death of a loved one may challenge the adequacy of the resulting equilibrium.

If there are any major resentments towards the deceased, they are usually unconscious. If the resentments were buried early in life, they may have grown unduly powerful. This can cause the patient to feel inexplicable guilt following the death of the relative towards whom he held ambivalent feelings. Such guilt can sometimes block adequate mourning for the loss. It is the hostile impulse, especially if it is unrecognized, about which the patient feels guilty. We have seen, for example, many migraineurs who were charged as children with taking care of a seriously ill younger sibling who eventually died; the patient's subsequent guilt inhibited mourning.

If the patient has generally tried to ignore or suppress his feelings, he is unlikely to be comfortable with the challenge to his sense of self-control posed by intermittent but overwhelming feelings of grief. He is, in short, just not in the habit of giving in to his emotions, even ones more modest in intensity. These personal qualities may also have placed him in a position in the family where he is relied upon to support and stabilize others through this period, giving further cause to inhibit grieving. Therefore he frequently does not allow himself to mourn; the loss is not acceptably resolved; and unresolved grief ensues.

INTERPERSONAL SAFEGUARDS WHICH ONLY SOMETIMES WORK

Although he may not fully recognize this as a motive, the migraine patient often tries to avoid getting himself into a position wherein the many feelings described earlier are likely to be triggered. He is observed to do so by arranging his life in such a way that he can avoid having to depend on the potentially fluctuating moods of others. He seeks work in which his discipline and diligence can be used and will be appreciated, and preferentially cultivates social relationships in which he has sufficient standing to predict or influence their direction. Often, he is most comfortable in social interchanges that are defined by clear technical, intellectual, or social guidelines. As most people, with good reason, try to put themselves in a situation wherein they can maximize assets and shelter their weaker side, this behavior is, in itself, not surprising. Although at times this is limiting, one can also see at work here the patient's innate sense of how to adaptively protect himself.

In line with the work he seeks out, the migraineur also commonly organizes his life so that it is filled with the types of tasks for which he either has a plan or can expect to develop one. This reduces unpredictability, and allows him to take comfort in the familiarity of form, if not of detail.

Such techniques may help shield the migraineur's vulnerabilities while emphasizing his assets; however, they have little influence on the superego. Thus the patient keeps striving to placate his superego in the old ways, as success in adulthood never obliterates the remembered atmosphere of the past or the feelings it engendered—unless and until they are understood.

The mechanism of transference causes the migraine patient to perceive unreasonably high demands coming from those around him, demands which bear an uncanny resemblence to the inexorable expectations he has of himself. Even when the demands upon him are great, the migraineur often chooses to tackle them alone, just as he is frequently reluctant to ask for help with his headache symptoms. If he can be reassured that the adaptive strengths inherent in this self-reliant approach to life will not be weakened, but rather are likely to be augmented by treatment, he may be willing to seek help in a more accepting and flexible manner.

TAILSPIN TO HEADACHE

When things are going well there are, as we have seen, many common elements underlying the equilibrium of the psychologically influenced migraineur. Four things can disrupt this status quo in ways that might potentiate migraine:

Roadblocks and Obstacles. Anything that intereferes with the patient's capacity to feel reassured that he is progressing apace at a given job, project, or task. Interference with all of these impedes the patient's ability to feel that he is satisfying his superego. Vacations, weekends, completion of jobs, or frustration that a job cannot be done "right" and, especially, a seemingly insoluble ambiguity about a situation all fall into this category. Important to note as well: it is the point at which the patient comes to an inner mental determination that the job is finished or is impossible to finish that is relevant to triggering the physiology of "letdown." This letdown may thus not correspond in time to external events, which may be confusing to doctor or patient: for example, the migraineur who has an attack during a large dinner party she is hosting at that paradoxical point in time when she feels sure that all the arrangements have worked out and is relieved of her concern that the evening might be a social disaster. The timing of the attack does not correspond to the period of anxiety and uncertainty beforehand, and neither does it need to await the actual conclusion of the actual party. It instead concides with the timing of her inner conclusion that all will be as planned, all will be well.

Anger and Resentment. Things that acutely stimulate anger or resentment, especially if the anger has been consciously inaccessible. For example: the patient is working on a team with others who feel little need to hold themselves to the standards of performance he has set for himself and, as a result, he is left with burdensome duties.

Increased Responsibilities. These call into play and question the adequacy or flexibility or the patient's adult coping capacity. The normal stressfulness of life's demands is also accentuated here by perfectionism, which magnifies both those demands and the expectations of the patient's superego. A sublimal awareness of perceived deficiencies—the feeling of being very competent in some ways, but the impostor in others—may cause the patient anxiety about how capable he is to fend in ambiguous situations, especially those for which he cannot construct a clear plan of action. Even when, as an adult, he in fact does have the capacity to do the job, these expectations can resurrect and push him back toward the memory of that anxious state of mind which was present when he was a "boy trying to do a man's job." This anxiety might not be visible or even conscious; but, the mild apprehension that everyone feels when facing responsibilities may, in him, evoke anxiety reminiscent of that which accompanied analogous circumstances in the past. This can be true even when, as in the case of Dr. Elkinton cited earlier, the patient's actual capabilities are exceptional. More importantly, when measured against the superego's perfectionistic standards, there are certainly areas in which the patient *fears* that his capacities will prove insufficient, and this is not a possibility which rests easily with him. The 25-year-old man who was a musical prodigy at age 7 may find that he is now his own hardest act to follow to get the same sense of accomplishment.

Undervalued and Unappreciated. This includes things which leave the patient feeling that, although he is doing what is expected, results—anticipated and even deserved—are not forthcoming. The patient is doing his part, keeping up the pace, but to his mind, still fails to receive recognition or appreciation: it is a frustrating, no-win situation. Perhaps he considers that the world has not "lived up to its end of the bargain." So much resentment is triggered that he "quits"

inside, and the accompanying physiological letdown leads to headache: for example, the attorney who did a conscientious and thorough job for a client who was unhappy with the case's outcome and argued about the bill.

All of these situations have the potential to flood the patient with feelings, both conscious ones and unconscious ones. To the psychologically influenced migraineur, for whom powerful feelings are often his downfall, this buildup carries the same inevitable consequences as a liter of roadside Chianti. Depending upon the underlying threshold for headache, influenced by factors as diverse as hormonal levels or amount of sleep, such noxious emotions either will or won't eventuate in an attack of migraine.

From a psychological standpoint, the patient may, at this point, be confronting a basic anger which he usually manages to keep repressed, that his desires are not given high enough priority. What is ironic is that it is now, in part, the patient himself who is not according them that priority. The migraine is likely to start before he can fully experience the anger, or just after he has started to. Physiological accompaniments of this contestation between affect and defense trigger it automatically. (If he instead uses verbal channels for discharging these feelings, their intensity is sometimes lowered, which, in turn, occasionally decompresses the physiology enough to abort the headache.)

CONCLUSION

In conclusion we might consider these reflections of Friedman (23):

During the past thirty years I have had the opportunity to follow many headache patients from young adulthood to middle age and from middle age to old age. I am constantly impressed with the variability not only of the clinical course but of the background as well . . . the patients I have seen represent all types of occupations and professions; some are extensive travelers experiencing great changes in climate. **They may have wide cultural experiences as well as varying nutritional intake. The one constant factor for all these individuals, however, is their personal environment, i.e., their attitudes towards life and life situations and their genetic inheritance.**

In the preceding chapters we have seen abundant evidence to support the contention that subdiagnostic psychodynamic factors—predisposing, triggering, and resultant—are, along with genetics, the most important ones to look at for understanding and treating the therapeutically stalemated migraineur. The prospect of accepting this observation is actually an encouraging one, as it gives the clinician a concrete target, and one potentially amenable to change. Furthermore, if he is successful in helping the patient effect even modest psychological gains, it may eventually benefit not only treatment of the migraine, but also the patient's overall satisfaction with life.

There is another cause for optimism hidden within this psychological analysis of migraine: the same psychological defenses which were at first adaptive, but later locked the psychologically influenced migraineur into a life pattern which aggravated headache, often prove the very assets he ultimately uses to modulate the headache propensity. The strengths which are part and parcel of the liabilities in these patients can also be applied, in other words, to psychotherapy and to growth.

REFERENCES

1. Graham JR: Migraine: clinical aspects. In Vinken PJ, Bruyn GW (eds): *Handbook of Clinical Neurology.* Amsterdam, North-Holland, 1968, pp 45–58.

2. Elkinton JR, Graham JR: Forty-five years of migraine—observations and reflections "from the inside" by a physician-patient. *Cephalalgia* 5:187–195, 1985.

3. Heberden W: *Commentaries on the History and Cure of Diseases.* London, T. Payne, 1802, p 97.

4. Ottaviano S, Guidetti V: Functional bent of central nervous system: neonatal hyperreactivity and developmental disorders. A 10-year follow-up study. *Funct Neurol* 1:21–27, 1986.

5. Kolb LC: Psychiatric and psychogenic factors in headache. In Friedman AP, Merritt HH (eds): *Headache, Diagnosis and Treatment.* Philadelphia, F.A. Davis, 1959, pp 259–298.

6. Frazier SH: Complex problems of pain as seen in headache, painful phantom, and other states. In Arieti S, Rieser MF (eds): *The American Handbook of Psychiatry.* ed 2. New York, Basic Books, 1975, vol 4, pp 838–851.

7. Frazier SH: The psychotherapeutic approach to patients with headache. *Mod Treatment* 1:1412–1424, 1964.

8. Friedman AP: Mechanisms in development of migraine and muscle-contraction headaches. In Nodine JH, Moyer JH (eds): *Psychosomatic Medicine.* Philadelphia, Lea & Febiger, 1962, pp 129–133.

9. Furmansky AR: Dynamic concepts of migraine. A character study of one hundred patients. *Arch Neurol Psychiatry* 67:23–31, 1952.

10. Knopf O: Preliminary report on personality studies in thirty migraine patients. *J Nerv Ment Dis* 82:270–285, 400–414, 1935.

11. Touraine GA, Draper G: The migrainous patient: a constitutional study. *J Nerv Ment Dis* 80:1–204, 1934.

12. Wolff HG: Personality features and reactions of subjects with migraine. *Arch Neurol* 37:895–921, 1937.

13. Featherstone HJ, Beitman BD: Marital migraine: a refractory daily headache. *Psychosomatics* 25:30–38, 1984.

14. Selinsky H: Psychological study of the migrainous syndrome. *NY Acad Med Bull* 15:757–763, 1939.

15. Adler CS, Adler SM: Existential deterrents to headache relief past midlife. In Critchley M, Friedman S, Gorini S, Sicutui F (eds): *Advances in Neurology, Headache: Pathophysiological and Clinical Concepts.* New York, Raven Press, 1982, vol 33, pp 227–232.

16. Wolberg LH: Psychosomatic correlations in migraine: report of a case. *Psychiatr Q* 19:60–70, 1945.

17. Friedman AP, von Storch TJC, Merritt HH: Migraine and tension headaches, a clinical study of two thousand cases. *Neurology* 4:773–778, 1954.

18. Harlow HF: The nature of love. *Am Psychol* 13:673, 1958.

19. Pavlov JP: *The Work of the Digestive Glands.* London, Charles Griffin, & Company Ltd, 1902.

20. Freud A: *The Ego and the Mechanisms of Defense.* New York, International Universities Press, 1946, p 121, 129.

21. Friedman AP, Merritt HH: Migraine. In Friedman AP, Merritt HH (eds): *Headache; Diagnosis and Treatment.* Philadelphia, F.A. Davis, 1959, pp 201–249.

22. Piaget J: *The Grasp of Consciousness,* Cambridge, MA, Harvard University Press, 1976.

23. Friedman AP: Migraine: an overview. In Pierce H: *Modern Topics in Migraine.* London, William Heinemann Medical Books, 1975, p 159.

24. Bille B: Migraine in school children. *Acta Paediatr* (Suppl. 136) 51:14, 1962

25. Adler SM, Adler CS: Psychiatric treatment of the headache patient." *Panminerva Med* 24:145–149, 1982.

Psychiatric and Mental Presentations of the Migraine Prodrome, Aura, and Attack

GEORGE W. BRUYN, M.D., D.Sc.

. . . to expect ever to treat the head by itself, apart from the body as a whole, is utter folly.

PLATO, *Charmides,* 156 B.C.

Even those who consider migraine a reality, whether patients (through anguish) or doctors (through vocation) generally concede their uncertainty about the precise identity of the disorder. Its transient and episodic nature, the absence of a well-established structural basis or pathognomonic biochemical test, its inability to be reproduced in animal experiments, its multifaceted and moire-patterned clinical manifestation—these all render unto migraine an air of nebulosity, one which even modern medicine finds itself taxed to dispel.

One might find sufficient justification in these considerations to question the utility of a treatise on migrainous phenomena which are even more evanescent, elusive, and incomprehensible than its somatic ones. Will such a treatise *eo ipso* not ultimately prove the precarious concept of a migraine to be a chimera, an aberration of medical thought?

Before delving into these exotic matters, then, it will perhaps reassure the reader to state that the author views migraine as a dysfunction of the central nervous system, and as such, one clearly rooted in matter. It is the manifestation of a dynamic disturbance in the relationship between two partially interdependent systems: the cerebrovascular and the neuronoglial. (This author outlined a synopsis of this model at the 1983 International Migraine Symposium in Beerse, Belgium.) Inasmuch as migraine is produced by a derangement in living matter (the brain) and, insofar as, empirically, mind is only perceptible in the presence of its living brain substrate, the mental, emotional, and volitional abnormalities that occur in migraine are ultimately referable to the matrix of cerebral matter. Psychiatric migrainous phenomena are, therefore, inherently organic. The patient, in mind and mat-

181

ter, in soul and soma, is a whole, an integrated entity.

Migraine is usually overdiagnosed. Conversely, as soon as migraine manifests itself mainly or exclusively with psychiatric phenomena, migraine becomes underdiagnosed. The diagnosis is missed because many physicians are unfamiliar with migraine's ability to come in this guise—and what one does not know, one cannot diagnose. Mental migrainous variants may instead entice the diagnostician to leave the straight and narrow path of diagnostic rectitude, which for the great majority of physicians is marked by such familiar signs as "common" or "classical," but which, beyond these two signs, leads into poorly charted and, at any rate, disquieting territory.

Finally, from the semantic point of view, the following should be pointed out. The term "migraine-variant" denotes any form of clinical migraine other than the common or classic types; as such, the term delineates episodes of dysfunction of an organ or system in a migraine sufferer which are closely associated with or relatable to the typical migraine attacks of the patient. The adjective "variant" emphasizes that symptoms arise in addition to the usual prodromes, aura, scintillating scotomata, headaches, and vegetative syndromes. Also, the temporal link between the migrainous aura (usually comprising the various symptoms of neurological deficit) and the actual headache may loosen up, so that considerable lapse of time may be present between the two. Such a case is termed "dissociated migraine." The time interval may be so considerable as to completely separate the original components of the attack: the neurological deficit component and the pain-vegetative syndrome component. In such instances, the exclusive appearance of a transient neurological deficit (or mental dysfunction!) is termed "migraine sine hemicrania."

Every migrainologist knows from personal clinical experience that there are headache-free neurological episodes of a migrainous nature. It is nevertheless hard to convince those unfamiliar with the concept that the underlying cause of such transient states of neurological dysfunction is not something quite different from migraine, such as epilepsy, microembolism from prolapsed mitral valves, or an internal carotid artery plaque. The fundamental prerequisites for correctly interpreting these neurological episodes as migrainous (i.e., as migraine sine hemicrania) is that they occur in a migraine sufferer; next in importance is a history of symptoms alternating between sides. Other clues to their migrainous nature include an episodic time sequence, response to antimigraine medication, occurrence of migraine in the patients' family, and an absence of epileptic or cerebral-ischemic EEG signs. Essentially, it is an isolated aura that occurs without the full constellation of symptoms that defines the classical migraine attack: prodrome, pain, and vegetative symptoms. One might term such partial attacks "abortive migraine" or "forme fruste" attacks. This author has clinically witnessed cases of headache-free transient homonymous hemianopsia, transient hemiplegia, and transient paresthesias in migraineurs (also documented by Barolin) (1); and he has had personal experience with isolated scintillating scotomata since age 35. With respect to the latter phenomenon, the occurrence of isolated scintillating scotomata in migraineurs from middle age onward, has as a *pars pro toto* for the complete migraine attack, been repeatedly documented (2–6). It does not need to be emphasized that before settling on this diagnosis the conscientious physician excludes, by performing all appropriate procedures, other possible causes.

Therefore, when a migraine patient has clinical, episodic dysfunction of an organ or system temporally dissociated from headaches, or when it indeed substitutes for or replaces the headache, the term "migraine equivalent" is justified. With regard to this chapter's topic: these terms cover not only somatic symptoms, but are also applicable to migraine's psychiatric manifestations.

Minor symptoms of psychic dysfunction during migraine attacks (apart from the increased occurrence of somnambulism and left handedness in children with migraine (7, 8) are familiar to most migraine patients, and to many physicians. These symptoms are typically bothersome but not disquieting. They involve both the cognitive and emotional domains of higher nervous function and, occasionally, volitional and temperamental aspects as well. The slight-to-mild cognitive changes generally include diminished concentration (referred to in the German literature as "Schwerbesinnlichkeit," bradyphrenia, impaired ability to grasp the meaning of a text or conversation, indecisiveness, dysgraphic errors (such as writing p's for q's, d's for b's, and *vice versa;* or inverted 3's and 5's), slight paraphasias with the use of wrong words or mixing up of multisyllabled words, right-left and body-scheme errors, and memory lapses. The gamut of mental dysfunction included is too wide and varied to allow one to describe exhaustively all the irritating, incessant lapses the patient realizes that he makes. He may have to try four or five times before he succeeds in dialing a familiar telephone number in proper sequence; a simple memo written to a colleague may contain numerous spelling errors; the gist of a discussion at a meeting may completely escape a patient otherwise known for his quick intelligence. Recently, migrainous alexia without agraphia has been documented (9, 10). Emotional and mood changes range from feelings of elation, exhilaration, excitation, euphoria, and jocularity, to anxiety, phobias, dejection, weeping spells, a sense of impending doom, or even straightforward depression. The loquacious patient may become taciturn; the patient with a friendly, open-minded disposition may become mentally reserved or even slightly paranoid. Blau (11), in describing "complete migraine," pointed out that the poet-writer George Eliot felt "dangerously well before an attack," and that Sir John Forbes had an irresistible and horrid drowsiness. The classic migraine texts by Liveing (12) Möbius (13), and Flatau (14) contain many more examples.

Volitional and temperamental changes may range from unusual restlessness, hyperactivity, irritability, ebullience, irascibility, or irresponsibly enterprising zest, to lassitude, listlessness, apathy—even to mutism and stupor.

When the disturbance of mental functions in—and due to—migraine assumes major proportions, it is legitimate (and at least time-honored continental usage) for the clinician to speak of a predominantly mental migraine variant, called "hemicrania dysphrenica," or "dysphrenic migraine" (a term coined by Mingazzini (15). This type of migraine received particular attention from neurologists in the last quarter of the previous and first quarter of the present century. Lengthy, detailed, but nonetheless fascinating histories of severe cases of dysphrenic migraine, as well as of full-blown migraine psychoses, were published. Episodes of transient migrainous twilight states, hallucinations, somnambulism, suicide attempts, ideas of reference, religious and persecutional delusions, aggression and violence, dream-like states, confusion and stupor, all of them conspicuously followed by complete amnesia afterwards, were reported by Liveing (12), Lowenfeld (16), Mitchell (17), Zacher (18), Mingazzini (15, 19), von Krafft-Ebing (20, 21), Féré (22), Buringh Boekhoudt (23), Brackmann (24), Forli (25), Guidi (26), Flatau (14), Curschmann (27), Ranzow (28), Jahrreiss (29), Rümke (30) and, in exhaustive theses by van der Does de Willebois (31) and Vallery-Radot and Bamberger (32), respectively.

Flatau (14) collected 60 cases of such "migraine psychoses"; of these, three-quarters were in retrospect correctly diagnosed, and the remaining cases would today be diagnosed as epilepsy. Curiously, during this epoch, dysphrenic migraine remained a European affair, the only American sources being, to this author's awareness, Norsher (33), Moersch (34), and Nielsen (35). Weir Mitchell (17) reported on a patient who seems to have actually have been suffering from epilepsy. American interest in dysphrenic migraine arose later (28, 36–38) and in recent years has become the major source of information on the subject.

The phenomenological variety of higher nervous system disturbances in dysphrenic migraine is so rich as to bewilder the uninitiated. In order to facilitate orientation with regard to mental migrainous phenomena, the

TABLE 17.1.
TAXONOMIC DIAGRAM FOR MIGRAINE TYPES AND VARIANTS

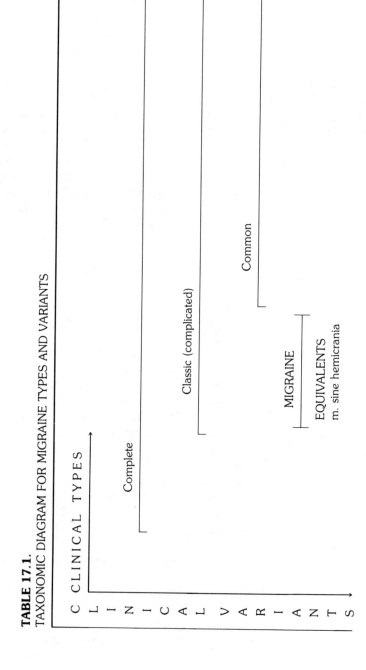

Table 17.1—*continued*

TYPE	PRODROME	AURA	HEADACHE	AUTON/VEGET. DYSFUNCTION
Classic (ophthalmic)	MOOD ACTIVITY YAWNING	Scintill. scot. Hemianop.	Photophobia	Nausea Vomiting Tachycardia Polyuria Diarrhea Fever Shivering (body temperature) Lassitude Inactivity SLEEP
Ophthalmoplegic		Oculomot. } palsy Abduc.		
Facioplegic		Facial palsy		
Cheiro-oral		Paresthesias		
Famil. hemipl.		Hemiplegia		
Basilar		Amnesia Vertigo Syncope Coma		
		Higher nervous system dysfunction Mental		
Dysphrenic	MENTAL			mental

present writer proposes a classification that, without claiming to be definitive, at least attempts to create provisional order from apparent chaos. Migrainous mental disturbances may be categorized as: (a) perceptual/cognitive, (b) emotional/affective, (c) volitional or (d) all-encompassing (see Table 17.2). Migrainous mental dysfunction can also be divided according to its severity, into minor and major versions.

In this sliding scale one can see progressively more facets of the personality become involved, ultimately ending with a full-blown migraine psychosis. In this last condition one may observe a true disintegration of the personality (see Table 17.2).

Characteristically, dysphrenic migraine is transient, repetitive, followed by postictal (retrograde) amnesia and, in the majority of patients, occurs in the prodromal or aural stage of a migraine attack (if it does not substitute for one.)

The perceptual disorders are most frequent. Objects may be seen as much smaller

TABLE 17.2.
DYSPHRENIC MIGRAINE

	DYSPHRENIC MIGRAINE			
	PERCEPTION, COGNITION, MEMORY, CONSCIOUSNESS	EMOTION, AFFECT/MOOD	VOLITION, TEMPERAMENT	ALL-ENCOMPASSING
MINOR	*Visual:* photophobia, micropsia, macropsia, teleopsia metamorphopsia, autokinesis, asthenopic scotoma, corona, optic alloasthesia, pulsation, perseveration, illusionary falsification	Elation Euphoria Laughing spells Loquacity	Lassitude Indolence Apathy	
	Olfact.: dysosmia			
	Acoustic: phonophobia, echo-acusia	Dysphoria	Restlessness	
	Dysgraphia: letter inversion, syllable mutilation	Weeping spells	Excitation	
	Dysphasia: alexia without agraphia		Poriomania	Transient
	Body scheme: disturbances	Anxiety, terror	Ebullience	Global
	Judgment: errors, indecisiveness	Dejection	Irritability	Amnesia
	Memory: lapses, forgetfulness, global amnesia, déjà vécu	Doom	Irrascibility Agitation	
	Consciousness: twilight state dreamy state automatism delirium confusion		Kleptomania Aggression Anger Violence	Acute Confusional State
MAJOR	stupor			
	Heautoscopia, environmental duplication, coenesthopathias	Depression	Suicide	Psychosis
	Hallucinations, incoherence of thought, delusions, paranoid state	Mania	Homicide	

(micropsia, Lilliputian), or much larger (macropsia), or much farther away (teleopsia) than they are. Rooms may seem enormously spacious, or the people in them gargantuan. Alternatively, the object may be perceived as partially or completely distorted (metamorphopsia (39), or experienced as situated in a part of space where it is not (optic alloaesthesia (40, 41). One patient of mine, some hours before her attack, saw people as cut longitudinally into two halves (right and left); they would subsequently become rejoined, but not until the left half had been caudally displaced over 20 cm (so that left half of the face was opposite the right half of the neck, and left half of the neck opposite the right half of the chest, etc.) Lippman's seventh case is similar to this (42). The phenomenon is somewhat analogous to the splitting of images in a camera's viewfinder. In other patients, immutable objects such as houses, shelves, etc. seem to move (autokinesis), or part of objects are lost to perception (asthenopic scotoma); or things become tilted from the true vertical or horizontal, or get turned upside down (43); or all sense of direction is lost (44). During this state, the migraineur's world turns surrealistic, Picassoan.

Spatial distortion may also be experienced acoustically, with discordant, disagreeable sound perceptions, with reverberations, or as with music played at the wrong number of revolutions of the turntable.

Similar things may happen in the sensory domain: this author knows of many patients who experience dysmorphesthesia, in which they develop distortions of body image. This includes the perception of having an inordinately thick and long finger, thumb, leg, or ear, or the feeling of water droplets running through the brain, or of a creek running through the abdomen; or they feel as if there were "nothing" where the liver or intestines should be, or as if they had a third buttock or an immense, ballooning hip, or they feel their head swelling and floating up to the ceiling—so much so that patients have even grabbed their heads in both hands to prevent this from happening (cenesthopathia) (42).

The self (or the environment) may appear as partially duplicated or even as completely doubled (33, 45). Partial duplication of the head was reported by Todd (38). In one case of mine, the patient would see his double on his left side, walking always one pace behind him (the so-called doppelganger, or heautoscopia; and, in case 10 of Hachinski et al (43). In Lippman's sixth case (42), the patient's double was "astrally floating" above him, and in others the "double" felt chilly (45). Todd's fourth case, a girl of 17, felt that her double, who was a yard away on the left, contained her mind. At 5 years of age she often cried out, "Mommy, come back to me" as she saw her mother receding into the distance. The duplication perception appears to be generated in the thalamus (46).

The size disturbances of body parts belong, of course, to disturbances of body scheme or body image. These "hallucinations" or, rather, illusionary falsifications, were most vividly described by Charles L. Dodgson, better known as Lewis Carroll, in his *Alice's Adventures in Wonderland*. Dodgson suffered from migraine; accordingly, Todd (38) epitomized these migrainous mental phenomena, calling them the "Alice in Wonderland syndrome". Golden (47) recently provided beautiful examples of the above mentioned disturbances as experienced during migraine in his description of attacks in two youngsters, in whom time sense also seemed to get speeded up.

Occasionally, patients see an object surrounded by a halo or corona, or see afterimages of the object after it has disappeared (perseveration or palinopsia). Elaborate visual hallucinations have been reported by Atkinson and Appenzeller (48). Olfactory "hallucinations" are much rarer than visual ones; Flatau described one such case (14), as did Wolberg and Ziegler (49), while Sacks, in his monograph on migraine (50), reported seeing several.

Disturbances of memory and consciousness in migraine fall into two major categories: migrainous transient global amnesia (MTGA) and migrainous acute confusional state

(ACS). Impaired consciousness is a well-known accompaniment of Bickerstaff's basilar artery migraine—indeed, one of its diagnostically clinching features (51, 52)—as is, to a much smaller degree, violence (53).

Not only with these two rather well-defined states of migrainous mental derangement, but also with the minor dysfunctions dealt with in the earlier paragraphs, the treating physician should remember that most patients experiencing these symptoms tend to conceal them out of fear of being declared "nutty." One would do well to ask specifically about mental symptoms.

Transient global amnesia is a disorder conspicuously associated with migraine, in both the author's experience and in the literature (35, 44, 54–80). In this disorder, which lasts from several hours up to a few days, recent memory is lost completely, though consciousness is apparently unimpaired; complex acts can be well executed; and self-awareness, and even insight into the condition, is maintained to some measure. Orientation to time and occasionally to place is, however, impaired, and the patient is often anxious. Retrograde amnesia for the episode

follows it. During a TGA episode, patients have been known to drive their car perfectly correctly through a city or, as was the case with the nurse/patient reported by Nielsen and Ingham (39), to correctly make all chart entries for her ward, without any recall of having done so after the attack passed. In 1972, after a Migraine Congress, this author had the experience of driving from Rotterdam to his home, a distance of 50 miles, through a pitchblack, rainy night at 4 AM, only to regain his senses in unfamiliar territory—at the Dutch-German border, 180 miles away to the east.

EEGs obtained during episodes of transient global amnesia reveal mostly temporal slow wave activity. Bilateral involvement of (para-) hippocampal, lingual, and fusiform convolutions, and of thalamus, provide the anatomical substrate (see Fig. 17.1); ischemia or metabolic impairment of that area is the pathophysiological mechanism. The area is supplied by branches from the posterior cerebral artery (see Fig. 17.2).

Migrainous TGA may occur at any age, but is predominantly seen in those over 40 years. It is identical to what, in earlier times, was called a "migrainous twilight state."

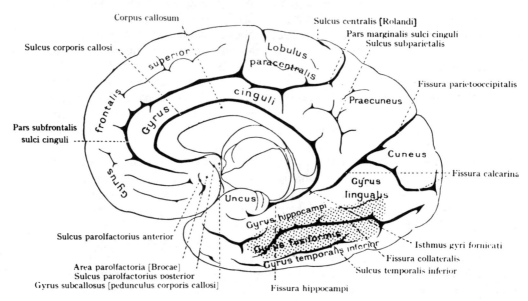

Figure 17.1. *Bilateral involvement of (para-) hippocampal, lingual, and fusiform convolutions, and of thalamus, provide anatomical substrate.*

Damasio et al (81) recently described a patient with migrainous transient *partial* amnesia who could not only remember some of what happened after the episode, but who wrote, during it, a detailed account of what he was experiencing.

The other main syndrome of migrainous mental dysfunction is the migrainous acute confusional state. It is characterized by acute onset, definite impairment of consciousness, loss of selective attention, disorientation in time and space often combined with agitation; severe impairment of abstract thought, judgment, and immediate memory; and purposeless, irrational behavior. In contrast to MTGA, this syndrome favors younger people. It is often accompanied by classic migraine symptoms, especially neurological ones, such

as extensor plantar reflexes, ataxia, slurred speech, vertigo, and sometimes coma. Migrainous transient ACS (MTACS) is also followed by retrograde amnesia. The condition has been reported in many studies (44, 52, 69, 82, 83). It has been seen to be precipitated by trivial trauma (72, 84, 85) and to accompany familial hemiplegic migraine (86).

Although not unequivocally and sharply delimitable *vis-à-vis* MTGA, the condition therefore exhibits a sufficient number of features to afford the physician a differential diagnosis: preferential manifestation in young patients, agitation, confusion, impairment of consciousness, and classic or complicated migraine symptoms. MTACS borders on the full-blown migraine psychosis, as described by numerous authors (19, 22, 31, 86–88).

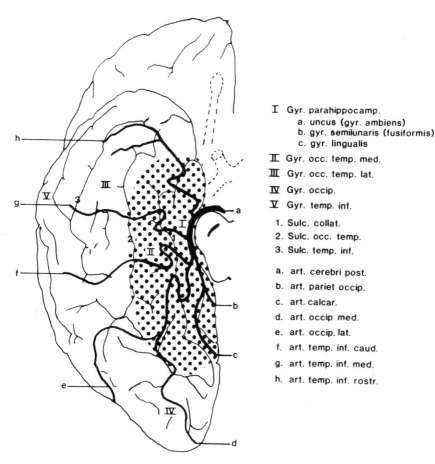

I   Gyr. parahippocamp.
    a. uncus (gyr. ambiens)
    b. gyr. semilunaris (fusiformis)
    c. gyr. lingualis
II   Gyr. occ. temp. med.
III   Gyr. occ. temp. lat.
IV   Gyr. occip.
V   Gyr. temp. inf.

1. Sulc. collat.
2. Sulc. occ. temp.
3. Sulc. temp. inf.

a. art. cerebri post.
b. art. pariet occip.
c. art. calcar.
d. art. occip med.
e. art. occip. lat.
f. art. temp. inf. caud.
g. art. temp. inf. med.
h. art. temp. inf. rostr.

Figure 17.2. *Posterior cerebral artery branches supplying involved hippocampal, lingual, and fusiform convolutions.*

The migraine psychosis, too, is followed by postpsychotic amnesia.

Recent research suggests that in spite of earlier data (88) implying inferior orbital and cingulate cortex ischemia in these syndromes, it is ischemia in the basilar/posterior cerebral artery territory which underlies both MTGA and MTACS. Areas most affected are infero-mesiotemporal, and include the fusiform, lingual, and hippocampal convolutions (85, 89, 91) (see Fig. 17.2).

Horenstein et al (89) extensively reported on nine cases with agitation, extreme distractibility, exaggerated responses to stimuli, shouting, grossly impaired time orientation, poor judgment, and occasional hallucinations—in short, patients with delirium. They also had regressed reflexes, such as sucking and grasping reflexes, and had homonymous hemianopsias. Autopsies showed these patients to have infarctions of the calcarine, fusiform, and lingual gyri, occasionally extending to the hippocampal or inferior temporal convolution, but sparing the uncus. Medina et al (90) described a patient with delirium (followed by agitated dementia), burst of rage, and shouting who was shown to have an infarction of the hippocampus, lingual and fusiform gyri, and pulvinar. Again, these same areas were involved in patients reported by Conomy et al (92) to have a clinical picture of agitated delirium, memory disturbance, profane loquacity, and visual defects. Brust and Behrens (91) observed metamorphopsia and palinopsia in posterior cerebral artery occlusion, and their article reviews the pertinent literature.

It would therefore appear that MACS is based upon ischemia in the mesencephalic, or thalamosubthalamic branches of the basilar/posterior cerebral artery system. The acute confusional state has, however, also been described in patients with nondominant middle cerebral artery infarctions (inferior parietal, inferior frontal), although such patients are much less agitated and distractible, and do not shout (88). A similar picture has been seen with anterior cerebral artery infarctions involving the mesiofrontal cingulate cortex, but patients with these lesions also exhibit sexually inappropriate behavior (93).

Interestingly, the hallucinations of environmental reduplication (46, 94–96) appear to develop when the nondominant hemisphere and thalamus are involved.

When one considers that migrainous alexia with agraphia has precise anatomical substrata (viz. the left mesiotemporooccipital white matter and cortex) (97) and that the various visual hallucinations of migraine, as well as MTGA and MACS, flourish upon involvement of the same mesiotemporooccipital area, it fits quite snugly with the concept that the posterior cerebral artery territory is the main scene for migraine. Also, that the cortex of the medial and basal temporal/occipital lobes apparently has much greater significance for the mind-matter entity of personality than has been realized up to now.

The phenomena of mental dysfunction in some patients with migraine presses home the inseparability of mind and brain, a conviction courted not only by the clinical neurologist. Conscientious observation and careful analysis of such phenomena therefore hold the promise of deeper insights into fields wider and more profound that the elucidation of migraine alone.

REFERENCES

1. Barolin GS: Familiäre paroxysmale Halbseitenausfälle mit und ohne Kopfschmerzattacken. *Schweiz Arch Neurol Psychiatr* 99:15–28, 1967.

2. Mitsui Y, Kochi Y: Diamox in treatment of scintillating scotoma. *Ophthalmology* 144:341–345, 1962.

3. Alvarez WC: Aberrant types of migraine seen in later life. *Geriatrics* 13:647–652, 1958.

4. Whitty CWM: Migraine without headache. *Lancet* II:283–285, 1967.

5. Riffenburgh RS: Migraine equivalent: the scintillating scotoma. *Ann Ophthalmol* 3:787–788, 1971.

6. Rau H, Vetterli A: Über die kopfschmerzfreie Migränevariante. *Arch Psychiatr Nervenkr* 225:325–332, 1978.

7. Geschwind N, Behan P: Left-handedness: as-

sociation with immune disease, migraine, and developmental learning disorder. *Proc Natl Acad Sci USA* 79:5097–5100, 1982.

8. Barabas G, Ferrari M, Schempp Matthews W: Childhood migraine and somnambulism. *Neurology* (Cleveland) 33:948–949, 1983.

9. Bigley GK, Sharp FR: Reversible alexia without agraphia due to migraine. *Arch Neurol* 40:114–115, 1983.

10. Fleishman JA, Segall JD, Judge FP: Isolated transient alexia. A migrainous accompaniment. *Arch Neurol* 40:115–116, 1983.

11. Blau JN: Migraine prodromes separated from the aura: complete migraine. *Br Med J* 281:658–660, 1980.

12. Liveing E: *On Megrim, Sick- Headache, and Some Allied Disorders*. A Contribution to the Pathology of Nerve-Storms. London, Churchill, 1873.

13. Möbius PJ: Die Migräne. In H. Nothnagel Spec Pathol Ther Bd XII, T3, 1ᶜ Abt., Wien, A Hölder, 1894.

14. Flatau E: Die Migräne. Monogr a d ges Gebiet d Neurol u Psychiat. 2. Berlin, Julius Springer, 1912.

15. Mingazzini G: Sui rapporti tra l'emicrania oftalmica e gli stati psicopatici transitori. *Riv Sper Freniatria* 19:110–119, 1893.

16. Löwenfeld L: Zur Casuistik der transitorischen psychischen Störungen. *Neurol Zentralbl* 1:268–272, 1882.

17. Weir Mitchell S: Neuralgic headaches with apparitions of unusual character. *Am J Med Sci* 93(4):415–419, 1887.

18. Zacher: Über einen Fall von Migraine ophthalmique mit transitorisch-epileptischer Geistesstörung. *Berlin Klin Wochenschr* 28, 1892. (Neurol Zentralbl nr 1, S 21, 1893).

19. Mingazzini G: Klinischer Beitrag zum Studium der cephalalgischen und hemikranischen Psychosen. *Z Neurol Psychiatr* 101:428–451, 1926.

20. Krafft-Ebing R von: Über Migräne und akute Geistesstörung. *Neurol Zentralbl* 21:1895. Nr 46, S 721.

21. Krafft-Ebing R von: Über Migränepsychosen. *Jahrb Psychiatrie* 21:38, 1902.

22. Féré Ch: Note sur un cas de psychose migraineuse. Rev Méd (Paris) 17:390–395, 1897.

23. Buringh Boekhoudt H: Psychische afwijkingen bij migraine. *Psychiatr Neurol Bl (Festschrift)*:63–72, 1896.

24. Brackmann H: Migräne und Psychose. *Allg Z Psychiatr* 53:554–561, 1897.

25. Forli V: I fenomeni psichici nell'emicrania. *Riv Sper Freniat* 33:220–241, 1907.

26. Guidi G: Sintomi psichici premonitori dell'attacco emicranico. *Riv Sper Freniat* 33:440–448, 1907.

27. Curschmann H: Öber einige seltene Formen der Migräne. *Dtsch Z Nervenheilkd* 53(4):184–205, 1915.

28. Ranzow E: Über Migränedämmerzustände und periodische Dämmerzustände unklarer Herkunft. *Monatschr Psychiatr Neurol* 47:98–118, 1920.

29. Jahrreiss: Über Migräne-Dämmerzustände. *Zentralbl Neurol* 48:63–64, 1927.

30. Rümke HC: Migrainepsychosen. *Ned T Geneesk* 43:5346, 1931.

31. van der Does de Willebois JJM: Over migraine, in het bijzonder over hemicrania psychica. Thesis, Utrecht. Kemink Zn, 1932.

32. Vallery-Radot P, Hamberger J: *Les Migraines*. Paris, Masson et Cie, 1935.

33. Norscher JM: Mania transitoria and epileptiform migraine. *Albany Med Ann* 62:255, 1921.

34. Moersch FP: Psychic manifestations in migraine. *Am J Psychiatry* III: 697–716, 1924.

35. Nielsen JM: Migraine equivalent. *Am J Psychiatry* 9:637–641, 1930.

36. Slight D, Morrison DAR: Migraine equivalents. *Am J Psychiatry* 97(I):623–632, 1940.

37. Vance FV, Klingman WO: Subtypes of migraine. *Virginia Med Monthly* 79:363–366, 1952.

38. Todd J: The syndrome of Alice in Wonderland. *Can Med Assoc J* 73:701–704, 1955.

39. Critchley M: Metamorphopsia of central origin. *Trans Ophthalmol Soc UK* 69:111–121, 1949.

40. Klee A, Willanger R: Disturbances of visual perception in migraine. *Acta Neurol Scand* 42:400–414, 1966.

41. Klee A: Perceptual disorders in migraine. In Pearce J (ed): *Modern Topics in Migraine*. London, W. Heinemann Med Books Ltd, 1975, pp 45–51.

42. Lippman CW: Certain hallucinations peculiar to migraine. *J Nerv Ment Dis* 116:346–351, 1952.

43. Hachinski VC, Porchawka J, Steele JC: Visual symptoms in the migraine syndrome. *Neurology* 23:570–579, 1973.

44. Nielsen JM, Ingham SD: Evidence· of focal vascular disturbance in migraine equivalent. Report of four cases. *Bull Los Angeles Neurol Soc* 5:113–119, 1940.

45. Lippman CW: Hallucinations of physical du-

ality in migraine. *J Nerv Ment Dis* 117:345–350, 1953.

46. Leiguarda RC: Environmental reduplication associated with a right thalamic haemorrhage. *J Neurol Neurosurg Psychiatry* 46:1154, 1983.

47. Golden GS: The Alice in Wonderland syndrome in juvenile migraine. *Pediatrics* 63:517–519, 1979.

48. Atkinson RA, Appenzeller O: "Deer Woman." *Headache* 17:229–232, 1977 and 1978.

49. Wolberg FL, Ziegler DK: Olfactory hallucination in migraine. *Arch Neurol* 39:382, 1982.

50. Sacks OW: *Migraine.* London, Faber and Faber, 1970.

51. Lees F, Watkins SM: Loss of consciousness in migraine. *Lancet* II: 647, 1963.

52. Lee CH, Lance JW: Migraine stupor. *Headache* 17:32–38, 1977 and 1978.

53. Brott T, Leviton A: Violence. *Headache* 16:203–209, 1976.

54. Fisher CM, Adams RD: Transient global amnesia. *Trans Am Neurol Assoc* 83:143–146, 1958.

55. Fisher CM, Adams RD: Transient global amnesia. *Acta Neurol Scand* 40 (suppl 9): 7–82, 1964.

56. Nielson JM: *Memory and Amnesia.* Los Angeles, San Lucas Press, 1979, vol 6, p 159.

57. Fisher CM: Migraine accompaniments versus arteriosclerotic ischemia. *Trans Am Neurol Assoc* 93:211–213, 1968.

58. Fisher CM: Cerebral ischemia: less familiar types. *Clin Neurosurg* 18:267, 1971.

59. Fisher CM: Late-life migraine accompaniments as a cause of unexplained transient ischemic attacks. *Can J Neurol Sci* 7:9–17, 1980.

60. Poser CM, Ziegler DK: Temporary amnesia as a manifestation of cerebrovascular insufficiency. *Trans Am Neurol Assoc* 85:221–223, 1960.

61. Evans JH: Transient loss of memory: an organic mental syndrome. *Brain* 89:539–548, 1966.

62. Gilbert JJ, Benson DF: Transient global amnesia: report of two cases with definite etiologies. *J Nerv Ment Dis* 154:461–464, 1972.

63. Godlewski S: Les épisodes amnésiques (transient global amnesia). *Sem Hôp (Paris)* 44:553–569, 1968.

64. Mumenthaler M, von Roll L: Amnetische episoden. Analyse von 16 eigenen Beobachtungen *Schweiz Med Wochenschr* 99:133–9, 1969.

65. Croft PB, Heathfield KWG, Swash M: Differential diagnosis of transient amnesia. *Br Med J* 4:593–6, 1973.

66. Laplane D, Truelle JL: Le mécanisme de l'ictus amnésique. A propos de quelques formes inhabituelles. *Nouv Presse Méd* 3:721–5, 1974.

67. Flügel KA: Transient global amnesia: a paroxysmal amnestic syndrome. *Fortschr Neurol Psychiatr* 43/9:471–485, 1975.

68. Frank G: Amnestische Episoden bei Migräne—Ein Beitrag zur Differential-diagnose der transienten globalen Amnesie (Ictus amnésique). *Schweiz Arch Neurol Neurochir Psychiatr* 118(2):253–274, 1976.

69. Emery ES: Acute confusional state in children with migraine. *Pediatrics* 60:110–114, 1977.

70. Caplan LR, Chedru F, Lhermitte F: Transient global amnesia and migraine. *Neurology* 28:387, 1978.

71. Caplan L, Chedru F, Lhermitte F, Mayman C: Transient global amnesia and migraine. *Neurology (N)* 31:1167–1170, 1981.

72. Ehyai A, Fenichel GM: The natural history of acute confusional migraine. *Arch Neurol* 35:368–369, 1978.

73. Boeri R, Boiardi A, Bussone G: Transient global amnesia as a confusional episode in complicated migraine. *Ital J Neurol Sci* 1:53–54, 1979.

74. de Fine Olivarius B, Jensen TS: Transient global amnesia in migraine. *Headache* 19:335–338, 1979.

75. Jensen TS, de Fine Olivarius B: Prognosen for transitorisk global amnesi ved migraene. *Ugeskr Laeg* 142(21):1344–1345, 1980.

76. Jensen TS: Transient global amnesia in childhood. *Dev Med Child Neurol* 22:654–667, 1980.

77. Jensen TS, de Fine Olivarius B: Transient global amnesia—its clinical and pathophysiological basis and prognosis. *Acta Neurol Scand* 63:220, 1981.

78. Ferguson KS, Robinson SS: Life-threatening migraine. *Arch Neurol* 39:374–376, 1982.

79. Crowell GF, Stump DA, Biller J, McHenry LC, Toole JF: The transient global amnesia-migraine connection: yet another intracerebral steal syndrome? *Neurology (N)* 32(2):A90, 1982.

80. Crowell GF, Stump DA, Biller J, McHenry LC, Toole JF: The transient global amnesia-migraine connection. *Arch Neurol* 41:75–79, 1984.

81. Damasio AR, Graff-Radford NR, Damasio H: Transient partial amnesia. *Arch Neurol* 40:656–657, 1983.

82. Symonds Ch: Migrainous variants. *Trans Med Soc Lond* 67:237–250, 1951.

83. Gascon G, Barlow Ch: Juvenile migraine,

presenting as an acute confusional state. *Pediatrics* 45:628–635, 1970.

84. Finelli PF: Confusional state and basilar artery migraine. *Neurology* 28:1201, 1978.

85. Walser H, Isler H, Hess R: Rezidivierende Bewusstseinsverluste mit Mittelhirnsymptomen bei Migräne. *Schweiz Med Wochenschr* 109:472–447, 1979.

86. Feely MP, O'Hare J, Veale D, Callaghan N: Episodes of acute confusion or psychosis in familial hemiplegic migraine. *Acta Neurol Scand* 65:369–375, 1982.

87. Klee A: A clinical study of migraine with particular reference to the most severe case. Copenhagen, Munksgaard, 1968.

88. Koeppen A: Ueber Migräne-Psychosen. *Zentralbl Nervenlk Psych* 21:269–270, 1898.

88. Mesulam MM, Waxman SG, Geschwind N, Sabin ThD: Acute confusional states with right middle cerebral artery infarctions. *J Neurol Neurosurg Psychiatry* 39:84–89, 1976.

89. Horenstein S, Chamberlin W, Conomy J: Infarction of the fusiform and calcarine regions: agitated delirium and hemianopia. *Trans Am Neurol Assoc* 92:85–89, 1967.

90. Medina JL, Rubino FA, Ross E: Agitated delirium caused by infarctions of the hippocampal formation and fusiform and lingual gyri: a case report. *Neurology* 24:1181–1183, 1974.

91. Brust JCM, Behrens MM: "Release hallucinations" as a major symptom of posterior cerebral artery occlusion: a report of 2 cases. *Ann Neurol* 2:432–436, 1977.

92. Conomy JP, Laureno R, Massarweh W: Transient behavioral syndrome associated with reversible vascular lesions of the fusiform-calcarine region in humans. *Ann Neurol* 12:P2, 1982.

93. Amyes EW, Nielsen JM: Clinicopathologic study of vascular lesions of the anterior cingulate region. *Bull LA Neurol Soc* 20:112–130, 1955.

94. Weinstein EA: Patterns of reduplication in organic brain disease. In: Vinken PJ, Bruyn GW (eds): *Handbook of Clinical Neurology.* Amsterdam, North-Holland, 1969, vol 3, pp 251–258.

95. Benson DF, Gardner H, Meadows JC: Reduplicative paramnesia. *Neurology* 26:147–151, 1976.

96. Ruff RL, Volpe BT: Environmental reduplication associated with right frontal and parietal lobe injury. *J Neurol Neurosurg Psychiatry* 44:382–386, 1981.

97. Damasio AR, Damasio H: The anatomic basis of pure alexia. Neurology 33: 1573–1584.

98. Willanger R, Klee A: Metamorphopsia and other visual disturbances with latency occurring in patients with diffuse cerebral lesions. Acta Neurol Scand 42:1–18, 1966.

99. Menken M: Transitory confusion after minor head injury. A Migraine Variant Syndrome. Clin Pediatr 17:421–2, 1978.

100. Müller D: Rational twilight state following minor head injury or isolated traumatic amnesia. *Z Arytl Fortbild (Jena)* 69(20):1054–1056, 1975.

CHAPTER EIGHTEEN

Conversion Headache

A. DIXON WEATHERHEAD, M.D.

If the uterus lodges in the loins the woman feels a hard ball or lump in her side. But when it mounts as high as the head it causes pains around the eyes and the nose, the head feels heavy and drowsiness and lethargy set in.

HIPPOCRATES (1)

It has been quite some time, since the "wandering uterus" referred to by Hippocrates (from which "hysteria" takes it's etymological origins) was considered the cause of conversion disorders. Today, a conversion headache is generally defined as one in which the causative disorder is a conversion reaction, and a peripheral pain mechanism is nonexistent. Although this description conforms to the categories proposed by the Ad Hoc Committee on Classification of Headache (2), it still leaves us with both theoretical and diagnostic problems. For one thing, some physicians still consider it an open question whether or not there are any local physiologic changes in this disorder (3). Another difficulty is that conversion headaches usually do not stand out in any clear or remarkable way from certain other types of headache, such as muscle contraction or posttraumatic headache. Most headache patients of all types have normal neurological exams and lab studies. Yet another problem has been the confusing and often ambiguous terminology used to describe headaches of emotional origin.

TERMINOLOGY

A conversion headache is, most simply, a headache that arises without any organic cause. It is a psychogenic headache of emotional origin, and is the major symptom of an underlying psychiatric disorder (4). Difficulties arise with these definitions, however, because different authors use these terms in different ways. "Psychogenic," "nervous," "tension," and even "conversion" have at times been used interchangeably by some authors. A number of general reviews and symposia dealing with psychogenic headache have either left it undefined or defined it differently in each case (5–7).

In 1976, a survey of physicians at a large medical center (8) asked them to define "psychogenic headache." Their 105 responses varied considerably. "Tension headache" was the most common response, with "no organic basis" the second most common. But it became apparent that the term "psychogenic headache" was neither precise nor diagnostic.

194

In 1980 the American Psychiatric Association's *Diagnostic and Statistical Manual III* was published. It added a new diagnostic category, that of somatoform disorders. Included in it were the diagnoses of hypochondriasis, somatization, conversion, and psychogenic pain disorders. These were accompanied by diagnostic criteria which technically changed the diagnostic evaluation of headaches. (Whether these changes have also amplified our understanding of such headaches is another question.)

The hypochondriacal patient complains insistently of physical symptoms for which organic findings are either minor or nonexistent. Physical symptoms are the patient's way of interacting. The patient's behavior is frequently insistent and demanding, with overt or barely submerged anger. Current or past physicians may be devalued, and blamed for inadequacies in diagnosis and care. Hypochondriasis typically comes in middle or old age, and is equally common in both sexes. The feelings and responses of those who work with such patients are often equally intense, since the patient seems unable to make constructive use of the physician's time and effort.

Patients with either somatization disorders or hypochondriasis have many somatic complaints in addition to preoccupations and fears that they might have a serious physical illness. A somatization disorder usually begins before age 30 and is almost always seen in women.

Both groups of patients often have complaints involving almost every organ system, even though the chief complaint may be headache. Patients with either disorder may go from physician to physician receiving many vague or contradictory evaluations and an equal number of unnecessary exploratory surgeries. Some become addicted to the drugs they are given for symptom relief.

The conversion disorder is characterized by some loss or alteration of physical functioning which cannot be explained by the findings on physical and neurological examination. This is a difficult concept in the headache situation. Most conversion disorders involve motor or special sensory symptoms, such as paralysis, aphonia, pseudoseizures, or visual disturbances (9). When, instead, the symptom is that of persistent pain without findings adequate to explain it, the diagnosis is now termed "psychogenic pain disorder." Yet the habit in medicine of calling headaches based on this mechanism "conversion headaches" persists.

Somatoform disorders of any type must be distinguished from organic illness that initially presents with vague or confusing symptoms. Particularly difficult is the patient with both headaches and a long-standing history of physical complaints. A distinction also needs to be made between the involuntary nature of symptoms seen in patients with somatoform disorders and the voluntarily controlled symptoms, complaints, and behavior of the patient who is malingering or has a factitious disorder.

In this chapter, conversion headache will be defined according to the Ad Hoc Committee criteria cited at the start of the chapter. The author will also give examples to support his contention that a conversion mechanism is present and to clarify it.

CLINICAL APPROACH

Although one can use the criteria just described to diagnose a patient who presents with headache of emotional origin, it is often even more useful clinically to think of certain functional characteristics including the quality of the patient's relationships with other people, his or her ability to work, the capacity to experience pleasure, the degree of self-destructiveness, the persistence of the complaints when in a supportive relationship, and the ability to test reality (10). Evaluating conversion headache patients along such a continuum often leads to important prognostic as well as diagnostic information.

A conversion headache is so called because anxiety is "converted" into a headache. Anxiety, then, plays an important part in producing the headache; yet the anxiety is itself not clinically manifest in the patient with a true conversion headache. By contrast, anxiety is overt and evident in other types of psychologically influenced headache noted above.

What does it take to develop a conversion headache? First it requires an emotionally stressful or conflictual situation, either acute or chronic, which the individual can neither solve nor shelve. The headache honorably allows the patient to avoid what might be a stressful or anxiety-laden experience.

In a true conversion reaction the source of this anxiety is repressed. This repression into the unconscious is called the "primary gain," and a conversion symptom, such as headache, appears in consciousness instead; a physical symptom, devoid of anxiety, replaces a psychological one. The entire process occurs outside of awareness. Indeed, the hallmark of the conversion reaction is the patient's apparent lack of concern about a symptom that normally would and should cause concern. Janet (11) described this as "la belle indifference." The patient may describe the headache in a dramatic but not altogether convincing manner. "Would you mind coming back later as I have the most terrible headache?" says this often scantily clad young lady from her bed. She may then continue to answer questions or embark upon a lengthy monologue about anything and everything except her headaches unless directly questioned about them. When asked to describe her headaches the patient will use vivid, descriptive adjectives. She says "It is a stabbing pain," or "it is a burning pain behind my eyeballs," or "a sort of pressure all over my head."

In obtaining a history from such a patient, careful inquiry has to be made as to the *nature* of the headache. The interviewer can refer to the patient's often dramatic description of his headache, which may be accompanied by expansive gesticulations and mannerisms, and can cautiously point out the paradox that, through all this, he (or, more often, she) does not appear to be in acute distress. For example, the patient may vigorously assert that bright light intensifies the headache, and be lying in bed with the curtains drawn. If the examiner then opens the curtains, the patient may at first protest, and dramatically cover his head and eyes; but this is soon followed by his seeming quite content to be examined in the bright light of day. The *quality and location* of the headache may also vary. The patient may describe the headache as a pressure sensation, like having his head in a vise, or as a crawling, burning, or stabbing sensation, or as "pins and needles." Or it may be a dull pain like a toothache. It may be localized to one part of the head or may be more generalized; unilateral or bilateral or migratory. It may or may not be associated with visual disturbances, diplopia, difficulty focusing, photosensitivity, etc. Also, it may or may not be associated with nausea and vomiting. Indeed, the only characteristic universally seen in conversion headache is that the patient's affect does not coincide with the description of pain. This may lead to delay in diagnosis. If the symbolism is good enough to fool the patient, it is often good enough to fool the physician, at least for a time. Frequently, this air of disconcern by the patient will "throw off" the physician, rather than be used by him as the single most important diagnostic observation.

A 20 year old Navy serviceman was admitted to the hospital with a three month history of "constant, squeezing, tense pain." This pain was described as worse than anything he had ever had. Multiple medications had been prescribed by multiple physicians without affording the slightest relief. Several previous neurologic examinations and angiography were normal. He stated his symptoms became worse with prolonged standing and were completely relieved by lying down for fifteen minutes. During the neurological examination, he held his head and insisted on lying down, but frequently smiled and joked with the examiner. Also, despite the "terrible pain," he never requested pain medication during his hospital stay, but continually pressed his doctor for a change in duty station, which he felt

was the only thing that would relieve his headache.

Significant background information included the statement that his father had such severe headaches he had to miss work, and would lie in bed without moving his head. Because the father refused to go to the doctor, the patient's mother had to take care of him. The father died four years before the patient was admitted. The patient's mother had remarried three months prior to the onset of the headaches. With a thinly disguised disgust, he said, "my stepfather is an okay guy." However, he no longer wished to visit his mother or her home. During the initial interviews the patient insisted on only talking while lying in bed. He appeared surprised when the examiner suggested that his behavior resembled the symptoms he had reported in his father. After this session, the patient tried to sit up in the doctor's office and started to show improvement. It became apparent that this patient had unconsciously identified with his father's symptoms. In addition, he felt abandoned and alone when his mother remarried, and displaced many of these feelings onto his job, where he no longer thought he was getting anywhere, or was being sufficiently noticed.

The *duration* of pain in conversion headache also varies. Some patients date the onset of their headaches to a particular event, often traumatic, such as an automobile accident. Conversion headache may, therefore need to be differentiated from true posttraumatic headache. Careful inquiry is necessary to ascertain: (a) the exact time relationship between the accident and the onset of headaches; (b) the nature and extent of any head or neck injuries; and (c) whether or not the patient lost consciousness and, if so, for how long.

The initiating event is often psychologically rather than physically traumatic—although it may have been both, as the following case illustrates:

A young, married woman was seen for headaches associated with blurring of vision, nausea and vomiting. No organic basis for these symptoms could be found, although an older sister was noted to have migraine. The problem would become worse after she had been driving in the country. During narcoanalysis using intravenous sodium amytal the patient tearfully and painfully recalled an incident in which her husband, a Viet Nam veteran, had by chance driven home by a different route, one that took him through the park. Noticing his wife's car parked in a wooded area some distance from the road, and thinking she possibly had car trouble, he walked over to offer assistance. To their mutual surprise he found her locked in the arms of an older man, whom he later learned was her boss. She immediately leapt out of the car and holding her hands over her eyes, tearfully complained of a lancinating pain behind her eyes which made it impossible for her to see. This was followed by nausea and vomiting. Her husband "rescued" her and took her home.

In subsequent psychotherapy sessions, this emotionally traumatic experience with its attendant anxiety, guilt, and shame were explored. The patient's symptoms (transient blindness) symbolically represented her wish "not to see" herself being caught in this compromising circumstance, and an inability "to stomach" the idea of being unfaithful led to nausea and vomiting. Her infidelity, and its humiliating manner of detection, was the source of much subsequent mental anguish. Furthermore, her symptoms automatically removed her from an emotionally stressful situation which she did not think she could otherwise resolve. The headaches had the added bonus of ensuring her husband's full attention, if not his full support and sympathy. Yet she was not consciously aware of either her motives or of their relationship to her symptoms.

This example demonstrates that, whatever the precipitating event, and its accompanying acute emotional state—which is relieved by "conversion" into a headache—the process is consciously unrecognized by the patient. For example, a man who presents with a history of daily headaches which started at the exact time his wife delivered their first child deserves further evaluation of his feelings about this situation, however strongly he may deny any connection between his headaches and his child's birth (12).

Secondary gain, though never the originating cause of conversion headache, may vary considerably in degree. The patient may show marked sick role behavior and may seek extensive if not exhaustive medical attention to supplement the attention already being demanded from loved ones. Although this pattern will markedly limit the patient's activities and his ability to enjoy life, it may also shield him from anxiety-laden situations. He may become practically bedridden and totally disabled, so that he is unable to work or even leave the house except for visits to the doctor.

Other patients, although their adjustment is suboptimal because of headaches, are still able to function in a limited fashion and pursue activities which they enjoy. For example, one young woman came to the physician complaining of headaches, constant nausea, and vomiting. Although 23 years old, she was accompanied by her mother, who insisted that the patient be hospitalized. Because the persistent nausea and vomiting had allegedly led to significant weight loss, her admission for that afternoon was arranged. However both patient and mother requested that she be admitted later that evening; they wished to go shopping first!

Conversion disorders, including conversion headaches, are more common in patients with hysterical personality disorder, but they are not limited to these patients. (The terms "conversion hysteria" or "hysterical headaches" are no longer used.) In patients who also have an hysterical personality there may be an abnormally strong and conflicted tie to the parent of the opposite sex, and this may lead to psychosexual immaturity. Further evaluation of the personal history often reveals an unstable marriage in which the emotionally immature patient has married a considerably older person who then serves as mother or father substitute. This may result in sexual problems, often originating from the combined wish and fear of transgressing—

symbolically—the incest taboo. These sexual problems are usually superimposed upon, and act as a smoke screen for, powerful dependency urges which the patient attempts to satisfy through these relationships.

Why does the patient develop a headache rather than a hysterical seizure of some other conversion reaction? The answer is often to be found in the patient's personal history: there is frequently a family history of headaches in important relatives. An emotionally immature, histrionic person may unconsciously identify with a headache sufferer. The more sophisticated the patient is, and the more symbolically significant the symptom is in extricating the patient from her predicament, the more closely the conversion symptom will mimic an organic symptom or disease.

An attractive young registered nurse who had been working on a neurological floor for some months, developed a clinical picture which closely resembled multiple sclerosis. She was admitted to the same neurological floor where she had been previously working. She was studied extensively. There were some equivocal neurological findings, including the sudden onset of her paralysis, equivocal Babinski responses, and most importantly, an unconcerned demeanor—in fact a beautiful indifference. Subsequent psychiatric interviews revealed the underlying psychodynamics of her conversion reaction. Her long-time overprotective friend and companion, upon whom she had been overly dependent for years and with whom she had had a long-standing homosexual relationship, had forsaken her in favor of another. The patient became "paralyzed with fear," and wondered how she could survive in a hostile world without the support of her long-time friend.

DIFFERENTIAL DIAGNOSIS

Although conversion reactions usually occur as a single psychiatric illness, they can also accompany or complicate any other illness, either physical or psychiatric. Charcot's "hysteroepilepsy" patients were known to have both hysterical and true, idiopathic, grand mal seizures. The same is possible with conversion headaches.

It does not matter how flamboyantly the patient may describe the headaches or how strongly the examiner may feel that the headaches are psychogenic: every patient with a recent onset of headaches is entitled to a complete physical and neurological examination, with appropriate ancillary studies, before the headaches are diagnosed as conversion. Also, a complete psychiatric evaluation is necessary to establish a positive diagnosis of a conversion headache, and to differentiate it from other types of headache influenced by psychological factors.

The differential diagnosis of conversion headache could easily be made (a) if the patient was a young woman with (b) an emotionally immature or hysterical personality (c) whose headaches developed abruptly after an acute, emotionally stressful experience, and (d) who described a terrible head pain, while maintaining a calm indifference. A history of sexual or aggressive impulses being struggled against and producing covert anxiety would also contribute to the diagnosis. Unfortunately, such a "pure" conversion headache is rarely encountered. More often, the anxiety from the underlying impulses and precipitating stimuli is not entirely converted into the headache symptom. The somatization of affect is only partial.

In such instances the patient remains anxious, and the headache assumes many characteristics of a muscle contraction or tension headache. In these patients other signs of anxiety are apparent, and the premorbid personality is more likely to be of the inadequate or passive type (13).

Patients with conversion headaches must also be differentiated from patients with depression where the headache represents a depressive equivalent. In such cases headache may be the only symptom of depression (14). However careful inquiry may sometimes uncover other physical and emotional concomitants of depression. Unlike the patient with a conversion headache, however, these pa-

tients *are* greatly concerned about their headaches.

Although conversion headaches were previously classified together with headaches of delusional or hypochondriacal states (2), it is rarely difficult to differentiate between the conversion headache and the head pain described by the psychotic patient, as the psychotic patient invariably shows other manifestations of psychosis. The hypochondriacal patient will be noticeably anxious, not only about the headaches, but about many additional body functions which he fears are malfunctioning, while the conversion headache patient will usually only complain about headaches. Patients with somatization disorders (3) (Briquet's syndrome) also have a multiplicity of complaints affecting many organ systems. Their symptoms are usually chronic, and are accompanied by anxiety and depression.

TREATMENT

Although every patient with chronic headache should have a complete physical and neurological examination, these examinations should preferably be performed once only, with the findings conveyed promptly, but not perjoratively, to the patient. Repeated examinations by the same physician may cause the patient to lose confidence in the examiner, while at the same time reinforcing his concern that "something is being missed."

Some patients with conversion reactions and functional symptoms seem sad, and occasionally even burst into tears when told that there is no organic basis for their symptoms. This is confirmatory of the diagnosis, and an entré into discussing the feelings behind the conversion defense. Other patients may turn on the examiner and angrily denounce him, contending that his examination has been inadequate or incomplete or even incompetently performed, and their previous apparent "belle indifference" is temporarily lost. In these cases the patient feels that the conversion defense is necessary, and fears that the physician may snatch it away prematurely.

Sometimes psychological testing can aid in the diagnosis or treatment. Discussing test results with the patient occasionally helps him open up about problems or realize that he has been denying a conflict. The test may also reveal the patient's premorbid personality or, especially with projective tests, may hint at underlying psychodynamics.

Initial treatment of the conversion headache patient is often supportive, and utilizes principles discussed elsewhere in this book. A good patient-physician relationship needs to be established, and this often takes both time and patience. At times, antianxiety or antidepressant medication will be helpful. Instruction in relaxation techniques, biofeedback training, or self-hypnosis sometimes puts the patient more in touch with his underlying feelings by reducing his anxiety.

In well-motivated patients, dynamic psychotherapy with a psychiatrist or clinical psychologist is the treatment of choice. The key to relinquishing the conversion defense is, after all, finding out what is being defended against and making peace with it. With a conversion headache problem, the effort of the psychotherapist must be to modify the communicative process so the patient can speak directly of the underlying impulses and anxieties. Reviewing the triggering event and helping the patient make associations to similar past experiences is psychotherapeutically beneficial, as it enables the patient to cope more effectively with subsequent anxiety and stress through insight gained in therapy.

One should not forget to take pleasure from the vitality frequently seen in such patients and their symptom dynamics, dynamics which, with increasing experience, often become increasingly, sometimes charmingly, transparent.

REFERENCES

1. Veith I: *Hysteria: The History of a Disease.* Chicago, University of Chicago Press, 1965. p 10.
2. Ad Hoc Committee on Classification of Headache: Classification of headache. *JAMA* 179:717–718, 1962.
3. Boag, TJ: Psychogenic headache. In Vinken PJ, Bruyn GW (eds): *Handbook of Clinical Neurology,* Amsterdam, North Holland Publishing Co, 1968, vol 5, pp 247–256.
4. Weatherhead AD: Headache associated with psychiatric disorders. *Psychosomatics* 21:832–840, 1980.
5. Kolb LC: Psychiatric aspects of the treatment of headache. *Neurology* 13:34, 1963.
6. Rosenbaum M: Symposium: psychogenic headache. *Cincinnati J Med* 28:8–16, 1947.
7. Warpman B: Symposium: psychogenic aspects of headache. *J Clin Psychopathol* 10:3–20, 1949.
8. Packard RC: What is psychogenic headache? *Headache* 16:20–23, 1976.
9. Lazare A: Hysteria. In Hackett TP, Cassem, NH (eds): *Massachusetts General Hospital Handbook of General Hospital Psychiatry.* St. Louis, CV Mosby, 1978.
10. Adler G: The physician and the hypochondriacal patient. *N Engl J Med* 304:1394–1396, 1981.
11. Janet P: *The Major Symptoms of Hysteria,* ed 2. New York, Macmillan, 1920, pp 160–163.
12. Packard RC: Conversion headache. *Headache* 29:266–268, 1980.
13. Weatherhead AD: Psychogenic headache. *Headache* 20:47–54, 1980.
14. Packard RC: Emotional aspects of headache. In Packard RC (ed): *Neurologic Clinics Symposium on Headache.* Philadelphia, WB Saunders, 1983, vol 1, pp 445–457.

CHAPTER NINETEEN

Psychiatric Aspects of Posttraumatic Headaches

WILLIAM G. SPEED, III, M.D.

The topic of psychiatric aspects of posttraumatic headaches is surrounded by controversy. Although the etiological relevance of psychological factors has been extensively compared to the relevance of organic ones, the relative role of each in the production of emotional symptomatology and chronic headache remains unsettled. It is probable that these two factors can never be clearly separated (1). The patient's personality before injury is seldom a major or specific factor in determining whether he will develop posttraumatic symptoms (2). However, the general observation that the stable, mature, successful, and responsible person with good coping abilities is more likely to bounce back from an illness, infection, or operation than is the anxious, depressed, or insecure person probably holds equally true for an individual's response to head injury. Or, expressed in other words, preexisting personality disorders may color the symptoms of the posttraumatic state but are not the cause of it. Moreover, patients who have previously had stable personalities may develop, along with posttraumatic headaches, anxiety, depression, and insecurity which may persist for weeks, months, years, or in some instances, indefinitely.

Chronic posttraumatic headache occurs in 30–50% of head-injured patients. It is considered to be present when the headache continues for more than 2 months following an injury (3, 4).

Surprisingly, there is no correlation between the severity of the headache and the severity of the head injury as evidenced by the presence of coma or its duration, amnesia, signs of focal brain damage, subarachnoid hemorrhage, increased intracranial pressure, or EEG abnormalities (3, 5). In fact, chronic headache may be less frequent after major cerebral injury than after minor concussion. Some of the most intractable cases of posttraumatic headache occur after trivial injury (6).

The most commonly reported symptoms following head injury are headache, lightheadedness or true vertigo, tinnitus, impairment of memory, reduced attention span, insomnia, easy fatigability, reduced motivation, decreased libido, as well as personality changes such as mood swings, anxiety, depression, and inability to tolerate frustration. Most of these symptoms, particularly the headaches, develop almost immediately after the injury. Appearance of some of the personality changes may be delayed by up to a few weeks.

STRUCTURAL AND METABOLIC FACTORS

Although it is generally agreed that constitution, personality, intelligence, age, preexisting neurosis, and life situation at the time of the injury contribute something to the posttraumatic problem there is less than total agreement on the extent of this contribution. However, the weight of evidence now tends to swing the pendulum towards the organic point of view. Studies on cerebral blood flow of head-injured patients have shown regional or generalized abnormalities (7). Other studies have shown evidence of faulty processing of information (8) and abnormalities of labyrinthine and vestibular function tests.

Damage to nerve fibers is prominent in head injury, and there is little doubt that it often occurs in cases of mild as well as severe injury (9–11). Striking, swirling movements of the brain have been demonstrated following even subconcussive blows to the head of rhesus monkeys whose skullcaps were replaced with transparent material (12).

From the standpoint of explaining the curiously prolonged posttraumatic symptomatology seen in some patients, perhaps those studies demonstrating a slowing of cerebral circulation lasting months or years after head injury are of considerable significance (7,13,14). It remains unclear as to why cerebral trauma is followed by such persisting circulatory delays. It is known that months after even a nonserious deceleration injury, multiple, old, circumscribed infarcts and widespread axonal tearing can be found, but what role, if any, these might play in the altered circulation is not known. Therefore, no explanation can currently be given for the observed prolongation of circulation time in patients with head injuries. Available evidence suggests a continuing metabolic abnormality, possibly one of carbohydrate oxidation and acid-base regulation, as the most likely underlying cause (15).

The purpose of devoting space to the material in the above paragraphs is simply to emphasize that accumulating data strongly points towards an organic basis for most, if not all, symptoms observed in post-traumatic headache syndromes. This "organicity" is probably the result of a combination of structural and biochemical abnormalities.

CLINICAL CHARACTERISTICS

Posttraumatic headache may mimic almost any type of chronic recurring headache. It may be constant or intermittent and may involve any areas of the head (e.g., frontal, temporal, vertex, occipital, in any combination) or involve the entire head. Depending on the mechanism producing the headache, there are a variety of descriptive terms used by patients. Patients with muscle contraction or nerve entrapment components may describe a broad band around the head, an ache deep inside the head or, more commonly, aching, pressing, squeezing, expanding, burning, and stabbing. Those who experience a vascular component are most likely to describe pounding or throbbing that may be aggravated by bending over, coughing, sneezing, straining, jarring of the head, exposure to loud noises and bright lights, ingestion of alcohol, physical exertion, stress, and anxiety. In other words, there is nothing about the clinical features of these headaches that separates them from other well-known headache syndromes (16).

A variety of mechanisms are responsible for posttraumatic headaches, and these may occur individually or in various combinations.

The muscle contraction headache is clinically indistinguishable from the chronic muscle headache that is unrelated to trauma. It is a constant, nonthrobbing, dull pressure pain that may be posterior cervical, occipital, vertex, temporalfrontal, or almost any combination of these. The pain may be a result of an accumulation of noxious metabolites in ischemic muscle (17, 18) acting in concert with sustained muscle contraction. The basis for posttraumatic muscle contraction headaches appears to be a malfunction in the control of normal muscle tone. Because the maintenance of normal muscle tone is dependent on a properly functioning gamma-efferent system and its interconnections with the brain (19), a malfunction somewhere in this complex system appears to permit excessive muscle contraction. There are no studies that shed light on the mechanism of this malfunction.

Vascular headaches, commonly seen in some posttraumatic headaches, are produced, at least in part, by vasodilation. These are usually pulsating, pounding, and throbbing headaches. Although many of these headaches are nonmigrainous vascular headaches, it is apparent that the migraine process can be triggered by head injury (20–22). Both classic migraine and common migraine have been precipitated by head injury. Another variety thought to be a vascular headache was described by Vijayan (23) as a posttraumatic dysautonomic cephalalgia. This is a rare variety of posttraumatic headache. He reported several cases, all of which involved injuries to the neck. Following these injuries there were recurrent ipsilateral headaches, accompanied by ipsilateral pupil dilation and excessive sweating, occurring 3–12 times a month and lasting 8–12 hours. He postulated that these symptoms were manifestations of localized sympathetic hyperactivity, presumably resulting from injury to the carotid artery.

Muscle contraction and vasodilation may coexist in the same patient, and the term "posttraumatic mixed type headache" is used to describe this combination.

If the soft tissues of the head are injured a visible and palpable scar in a localized tender area may result. Or, a localized tender area without a scar may result from injury. Both situations produce symptoms based on the entrapment of sensory nerve endings at the site of the scar or on the stimulation of nerve endings from the locally damaged tissue (24). It is suggested that scarring results from traumatic myositis, fibrositis, or periostitis. The headache is felt at the site of injury, and the pain may be intermittent or continuous. The area involved is always strikingly tender to finger pressure.

Muscle contraction, vasodilation, and scar formation may coexist in the same patient and will give a mixture of symptoms characteristic of each component.

Injury to the superficial and deep structures of the neck, involving muscles, ligament, bones, discs, or nerve roots can produce cervical pain that may be referred to the head.

The popular term "whiplash injury" describes a sudden hyperextension of the neck followed by hyperflexion, and is usually the result of a rear end automobile collision. Shortly after such an accident, most patients complain of diffuse muscle soreness followed by neck and head pain. Their headache may be limited to the occipital area, or may spread to involve the vertex, temporal, frontal and retro-ocular areas as well. The pain may be a dull pressure or squeezing sensation with, at times, pounding and throbbing components. The neck pain is aggravated by movements of the neck. Pain in the head and neck persist for days or weeks and in some cases becomes chronic, lasting many months or longer. Exacerbation of preexisting arthritis or discogenic disease may also occur. In some cases, the occipital neurovascular bundle—made up of the occipital nerve, artery, and vein—may be traumatized at the level of the occipital ridge at the time of the original injury, or may become traumatized secondary to prolonged muscle contraction or chronic recurring vascular dilation impinging on the occipital nerve itself. The term "occipital neuralgia" is used to describe this condition.

PSYCHOLOGICAL FACTORS

There is no doubt that when psychological disturbances are present to a degree sufficient to interfere with the patient's quality of life, the physician must address them in treatment, just as he would in patients with any other diagnoses, even if there is an organic basis for many or most symptoms. Unfortunately, cynicism of some physicians towards patients suffering from posttraumatic symptoms, particularly when they are dominated by symptoms appearing to be "psychological," may contribute to chronicity, and may enhance feelings of hopelessness and helplessness in those patients (25). Physicians must relate to patients, of course, but when treating posttraumatic headache they may also be obliged to relate to insurance companies, Workmen's

Compensation Commissions, lawyers, judges, and juries.

A dilemma faced by physicians is that of distinguishing the legitimately psychologically impaired patient, whose symptoms are produced or aggravated by trauma, from the patient in whom continuation of symptoms is motivated by revenge, greed, or the wish to avoid responsibility. In my experience malingering is rare in the posttraumatic situation, and as physicians we must guard ourselves against adopting a cynical attitude towards trauma patients because of fear of being duped by a clever malingerer. An in-depth history and detailed examination, done by a physician experienced in posttrauma syndromes, will make this distinction in the vast majority of the cases. Remember that legal settlements do not necessarily produce a cessation of symptoms or a return to work (26), and the same symptoms may develop when no litigation is pending (26).

It is easy to understand how the individual who has been functioning well in life and is suddenly brought to a standstill by headache, mental impairment, reduced attention span, inability to concentrate, memory loss, dizziness, depression, etc., after what may have been a relatively minor injury, will often begin to experience emotional symptoms as well. It is also easy to understand how, when these symptoms persist for many months or years and the patient remains incapacitated, a physician may feel that adding the diagnostic label "conversion reaction" is appropriate. This implies, or at least suggests, that the patient is himself responsible for the symptoms, even though a true conversion reaction is always subconscious and, therefore, is beyond the patient's conscious control.

As stated earlier, a growing body of evidence suggests that organic factors are probably operating in such patients. This may be disturbing to some physicians because our present state of knowledge does not permit us to understand how a movement injury or momentary blow to the head can produce alterations in brain function which persists for such long periods. Only time will lead us out of this

dilemma. Meanwhile, these patients need the understanding of their physician, as well as his patience and persistence in rendering help.

TREATMENT

The headache itself results from malfunctioning of the normal regulatory control of cranial vasculature and musculature, and sometimes from the formation of local scarring. Pharmacotherapeutic measures and biofeedback training may be useful in decreasing the extent of the malfunctioning regulatory systems. Malfunction of these symptoms is further aggravated by underlying anxiety, fear, apprehension, frustration, and depression. It is essential that the physician devote his efforts to ameliorating these symptoms as well as to stabilizing the vascular and muscle regulatory systems.

The type of pharmacological management selected depends on the primary physiological disturbance. Muscle contraction headaches may be helped by the use of tricyclic compounds such as amitriptyline, imipramine, doxepin, etc. The average dose is 50–100 mg per day, but may vary from 25 to 150 mg depending on the patient's response and tolerance. Occasionally the tricyclic compound dyclobenzaprine, which has no antidepressant effect but may have muscle relaxant properties, may be used. The dosage is 10 mg tid.

When muscle contraction and vascular dilatation coexist, one should add a beta blocking agent, such as propranolol, to the tricyclic compounds. The average dose for propranolol is 20 mg qid but higher doses may be used depending on the patient's response and tolerance.

Some posttraumatic headaches have, alone or in addition to muscular and vascular components, what is called a "nerve ending entrapment syndrome." This syndrome is readily identified by the presence of localized tenderness, which can be brought on by thumb or finger pressure. Pain of this origin may subside following Xylocaine injections directly into the areas of tenderness. As much as 7–8 ml of 1% Xylocaine can be used.

Treatment of neck and head symptoms associated with the so-called whiplash injury should be conservative; a cervical collar may be tried along with heat and massage. Sometimes a home traction unit is useful for short periods. There may also be localized areas of muscle tenderness which may respond to Xylocaine injections.

Techniques for teaching general body relaxation, including electromyographic (EMG) biofeedback for specific muscles and thermal biofeedback (hand warming) for vascular components, can benefit many posttraumatic headache patients. An adequate degree of motivation, and ability to concentrate despite the symptoms, are attributes of those who respond to this training program. Luthe (27) has advocated autogenic neutralization techniques to reduce and progressively eliminate any functionally disturbing posttraumatic symptoms. In this technique, a patient who, for example, "just can't get moving" may, by "reliving" the accident in detail, realize he is still going around "with a foot on the brake," or with a fear of dying.

In addition to these measures, other psychological interventions, including traditional psychotherapy or behavior modification, may be required for some patients. Posttraumatic headache and its related symptomatology have an impact not only on the patient, but on the patient's family, friends, employer, and work colleagues as well. In addition to the emotional symptoms resulting from organic disturbances sustained in the injury, powerful forces enhancing these symptoms can be generated by continuous head pain, impaired memory and concentration, reduced attention span, insomnia, easy fatigability, decreased libido, and pronounced frustration resulting from enforced change in routine. This can cause a "merry-go-round" effect, in which organically induced physiological malfunctions produce symptoms which in turn lead to anxiety, depression, and frustration, which in turn further enhances the physiological malfunction, etc.

Appropriate management involves consideration of all these factors. In addition to pharmacotherapy, biofeedback, and the usual modalities of psychotherapy, the physician must address the impact of these symptoms on the patient's immediate family. Both the patient and his family must be educated about the forces which produce the devastating chain of events in which the patient finds himself. When possible, employer, lawyer, and disability agencies should be included in the educational process; this is usually a difficult if not impossible task. Patience, persistence, understanding, empathy, and compassion are important attributes for the physician, in addition to his medical and psychiatric expertise.

REFERENCES

1. Lewis A: Discussion of the differential diagnosis and treatment of post-contusional states. *Proc R Soc Med* 35:607–614.

2. Kozol H: Pre-traumatic personality and psychiatric sequelae of head injury. *Arch Neurol Psychiatry* 53:358–364, 1945.

3. Brenner CT, Friedman AP, Merritt HW, Denny-Brown DE: Posttraumatic headache. *Neurosurgery* 1:379, 1944.

4. Merritt HH, Friedman AP, Brenner CT: Headache and posttraumatic syndrome. *Trans Am Neurol Assoc*:70–77, 1944.

5. Friedman AP, Merritt HH: Relationship of intracranial pressure in the presence of blood in the cerebrospinal fluid to the occurrence of headache patients with injuries to the head. *J Nerv Ment Dis* 102:1–7, 1945.

6. Miller H: Accident neurosis. *Br Med J* 1:919–925, 992–998, 1961.

7. Taylor AB, Bell TK: Slowing of cerebral circulation after concussional head injury. A controlled trial. *Lancet* 2:178–180, 1966.

8. Gronwell D, Wrightson P: Delayed recovery of intellectual function after minor head injury. *Lancet* 2:605–609, 1974.

9. Oppenheimer DR: Microscopic lesions in the brain following injury to the brain. *J Neurol Neurosurg Psychiatry* 31:299, 1968.

10. Strich SJ: Diffuse degeneration of the cerebral white matter and cerebral dementia following head

injury. *J Neurol Neurosurg Psychiatry* 19:163, 1956.

11. Strich SJ: Shearing of nerve fibers as a cause of brain damage due to head injury. A pathological study of 20 cases. *Lancet* 2:443, 1961.

12. Pudenz RH, Sheldon CH: The lucite calvarium. A method for direct observation of the brain. Cranial trauma and brain movement. *J Neurosurg* 3:487, 1946.

13. Oldendorf WH, Kitano M: Radioisotope measurement of brain blood turnover as a clinical index of brain circulation. *J Nucl Med* 8:57, 1967.

14. Skinhoj E: Determination of regional cerebral blood flow in man. In Caveness WF, Walker AE (eds): *Head Injury Conference Proceedings.* Philadelphia, Lippincott 1966, p 431.

15. Taylor AR: The cerebral circulatory disturbance associated with delayed effects of head injury. In Caveness WF, Walker AE (eds): *Head Injury Conference Proceedings.* Philadelphia, Lippincott, 1966, p 52.

16. Speed WG: Posttraumatic headache. *The Practicing Physician's Approach to Headache,* 1986, pp 113–119.

17. Dorpat PL, Holmes TH: Mechanism of skeletal muscle pain and fatigue. *Arch Neurol Psychiatry* 74:628–640, 1955.

18. Perl SP, Markoen LN: Factors involved in the production of skeletal muscle pain. *Arch Intern Med* 53:814–824, 1934.

19. Chausid JT: Neurological basis of muscle tone. In *Correlative Neurological Anatomy and Functional Neurology,* ed. 17. Lente Medical Publication, p 167.

20. Bennett ER et al: Migraine precipitated by head trauma in wrestling. *Am J Sports Med* 8:202–205, 1980.

21. Haas DC, Pineda HL: Juvenile head trauma syndrome and their relationship to migraine. *Arch Neurol* 32:727–730, 1975.

22. Kalenak A, Petro DJ, Brennar RW: Migraine secondary to head trauma in wrestling. *Am J Sports Med* 6:112–113, 1978.

23. Vijayan N: A new posttraumatic headache syndrome. Clinical and therapeutic observation. *Headache* 17:19–20, 1977.

24. Jones OW, Brown HA: The measurement of posttraumatic pain. *J Nerv Ment Dis* 99:668, 1944.

25. Kelly R: Posttraumatic syndrome: An iatrogenic disease. *Forensic Sci* 6:17–24, 1975.

26. Balla JI, Moratis S: Knights in armour. A follow up study of injuries after legal settlements. *Med J Aust* 2:255–261, 1970.

27. Luthe W: *Autogenic Therapy.* vols. V and VI. New York, Grune & Stratton, 1973.

CHAPTER TWENTY

Psychometric and Descriptive Aspects of Cluster Headache

LEE KUDROW, M.D.

Cluster headache is generally recognized as a distinct syndrome characterized by a stereotypic clinical presentation, specific vascular changes, and response to unique treatment modalities. Psychological symptomatology observed during the cluster period may be more a function of the pathophysiology of cluster headache than a function of personality dynamics of characterological structure. Emotional change associated with the acute attack, however, is certainly reactive and not unexpected in view of the excruciating and debilitating quality of the pain.

CLINICAL PICTURE

Cluster headache is classified as episodic or chronic. In the former type, attacks occur only within a specific period (the cluster period) of 1–3 months' duration, followed by a remission period of approximately 12 months on the average. The chronic type is distinguished by an absence of remission periods.

Attacks during the cluster period are extremely severe, of 30–90 minutes in duration, located around the eye and temporal region unilaterally, and associated with symptoms referable to the autonomic nervous system. Thus, during attacks, patients generally experience ipsilateral lacrimation, rhinorrhea or nasal stuffiness, conjunctival suffusion, and ptosis and miosis. A typical cluster headache attack is best described in the following first person account (1):

Following a period of perhaps several hours of feeling quite elated and energetic, I experienced a fullness in my ears, somewhat more on the right side than the left, and having a character similar to that which occurs during rapid descent in an airplane or elevator. I then become aware of a dull discomfort, an extension of ear fullness at the base of my skull—further extending over the entire head, on both sides, though somewhat more on the right. At this point, two or three minutes have elapsed; seemingly short but long enough for me to know that a 'cluster' has indeed begun and will ultimately get worse. Such anticipation causes me considerable consternation regarding any decision to continue my activities, or cancel plans and find a place to be alone, giving way to a slowly increasing anxiety, fear, panic, and withdrawal. I become aware of myself 'listening' for changes in my head. Is the cluster prematurely aborting itself, progressing further, or unchanging? A sudden stab, only fleeting, strikes my temple, then again—somewhat near the apex of my skull and upper molars in my face, always on the right side. It strikes me again, deep into the skull base, and as quickly, changes location to a small area above my eyebrow. My nose is stuffed and yet runs simultaneously. If I could sneeze I feel the attack would end. Yet in spite of all tricks, I find myself unable to induce sneezing. While the sharp stabs continue in this fashion, a slow crescendo of dull pain presents itself in an area of a hand's length and breadth over the eye and temporal region. The pain area narrows into a smaller area, and yet, as if magnified, enlarges in intensity. I find myself bending my neck downward, though slightly, as if my head is being gently pushed from behind. My neck, up to the base of my skull, is tight and feels as if I were wearing a neck collar. I feel compelled to remove my tie and loosen my shirt collar even though I know that it will not offer me even a modicum of relief.

In an effort to alter this persistent discomfort, I drop my head between my legs while seated. My face and eyes seem to fill with fluid, but the pain remained unchanged. Despite my suntan, as I look into the mirror, a gaunt, sickly, pale face peers back. My right lid is only slightly drooping and the white of my eye is charted with many red vessels, giving the eye an overall color of pink. Right and left pupils appear equal and constricted, as is usual for light-eyed people. Having difficulty standing in one place too long, I leave the mirror to continue alternating my pacing and sitting.

As usual, I am struck with the additional fear that the pain will never end, but dismiss it as impossible since even if that were the case, I would surely kill myself.

The pain, now located somewhere behind my eye and slightly above it, worsens. The pain is best described as a 'force' pushing with such incredible power through my eye that my head appears to be moving backward, yielding to its resistance. The 'force' wanes and waxes, but the duration of successive exacerbations seem to increase. The cluster attack is at its peak, which is celebrated by an outpouring of tears from only my right eye. I have now been in cluster for thirty-five minutes—ten minutes at its peak.

My wife peeks into the room where I hold forth. I look up and see her expression of pity, frustration, and helplessness. She sees my tortured face as I have seen it in the mirror at this stage before; a drooling mouth, agape, gray face wet on one side, an almost closed eyelid, and smelling of pain and anguish. She closes the door and leaves, feeling hurt for me, anger for the stupidity of medical science, and guilt—since deep within her mind is the suspicion that she is the cause for my suffering.

I cry for her, but cry more for myself. The pain is so incredible. Suddenly I am overwhelmed by a fury. I lift a chair high over my head and crash it to the floor. With a doubled fist I strike the wall. The pain persists.

Waning periods soon become longer in duration and I allow myself to suspect that the peak is behind me—but cautiously, since I have been too often disappointed.

Indeed, the pain is ending. The descent from the mountain of pain is rapid. The 'force' is gone. Only severe pain remains. My nose and eye continues to run. The road back, as with all travel, covers the same territory, but faster. Stabbing, easily tolerated pain is felt. Then gone. Dull, aching fullness, neck stiffness, all disappear, replaced in turn by a welcome sensation of pins and needles over the right scalp area—similar to the way one's leg feels after it has been 'asleep.' Thus, my head has awakened after a nightmare of torment.

Eye and nose dry, I let out a sigh. I collect my pile of wet tissues that are strewn all over the floor and deposit them in a wastepaper basket. The innocent chair, now uprighted, I rub my slightly bruised fist.

Thus, having ended the battle and cleaned up its field, I open the door and enter my pain-free world—until tomorrow.

The preceding account of an acute attack describes the intense anguish experienced by the cluster victim. Thus, during the cluster period, the patient is not only subjected to episodes of terrifying pain but must also endure the terror of anticipation. Anticipatory anxiety in this case, therefore, is an appropriate psychological response.

PERSONALITY TESTING

Although earlier literature depicted cluster headache groups as neurotic (2–4), recent studies have not corroborated these findings (5–8). Indeed, personality profiles of cluster patients differed little from those of control groups. This does not suggest that all cluster patients are emotionally stable; there appears to be a subgroup of treatment-resistant patients who manifest symptoms and test scores characterizing neuroticism.

Concerning the Minnesota Multiphasic Personality Inventory (MMPI) test, Harrison (2) stated that conversion "v" patterns were consistently found in all headache patients, including cluster. Steinhilber et al (3) found that cluster patients had scored similarly to an "other headache" group on all scales of the MMPI. Both groups scored significantly high on the *hypochondriasis* and *hysteria* scales, and lower on the *depression* scale. Rogado et al (4) obtained similar results in comparing MMPI profiles between 50 cluster patients and matched migraine groups.

In 1977, Sutkus and I (5) obtained MMPI results from 41 patients with cluster headaches, 32 men and 9 women. This group was compared to five other headache groups: migraine, combination headache (migraine + scalp muscle contraction headache), posttraumatic cephalalgia, conversion cephalalgia,

and chronic scalp muscle contraction (CSMC) headache. A control group of 30 nonheadache subjects was included. With the exception of the conversion group, the mean ages of all other groups were similar.

We found that migraine and cluster groups scored similarly on all scales and, contrary to previous reports, there was no evidence of a conversion "v" configuration. Abnormal profiles, however, were noted for other headache groups (Fig. 20.1). The mean of five MMPI scales (scales 1, 2, 3, 7, 8) were averaged for a single value of psychopathology. This value was calculated for each headache category, including controls, and was

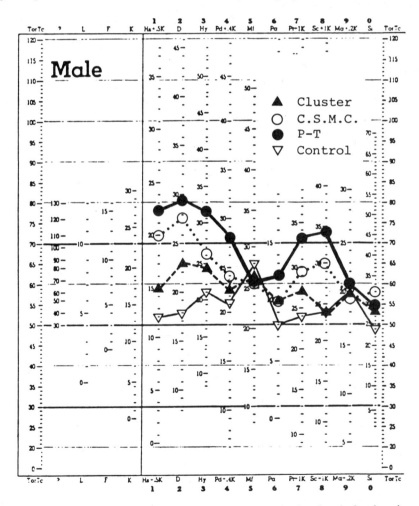

Figure 20.1. *MMPI patterns of males with cluster headache and other headache disorders. (Modified from Kudrow L, Sutkus BJ: MMPI pattern specificity in primary headache disorders. Headache 19:18–24, 1979.)*

plotted. As seen in Figure 20.1, this score for cluster patients did not differ significantly from that of controls, in contrast to other headache disorders. Indeed, our findings suggested a continuum of psychopathology, with post-traumatic and conversion groups scoring most severely (Fig. 20.2). In conclusion, we had demonstrated little evidence of psychopathology among cluster patients as a group (5).

In a subsequent study, Cuypers et al (6) also reported an absence of neuroticism among cluster or migraine groups, as measured by the Freiburg Personality Inventory (FPI). Our results were further corroborated by Andrasik et al (7). In a cross-validation analysis they found little difference between control and cluster or migraine groups when assessed by neurotic scales of the MMPI. There was less agreement, however, concerning other headache categories. Similarly, Sternbach et al (8) found that vascular headache patients scored less neurotically on MMPI examinations than other headache groups. They made no mention, however, of whether cluster patients were included in the vascular group.

It would appear from the aforementioned studies that patients with cluster headache differ little from nonheadache controls on certain personality inventories; yet among cluster patients we are finding a subgroup which exhibits significant neuroticism and addiction-proneness, as measured by MMPI evaluations.

ADDICTION-PRONENESS

In two surveys, done in 1974 and 1980, respectively, (9, 10) we reported that cigarette smoking and alcohol use occurred with a significantly greater frequency in a cluster population than in migraine or nonheadache control groups. We speculated that this high frequency of substance abuse was related more to personality factors of cluster patients than to the disorder itself. We could not, however, identify this personality trait by analysis of conventional MMPI scales.

In an ongoing study we are currently evaluating cluster patients in an effort to define a clinical subgroup which exhibits neurotic behavior, substance abuse, and resistance to conventional anticluster therapy. Using the MacAndrews Scale (on the MMPI) for addiction-proneness (ADD), we are beginning to understand this treatment-resistant subgroup of cluster patients. We have, up to

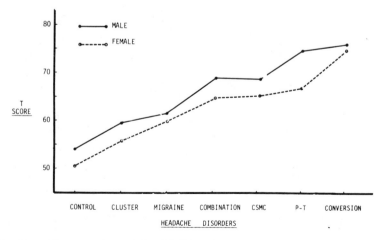

Figure 20.2. *Mean T-score values of five MMPI scales in each headache disorder. (From Kudrow L, Sutkus BJ: MMPI pattern specificity in primary headache disorders. Headache 19:18–24, 1979.)*

TABLE 20.1.
ADDICTION-PRONENESS (ADD) AND NEUROSIS IN MMPI PROFILES OF 13 CHRONIC AND 21 EPISODIC CLUSTER PATIENTS

	Neurotic		Nonneurotic		N	(%)
	Chronic	Episodic	Chronic	Episodic		
Add	6		3		9	(69.2)
		2		7	9	(42.9)
Non-add	2		2		4	(30.8)
		1		11	12	(57.1)
Total	8(61.5)	3(14.3)	5(38.5)	18(85.7)	34	(100)

date, tested 34 patients with cluster headache and 60 migraine controls.

Addiction-proneness was found in 52% of the cluster group and in only 16.9% of the migraine control group. These frequencies were remarkably similar to those for alcohol abuse in an earlier report: 51% frequency for cluster, and 19% for migraine (10). These results lend support to the validity of the MacAndrews Scale and also suggest that half the patients with cluster headache are indeed prone to substance abuse.

The MMPIs from 34 cluster patients were also analyzed for neurotic profiles, particularly in relation to addiction-proneness. Of this group, 13 were chronic and 21, episodic. Almost 70% of chronic patients were found positive for ADD. Sixty-one per cent also had neurotic profiles. Nonneurotic profiles were found in 86% of episodic patients. Frequency of ADD among episodic patients, however, was increased (43%), but was lower than in the chronic group (Table 20.1).

We are tempted to conclude from this survey that the high alcohol abuse rate in cluster populations is reflected in the increased frequency for ADD; also, the higher frequency of neuroses and ADD among chronic patients may be related to pathogenesis of chronicity and to treatment resistance. Our final conclusions, however, await completion of these studies.

REFERENCES

1. Kudrow L: *Cluster Headache: Mechanisms and Management.* London, Oxford University Press, 1980, pp 25–27.
2. Harrison RH: Psychological testing in headache: a review. *Headache* 13:177–185, 1975.
3. Steinhilber RM, Pearson JS, Rushton JG: Some psychological considerations of histaminic cephalgia. *Mayo Clin Proc* 35:691–699, 1960.
4. Rogado A, Harrison RH, Graham JR: Personality profiles in cluster headache, migraine and normal controls. Presented at the 10th International Congress of the World Federation of Neurology, September 1973.
5. Kudrow L, Sutkus BJ: MMPI pattern specificity in primary headache disorders. *Headache* 19:18–24, 1979.
6. Cuypers J, Altenkirch H, Bunge S: Personality profiles in cluster headache and migraine. *Headache* 21:21–24, 1981.
7. Andrasik F, Blanchard EB, Arena JG, Teders SJ, Rodichok LD: Cross-validation of the Kudrow-Sutkus MMPI classification system for diagnosing headache type. *Headache* 22:2–5, 1982.
8. Sternbach RA, Dalessio DJ, Kunzel M, Bowman GE: MMPI patterns in common headache disorders. *Headache* 20:311–315, 1980.
9. Kudrow L: Physical and personality characteristics in cluster headache. *Headache* 13:197–201, 1974.
10. Kudrow L: *Cluster Headache: Mechanisms and Management.* London, Oxford University Press, 1980, p 42.

CHAPTER TWENTY ONE

Psychodynamics of Cluster Headaches

CHARLES S. ADLER, M.D.
SHEILA MORRISSEY ADLER, PH.D.
JOHN R. GRAHAM, M.D.

The mighty Mars did oft for Venus shreek, privily moistening his horrid cheek with womanish tears . . .

ROBERT BURTON, *The Anatomy of Melancholy* (1)

SOME OBSERVATIONS

In the preceding chapter, Kudrow vividly describes the anguish of those who suffer cluster, through the words of a cluster patient. Clearly, each attack brings a cascade of events both familiar and excruciating, and the pain is neither imagined nor symbolic. As with migraine results of psychometric testing do not consistently correlate this syndrome with formal psychiatric diagnoses. Therefore, the first question we must address is this: Is cluster headache an issue for psychiatry? Wouldn't anyone in such pain react the same? In short, why write a chapter on it?

Traditionally, the most popular view in medicine has answered these questions on cluster in the safety of conservatism: because the illness is "real," any emotional concomitants are the result of the illness, or somatopsychic. Such influences in cluster are, as Kudrow has aptly pointed out, powerful indeed. Yet significant observations about these patients' psychological status and life style have also been made, observations which concern his modus vivendi between attacks as well as during them. For example, Lesse (2) observed 50 of 53 cluster patients to be depressed; Violon (3) found that not only were 84% of his cluster patients depressed during the headache siege, but 61% were also depressed during the headache-free interval. Because similar observations appear so consistently, it would be irresponsible to ignore what cluster patients relate over and over in their histories, or the behavioral patterns clinicians have observed repeatedly in their offices. The quantity of raw data has now passed the stage of anecdote. A conclusion of the Headache Research Foundation Cluster Conference (4) phrases this thought sparsely: "Some attributes of the personality structures of these patients begin to stand out. Further documentation and relation of these to the physiology of the attacks seems indicated."

There is precedent for looking beyond the bounds of the usual type of information collected to understand a disorder in a way that can radically supplement our existing knowledge without rejecting it. Kuhn (5), in *The Structure Of Scientific Revolutions*, makes the following point:

Sometimes a normal problem, one that ought to be solvable by known rules and procedures, resists the reiterated onslaught of the ablest members of the group . . . And when it does—when, that is, the profession can no longer evade anomalies . . . Then begin the . . . investigations that lead the profession at last to a new set of commitments . . . Each produced a consequent shift in the problems available for scientific scrutiny and in the standards by which the profession determined what should count as an admissible problem or as a legitimate problem-solution.

Valid psychological information about a disorder is important whether or not it corresponds in degree or type to a formal psychiatric diagnosis. Psychodynamic patterns emphasized in this chapter—or, for that matter, any psychological patterns—will not necessarily be found in all patients with cluster. The typical distribution curve for illnesses subject to emotional influence is that psychological contributions are absent in some patients, and present to varying degrees in others. For those patients who do show them, however, a full delineation of the elements involved can be crucial, not only to understanding the pathogenesis and triggers of this illness, but to successfully treating it.

The reader should assume that this chapter only concerns itself with patients who have psychologically influenced cluster headaches, even when that rather cumbersome phrase is not specifically employed. We hope our observations will stimulate the reader to reflect upon his own experiences, and see if any of the traits described spark in him a sense of familiarity or of recognition. By thus joining forces we may ultimately refine the details of what has so intrigued many of our colleagues about this disorder.

SOME BACKGROUND

In 1684 the venerable Thomas Willis (6) made the first written reference to what was likely a cluster headache. Since then, the physiological aspects of the disorder have been focused on almost exclusively; while psychological observations are at times alluded to, it is usually not considered within the scope of the paper or followed up upon.

Wolff (7) believed that cluster, like migraine, is related to a patient's emotional conflict and life stresses. In 1958 Friedman and Mikropoulos (8) reported on 50 cluster patients, about whom they stated: "Although it was not possible in many of these patients to verify the primary etiology is psychogenic, the importance of psychological factors in their headaches could not be minimized."

In 1968, John R. Graham (4) and the Headache Research Foundation organized a conference on cluster at the Faulkner Hospital in Boston at which the significance of the link between a cluster patient's psyche and headache period was one major focus of presentation and discussion.[1] Rushton (4) summarized the beliefs of many conference participants: "One reason I am convinced of [common character traits in cluster] . . . is that when you see a person who does not fit the category . . . it comes as rather a shock, and you recognize these people as being exceptional in this group."

INSIDE THE BIOLOGICAL CLOCK: OBSERVATIONS ON TIMING

The most simple and direct evidence that psychological factors are operative in a given headache type is that the headaches coincide with or follow psychosocial misfortune or distress. This relationship was apparent to Wolff (7) in his observations of cluster patients. To determine whether this impression held up under more careful scrutiny, Hinkle (9) obtained biological and social histories of cluster patients coming to the New York Hospital. To this end he amassed data from 40 consecutive cluster patients. In this way he investigated whether patients' activity patterns bore any relationship to their headaches. Hinkle found several common patterns. First was the presence of a driving personality in restless

---

[1] In 1983 the authors also participated in a symposium on cluster organized by Hansrudi Isler at the University of Zurich in which there was a lively debate about the relevance of psychological factors to cluster.

pursuit—and usually achievement—of success. He also found:

The patients' stories suggest that the relationship between the biological phenomena of alertness, activity, and sustained, goal directed effort which is a feature of other forms of vascular headache is a feature of this form of headache also. The fact that the activity is sustained over such a long period of time and with such evident success often leads the patients to deny that they have any problems or difficulties; and the fact that the clusters often appear during periods of vacation, retirement, or well deserved relaxation tends to make the patient forget all that had gone before.

In other words, if one looks not at each headache but at an entire cluster period he is likely to see that the latter follows a letdown period which in turn has been preceded by intensively sustained purposeful activity. He gives the following examples:

- A pediatrician who struggled endlessly to cover up for his alcoholic wife and carry out her responsibilities. He developed severe clusters when the demands on him were suddenly reduced.
- A field boss for a large construction company routinely had clusters after finishing a large job.
- Cluster headaches in three patients came when they joined the Navy and were assigned to a leisurely but boring tour of sea duty.
- A widowed tailor struggling to put his children through college was headache free while he worked from morning until late night, but developed clusters during the relaxed periods in this seasonal business.
- A man who leased oil tankers came down with cluster headaches after concluding his most successful deal ever.
- A wealthy entrepreneur and successful developer had his first series of clusters when he finally retired at age 55.
- The sales director of a major company who had risen through the ranks had his first

cluster right after his most successful business show.

If drive and letdown wind the biological clock, what mechanism sets—and so precisely—the alarm? While it would appear that the factors setting it are physiological and, although there is no evidence at this point that the unconscious significance of a particular time determines this rhythmicity, Stroebel (10) found that most people can waken themselves at a specific time through self-suggestion, without a clock, yet with great accuracy. Smith (11) described a patient wakened by a cluster headache each night at 11:00. The patient related it to the noise his stepson, with whom he did not get along, made in the shower at that hour. Most curious, though, when daylight savings time began, the headaches shifted an hour to catch up. It has been pointed out (4) that a patient may have these headaches within 5 minutes of each other every single day, a timing which will even adjust for time zones if he flies across the country.

A PSYCHOANALYTIC CONSULT

At the Headache Research Foundation conference Howard Corwin, a psychoanalyst, discussed the character structure and psychic conflicts he observed in cluster patients (12). The three patients whom he presented reflect many characteristics commonly seen in psychologically influenced cluster patients.

CASE 1

The first patient, 44-years old, alternated between working as a male nurse and a sandblasting foreman. He

nurtured an intense hatred for his vicious, alcoholic, irresponsible father, whose family suffered because of his alcoholism. Father ignored the patient and nine other children, and the patient felt he never gave them anything. Despite this picture, when father devel-

oped a cerebrovascular accident the patient, after many years of no contact with father, was compelled to give father many months of intensive nursing care to rehabilitate him."

The father had promised to stop drinking if he recovered, but later broke that promise, leading to a resumption of the rift between them—and to the onset of cluster headaches in the patient.

The parents were divorced. "Mother relied upon the patient as the man of the family" through his early life. She was described as hard working, long suffering, and masochistic. "During his formative years, the patient had the feeling that he had always had to do everything on his own. He fought for everything he had, worked after he had left school in tenth grade to support mother, but nevertheless was constantly belittled and ridiculed by father." While in the military he transferred jobs from medic to paratrooper, but developed hysterical aphonia immediately before combat, and was therefore discharged. He then underwent intermittent psychotherapy. Nevertheless, he continued to present, on a superficial level, an air of hypermasculinity, and remarkable independence.

He has been given to violent physical aggressive outbursts, in which he becomes almost uncontrollable and regards himself as a Dr. Jekyll and Mr. Hyde. He has struck many authority figures both in civilian and military life. Despite this he wishes to be known as a "good guy," strives to control himself and his moods at all times, regards himself as careful, attentive to details, perfectionistic, and always fights rage at the ineptitude of others . . . currently in his job he has not only worked his way up to foreman but is union representative for the group. He has never missed a day's work even during the worst of his headaches. Initially his mental status exam revealed that he was 'hale fellow well met.' He was in constant need in the interview to prove his strength and masculinity to me. Despite this hypermasculine stance he revealed an inner sense of desperation about himself and an intense dependency on wife and doctors . . . though he was not overtly depressed he did speak of killing himself if there was no posi-

tive result or relief. His mental content revealed a fantasy he had always had. He felt that he could essentially lose everything in a short period, that his security was flimsy at best, and prolonged illness could certainly fulfill his worst expectations.

This patient displays many of the characteristics commonly seen in patients with cluster headaches. Corwin characterizes him as having:

latent passive dependent features, and serious problems in identification. There had been lifelong striving to be independent, aggressive, forceful, and respected. His identification with father had been pathological, and is evidenced as an identification with the uncontrolled aggressor. He has little inner sense of solid masculine identification. He does have an identification with mother, as seen in his nutritive nursing side.

Although his basic character structure seemed to be compulsive, there was also available to him the defense mechanism of somatization of his anxiety, which was demonstrated by the conversion aphonia. At other times he handles his feelings in a more stable fashion through the defenses of "prominent reaction formation, compensatory hypermasculinity, obsessional perfectionism, with an accent on control at all times. These at no time work well enough to negate his deep insecurity, whose nature is most clearly seen through the fantasy that he could lose everything at any time. His greatest struggle has been to control his hostility. His latent yearning for a supportive person to help him be a man may provide a toehold for psychotherapy in such a patient."

CASE 2

The second case was a 31-year-old business executive with a 6-month history of clusters who "made clear that headaches or pain could not keep him from working on his job as the job was the most demanding and significant part of his life at present." He was unable or unwilling to give any significant past history, instead simply characterizing all questions about his background and early life as having been "typical." This was especially true when it came to questions about personal situations. From the comments he made, however, it was evident that this patient felt extreme competitiveness towards his father, a relationship the patient believed he had lately dominated on all fronts: he simply said he has a better house than his father, will make more money than his father, and "is involved in a different and more important world."

The patient stated that he was working for his father-in-law, a self-made magnate and an absolute tyrant. That his involvement with business was a driving preoccupation was seen to be no exaggeration when he gave details. He described his father-in-law as a cutthroat man who "works by essentially overwhelming everyone; gambles heavily in his enterprises; and 'knocks down' his competition. He outshouts, outfinances, and outmaneuvers with extraordinary skill. He wins by overpowering his opposition, moving his money more quickly, and essentially makes others concede his superiority." In his job, the patient was "under the constant surveillance of his father-in-law who rides, harasses, ridicules and belittles all of his employees." Nevertheless the patient has some compelling attraction towards this situation and could not see it for what it was. Instead he admired his father-in-law for "fighting for his rights and his basic ability." Even the patient's wife saw what a no-win situation the patient was in and pleaded with him to find work elsewhere. But he wouldn't listen.

Some years back he tried to leave this employ, but his ultimate return only demonstrated his magnetic attraction to the relationship. Indeed, the marriage itself was getting wounded, perhaps mortally, by the patient's obsession with succeeding in father-in-law's business; he hardly ever saw his wife and children, or recognized the unhappiness he caused them; and, he rationalized his treatment of them as though they were of minimal importance. The headaches began 6 months

earlier, when he finally started turning a profit and feeling more confident about his work.

He had an air of business and busyness about him. Appointments were hard to make because of his more important duties. He had to be on the run the moment the hour was over. He denied depressive feelings and focused all of his difficulty on his headaches alone. The most striking aspects about him are his tense compulsivity, his capacity to isolate his conflicts, his driven quality, his extreme competitiveness, and the extent to which he was caught up in the situation wherein he is undergoing a metamorphosis from a more easy going, and somewhat introspective fellow to an aggressive, father-in-law type person.

Corwin described the patient's character structure as compulsive, with latent rivalry and dependency. Conflict centered about his wish to identify with the aggressor (father-in-law) whom he nevertheless also despised. At a very basic level, it was the competitive feeling towards his father which were being reenacted in this arena, though not consciously. The identity for which he struggled did not sit comfortably within him, and lead to an inner warring of differing parts of his personality.

Peculiarly too, he was a very fearful person. Again, the dependency characteristic. He felt shaky, needed to over ensure his security, and also had this fantasy that he could lose everything if he let down. Physical impairment was hazardous as it could easily jeopardize his job. Any suggestions made by others that he change his job aroused conscious anxiety, as it meant to him that he would lose everything.

CASE 3

The final patient was a 52-year-old contracting entrepreneur, who displayed hypermasculine speech and mannerisms, "attention to detail, sharpness, compulsive ability, and skill at manipulating business deals." He too had a history of a hostile dependent relationship

. . . with an 'entrepreneurial,' self-made-man-type father, with whom he was deeply identified. The father was vicious in business deal-

ings, a ruthless, reckless, heavy gambler. When the patient went into business with him, father had applied some of his same techniques to the patient as he had to others. Despite this the patient, out of feelings engendered by his mother that the family should remain close together, could constantly forgive his father's misdeeds.

Nevertheless, he had "a strong need for being admired and loved and held closely in the family . . ." and "a strong but ambivalently held identification with his father, and a dependency whose core is not clear to us . . ."

In closing, Corwin concluded that there were certain communalities in these three cases. (With regard to these and other attributes, Hinkle, Friedman, and Carroll (4) found no differences between cluster patients seen in public clinics and those seen in private practices, or between patients from different socio-economic levels.) As Kunkle et al (13), Wolff (7), Robinson (14), Friedman and Mikropoulos (8), and Symonds (15) had previously noted in cluster patients, Corwin saw in these three gentlemen compulsive character defenses. He also observed in all three the possibility of some very high level, pre-verbal "hysterical vulnerabilities." What he asserted that was most clear, however, was this: ". . . underlying conflicts that these patients present deal with issues of dependency, control of aggression, and instability of masculine self image based on impaired male identifications."

UPWARD MOBILITY, HIGH ENERGY LEVELS, "DRIVEN" QUALITY OF LIFE

The afterimage these three gentlemen leave, not of merely having been diligent in toiling, like migraine patients, down the road to success, but of speeding down it in frenetic pursuit, has been seen in many cluster patients. As Graham (16) notes: "These patients are ambitious, hard working, and have a strong sense of upward social mobility. They push and push until they break with symptoms, or reach the goal and drop exhausted into a batch of headaches." This "driven" quality is more than an epiphenomenon of pain, as it also occurs between cluster periods. Hinkle (9) only found one of 40 patients who didn't show long periods of being filled with alert and purposeful activity between cluster periods. He defines purposeful activity as intensive behavior "pursued for a purpose and not as an end in itself." This activity is most commonly directed toward business and professional achievements, but can have other apparent objectives as well. Hinkle leaves no doubt about the intensity of this "purposeful activity":

These are people who get up early in the morning; who go to work and work steadily, who often say they do more work than anyone else around them; who may take little time off for lunch; who may work beyond the regular time in the evening; and who frequently bring work home or continue in the evening with other activities of a purposeful nature that are related to their occupation. They will do this on weekends; they will do it twelve months of the year; and they very often go without vacations. Frequently they are involved in not one but two, three, or more activities of an occupational nature. This has been the case in 30 of our 40 people.

Hinkle pointed out that, although these patients worked as long as possible, at its peak the cluster period often becomes irresistibly disabling, and they must stop. But as soon as they are at all able to, they are back in action. Cluster patients generally take few vacations, or none at all. "They were sort of one man businesses. They felt they just had to keep going" (17). Blumenthal (4) has commented that even when a cluster period begins, it is often the patient's wife who calls to make the appointment, with the patient saying he is working too hard to stop and call himself. This has also been a common experience of the authors. Sweet (18), a surgeon, observed: "Cluster patients tend to be a very stoic group and . . . don't get submitted to surgery because they put up with this intense pain."

We should emphasize that these traits in the cluster patient are seldom viewed as problems by his acquaintances, neighbors, and business associates. "The capacity of these people to attain their goals, to maintain their families, to feel that they are doing this successfully and not to express to the physician any sentiment other than happiness or pride in what they are doing has been an outstanding feature . . . They have not often regarded themselves as being people who have 'problems'. Quite to the contrary, in many instances they are viewed as outstanding, successful people who can do more work than anyone else in the office"(9).

Just how successful are these patients? Extremely, in many cases. Yet while many are as "successful as one can be," the story of a struggle or fight to get there, sometimes from poor beginnings, is just as common. They often refer to themselves as Horatio Algers. Some examples from Hinkle:

- A man with three years of schooling who began as a rural store clerk. He advanced to ownership of several banks and the largest hardware chain in his state; he was debating whether to run for Lieutenant Governor of that state.
- An oil well rigger who rose to construction boss for one of the largest international construction firms.
- A patient from rural community with four years schooling who started out as gas station attendant and door to door salesman; his success was so great it accounted for half of all sales, and he became vice president of the corporation.
- An illiterate dishwasher who became manager of one of the largest hotels in New York.
- A vice president of one of the largest automobile manufacturers in the nation.
- One of the youngest floor brokers on the New York Stock Exchange.
- One of the most successful brokers in the international business of leasing tankers.

Working class men who do not rise as dramatically are, nevertheless, often considered successful and energetic in other areas. Fried-

man (4) cites, as an example, a janitor attending night school in order to get a degree.

As with the migraineur, the cluster patient deserves respect for his "real world" accomplishments. Nevertheless, this inflexible behavior pattern typically puts him under too much pressure.

Another observation that calls into doubt the belief that this tendency is merely red-blooded corporate ladder climbing is that of Carroll (4):

It is my experience that patients with this condition are full of drive, obsessional, perhaps a little rigid and very anxious to achieve success in life. However, having reached a certain point of success, one finds that after an interval they become restless and are anxious to achieve more so that their life, as it were, becomes a vicious circle with a continuously underlying current of stress.

It's as if they reach many possible stopping points on the road of success, but none are ever quite what they are looking for. Carroll goes on to describe a side to these patients not seen in the boardroom:

Another feature which I have noted is their ability to present a calm exterior and so give the impression of being in full control of the situation. However, when you interview the relatives, particularly the wife, they often tell you that the patient reacts badly to stress, and one also finds that they are dependent on their wife, and sometimes on other people, even their children.

Hinkle (9) found that cluster periods were associated with being "successful in business" in 32 patients, and were only clearly unrelated to success in two of them; yet, by and large, sustained interpersonal conflicts tended to be present, conflicts which took something away from these victories. Other, less well-defined factors, seemed to interfere with feelings that should accompany success, and cluster patients were rarely found basking in the afterglow of their achievements. Even when they had beaten the competition, the competitiveness remained, restlessly searching for a new objective. Interestingly, this competitiveness is often hidden behind a veneer of affability which in part may be an attempt to disguise the scale of the patient's competitive motivations from himself. As part of that posture, occasional patients display a dry, finely tuned sense of humor. It is humor of the "It only hurts when I laugh" genre, drawing it's comic effect from the appearance of being impervious to what should have been painful blows, of absorbing them with a seemingly wry diffidence.

The cluster patient is not only active, but he often also feels an inner pressure toward activity which can't be shut off. Many stay awake and alert late into the night, busying themselves with activities. Usually, the cluster patient simply cannot stop such behavior; he interprets rest as "doing nothing," an anticipation which in turn only triggers more restless anxiety—and before long, further action.

It is often difficult to fathom these patient's inner mental life, as their hopes, fears, and fantasies seem inextricably bound up in external "reality situations." The patient experiences his problems as being on the outside; solutions are also seen as coming primarily from the outside. Attempts to draw the patient in the direction of introspection frequently lead to his becoming confused or distrustful. This commitment to seeing things through concrete external events, actions, and interactions is often striking. Similarly striking is the related tendency in cluster patients to show significant impulsivity.[2]

---

[2] While not identical to them, these personality characteristics have features reminiscent of certain other character types described in the literature. One such type is the "hypomanic character", in which a relatively stabilized, low level manic behavior pervades the personality. (This may be relevant to the usefulness of lithium in treating cluster). "Type A" personality characteristics are also close enough to features seen in cluster patients to one day warrant more detailed comparison. Similarities include a driven quality of life, a preoccupation with time, and an underlying anticipation that people will ultimately let one down. A standardized interview to test for the Type A personality pattern has been devised and validated, and might be used to more specifically outline differences between these two predispositions.

DENIAL

The cluster patient's success in business or community ventures often makes the physician less alert to potential psychological difficulties in him. Another factor that encourages one to underappreciate psychological difficulties is the vigorous manner in which the cluster patient typically denies significant past problems.

Graham (17) reported that cluster patients "show massive reluctance to divulge to an outsider, including the doctor, disturbing and powerful feelings of anger, guilt, and inadequacy . . . . We found them very loathe to give up the secrets of their psychiatric problems . . . . Sometimes they tell you two years later what was really happening two years before, when they had the last cluster." Rushton (4) stated: "Most of these patients will never experience or never consent to prolonged psychiatric investigation . . . ," while Steinhilber et al (19) found that "Initially most patients totally denied any emotional difficulties in their life and saw no correlation between their headaches and the adaptive mechanisms utilized to handle life's stressful encumbrances." Finally, Adler and Adler (20) have written: "The cluster patient will typically deny deep seated emotional difficulties; he is an iron clad man." Even when the cluster patient does describe troublesome events from his past, the manner in which he conveys this information implies that he has dealt with his past in his own way, and to his satisfaction. This implication is communicated even when he acknowledges that such events might have been important. Why not take him at his word?

The implication that the cluster patient's past was untroubled does not hold up to scrutiny, no matter how vigorous its assertion. Violon (3) found that 92% of his sample of cluster patients had childhoods characterized by early affective deprivation. Graham (17) has collected the surprising statistic that 35% of 100 cluster patients had at one time consulted a psychiatrist. (Nevertheless, the absolute number of such patients is so small that any individual psychiatrist rarely has occasion to know more than several.) This contrasts with 26% of migraineurs and 12% of a control group. The figure is even striking considering such patients' frequent reluctance to either see their problems as partly psychological, or to tolerate psychotherapeutic probing.

What is most inconsistent with the "All's well" assertion is the patient's common description of a severe blow to his psychological equilibrium in childhood, usually in latency; it is of a type which could not help but have massively stunned him. Their backgrounds and experiences often read as though from a Dickens novel. Sometimes there was an abrupt and marked change in family circumstances. Overwhelming losses were common, often of a parent or sibling and, often, set in a context of further tragedy or resulting in it. Yet when describing these occurrences, the typical cluster patient might just as well be reading a railroad schedule for all the outward feeling he betrays. It's as if he has placed the most upsetting emotional experience in his life behind a door of steel. The principal function of that door is to keep the feelings about the event hidden from himself.

The patient frequently describes his reaction to the catastrophe in a way that makes that reaction appear either insufficient or bizarre. Typical is the example of the youth who came home to find that his father, a professor, had abandoned the family, without so much as a goodbye. As an adult the patient insisted that he was totally unmoved by the event, but that he had been "very clever," as he used the opportunity to ask his distraught mother whether he could have a pet dog he'd been wanting—in his father's place—and that he was "lucky" enough to have his wish granted. He had not shed a single tear for his father in the years since.

Violon (3) found that "most patients complained of having been . . . battered, rejected, abandoned or having lived in a cold atmosphere without any demonstration of affection." A greater than average number of cluster patients seen at the Headache Research Foundation directly report having

been subjected to physical or emotional violence at the hands of a childhood caretaker, usually the father. One patient's father would come home drunk and bitter and try to physically vent his frustrations on the patient. The boy "with the cleverness of Ulysses escaping from the Cyclops by clinging to the underbelly of a sheep" would hide under his bed, pulling himself up against the springs so the father's groping arm would not find him.

Another clue to the power of repressed memories in a cluster patient may come through a study of his dreams. In one investigation, 39 of 100 cluster patients were found to remember their dreams frequently, compared to 35 migraineurs and 21 controls. Thirteen of these cluster patients were prone to "very bad night terrors [which] on various occasions . . . precipitated a headache" (16). Friedman (4) reported: "In our experience night terrors and nightmares are more common and more severe in this group than in persons with the usual forms of migraine." Some patients remember a greater percentage of dreams during cluster periods than at other times.

ATTEMPTED RESOLUTION OF LOSS AND SEPARATION

The mothers of cluster patients are often described in either bland, general terms or are portrayed as having been strong-willed. Sometimes they are capable, determined, or dominant, traits which they must occasionally use to hold the family together through adversity. Nevertheless, the images of their mothers that cluster patients convey tend on the whole to be more vague and variable than those of their fathers. Therefore, we will describe the paternal relationship in somewhat more detail.

Difficulties in the relationship between the patient and his father seem to be a recurring theme with male (and possibly female) cluster headache patients. In its extreme form, this involves actual loss of the father through death or abandonment; more common is the sense of loss experienced in the absence of his loving contact, resulting from abusiveness, indifference, unavailability, alcoholism, or intense rivalry. Occasionally, the patient's father is also described as having the characteristic of aggressive striving for success, or also has characteristics of the self-made man. With a number of patients, these traits were decidedly present in close grandfathers or uncles. Examples of the types of separation from or disillusionment with father can be seen in the following unselected, consecutive series of cluster patients:

- A man whose mother, in his presence, died suddenly of a heart attack when he was a young boy. The father, to whom the patient had previously been extremely close, quickly remarried a powerful, selfish woman who brought her children to the house and insisted on most of the father's attention. Father, a prominent attorney, would not fight to keep the relationship with his son strong, but instead exiled him to a room over the garage, and later sent him out of state to boarding school. Try as he might, he was never really able to break back into his busy father's attentions.

- Patient whose father worked for a multinational company and was frequently gone, leaving the beleaguered mother with 10 children. One day, when he was in the Far East, the mother just disappeared, abandoning the family. The father came home, put the patient in an orphanage (where he grew up), and returned to his travels.

- Patient whose father died precipitously when patient was young. No opportunity for grieving.

- Patient who was doing well, having friends in school, but "my father had higher hopes for me." Domineering father was disparaging of this child, looked at him as mental and physical reject. Sent him off to a military academy for sixth to ninth grade which "turned me into an intensely shy person." Father himself had wanted to go to the military academy but had been unable. Father was a traveling salesman, never home, subject to fits of rage; never showed interest in patient. Father died when patient was 15 and still at the military academy.

- Young man whose parents put him up for adoption at an early age. Adoptive father was self-made executive of national corporation. Mother had several operations for cancer. When patient was latency age, he was told he was adopted. Denied any feelings about this . . . thought "everyone was." Nevertheless, maintained secret fantasies of developing a "special relationship" with male talk show host. Similar relationships repeatedly sought elsewhere, notably in sports coaching, at work, and in therapy.

- Man whose father was self-made executive. Father unrealistically refused to declare bankruptcy during depression when patient was a child, and simply had everyone in the family working morning until night; presumably, he was unavailable.

- President of a major international corporation whose depressive father quietly left town one day for a "business trip" and committed suicide.

- Patient, previously described, whose alcoholic father abandoned the family precipitously.

- Patient with obvious characterological difficulties who stated: "I have a good marriage, my parents are super people, and I had a good childhood." When pressed would only say, "Father owned restaurants and was always pursuing the almighty dollar. I do too, and I am in the same kind of work he was."

- Female patient. Father was wealthy immigrant who established large construction company. He then developed severe T.B. and became a bedridden invalid. Distant and autocratic, he had little to do with the children, turning them over to governesses. Grandiosely refused to acknowledge the business failure that resulted in their "losing everything." Mother had to sneak in laundry at night to survive. Father felt children were beneath him, and told them to "deal with the servants." Father had a bad temper and patient was afraid of him, yet he was idealized by mother. Patient felt it was her obligation "to redeem the family name."

- Female cluster patient of poor immigrant parents. Expected to do heavy labor as child. At age 13 father had CVA, was paralyzed. All responsibility for caring for father fell on her. The situation became "tyrannical"; nothing she did pleased him.
- Female patient whose father was prominent professor. He was generally indifferent to the patient, but raped her at time of puberty. She had relied on him to be a counter-point to a borderline mother. Father died during patient's mid-adolescence.

Typically, the cluster patient does not mourn his loss or make peace with it, and this interferes with his going on to consolidate his identity in the context of another relationship. Nor does he want to again be vulnerable to similar emotional injuries from relationships. Thus, the patient's yearning to be close to such a father often conflicts with the need to be protected from the emotional or even physical hurt that can follow attempts to actualize his wish for such a relationship.

The patient often shields himself from his past by denying its importance, by not allowing himself introspection or self-reflection, by devoting all of his attention to the action-oriented present and future rather than the past, and by keeping his relationships broadly based—not putting all of his eggs in one basket. Working at three jobs allows any one of them to be relatively expendable. The future patient often imagines that if he were to give up hope to be close to and like his father he would in essence be resigning himself to an identification with mother, which would be, in his mind, a defeat. In the future psychologically destabilized cluster patient, what often results is a failure to integrate these competing identities (with the mother and with the father) in a healthy fashion. Instead, they alternate with each other in terms of their power to define the patient's sense of self.

With cluster patients, as with other people, the repetition compulsion often causes one to pass problems on to the next generation. For some cluster patients this means re-enacting an unfulfilling father-son relationship, this time in the role of the father. Considering the active lives cluster patients lead, it is clear that they frequently have limited time for their families. Even when father does get home from the office, his children may find him irritable and exhausted from the pace he keeps. Hinkle (9) described an alternate pattern, however, one in which the zeal more typically devoted to business is directed instead towards family "accomplishments." As examples, he cites a young widow immigrant who, by working 70 hours a week as a practical nurse, supported one child through college and two more through medical school; a widowed tailor who worked extensive hours to put his children through college, even though he himself had not been; a physician who spent all of his spare time caring for home and children—and his alcoholic wife; and, a woman who supported her family through her husband's recuperation from carcinoma, while at the same time putting their children through college. Headache clusters often followed successful completion of such family commitments.

In many cases, this second pattern Hinkle cites probably reflects the patient's wish to protect his own children from the types of painful experience which he himself endured. Ironically, in working so hard to provide for their offspring, some of the widowed parents described above may have inevitably repeated this familiar pattern of unavailability.

UNDECLARED DEPENDENCY, UNACKNOWLEDGED PASSIVITY

In most of his encounters, the male cluster patient is an energetic and virile individual, often athletically inclined, and assertive or even aggressive in his interactions. Some patients are even characterized as having "hypermasculine" attributes. This perception is intensified when the patient also has the large stature and rugged physiognomy which frequently accompanies this condition. As Graham (16) points out, however, closer examination reveals that this presentation often tells only part of the story. Human nature involves dependent as well as assertive strivings. The more the former are denied outwardly, the stronger they may grow within. Such dependent feelings, wishes, attitudes, and behaviors are often split off from the cluster patient's more rugged characteristics and are seen to alternate with them, or come to out in secretive ways. This can be observed most clearly in the relationships that some patients have with their wives. Graham (17) invokes the image of MacBeth and his "Lady," and notes the resemblance of their relationship (though not of their deeds) to cluster couples. *He* in deadly and guilt-inducing competition with the King (a universal symbol for father), yet *she* commandeering all initiatives behind closed moats. The wives are often the ones who make the appointments, put out their hands for the prescriptions, or even describe "how the patient is doing."

The dichotomy described above is brought alive by the following comments from an initial interview. The patient was a burly, intermittently animated, 58-year old shopteacher at a juvenile detention center:

- "I can break my arm and I would go ahead and play football. I am not sensitive to pain. I used to drive my head into a wall. I have a scar and if I could have found something I would have killed myself."
- "My wife wanted me to come and see you."
- "I used to have quite a temper. I probably could lick six kids at a time when I was young. I love to fight. I would rather fight than eat. I fought in the Golden Gloves once."
- "I don't know the names of the pills I was taking, but my wife would remember them."

- "When I do lose my temper I have absolutely no control over it. I don't care if I live or die. I would die protecting someone. I get threats all the time in juvenile hall. There were some kids driving fast around the neighborhood and could have hit someone, so I leaped at the car and grabbed the wheel when it was going 35 miles an hour. I got all bruised up in that incident, but I just didn't think about it."
- "I do cry at times. I cried when my wife was in surgery, and I cried when a friend had to have surgery, and in movies. I could cry at Bambi."
- "I have guns all over. Under my bed, in the drawer, and in the car. I never get frightened. I had six murderers in my class at one time. One time I saw a robber going into my neighbor's house and I got so angry that I pointed a finger at him from under my jacket, and shouted 'Stop or I'll blow you apart.' Fortunately, he did. I just did it without thinking."

Another hearty and aggressive man with clusters said: "I don't have affairs now. My wife would beat me."

When present, one reason for this passive stance with women might be that the patient has never allowed his relationship with his mother to fully mature because his emotional energy is still invested in seeking to recapture his relationship with his father. As a result, he vacillates between flight into hypermasculine identification with an idealized father image, and resignation to the ties with women when this falters.

ADDICTIVE BEHAVIORS: URGENCY, ANXIETY, AND ORALITY

Cluster patients are far more likely to smoke and drink than are controls (21). These are strong and determined habits. Many drink to the point of abuse, and suffer the physical consequences of that abuse.[3] Quite strikingly, 21% of patients continue their drinking (24) through a cluster period, even though alcohol often initiates attacks. This behavior is testimony to the strength of the habit and to anxious, impulse-ridden characteristics buried in the personalities of those unable to stop.

Caffeine, in the form or coffee and colas, is also used to excess. It has been observed (4) that the caffeine encourages these hardworking people to keep up their excessive pace and to feel on top of things. Although limiting caffeine or tobacco use can reduce frequency of attacks, the number of patients willing to do this turns out to be small.

LETUP OF PACE, BUILDUP OF ANGER, LEAD-IN TO HEADACHE

Hinkle's study found, in all but 5 of his 40 patients, that a sudden slowing of pace typically preceded cluster periods. The slowdown might have occurred because of a vacation, retirement, the successful attainment of a goal, the rest imposed by an intervening illness, or cumulative fatigue.

Another view of the period before clusters holds it to be a time when the patient is undergoing a buildup of resentment or anger. Saper (21) cites evidence that "the presence

---

[3] The nature of the diseases whose prevalence is increased in cluster patients goes along with the dichotomous identification frequently seen. These include atherosclerotic coronary artery disease which, in many young individuals, is clinically associated with hypermasculine, restlessly impatient ("Type A") behavior patterns. It is seen more often in males who struggle with an overabundance of hostile impulses, and who have trouble letting themselves trust others (22). Perhaps these attitudes are related to the patient's state of mind when he is trying to forge his masculine identity. Peptic ulcers are also significantly more common in cluster patients, and these are frequently associated with a struggle to repress strong dependency longings (23); this is possibly correlated to the state of mind accompanying denial of the maternal identification. Naturally, the coffee, alcohol, cigarette smoke, and pressured life styles directly contribute to these two diseases as well.

of sustained stress and/or rage may provoke a bout of episodic clusters, and a disturbance of sleep and mood may also occur prior to the onset of the headaches." Although the cluster patient is normally proud of his accomplishments, he may harbor various resentments about the frustration he encounters at home and work. Nevertheless, cluster patients "may be able to express feelings of hostility or resentment towards the person with whom they are involved in the conflict" (9). Others (20, 21) find that cluster patients do have difficulty expressing anger, and believe that when this anger is suppressed too long it may contribute to the onset of a burst of cluster headaches.

Perhaps the contradictory impression that the cluster patient both expresses anger and has difficulty expressing it can be resolved. Consider: although he often exhibits significant anger, it might be directed at someone other than his true primary target. This brings up the concept of transference, and the difficulty in unburdening deep-seated anger at an internalized figure from the past by means of venting displaced anger at someone in the present. Even if they have realistically erred, how much arguing with one's boss does it take to get feelings of rage at, say, a bullying parent off one's chest? Such actions inevitably fail to cure the underlying problem fueling the anger. In any event, the cluster patient's anger, when it does emerge, can be both severe and abrupt, riding as it does, on the coattails of impulsivity.

McNeil (25) observed that when a cluster period is blocked pharmacologically, many patients develop chronic tension headaches instead. He believes that this shows that cluster headaches fill a psychological need. Specifically, McNeil suggests that "then you have to delve into their hostilities and find out why they hate the person they do. . . ."

THE ATTACK: BREAKTHROUGH OF SYMPTOMATIC BEHAVIOR AND FEELINGS

The pain of cluster is excruciating. Along with it the patient must endure dread generated by foreknowledge of what is still to come. Such a patient can be expected to act highly distressed by his condition; indeed, it would be abnormal for him not to be. Yet the behavior of a cluster patient during an attack often transcends even this expectation.

During actual attacks 64 percent pace the floor, 71 percent shut out the family, 32 percent weep, 37 percent yell out loud, 16 percent bang their head on the wall, 14 percent roll on the floor, 7 percent go into a 'trance,' 7 percent 'become unconscious' " (16).

This common observation—that the typical reaction to cluster headache pain is unlike the reaction to other types of intense pain—should arouse clinical curiosity and stimulate scientific investigation, as would any repeated observation. One will find, in any emergency room, many patients waiting in pain, much of it acute and severe. Despite the combination of all variety of personalities with the pain of massive trauma, carcinoma, tic douloureux, slow subarachnoid bleeding, peritonitis, renal calculi, herpes zoster, or causalgia, florid reactions to pain that equal those observed in patients suffering a cluster attack are rare. And, many of these other conditions have a greater burden of anxiety, as their clinical course is unfamiliar to the patient, and they may have ominous prognostic implications. Consider now some further behaviors observed during a cluster attack:

We have observed very wild behavior in some of them . . . one man puts his head in a hot oven. Another one complained of passing out, though he wasn't really unconscious. Many of them scream. A good many of them cry. One man in the hospital really got himself practically upside down and kept biting the pillow. Other men lock themselves in the bathroom so that their family and children will not see them in this terrible state of crying or breaking down; or they get in their car and drive around so that nobody will catch up with the fact that they are having this trouble. During attacks in the hospital one man in the midst of a very bad attack just got sort of frantic and he took a little student nurse and hugged her and kissed her during this attack. Another one

'passed out' seemingly and cast his eyes up to the ceiling in a very wild sort of way . . . they do very strange things. . . ." One patient, a frequent hunter, "gets frantic in his attacks, loses his memory, and wonders whether 'to jump in a lake himself or shoot another hunter' " (17).

Saper found that a full 41% of 101 cluster headache patients admitted to suicidal ideation during headaches. "Violent emotions during cluster attacks may represent deeply repressed emotions . . ." (24).

Patients with cluster headaches demonstrate rather overt acts of hysteria during attacks in which they do bizarre things such as go into a trance, scream, or jump out of a car. Between clusters when they are not having headaches we have observed several interesting episodes of hysterical deafness, hysterical aphonia, and writer's cramp" (17).

CLUSTER HEADACHES AND CONVERSION REACTIONS: A FALSE EQUATION

A number of factors have caused investigators to question whether conversion mechanisms are relevant to cluster headache episodes. The frequent presence in MMPIs of a "conversion v" configuration, the dramatic behavior, and, in many patients, a seeming indifference to the headaches between cluster periods, and sometimes even between headaches, have aroused these doubts.

The relevance of the "conversion v," which is also seen in other types of headache, was disclaimed by Rushton (4), who participated in an early study which showed its presence in patients with cluster. He believed:

[The conversion v] should not be taken as any evidence of profound insight. I think it does represent, oftentimes, a person who has symptoms, but he thinks about them a great deal even though he doesn't let them particularly influence what he really wants to do. That's where the notion of indifference comes in . . . so that the term conversion v is more or less a superficial psychiatric term, and I don't think it would stand up under prolonged and detailed probing. (**The present authors would concur with these conclusions.**)

The primary question with regard to the phenomenon of indifference is whether this truly represents the "La Belle Indifference" which is the type specifically associated with conversion reactions. It has seemed otherwise to most psychiatrists observing this phenomenon in cluster (12), and does not appear to represent the French variety of "indifference" to the authors either. Indeed, the comments in Table 21.1 represent the height of attentiveness! The blasé facade observed between cluster periods and sometimes between attacks should be considered in light of personality type: these are patients who try to rapidly

push from their minds and deny unpleasant experiences, focusing instead on tasks of the present and hopes for the future. They hope that by ignoring their condition they will disallow it to interfere with their functioning . . . maybe it will even go away. Theirs is an attempt to divert attention, to distract, and to struggle on in spite. This can be misread as indifference.

The nature of the personality also sheds light on the dramatic behavior, although it does not illuminate it entirely. Recall, these are patients who have repressed and avoided pain throughout their lives. They have always been able to parry reminders of emotional wounds by throwing themselves into work, or by becoming more physically active. Such

TABLE 21.1
REPRESENTATIVE STATEMENTS BY PATIENTS ABOUT THEIR FEELINGS AND BEHAVIOR DURING CLUSTER HEADACHES

Patient 1:	"I get annoyed really easily during an attack. Everything is chaotic and I want to be left alone. It will go away quickly if I am just left alone. I am extremely irritable during the attacks. I go downstairs and turn the lights off and drift around real slow in a ten-foot area. I don't want anyone around me. When the attack is over I don't think about it, don't dwell on it."
Patient 2:	"It's untouchable pain like something trying to burn out inside of me like a fire. Sometimes I would beat my head against the wall from pain. I eat Midrin (a medication) like popcorn, but after a time it doesn't help. I pace. The pain just consumes me. Once when I was in pain I wanted someone to shoot me."
Patient 3:	"I used to drive my head into a wall. I have a scar and if I could have found something I would have killed myself. I have laid down with my feet up so the blood runs to my head."
Patient 4:	"When the headache comes I feel like I want to pull my eyeball out. On occasion I would feel restless and thrash around, moan, groan, yell and cuss."
Patient 5:	"The severity of this headache . . . I just don't believe that some people could survive them. It's hard not putting your hand through the wall they're so terrible. I almost thought of hurting myself during them. If something didn't happen I probably would. I will lose all contact with what I am taking in terms of medication. I will take whatever anyone gives me. I pace the floor. I get on the floor on my knees like in prayers or lay on a certain side. I just have to walk during a headache or cry, sometimes uncontrollably. I cry out 'what have I done to deserve this headache?'. And I am not a crier. It hurts so bad you want to die. I just have to cry. The crying doesn't help it though. It seems like it's got a course it's going to run. I have been to the point where I damn near wanted to pass out. Sometimes I smash things. My first headache was when I was 18 and I tore the towel racks off the wall. I have had some diarrhea with it and that's good because it takes my mind off it. I once rubbed some DSMO on my face and forehead as a last resort, and I could have rubbed cow dung on it."
Patient 6:	"I lean up against the wall with the top of my head, especially against the refrigerator. I use a hot steam kettle over my nose. I lay on my back on the left side. I twist my neck and my spine. I push on a certain spot on the right side of the back of my neck. I push on the scalp. I urinate or defecate to avoid the headache. I pull on my head or push on my nose."

strategies prove insufficient, however, against the pain of cluster. It is this pain which so threatens the brittle retaining wall the patient may have constructed around his memories and feelings. If the intensity of this pain shatters the patient's defenses, a host of feelings surge through. These may include grief, agitated depression, suicidal impulses, and extreme anger.

The patient responds first with a series of increasingly frantic attempts to repair the breach, similar in type to ones that have worked for him in the past. They involve action, but under these circumstances it is imperative that the actions be of the most intensive sort. These may include attempts at acute distraction, self-exhaustion, or counterirritation—one patient would go to the basement and rock so furiously that her rocking chairs would repeatedly wear grooves into the cement floor. These defensive maneuvers mingle with the outpouring feelings which had been repressed, presenting for the clinician a combined picture of symptomatic affect and defense, all of it superimposed upon the pain itself. Thus, many forms of extreme or bizarre behavior may be observed.

When the pain subsides—often, even when the patient knows it is starting to—he is able to reconstitute his defenses again. If the degree of pain experienced or the power of the feelings being held in are not great, the patient may be able to block such an external reaction entirely. Therefore, despite this potential for extremes, cluster patients sometimes report continuing to work on their jobs right through the attacks.[4]

Factors of which we are unaware may also contribute to the quality of the patient's reaction to his headache. Kudrow (26), for example, has hypothesized that the mechanism of cluster may include an intermittently manifested disorder of the carotid body—hypothalamic axis, resulting in a cyclical cerebral hypoxia which then initiates attacks. Physiological changes which begin during the attack ultimately compensate for the triggering hypoxia. The sense of panic that accompanies hypoxia, and the sense of urgency to find anything to do that will reverse the situation, may thereby also have reflexive neurological roots. Desperate activity would not be strange behavior for someone who had aspirated a piece of meat, or who fears he is drowning. Conceivably, diffused elements of this reflex which, perhaps as a result of some perceptual blunting inherent in the disease, are cognitively dissociated from the respiratory apparatus, and are thus unidentified as respiratory by the patient, may contribute to the experience of desperation.

Based on current evidence, it appears unlikely that the cluster episode is a form of conversion reaction, "preverbal" or otherwise.

DEPRESSION

The pain of unfinished business from the past—grieving is a prime example—appears to motivate the depression from which many of these patients, through frenetic activity, are trying to escape. As noted before, Lesse (2) and Violon (3) found depression in 97% and 85% of cluster patients, respectively. Hinkle (9) found overt depressive symptoms in over half of his patients during a cluster period:

Yet aside from their focusing on the pain they have a general feeling of hopelessness and of lack of meaningful outlook on life. They say 'yes, I am very depressed' even though they often say also, 'it's the pain that has been getting me down, not anything else.' Difficulties with the sleep cycle have been features in about half of our cases.

Hinkle's experience parallels that of others. Adler and Adler (20) found that these patients incorrectly ascribed both the depression and the suicidal thoughts entirely to pain alone. In 1980 they noted that:

---

[4] When anger unites with head pain and the desperate impulse to "do something," one result may be the frequently seen attacks directly upon the painful head itself—hitting it into a wall, or in some other fashion assaulting it.

. . . clues to deeply repressed suicidal thinking can sometimes be seen during headache free intervals as well.

Graham found underlying depression "often centered and around ambivalent feelings of anger and dependency towards an overbearing parent or boss. Difficult father-son relations in business are particularly common and powerful" (17).

SUPERSTITIONS: SCANNING THE OUTSIDE FOR ANSWERS

Cluster patients frequently tend to seek relief in concrete or magical ways. Because they generally avoid introspection, cluster patients may see both their problems and any potential solutions as external. Smith (1) cites a case in which such externalization and "magical thinking" occurred:

He [the cluster patient] also reported on another occasion that with particularly severe headaches he would develop throbbing in his hands and forearms and the veins of the dorsum of his hand would appear greatly engorged, and at times he felt that his wrist had actually swelled. This brought him into another line of thinking as he would look down at his wrist and his wristwatch, which had a stainless steel band, he wondered if this had something to do with it. So he took the watch off and didn't wear if for several ways. He called me in great excitement saying that he had to come to see me right away with some astounding information. His headaches had ceased. He repeated the story to me. I was naturally rather skeptical but he agreed to try a little experiment. He would wear the watch for a few days and leave it off for a few days. This went on for two or three weeks, and he was convinced that on the days he wore the watch with the metal watchband he got the headaches and on the other days he didn't. He then thought back to the only period in two weeks since his cluster began that he was free of headaches and he recalled that this was a period when he had broken his watchband and had sent it off to the jewelers to be

repaired. As best he could recall he had not had any headache at all. Well, gradually, wristwatch or no wristwatch he got back into his usual pattern of headache.

A similar vignette is described by Friedman (4):

A man came to me with a history of long intervals between cluster headaches. He had been in California and had been treated there; after his last attack he had been told to take a half a pound of honey daily. The usual intervals between his attacks was about a year. When at the end of the year the headache did not occur he continued this regimen and remained headache free. He increased his daily consumption of honey to about a pound a day. After three and a half years he had a series of cluster headaches at which point he came to see me. He was 150 pounds overweight, had diabetes and hypertension.

OUTLINE OF A "TYPICAL" CLUSTER PATIENT'S STORY

As with migraine, though not as dramatically, possible hereditary patterns can be seen in the illness. Graham (17) has described a tendency for vascular headaches to be present in the family histories of cluster patients, and notes a "leonine facies" is common in the patients. Although there is debate about the role, if any, of heredity in this disorder, it is generally not considered the primary determinant.

When taking the history, one is likely to be impressed by the constant motion of these patients' lives, the restless, searching quality of their existence.[5] They are alert, active, striving, fighting David and Goliath fights and, with unusual frequency, ending up at the top.

---

[5] Because males so predominate in the finite number of patients seen with this condition, we should assume, for the time being, that these thoughts may or may not apply to females. From the authors' clinical impressions, they probably do have areas of congruence, but we simply lack the data to address this issue yet.

They will rarely be found in a chaise lounge. This is true even though many of these patients develop a compensatory reaction against these urges, and present a demeanor that is casual, even diffident. Depending upon their intelligence and sophistication, this facade may be more or less convincing; but the more the patient reveals about his life, the more often a far less placid "self" will be seen beneath this exterior. As noted earlier, when one listens further to the patient's history he is likely to hear of an event or series of events in childhood, most commonly in latency or early adolescence, of a type that would normally cause sharp disillusionment. These events characteristically occur in a harsh context, are of a profound nature, are unexpected, and are reacted to in characteristic ways by the patient—the normal emotional response is often truncated or absent. With some frequency, such an event involves the relationship with a parental figure. It is also usually a situation one would expect to trigger bitterness, cynicism, or anger. Major or sudden loss—or multiple losses—are representative of the type of incident giving rise to this, and are also frequently seen in fact. This can include abandonment, "abandonment" by death (which the young child does not always appreciate as involuntary), the de facto loss of a parent who works too hard or long (for example, the never home "traveling salesman"), or loss of the parent through lack of interest in or basic loyalty toward the child. For example, a number of patients describe their fathers as being temperamental, explosive, moralistic, or physically abusive—difficult people to get along with. The father may have put his time and energies into some idealized business venture or other activity, leaving the patient feeling relatively unimportant, and severely detracting from his self-esteem.

One consequence of such disillusionment in the patient is an underlying, usually well camouflaged, pessimism about life. It is an insecurity best characterized by the expectation that he could somehow "lose everything," precipitously. This same lack of faith that his world is secured is part of what fuels an anxious ambition to succeed; and the cynicism typically accompanying that lack of faith leads him away from participation in formal religion (17).

When the original trauma giving rise to this disillusionment is some form of "abandonment," the patient generally fails to acknowledge the loss emotionally, to mourn it, and rebuild his self-esteem elsewhere. Sometimes, this is partly because the loss is too unexpected and catastrophic to accept straight out; generally though, the youngster's previous personality development and the stressful context of the loss are equally important. Instead, there is still seen in adulthood a sense that the patient continues searching to repair that lost and sometimes idealized relationship, though not consciously. Vaillant (27) convincingly argues that the purpose of mourning is not only to gain distance from the grief of a loss, but to recover and retain the good parts of the relationship with the deceased, such as would be needed to establish or maintain a firm identification with the person.

When the patient fails to grieve, he is left with an underlying core of melancholy or even despair. Although such despair is vividly seen *during* many cluster attacks, when one listens carefully to the patient's verbal associations *between* cluster periods, intrusive images of suicide and evidences of related depression are often apparent then also. In some ways, the suicidal fantasies are metaphors communicating the intensity of the pain that life has inflicted which the patient is trying to elude.

Many a cluster patient can be seen to be in constant flight from this feeling state and the repressed memories which initiated it. He crowds his schedule to distract himself from things which might remind him of that feeling state, even though he is likely to attribute this behavior to other motives. He rarely looks back, especially toward feelings; is usually avoidant of introspection; and if he does focus on his history, does so in a stereotyped, behaviors-and-events sort of way.[6]

If the trauma experienced by the patient involved the relationship with his father, the patient has often consciously convinced himself that he has simply moved away from that relationship with no regrets. Underneath, he often feels a stubborn yearning to not disappoint or give up entirely on Dad, even to make his father proud or interested. Yet at the same time, there is often significant competition with the father. In part, this competitiveness may draw its energy from an underlying anger. One patient said: "I am a vengeful person. I keep a scorecard. I think 'every dog has his day.' And when it comes, I won't forget." When present, the intensity of such anger varies. In a few cluster patients, especially where there was physical abuse, it is quite strong. Evidence for excessive anger includes cluster patients' frequent preoccupation with aggressive·fantasies and imagery, use of violence-connoting words, strong emotional investment in gun collecting, and putting themselves in positions where violence could be observed or enacted. Sometimes the signs are less direct: when asked about his hobbies, one patient stated he "writes sarcastic letters to people for fun."

The cluster patient tends to avoid working out emotional problems by means of self-reflection, but tends instead to try his cases in the court of action. An action-oriented person, he often prefers to "do something" when—preferably even before—a feeling threatens to overtake him. Thus, he is more liable to vague restlessness in the place of depression when things become quiet, and he tries to prevent that restlessness from turning into depression by allowing it to catapult him into the next symbolic enterprise. The combination of an action orientation and powerful

feelings leads to impulsivity. Sometimes it seems that much in the psychologically influenced cluster patient's life is but an allegorical replaying of traumatic memories and reactions to them, in a way that substitutes for mental representations of his history, much as rearranging the figures in a dollhouse substitutes for a remembering of home.

Often uncovered in the psychologically influenced cluster patient is the expectation, at a deep level, that his best efforts are inherently and unpredictably vulnerable to failure, his achievements to utter reversal, in that heartless, inevitable, "lose everything" way. He fights to deny victory to fate, which he perceives not only to be indifferent and arbitrary but even perhaps inevitable. One patient, for example, after finishing college with excellent grades, very much wanted to go on to graduate school. He was assured by his faculty that he would have no trouble getting in somewhere. But when he was then turned down by his undergraduate college he simply withdrew all applications in discouragement and became a blue collar laborer. This energetic, intelligent young man then rose to a middle management level; but when he had to contend with frustrating events for a short time, suddenly became again discouraged, and asked for his old job back. When his request was granted he again felt trapped, and yearned to break free of that position. But sharp feelings that "nothing would ever work" kept him from taking effective action. Each of these "interruptions" was followed by a cluster period.

Another patient further illustrates the fatalistic expectations which so often underline the striving behavior. The patient is a married teacher of Asian-American descent, a police officer, and a stock market entrepreneur. While holding down these three professions, he completed an M.A. and Ph.D. in different fields and designed, and largely built, his own home. He hardly had time for his family, and even less to sleep. He felt unliked in the police department: "So I act a little standoffish. They are afraid to attack me because I will verbally beat them to death. Anywhere else I can go

---

[6] Many display as what is known as "alexithymia," an inability to put feelings into words. It is a personality style often described in patients prone to psychologically influenced physical disorders. The aim of this style when it is present in the psychologically influenced cluster patient seems straightforwardly defensive.

and be the life of the party, but I don't care about the police, maybe because they don't seem to care about me." Although he received his Ph.D. while working on the force full time, for a long period he kept it secret, afraid of his associates' reactions. He in fact became quite hurt, after he told them, that no one offered him a special job. Nevertheless, he reflected, "As soon as I had an education the newness of it wore off, and if someone had said, 'Doctor' right after that I wouldn't have even turned around." He also felt unappreciated or doomed in his other areas of endeavor. "I feel I am being pushed out of my old teaching job by being made uncomfortable by politics." About the house building he noted, "I had to go to twelve companies to get a loan, even though I had half the money. I'm doing the building myself because builders steal from you." Although he made money on the stock market, he eventually became restless and bored with it, and put his energies elsewhere. In his summary, it is noted that:

His pattern is that of trying to win people over, getting discouraged, hurt, and frightened and becoming cold and withdrawn. At that point he convinces himself that the goals he sought were not so important or interesting to him (sour grapes). He then moves on to a new field of endeavor, only to have the pattern repeat itself. He is terrified of his anger erupting if he were provoked and lost control. This has never happened and, though an extremely large man and strong, he is overcontrolled. However, during cluster attacks the opposite is true.

In both of the foregoing cases the underlying pessimism, mistrust, and suspiciousness about the possibility of establishing close and lasting human relationships is evident. So is the ambivalence about even trying, manifested as vigorous surges of hopeful behavior alternating with equally vigorous retreats into resignation and defeat. As can be seen in the last case, with such perceptions patients are often uneasy about making commitments. This fear also applies to the commitment of oneself needed in psychotherapy, and adds

to the fear of having to resurrect early traumas.

The psychologically influenced cluster patient does not necessarily recognize exactly what he is wanting for his accomplishments. More often he fails to really feel the pleasure of success largely because he never achieves what he is truly after. Also, anger is mobilized by the feeling that he tried so hard but to no avail. His outward success may bring with it an elusive aura of unfulfillment, something he didn't have while he was still striving and hoping.

What psychological conditions precede the cluster period? As noted earlier, the first is a slowdown of pace; this may be forced or natural. Because the distractions competing for the patient's attention during this slowup period are less, the pressure from unresolved memories and feelings increases. The patient tries to resist this by becoming restless and by quickly trying to get invested in some new venture. But sometimes it doesn't happen soon enough. A second psychological factor which often precedes the outbreak of cluster is the completion of the project without the patient having moved closer to his unconscious goal. At such times he simply stops because things seem pointless, he gives up in frustration. A third element is when specific events before the slowdown stimulate renewal of hurt or anger. Once the physiological events of a cluster period are finally called into play, however, they are then, like a duodenal ulcer or migraine headache, seemingly autonomous of psychological factors.[7] Nevertheless, when a headache does strike, the depression, along with the rage, the despair, the panic, and the suicidal impulses, comes through like a tidal wave. And at this point the

---

[7] It is unclear whether one unconscious "goal" of the headache is to catalyze the release of repressed emotion, or whether this is just an inadvertent "side effect." It would be theoretically very tidy to think that the headache had this "purpose," but such a proposition tiptoes around the edge of philosophical quicksand, and is finally stopped by simple empirical unknowns.

patient needs all the available help and comfort the physician can provide.

TREATMENT CONSIDERATIONS

The first consideration when treating a cluster patient is not to be deceived by the apparent casualness with which he may regard therapy when he is headache free: in the midst of a headache one would know they are treating a desperate man. The patient needs to feel reassured that the physician will make every effort to be available at the time a cluster strikes. Although this knowledge is extremely important to the cluster patient, this does not mean he will be continually testing its validity. To the contrary, a knowledge of the doctor's availability may be more important than his availability. Frequent office visits during a cluster period are also advisable to show the patient that one recognizes the acuteness of his situation. This is an important message to convey even if the patient himself is trying so hard to ignore his headaches that he makes scheduling appointments frustrating.

In supportive psychotherapy, the therapist can allow the patient to ventilate his resentments and situational dilemmas. Wolff (7) described specific cases wherein cluster periods abated in response to this sort of simple intervention. Friedman (4) found that: "The headaches have recurred in situations of tension, stress, or exhaustion. When therapeutic attention was directed towards these life situations, in some instances they were effectively modified, even as is the case with certain patients with common or classical migraine." The same difficulty in assessing treatment interventions of any sort with cluster, namely, that remissions occur spontaneously, must, of course, temper any enthusiasm. Yet no *more* skepticism is called for when contemplating the results of psychotherapy than when considering new pharmacological approaches.

The optimal treatment for a psychologically influenced cluster patient would be to engage him in psychotherapy. This might allow him to remember any aversive early experiences and the reactions which it stirred in him. He could then be helped to gain a true distance from and peace with his past, more perspective on his yearnings, a more stable self-esteem from an ability to integrate an identity involving both male and female components, moderate comfort with his fantasy life, and a more considered approach to solving his problems. This would be ideal. Yet suggesting this to the cluster patient directly will often fail.

These patients are frequently resistive to traditional psychotherapy, especially if it is recommended during an early encounter. They often slip away from insight, even if, at times, they have caught glimpses of their anguish, and even if a part of them recognizes the need for treatment. They more often prefer to avoid feelings, bypass talk, and go straight to action; and they are apprehensive about this "new method." The simplest "action" that anyone can invoke in a threatening situation is to leave. Therefore, in therapy, these patients often do, after hurriedly describing their desperate situation. They also feel too vulnerable for therapy; their elaborate but brittle safeguards could be ravaged by an insensitive therapist's well meaning but too aggressive interpretations. These and other fears suddenly remind the patient of what a busy man he is, and of how hard it is to schedule in time for an appointment just now.

Yet certain techniques can ease the patient's fears about this transition. The therapeutic process begins by offering the patient an interested and predictable role model, in the form of the therapist. This may be the only level on which therapy proceeds: but it is something that many a cluster patient is searching for anyway, and he often selects unworthy mentors on his own. In such a relationship the patient may want help with concrete problems of living. Eventually, transference elements of competitiveness, hurt, and anger will likely creep into the therapeutic situation; but when they do, the relationship may be strong enough for the therapist to point these out in a constructive way. It is wise to allow the patient latitude in controlling appointment times and even in starting up and stopping therapy. The patient may do this for some time before he decides whether he feels comfortable enough to stay.

It is important that the therapist avoid confronting the patient's rigid defenses in too forceful a fashion. Caution is also the rule when helping him to recall what happened in the past and how he reacted to it. Though the more direct approach might occasionally succeed, sooner or later the therapist is likely to misjudge underlying emotions, and to force the patient into a position where he becomes so threatened and anxious he feels he must abandon treatment. Instead, it is better to phrase interpretations in indirect ways which leave the patient free to accept what he is able to tolerate. Many times, things that could not be said any other way can be conveyed to the cluster patient via shared humor.

What we have described, then, are patients with character structures forged under high pressure, and in specific ways. These patients are seen to have a discrete, psychologically influenced physical disorder, one which often releases great bursts of repressed affect along with its intense pain. One of the keys to such a patient's treatment may be through uncovering and understanding those original forces which shaped, and continue to shape, his psychic structure. Many cluster patients will need to deal with traumatic memories and to discharge the emotions consequent to them in a therapeutic manner to help lay them to rest. Often, an essential element in treatment is assisting the patient to supplement, integrate, and unify his identifications, and this may require delving into those feelings and memories which have disrupted the process. While repairing these wounds is sometimes a complicated task, the illness is surely distressful enough to warrant a full measure of commitment towards its relief. For, as E. Charles Kunkle (28) has so catchingly put it, "This illness has special and fiendish qualities. . . . it has so many striking symptoms and signs that we ought by now to understand it better than we do."

REFERENCES

1. Burton R: *The Anatomy of Melancholy.* London, Thomas McLean, 1826, p 291.
2. Friedman AP: The psychological and behavioral aspects of the cluster headache patient. In Mathew NT(ed): *Cluster Headaches.* New York, Spectrum, 1984, pp 73–78.
3. Violon A: The onset of facial pain: a psychological study. *Psychother Psychosom* 34:11–16, 1980.
4. *Proceedings of the Conference on Cluster Headache.* Boston, Headache Research Foundation, 1968.
5. Kuhn TS: *The Structure of Scientific Revolutions,* ed 2. Chicago, University of Chicago Press, 1970, pp 5–6.
6. Isler H: *Thomas Willis.* New York, Hafner, 1968.
7. Wolff HG: Headache mechanisms. *Int Arch Allergy* 7:210–278, 1955.
8. Friedman AP, Mikropoulos HE: Cluster headaches. *Neurology* 8:653–663, 1958.
9. Hinkle LE: Clinical observations on some aspects of the behavior pattern of patients with cluster headache. In *Proceedings of the Conference on Cluster Headache.* Boston, Headache Research Foundation, 1968, pp 3–11.
10. Stroebl CF: Biological rhythms in psychiatry. In Kaplan HI, Sadock BJ (eds): *Comprehensive Textbook of Psychiatry, IV.* Baltimore, Williams & Williams, 1985, pp 67–70.
11. Smith HF: Case history. In *Proceedings of the Conference on Cluster Headache.* Boston, Headache Research Foundation, 1968, pp 52–54.
12. Corwin H: Psychiatric attributes of the cluster headache patient. In *Proceedings of the Conference on Cluster Headache.* Boston, Headache Research Foundation, 1968, pp 11–21.
13. Kunkle EC, Pfeiffer JB, Wilhoit W, Hamrick LW: Recurrent brief headaches in cluster pattern. *Trans Am Neurol Assoc* 77:240–243, 1952.
14. Robinson BW: Histaminic cephalgia. *Medicine* 37:161–180, 1958.
15. Symonds CP: A particular variety of headache. *Brain* 79:217–232, 1956.
16. Graham JR: Some physical and laboratory characteristics of cluster patients. In *Proceedings of the Conference on Cluster Headache.* Boston, Headache Research Foundation, 1968, pp 21–23.
17. Graham JR, Rogado AZ, Rahman M, Gramer IV: Some physical, physiological, and psychological characteristics of cluster headaches. In Coch-

rane AL (ed): *Background to Migraine*. London, William Heinemann, 1970, pp 38–51.

18. Sweet WM: Surgical therapy. In *Proceedings of the Conference on Cluster Headache*. Boston, Headache Research Foundation, 1968, pp 73–76.

19. Steinhilber RM, Pearson JS, Rushton JG: Some psychologic considerations of histaminic cephalgia. *Proc Staff Meeting Mayo Clin* 35:691–699, 1960.

20. Adler CS, Adler SM: Psychiatric aspects of headache. *Panminerva Med* 24:167–172, 1982.

21. Saper JR: *Headache Disorders*. Boston, John Wright, 1983, pp 99–114.

22. Gentry DW, Williams RB: *Psychological Aspects of Myocardial Infarction and Coronary Care*. St. Louis, Mosby, 1975.

23. Alexander F: *Psychosomatic Medicine: Its Principles and Applications*. New York, Norton, 1950.

24. Saper JR: Non-headache disorders and characteristics of cluster headache patients. In Mathew N (ed): *Cluster Headache*. New York, Spectrum, 1984, pp 39–42.

25. McNeal PS: Treatment. *Proceedings of the Conference on Cluster Headache*. Boston, The Headache Research Foundation, 1968, pp 60–63.

26. Kudrow L: A possible role of the carotid body in the pathogenesis of cluster headache. *Cephalalgia* 3:241–247, 1983.

27. Vaillant GE: Attachment, loss and rediscovery. *Psychiatr Times* 3:1–16, 1986.

28. Kunkle EC: The problem. *Proceedings of the Conference on the Cluster Headache*. Boston, The Headache Research Foundation, 1968.

SECTION FOUR

Psychobiology of Stress and Headache

The Physiology and Biochemistry of Stress in Relation to Headache

EGILIUS L. H. SPIERINGS, M.D., PH.D.

Stress affects the functioning of many tissues and organs in the body, and by so doing, influences many disease processes. Some diseases, however, are more sensitive to stress than others, and those that react to stress vividly are generally referred to as psychosomatic or psychophysiological. Included in these categories are the headache disorders that are caused by a derangement in function rather than in structure of the tissues or organs involved. The two prevailing types of these functional headache disorders are migraine and muscle contraction headache, with localized vasodilatation and sustained muscle contraction as the mechanism underlying the pain experienced with each, respectively.

Stress exerts a pronounced effect on the skeletal muscle tone through an activation of the reticular activating system (Fig. 22.1); the word "tension," as used in relation to stress, refers to this effect. However not all muscles of the body are affected by stress to the same extent; the reticular activating system primarily activates the antigravity muscles which are involved in maintaining our upright position. In particular these are the muscles of the neck, which support the head, and those of the lower back, which help prevent the pelvis from falling forward. The pronounced effect of stress on the tone of the former muscles may explain the sensitivity of muscle contraction headache to stress, as this headache is particularly caused by a sustained contraction of the neck muscles.

With migraine, however, the situation is much more complex. Migraine not only has a more intricate symptomatology than muscle contraction headache, but also occurs in a less direct time relationship to stress. A migraine attack triggered by stress follows the stress rather than occurs during it. In this respect, the migraine headache is diametrically opposed to the muscle contraction headache, which most often begins when the stress is at its peak (Fig. 22.2). Thus, muscle contraction headache may justifiably be called a "stress headache," while migraine, at least with regard to its timing, it typically a "relaxation headache."

In what follows, the physiological basis of the specific time relationship between migraine and stress will be explored against the background of what is known about the pathogenesis of the different symptoms that normally constitute a migraine attack. As the nature of the basic migraine process lying at the depth of the attack is still obscure, so also is the anatomical site of impact of the stress so often responsible for the occurrence of an attack.

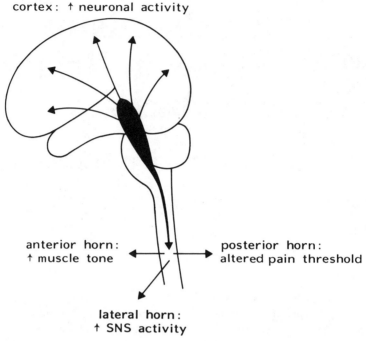

Figure 22.1. *The reticular activating system in the brain stem influences neuronal activity at the cortical level and at the spinal level, affects the pain threshold, changes the general (skeletal) muscle tone, and alters the activity of the sympathetic nervous system.*

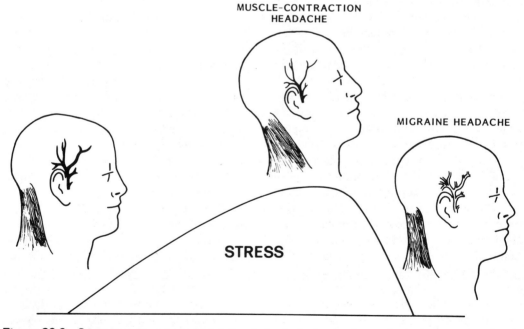

Figure 22.2. *Stress is an important precipitating factor for both migraine and muscle contraction headache, but while muscle contraction headache usually occurs during the stress, a migraine headache characteristically follows it.*

THE SYMPTOMS OF MIGRAINE

Migraine is a condition characterized by the occurrence of attacks which may last from several hours to 2–3 days. These attacks are usually composed of a multitude of symptoms, of which headache is the most constant. The headache is most often one-sided but it may alternate sides; or it may be bilateral. It most frequently localizes in the temporal or frontotemporal region. The pain often has a throbbing quality, if not continuously, then at least during activities which accentuate the distension of the blood vessels, such as physical exertion, bending over, coughing, or straining.

Symptoms which may accompany the headache during the attack, also known as "migraine accompaniments," can be classified into one of two categories: neurological and autonomic. The neurological accompaniments include such symptoms as the scintillating scotoma (also called teichopsia or fortification spectra); also common is the digitolingual or cheirooral syndrome. These are the two most characteristic neurological symptoms of migraine and may be considered highly specific for the condition. They are schematically shown in Figure 22.3, which also illustrates the typical progression of the symptoms in time, a progression which usually takes 20–30 minutes. The autonomic accompaniments of migraine are numerous, and include pallor, cold perspiration, cold extremities, anorexia, nausea, vomiting, diarrhea, and polyuria.

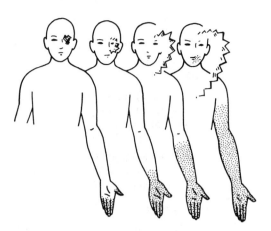

Figure 22.3. *The two most characteristic neurological accompaniments, or aura symptoms, of migraine, the scintillating scotoma or fortification spectra and the cheirooral or digitolingual syndrome, are shown in their successive stages of development, usually reaching completion in 20–30 minutes.*

The typical time relationship of the three groups of symptoms, that is, the headache, the neurological, and the autonomic accompaniments over the course of an attack is shown in Figure 22.4. Neurological accompaniments generally precede the headache, while autonomic accompaniments usually follow it. However, symptoms from all three categories are not necessarily present in every attack.

The most frequent form of migraine involves a headache which is *not* preceded by neurological symptoms, the so-called common migraine. When the headache is pre-

Neurological Accompaniments	→ HEADACHE →	Autonomic Accompaniments
scintillating scotoma		nausea
digitolingual		vomiting
syndrome		diarrhea
		polyuria

Figure 22.4. *The typical time relationship of the three groups of migraine symptoms, the headache, the neurological, and the autonomic accompaniments.*

paroxysmal headache with neurological (and autonomic) symptoms	Classical Migraine
paroxysmal headache with autonomic symptoms	Common Migraine
paroxysmal neurological symptoms without headache	Isolated Neurological Migraine Accompaniments

Figure 22.5. *The different combinations in which the three groups of migraine symptoms, the headache, the neurological, and the autonomic accompaniments, usually occur giving rise to the syndromes of classical migraine, common migraine, and isolated neurological migraine accompaniments (INMAs).*

ceded by neurological symptoms—an attack referred to as classical migraine—the autonomic symptoms are often only present in a mild form, or may even be totally absent. This may be because in classical migraine the headache itself is usually of a lesser intensity and shorter duration than in common migraine.

In relatively rare cases the neurological accompaniments of migraine appear without headache, and thus without autonomic symptoms. In such cases some speak of "migraine equivalents;" Fisher has proposed the term "transient migrainous accompaniment" (1). However, I believe a more precise term here is "isolated neurological migraine accompaniments" (INMAs). The clear recognition and precise definition of this migraine syndrome is important, because it often must be differentiated from transient ischemic attacks (TIAs), a diagnosis which leads to a different treatment and has a sharply different prognosis. The various combinations of migraine symptoms are summarized in Figure 22.5.

THE PATHOGENESIS OF MIGRAINE SYMPTOMS

The migraine headache is thought to originate from a dilatation of *noncerebral* blood vessels of the head, with a preference for the frontal branch of the superficial temporal artery, giving rise to a characteristic, throbbing pain in the temple. This notion is based on the following observations: (a) during the migraine headache the amplitude of pulsation of the superficial temporal artery is increased (2) and administration of ergotamine, the most effective and specific drug to treat a migraine headache, leads to a decreased headache intensity simultaneously with a parallel decrease in the amplitude of the temporal artery pulsations (Fig. 22.6) (3); (b) increasing the cerebrospinal fluid pressure by intrathecal injection of saline, thereby reducing the amplitude of pulsation of the *cerebral* arteries, does *not* reduce headache intensity (4). However, dilatation of blood vessels is probably not the only mechanism involved in generating the severe pain of migraine, and a decrease in pain threshold may also play a role.

There is some evidence that a substance with pain threshold lowering properties called "neurokinin" accumulates at the site of the pain (5). It has been shown to be released into the tissue fluid of the skin during antidromic stimulation of the dorsal root and during the axon reflex flare (6). It is possible, therefore, that release of this substance is initiated by the vasodilatation caused by stimulation of perivascular nerve endings and activation of the axon reflex. Because neurokinin also has vasodilating properties (5), this substance could incite a vicious circle of vasodilatation causing a decrease in pain threshold and also causing further vasodilatation.

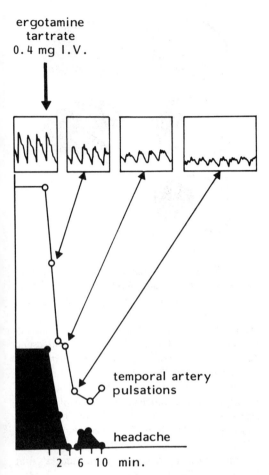

Figure 22.6. *The effect of ergotamine tartrate on the intensity of the migraine headache and on the amplitude of pulsation of the superficial temporal artery. Note the parallel course of the two effects, suggesting a causal relationship between them. (From Graham JR, Wolff HG: Mechanism of migraine headache and action of ergotamine tartrate. Arch Neurol Psychiatry 39:737–763, 1938.)*

THE NEUROLOGICAL MIGRAINE ACCOMPANIMENTS

It is generally believed that the neurological migraine accompaniments, or migraine aura symptoms, are caused by a localized constriction of cerebral blood vessels. This notion is based largely on the observations of Cahan (7), later confirmed by Hare (8), and the study of Marcussen and Wolff (9). Cahan and Hare studied the effects of the cerebral vasodilator amyl nitrite (10) on their own visual

migraine auras, and observed a transient regression of symptoms after inhalation of the drug (Fig. 22.7). Marcussen and Wolff studied the effects of carbon dioxide, another potent cerebral vasodilator, on the development of a migraine aura in 15 patients during 25 attacks. Inhalation of room air fortified with an additional 10% carbon dioxide resulted in a transient clearing of symptoms in all cases.

Measurement of man's cerebral blood flow in a relatively accurate way was not possible until the xenon-133 clearance technique was developed. This technique measures the rate of clearance from the brain of the freely diffusible and metabolically inactive isotope,

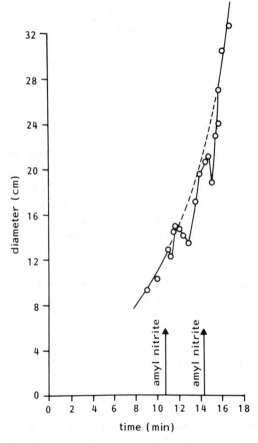

Figure 22.7. *The effect of amyl nitrite on the development of the scintillating scotoma. Note the immediate reduction in the diameter of the scotoma after inhalation of the drug. (From Hare EH: Personal observations on the spectral march of migraine. J Neurol Sci 3:259–264, 1966.)*

xenon-133, a rate which is proportional to the capillary blood flow. However, results from the initial studies of neurological migraine symptoms had been relatively disappointing: they showed a decrease in cerebral blood flow which was general, rather than focal, and bilateral rather than unilateral, despite the focal and lateralized nature of the symptoms (11–13).

Recent xenon-133 studies have used a more sophisticated technique, and revealed that the general decrease in cerebral blood flow is but the final stage in a series of changes. The changes include a focal increase in cerebral blood flow in the parietooccipital area, followed by a reduction to a level 20–30% below normal, and a gradual spreading of this reduction toward the fontal pole (Fig. 22.8) (14, 15). The decrease was described as oligemia rather than ischemia, because blood flow remained well above the threshold for producing neuronal dysfunction due to hypoxia.

The specific changes in cerebral blood flow observed during the neurological migraine accompaniments have shed new light on the hypothesis formulated by Milner in 1958 (16). This hypothesis suggests that the migraine aura symptoms are caused by a primary neuronal process, described by Leão as "spreading depression" (17). Grafstein (18) demonstrated that this phenomenon, which is a wave of inhibition of "spontaneous" neuronal activity, travels over the cerebral cortex at a rate of 2–5 mm/min. Grafstein also showed that the spreading depression is preceded by a short-lasting period of intense neuronal activity.

The particular rate of propagation of the spreading depression led Milner (16) to propose a link between this phenomenon and the migraine aura, as the process underlying the migraine aura had also been calculated to travel over the cerebral cortex at a rate of approximately 3 mm/min (19, 20). The further support Milner's notion gets from the recent cerebral blood flow studies is twofold: first, the cerebrovascular accompaniments of the spreading depression have been shown to

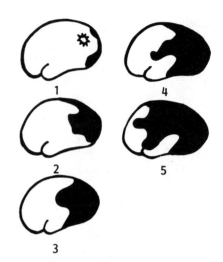

Figure 22.8. *The results of xenon clearance cerebral blood flow studies performed during the development of neurological migraine accompaniments. It shows that a short-lasting increase in blood flow (*) occurs in the parietooccipital area at the onset of symptoms, followed by a long-lasting decrease which gradually spreads towards the frontal pole. (Modified from Olesen J, Larsen B, Lauritzen M: Focal hyperemia followed by spreading oligemia and impaired activation of rCBF in classic migraine. Ann Neurol 9:344–352, 1981, and Lauritzen M, Olsen TS, Lassen NA, Paulson OB: Changes in regional cerebral blood flow during the course of classic migraine attacks. Ann Neurol 13:633–641, 1983.)*

consist of a short-lasting increase in cerebral blood flow followed by a long-lasting decrease (21). This decrease was described again as oligemia rather than ischemia, and was calculated to amount to 20–25%, which very well coincides with blood flow changes observed during migraine attacks; second, the rate of propagation of the "spreading oligemia" observed during a migraine attack has been calculated to be at least 2 mm/min (15), and this rate also coincides with that of "spreading depression" (18).

THE AUTONOMIC MIGRAINE ACCOMPANIMENTS

I have recently suggested that the autonomic symptoms of migraine, such as pallor, nausea, vomiting, diarrhea, frequent micturition, and coldness of the extremities are of sympathetic origin (22). There is ample evidence, especially biochemical, that activity of the sympathetic nervous system is increased during a migraine attack. Most directly indicative of this are Anthony's findings of a significantly higher plasma noradrenaline level and dopamine-β-hydroxylase activity during the migraine attack, when compared with the headache-free interval (23).

Noradrenaline is the major neurotransmitter of the sympathetic nervous system, and dopamine-β-hydroxylase is the enzyme responsible for its synthesis from dopamine. This enzyme is stored, together with the transmitter, in vesicles at the sympathetic nerve endings, and both are released whenever action potentials arrive at these nerve endings. After its release, most of the noradrenaline is rapidly reabsorbed into the nerve endings, so as not to continue stimulating the postsynaptic receptors. However, the dopamine-β-hydroxylase enzyme diffuses into the bloodstream, where it can be measured as a relatively accurate index of sympathetic nervous system activity (24).

Although reuptake by sympathetic nerve endings is the major means of inactivating noradrenaline which has been released, a proportion of this neurotransmitter is instead converted, by the combined action of catechol-0-methyltransferase (COMT) and monoamine oxidase (MAO), to vanillic mandelic acid (VMA). The VMA, in turn, is excreted in the urine. During a migraine attack the urinary excretion of this noradrenaline metabolite was found to be significantly increased by Sicuteri (25) and Curran et al (26) (but not by Kangashiemi et al (27)).

There are also changes in other biochemical variables which support the theory that sympathetic nervous system activity is increased during a migraine attack. One of these variables is the plasma level of free fatty acids, i.e., fatty acids not esterified by glycerol, cholesterol, or lysolecithin, and which are present in the plasma, loosely bound to albumin. In several studies (23,28–30) Anthony has shown that the plasma level of these fatty acids increases during a migraine attack. In addition, Hockaday et al (31) and Shaw et al (32) observed that the increase in plasma-free fatty acid level following administration of glucose is significantly greater during a migraine attack than before or after it.

In accord with the finding of an increase in plasma-free fatty acid level is the work of Anselmi et al (33), who found the plasma-free tryptophan level significantly higher during a migraine attack than in the attack-free interval. Tryptophan is found in the plasma, either free or bound to albumin, and free fatty acids compete with tryptophan for binding to albumin. A previous study by the same group at the same research center (34) found that the plasma-free tryptophan level was not significantly increased during an attack, when compared to the headache-free interval, but that it was significantly higher than that of a control group of healthy, nonmigrainous subjects. Because this increase in plasma-free tryptophan level was *not* accompanied by an increase in total plasma tryptophan concentration it indicates that the tryptophan shifted from the albumin-bound to the plasma-free state as can only be produced by an increase in plasma free fatty acid content.

Lipolysis is one metabolic effect of catecholamines, mediated through activation of adenylate cyclase and the formation of cyclic-adenosinemonophosphate (c-AMP) (as a second messenger). There is controversy about whether an increase in plasma c-AMP level occurs during migraine, a finding which would lend further support to the idea of increased sympathetic activity during an attack: Although Welch et al (35) could not detect any changes, Anthony (23) reported a two-fold increase (significant) in the plasma level of c-AMP compared to preattack levels.

Yet another biochemical observation supports the notion of increased sympathetic nervous system activity during migraine, namely, that of decreased insulin secretion in response to glucose administration. This finding was reported by Shaw et al (32). A biochemical change which may also be linked to activation of the sympathetic nervous system during an attack is the drop in platelet serotonin content, first reported by Curran et al (26) in 1965, and confirmed many times since (28–30, 36–42). This decrease in platelet serotonin appears to be the result of a change in plasma constitution (38, 40, 42, 43), and is due to the appearance in the plasma of a compound with a molecular weight of less than 50,000 daltons (40). Whether this plasma factor only affects platelets of migraineurs and has no activity against the platelets of nonmigrainous subjects remains a matter of dispute (refs. 42 and 43).

Serotonin is stored in the platelets in the form of aggregates with calcium, adenosine-triphosphate (ATP), and adenosinediphosphate (ADP). Platelet ATP content has also been shown to decrease during a migraine attack (37, 38, 44), although such changes never reached a level of statistical significance, and the same is true, to some extent, of platelet ADP content (37, 44). However, upon activation, platelets not only release serotonin,

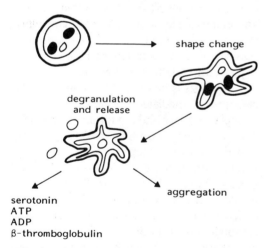

shape change

degranulation and release

aggregation

serotonin
ATP
ADP
β-thromboglobulin

Figure 22.9. *Schematic representation of the platelet release reaction. Upon activation, the platelets undergo a change in shape and degranulation, the latter being associated with the release of substances into the plasma. These include, among others, serotonin, ATP, ADP and β-thromboglobulin, a platelet-specific protein with prostacyclin inhibitory action. (From Gawel M, Burkitt M, Rose FC: The platelet release reaction during migraine attack. Headache 19:323–327, 1979.)*

ATP, and ADP, but also several specific and nonspecific proteins (Fig. 22.9). One of these platelet-specific proteins is β-thromboglobulin, which Gawel et al (45) have shown increases twofold during an episode of migraine. Together with the already mentioned platelet changes, this observation provides good evidence that platelets undergo a release reaction during a bout of migraine. It is likely, however, that this release reaction is restricted to the headache phase of the attack and that it does not occur during the aura. This is probably true because induction of a partial release reaction is typically followed by a drop in platelet sensitivity to the aggregating agents (46); and, while platelet aggregability is high during the aura (47), it is low during the headache phase (47).

As previously mentioned, and judging from the release of serotonin, platelet activation during migraine seems to be due to appearance in the plasma of a compound weighing less than 50,000 daltons. Many substances would fit into this category, ranging from simple molecules to small proteins. Fatty acids, which increase in the plasma during an attack (*vide supra*) and which are known to activate platelets and cause serotonin release (48, 49), have been implicated here. However, when I analyzed Anthony's data on the changes in plasma free fatty acid level and platelet serotonin content (28, 29) I did not find support for this notion (50).

The platelet activation cascade, however, may also be linked more directly to the heightened sympathetic activity during migraine, as both adrenaline (51, 52) and noradrenaline (51, 53) activate platelets. It is therefore tempting to postulate that the low molecular weight, proaggregatory plasma factor is a catecholamine. This possibility is illustrated in Figure 22.10, which summarizes the biochemical changes during a migraine attack and places them in relation to each other as discussed above.

The gastrointestinal symptoms accompanying migraine, particularly nausea and vomiting, can also be associated with an activation of the sympathetic nervous system. The

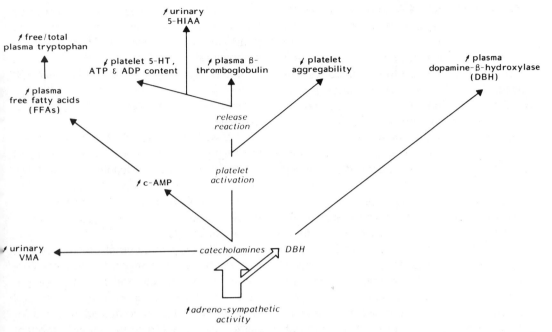

Figure 22.10. *Summary of the biochemical changes of the headache phase of migraine put in sequential relationship to each other. They suggest increased sympathetic nervous system activity during the attack. (Modified from Spierings ELH: The Pathophysiology of the Migraine Attack. Ph.D. thesis, Erasmus University, Rotterdam, The Netherlands. Alphen a/d Rijn, The Netherlands, Stafleu's Scientific Publishing Company, 1980.)*

mechanism here would include atony and dilatation of the stomach with contraction of the pyloric sphincter, processes which have in fact been revealed by radiological studies (54, 55) (Fig. 22.11). A similar depression of the gastrointestinal motility has also been observed in rats whose brains were selectively depleted of serotonin. In these rats, the exaggerated sympathoadrenal response to stress, which occurs after central serotonin depletion, was not ameliorated by extensive handling (56).

The aberration in gastrointestinal function during migraine is also probably responsible for the impaired absorption of orally administered drugs, as has been shown to be the case for acetylsalicyclic acid by Volans (57, 58) and for ergotamine by Orton (59). In support of this conclusion is Volans' observation that impaired absorption of acetylsalicyclic acid during migraine can be antagonized by prior administration of metoclopramide (58). Metoclopramide is a potent antiemetic drug which promotes gastric contraction and

antroduodenal synchronization (60), thereby increasing the gastric emptying rate (61). This effect is probably established by the facilitation of acetylcholine release from postganglionic parasympathetic neurons in the wall of the gastrointestinal tract (62).

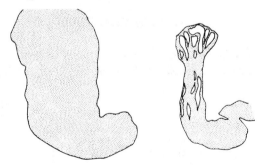

Figure 22.11. *Radiographic examination of the fasting stomach during (left) and after (right) the migraine attack. Note the dilatation and atony of the stomach with contraction of the pyloric sphincter during the attack. (Modified from Kaufman J, Levine I: Acute gastric dilatation of stomach during attack of migraine. Radiology 27:301–302, 1963.)*

PATHOGENESIS OF THE MIGRAINE ATTACK—A NEW THEORY

The symptoms of migraine attack have been described as falling into three categories: the *headache per se,* the *neurological* accompaniments, and the *autonomic* accompaniments. During the course of an attack the neurological accompaniments usually appear first, followed by headache and, after the onset of headache, by autonomic disturbances (Fig. 22.4).

The headache has been ascribed to a dilatation of blood vessels in the cranial noncerebral circulation in combination with a lowering of the patient's pain threshold. The neurological accompaniments have been conceptualized as being related to a primary neuronal process, known as Leão's spreading depression; the autonomic accompaniments can be explained on the basis of activation of the sympathetic nervous system, the ample biochemical evidence for which I have outlined in Fig. 22.10.

In what follows, I will bring the three symptom categories together in a novel concept of the pathogenesis of the migraine attack. Then, those features which determine, as I see it, migraine's characteristic time relationship to stress, i.e., the precipitation of attacks during periods of relaxation following stress, will be discussed.

WOLFF'S CONCEPT

The late Harold G. Wolff, professor of neurology at Cornell Medical School-New York Hospital, was the first to systematically study the problem of headache, and migraine in particular, in a scientific way. His view on the pathogenesis of a migraine attack (63), shown schematically in Figure 22.12, has become generally accepted and, after more than 2 decades, still dominates our thinking about migraine.

In Wolff's hypothesis the initial event of the migraine attack is a localized spasm of cerebral blood vessels leading to tissue hypoxia. The tissue hypoxia is thought to underlie the focal neurological symptoms, described above as neurological migraine accompaniments.

A dilatation of cerebral blood vessels is thought to occur as a reaction to vasoconstriction-induced hypoxia, and is also accompanied by dilatation of cranial noncerebral blood vessels; this, in combination with a localized decrease in pain threshold, is thought to cause the migraine headache. When the migraine headache is *not* preceded by focal neurological symptoms, as is the case in common migraine (Fig. 22.5), a phase of vasoconstriction-induced cerebral hypoxia is still believed to precede the headache—but in those instances it is in a so-called "clinically silent" area of the cerebral cortex.

With regard to the pathogenesis of neurological migraine symptoms, Wolff based his hypothesis on the observation that inhalation of a cerebral vasodilator, such as amyl nitrite (7, 8) or carbon dioxide (9), is followed by a transient regression in symptom development (Fig. 22.7). Wolff derived the notion that the headache itself is caused by dilatation of

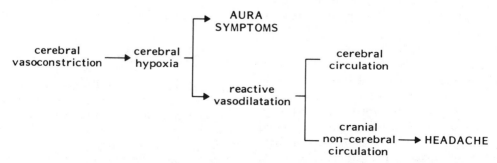

Figure 22.12. *Schematic representation of the vasoconstriction-cerebral hypoxia-vasodilatation concept of the pathogenesis of the migraine attack as suggested by Harold G. Wolff in the 1950s (63).*

blood vessels in the cranial noncerebral circulation both from experiments with ergotamine (3) (Fig. 22.6) and from the observation that, if one increases the spinal fluid pressure and thereby reduces the amplitude of cerebral artery pulsations, this does *not* decrease the intensity of the headache (4). However, the basis of Wolff's assumption that the dilatation of cerebral blood vessels which follows the vasoconstriction is also accompanied by a dilatation of noncerebral blood vessels, is unclear. Also, his hypothesis explains neither the autonomic symptoms nor the autonomic migraine accompaniments so often prominent, especially in common migraine.

SPREADING DEPRESSION

Measurements of cerebral blood flow using the xenon clearance technique have failed to support Wolff's concept of the pathogenesis of the migraine attack. Instead, they have provided evidence in favor of a primary neuronal pathogenesis of the aura symptoms, i.e., Leão's spreading depression (17), as originally suggested by Milner (16). The spreading depression is a wave of inhibition of "spontaneous" neuronal activity which travels over the cerebral cortex at 2–5 mm/min (18), a rate comparable to both that calculated for the process underlying a scintillating scotoma

(19, 20) and to that of the spreading oligemia of the migraine attack (14, 15) (Fig. 22.8).

Unfortunately, a simple incorporation of the phenomenon of spreading depression into Wolff's theory is impossible. There are two reasons for this: (a) spreading depression can be initiated by a number of stimuli, but *not* by ischemia, as Leão himself showed (64); and (b) there is no evidence that spreading depression can lead to cerebral vasodilatation; to the contrary, it has been shown to be followed by a long-lasting decrease in cerebral blood flow (21). Also, the supposition of cerebral vasoconstriction is not necessary with regard to the beneficial effects of carbon dioxide on an aura, as it has recently been shown that inhaling 10–15% carbon dioxide in oxygen will completely abolish a spreading depression (65).

AN ALTERNATIVE THEORY

As incorporation of the phenomenon of spreading depression into Wolff's concept of the pathogenesis of a migraine attack is impossible, an alternative concept is necessary, and the author suggests for consideration the one outlined in Figure 22.13. This concept not only accommodates the spreading depression as the phenomenon underlying neu-

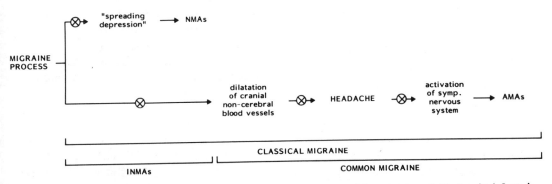

Figure 22.13. *The author's present concept of the pathogenesis of the migraine attack, in which Leão's spreading depression is incorporated as the process underlying the neurological migraine accompaniments (NMAs). Note that the neurological symptoms and the headache are considered here to be generated as parallel rather than, as Wolff suggested, sequential processes. This concept also offers an explanation for the autonomic migraine accompaniments (AMAs). The circled crosses indicate where the pathogenesis of a migraine attack is facilitated when the organism is in a state of relaxation (see text).*

rological migraine symptoms, but also incorporates an explanation of autonomic symptoms migraine, which is lacking in Wolff's theory. The crucial point of difference between the present concept and Wolff's, however, is that the former views the processes underlying both neurological migraine accompaniments and the headache as parallel, rather than as sequential. In viewing them as parallel, the current theory better explains the occurrence of neurological symptoms and headache *simultaneously* (as is sometimes seen in cases of classical migraine), the occurrence of headache without neurological symptoms (common migraine), and the occurrence of neurological symptoms without headache, for which the term, "isolated neurological migraine accompaniment," was suggested.

In the present concept, autonomic migraine accompaniments are considered to be a consequence of the headache, and this is based on the assumption that they are caused by heightened sympathetic activity. As shown above, there is ample biochemical evidence that the sympathetic nervous system is in a state of increased activity during migraine, and that this is probably related to the headache phase of the attack. Pain is a potent stimulator of the sympathetic nervous system, and the migraine headache is in general, undoubtedly, severe enough to account for the kind of vigorous sympathetic nervous system activation seen during migraine. (Fig. 22.14).

STRESS, RELAXATION, AND MIGRAINE

The migraine process is sensitive to stress, and when a migraine attack is triggered by it, the attack characteristically occurs when the stress is over and relaxation begins (Fig. 22.2). We do not know exactly what it is in the migraine process that makes it so reactive to stress, and neither can we pinpoint the structure or system that, like a capacitor, first accumulates stress, and then lets it go when overloaded. As the discharge of the "migraine capacitor" preferentially occurs during relaxa-

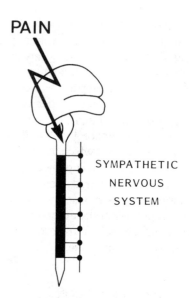

Figure 22.14. *Pain is a potent stimulator of the sympathetic nervous system, and during the migraine attack this probably accounts for the increased sympathetic nervous system activity.*

tion, this is when the steps through which the capacitor has to unload can be considered to show least resistance (these steps are indicated in Fig. 22.13 by circled crosses.)

Spreading depression, the phenomenon supposedly underlying the neurological symptoms of migraine, is considerably easier to initiate in an isolated slab of cortex than it is in an intact brain (18). Because activation of the cortex can completely arrest the spread of an oncoming depression, this enhanced "irritability" in the cortical slab has been attributed to its isolation from large amounts of spontaneous neuronal activity. Thus, a very active brain seems to present less fertile ground for the initiation of a spreading depression than does a resting brain. Through the reticular activating system (Fig. 22.1) stress increases, and relaxation decreases, the activity level of cortical neurons, which is reflected in cerebral blood flow changes accompanying these changes in the level of arousal (66). The fact that neurological migraine accompaniments most commonly announce themselves in the center of vision, as in the case of the scintillating scotoma, or in the hand or about the tongue or mouth, as in

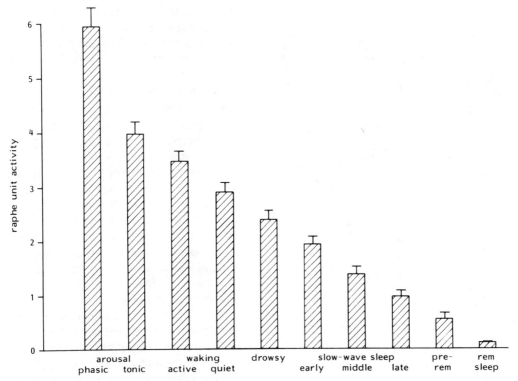

Figure 22.15. *Raphe unit activity across the different sleep-wakefulness states as observed in freely moving cats. Note the progressive decrease in raphe unit activity with decreasing level of arousal. (From Trulson ME, Jacobs BL: Raphe unit activity in freely moving cats: correlation with level of behavioral arousal. Brain Res 163:135–150, 1979.)*

the case of the digitolingual syndrome, may be explained by the fact that these areas represent the most excitable and massively represented portions of the visual and tactile fields, respectively.

With regard to the generation of migraine headache by the dilatation of extracranial blood vessels, it is relevant that, with the exception of those of the forehead, these blood vessels are innervated by sympathetic, noradrenergic fibers, which cause the arteries to constrict (67) when the nerve cells fire. Stress activates the sympathetic nervous system and, thus, when the stress level is high the cranial noncerebral blood vessels are in a relatively constricted stage; this disallows the migraine process to begin, by inhibiting excessive dilatation. Dilatation only becomes possible when the stress level is low, i.e., during relaxation.

Pain production initiated by vasodilatation is also facilitated by the relative decrease in pain threshold associated with relaxation. These differences in pain threshold between stress and relaxation are probably related to changed activity in the serotoninergic raphe neurons, which have been shown to produce during varying levels of arousal. This was demonstrated by Trulson and Jacobs in freely moving cats (68). Figure 22.15 reproduced from their study, and it shows how the activity of serontoninergic raphe neurons progressively diminishes as the organism's level of arousal decreases.

The serotoninergic raphe neurons have been shown to project to enkephalinergic neurons in the nucleus of the trigeminal tract and to its caudal extension, the dorsal horn of the spinal cord (Fig. 22.16). The enkephalinergic neurons are interneurons. They medi-

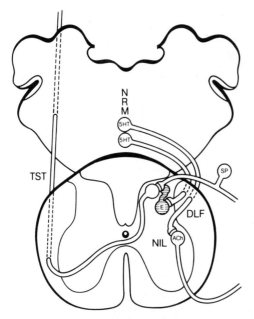

Figure 22.16. *Serotoninergic (5HT) fibers that originate from the raphe magnus nucleus (NRM) and descend down the spinal cord in the dorsolateral funiculus (DLF), exert an inhibitory influence not only on the transmission of pain signals to the spinothalamic tract (TST) but also on the activity of the sympathetic preganglionic neurons in the intermediolateral nucleus (NIL). The inhibition of the transmission of pain signals from the primary sensory efferents which release substance P (SP) at their terminals to the spinothalamic tract is mediated through enkephalinergic (E) interneurons and the mechanism of presynaptic inhibition.*

ate, through presynaptic inhibition, the inhibitory influence of serotoninergic raphe fibers on the transmission of pain signals from the primary sensory neurons to the trigemino- and spinothalamic tracts (69). Decreased activity of the serotoninergic raphe neurons during relaxation thus means that, on this level, pain transmission is facilitated as a result of the lessened activity of these enkephalinergic interneurons. That this may indeed be a mechanism involved in the pathogenesis of the migraine attack is further suggested by Anselmi's finding (33) that the met-enkephaline content of the cerebrospinal fluid is significantly lower during the migraine attack when compared to the attack-free interval. How-

ever, the changes observed in the cerebrospinal fluid concentration of the main metabolite of serotonin, 5-hydroxyindoleacetic acid, are not consistent and allow no conclusion (27, 70, 71).

As shown in Figure 22.16, the serotoninergic raphe neurons innervate not only the enkephalinergic interneurons in the dorsal horn of the spinal cord, but also the preganglionic sympathetic neurons in its lateral horn. These neurons are part of the efferent limb of the sympathetic nervous system, and synapse in the para- and prevertebral ganglia with neurons that ultimately go to the target organs. As shown by Cabot et al (72) raphe neurons exert an inhibitory influence on the activity of the preganglionic sympathetic neurons. This means that during relaxation, when the level of activity of these raphe neurons is low (Fig. 22.15), the sympathetic neurons are in a relatively dysinhibited state. This allows pain to cause an exaggerated activation of the sympathetic nervous system, which could explain the often abundant autonomic symptoms during a migraine. Thus, the final step in the pathogenesis of the migraine attack, shown in Figure 22.13, i.e., generation of autonomic migraine accompaniment, is also facilitated by relaxation and hampered by stress.

The serotoninergic raphe system may not only play a role in generating the symptoms of a migraine attack, but also in terminating these symptoms. One of the many biochemical changes that occurs during the migraine attack is an increase in the plasma level of free, i.e., nonesterified, fatty acids. This has been linked to the increase in sympathetic nervous system activity during the attack, and it occurs as a result of catecholamine-induced lipolysis (Fig. 22.10). The free fatty acids in the plasma compete with tryptophan for binding to albumin, leading to a rise in the level of plasma-free tryptophan. In contrast to albumin-bound tryptophan, free tryptophan can pass the blood-brain barrier, causing an increase in plasma-free tryptophan to be followed by an increase in brain tryptophan concentration (73). Tryptophan is the precursor amino acid of serotonin, and it is, therefore, not surprising that an increase in plasma-free tryptophan ultimately results in an increase in brain serotonin concentration (73).

The enzymes involved in the synthesis of serotonin from tryptophan are tryptophan-5-hydroxylase and aromatic amino acid decarboxylase. While the latter enzyme is widely distributed in the central nervous system, the former is only present in low concentrations, and its distribution is probably limited to the serotoninergic neurons. Furthermore, although the affinity of tryptophan-5-hydroxylase for its substrate is low, the concentration of tryptophan usually present in neurons that produce serotonin may still not be sufficient to saturate the enzyme. Thus, brain serotonin synthesis may normally be limited by the availability of tryptophan. On the other hand, this means that any change in brain tryptophan concentration is of significance in the functional activity of these neurons. In this way, the increase in plasma-free tryptophan, as occurs in migraine, would also potentiate the increased activity of the serotoninergic raphe system which is already being aroused by the pain. Suppression of pain signal transmission and inhibition of sympathetic nervous system activity may result from this to such an extent that a "spontaneous" termination of the migraine attack becomes a fact.

ACKNOWLEDGMENTS

I would like to thank my wife, Malina, for editorial assistance in the preparation of this manuscript and Ms. Monica van den Hoven for typing it. Also, I would like to thank The Audiovisual Service of the Faculty of Medicine of the Erasmus University, Rotterdam, for the preparation of the illustrations.

REFERENCES

1. Fisher CM: Late-life migraine accompaniments as a cause of unexplained transient ischemic attacks. *Can J Neurol Sci* 7:9–17, 1980.

2. Tunis MM, Wolff HG: Analysis of cranial artery pulse waves in patients with vascular headache of the migraine type. *Am J Med Sci* 224:565–568, 1952.

3. Graham JR, Wolff HG: Mechanism of migraine headache and action of ergotamine tartrate. *Arch Neurol Psychiatry* 39:737–763, 1938.

4. Hachinski VC, Norris JW, Edmeads J, Cooper PW: Ergotamine and cerebral blood flow. *Stroke* 9:594–596, 1978.

5. Chapman LF, Ramos AO, Goodell H, Silverman G, Wolff HG: A humoral agent implicated in vascular headache of the migraine type. *Arch Neurol* 3:223–229, 1960.

6. Chapman LF, Ramos AO, Goodell H, Wolff HG: Neurohumoral features of afferent fibers in man. *Arch Neurol* 4:49–82, 1961.

7. Schumacher GA, Wolff HG: Experimental studies on headache: A. Contrast of histamine headache with the headache of migraine and that associated with hypertension. B. Contrast of vascular mechanisms in preheadache and in headache phenomena of migraine. *Arch Neurol Psychiatry* 45:199–214, 1941.

8. Hare EH: Personal observations on the spectral march of migraine. *J Neurol Sci* 3:259–264, 1966.

9. Marcussen RM, Wolff HG: Studies on headache: 1. Effects of carbon dioxide-oxygen mixtures given during the preheadache phase of the migraine attack. 2. Further analysis of pain mechanisms in headache. *Arch Neurol Psychiatry* 63:42–51, 1950.

10. Sokoloff L: The action of drugs on the cerebral circulation. *Pharm Rev* 11:1–85, 1959.

11. O'Brien MD: Cerebral blood flow changes in migraine. *Headache* 10:139–143, 1971.

12. O'Brien MD: The relationship between aura symptoms and cerebral blood flow changes in the prodrome of migraine. In Dalessio DJ, Dalsgaard-Nielsen T, Diamond S(eds): *Proceedings of the International Headache Symposium,* Elsinore, Denmark. Basel, Switzerland, Sandoz, 1971, pp 141–143.

13. Mathew NT, Hrastnik F, Meyer JS: Regional cerebral blood flow in the diagnosis of vascular headache. *Headache* 15:252–260, 1976.

14. Olesen J, Larsen B, Lauritzen M: Focal hyperemia followed by spreading oligemia and impaired activation of rCBF in classic migraine. *Ann Neurol* 9:344–352, 1981.

15. Lauritzen M, Olsen TS, Lassen NA, Paulson OB: Changes in regional cerebral blood flow during the course of classic migraine attacks. *Ann Neurol* 13:633–641, 1983.

16. Milner PM: Note on a possible correspondence between the scotomas of migraine and spreading depression of Leão. *EEG Clin Neurophysiol* 10:705, 1958.

17. Leão AAP: Spreading depression of activity in the cerebral cortex. *J Neurophysiol* 7:359–390, 1944.

18. Grafstein B: Mechanism of spreading cortical depression. *J Neurophysiol* 19:154–171, 1956.

19. Lashley KS: Patterns of cerebral integration indicated by the scotomas of migraine. *Arch Neurol Psychiatry* 46:331–339, 1941.

20. Richards W: The fortification illusions of migraines. *Sci Am* 224:88–96, 1971.

21. Lauritzen M, Jørgensen MB, Diemer NH, Gjedde A, Hansen AJ: Persistent oligemia of rat cerebral cortex in the wake of spreading depression. *Ann Neurol* 12:469–474, 1982.

22. Spierings ELH: Migräne and sympathisches Nervensystem. In Pfaffenrath V, Schrader A, Neu IS (eds): Primäre Kopfschmerzen—Pathogenese, Diagnostiek und Therapie. München, Medizin Verlag, 1984, pp 53–66.

23. Anthony M: Biochemical indices of sympathetic activity in migraine. *Cephalalgia* 1:83–89, 1981.

24. Kopin IJ, Kaufman S, Viveros H, Jacobowitz D, Lake CR, Ziegler MG, Lovenberg W, Goodwin FK: Dopamine-β-hydroxylase. Basic and clinical studies. *Ann Intern Med* 85:211–223, 1976.

25. Sicuteri F: Vasoneuroactive substances in migraine. *Headache* 6:109–126, 1966.

26. Curran DA, Hinterberger H, Lance JW: Total plasma serotonin, 5-hydroxyindoleacetic acid and *p*-hydroxy-*m*-methoxymandelic acid excretion in normal and migrainous subjects. *Brain* 88:997–1010, 1965.

27. Kangasniemi P, Sonninen V, Rinne UK: Excretion of free and conjugated 5-HIAA and VMA in urine and concentration of 5-HIAA and HVA in CSF during migraine attacks and free intervals. *Headache* 12:62–65, 1972.

28. Anthony M: Plasma free fatty acid changes in migraine. *Proc Aust Assoc Neurol* 10:87–89, 1973.

29. Anthony M: Plasma free fatty acids and prostaglandin E_1 in migraine and stress. *Headache* 16:58–63, 1976.

30. Anthony M: Role of individual free fatty acids in migraine. *Res Clin Stud Headache* 6:110–116, 1978.

31. Hockaday JM, Williamson DH, Whitty CWM: Blood-glucose levels and fatty-acid metabolism in migraine related to fasting. *Lancet* 1:1153–1156, 1971.

32. Shaw SWJ, Johnson RH, Keogh HJ: Metabolic changes during glucose tolerance tests in migraine attacks. *J Neurol Sci* 33:51–59, 1977.

33. Anselmi B, Baldi E, Cassacci F, Salmon S: Endogenous opioids in cerebrospinal fluid and blood in idiopathic headache sufferers. *Headache* 20:294–299, 1980.

34. Salmon S, Fanciullacci M, Bonciani M, Sicuteri F: Plasma tryptophan in migraine. *Headache* 17:238–241, 1978.

35. Welch KMA, Chabi E, Nell JH, Bartosh K, Chee ANC, Matthew NT, Achar VS: Biochemical comparison of migraine and stroke. *Headache* 16:160–167, 1976.

36. Anthony M, Hinterberger H, Lance JW: Plasma serotonin in migraine and stress. *Arch Neurol* 16:544–552, 1967.

37. Hinterberger H, Anthony M, Vagholkar MK: Platelet 5-hydroxytryptamine and adenine nucleotides, serum arginylesterase and plasma 11-hydroxycorticosteroids in migraine. *Clin Sci* 34:271–276, 1968.

38. Anthony M, Hinterberger H, Lance JW: The possible relationship of serotonin to the migraine syndrome. *Res Clin Stud Headache* 2:29–59, 1969.

39. Anthony M, Lance JW: Histamine and serotonin in cluster headache. *Arch Neurol* 25:225–231, 1971.

40. Anthony M, Lance JW: The role of serotonin. In Pearce J (ed): *Modern Topics in Migraine*. London, W Heinemann Medical Books, 1975, pp 107–123.

41. Somerville BW: Platelet-bound and free serotonin levels in jugular and forearm venous blood during migraine. *Neurology* 26:41–45, 1976.

42. Mück-Seler D, Deanović Z, Dupelj M: Platelet serotonin (5-HT) and 5-HT releasing factor in plasma of migrainous patients. *Headache* 19:14–17, 1979.

43. Dvilansky A, Rishpon S, Nathan I, Zolotow Z, Korczyn AD: Release of platelet 5-hydroxytryptamine by plasma taken from patients during and between migraine attacks. *Pain* 2:315–318, 1976.

44. Rydzewski W, Wachowicz B: Adenine nucleotides in platelets in and between migraine attacks. In Greene R (ed): *Current Concepts in Migraine Research.* New York, Raven Press, 1978, pp 153–158.

45. Gawel M, Burkitt M, Rose FC: The platelet release reaction during migraine attack. *Headache* 19:323–327, 1979.

46. Harbury CB, Schrier SL: The effect of a partial release reaction on subsequent platelet function. *J Lab Clin Med* 83:877–886, 1974.

47. Deshmukh SV, Meyer JS: Cyclic changes in platelet dynamics and the pathogenesis and prophylaxis of migraine. *Headache* 17:101–108, 1977.

48. Shore PA, Alpers HS: Platelet damage induced in plasma by certain fatty acids. *Nature* 200:1331–1332, 1963.

49. Inouye A, Shio H, Sorimachi M, Kataoka K: Unsaturated fatty acids; platelet-serotonin releasers in tissue extract. *Experientia* 26:308–309, 1970.

50. Spierings ELH: *The Pathophysiology of the Migraine Attack.* Ph.D. Thesis, Erasmus University, Rotterdam, The Netherlands. Brussels, Stafleu's Scientific Publishing Company, 1980.

51. O'Brien JR: Some effects of adrenaline and anti-adrenaline compounds on platelets *in vitro* and *in vivo. Nature* 200:763–764, 1963.

52. Mills DCB, Robb IA, Roberts GCK: The release of nucleotides, 5-hydroxytryptamine and enzymes from human platelets during aggregation. *J Physiol* 195:715–729, 1968.

53. Haft JE, Kranz PD, Albert FJ, Fani K: Intravascular platelet aggregation in the heart induced by norepinephrine. *Circulation* 46:698–708, 1972.

54. Kaufman J, Levine I: Acute gastric dilatation of stomach during attack of migraine. *Radiology* 27:301–302, 1963.

55. Kreel L: Recent advances in the radiology of the gastrointestinal tract. *Arch Gastroenterol* 6:155–164, 1969.

56. Saller CF, Stricker EM: Gastrointestinal motility and body weight gain in rats after brain serotonin depletion by 5, 7-dihydroxytryptamine. *Neuropharmacol* 17:499–506, 1978.

57. Volans GN: Absorption of effervescent aspirin during migraine. *Br Med J* 4:265–269, 1974.

58. Volans GN: The effect of metoclopramide on the absorption of effervescent aspirin in migraine. *Br J Clin Pharmacol* 2:57–63, 1975.

59. Orton D: Ergotamine tartrate levels using radioimmunoassay. In Greene R (ed): *Current Concepts in Migraine Research.* New York, Raven Press, 1978, pp 79–84.

60. Johnson AG: Gastroduodenal motility and synchronization. *Postgrad Med J* 49(Suppl):29–33, 1973.

61. Howard FA, Sharp DS: The effect of intramuscular metoclopramide on gastric emptying during labor. *Postgrad Med J* 49(Suppl):53–56, 1973.

62. Hay AM, Man WK: Effect of metoclopramide on guinea pig stomach. Critical dependence on intrinsic stores of acetylcholine. *Gastroenterology* 76:492–496, 1979.

63. Dalessio DJ: *Wolff's Headache and Other Head Pain,* ed 4. New York, Oxford University Press, 1980.

64. Leão AAP: Further observations on the spreading depression of activity in the cerebral cortex. *J Neurophysiol* 10:409–419, 1947.

65. Gardner-Medwin AR: The effect of carbon dioxide and oxygen on Leão's spreading depression: evidence supporting a relationship to migraine. *J Physiol* 316:23P–24P, 1981.

66. Lassen NA, Ingvar DH, Skinhøj E: Brain function and blood flow. *Sci Am* 239 (4):50–59, 1978.

67. Spierings ELH: Craniovascular accompaniments of the vascular headache of the migraine type. *Headache* 19:397–399, 1979.

68. Trulson ME, Jacobs BL: Raphe unit activity in freely moving cats: correlation with level of behavioral arousal. *Brain Res* 163:135–150, 1979.

69. Basbaum AI, Fields HL: Endogenous pain control mechanism: review and hypothesis. *Ann Neurol* 4:451–462, 1978.

70. Poloni M, Nappi G, Arrigo A, Savoldi F: Cerebrospinal fluid 5-hydroxy-indoleacetic acid level in migrainous patients during spontaneous attacks, during headache-free periods and following treatment with 1-tryptophan. *Experientia* 30:640–641, 1974.

71. Hyyppä MT, Kangasniemi P: Variation of plasma tryptophan and CSF 5-HIAA during migraine. *Headache* 17:25–27, 1977.

72. Cabot JB, Wild JM, Cohen DH: Raphe inhibition of sympathetic preganglionic neurons. *Science* 203:184–186, 1979.

73. Fernstrom JD, Wurtman RJ: Brain serotonin content: physiological dependence on plasma tryptophan levels. *Science* 173:149–152, 1971.

CHAPTER TWENTY THREE

The Relationship between Headache Syndromes and Sleep

JAMES D. DEXTER, M.D.

SLEEP AND MIGRAINE

The effect of sleep on the patient with migraine is a paradox, for it will relieve a headache in many patients, but precipitate a headache in others.

Ever since Liveing (1) wrote about persons who had relief of migraine after periods of sleep of varying lengths, many people have suggested sleep as therapy, and many methods of sleep induction have been tried. Gowers (2) recommended use of opiates, alcohol, bromides, and tincture of cannabis as "sleep inducers," helpful in the acute attack.

The restorative nature of sleep has been further substantiated by the studies of Wilkinson et al (3), who showed that sleep, after the administration of an antiemetic and analgesic, was a significant factor in the relief of acute migraine. Blau (4) reported that 14 (28%) of 50 patients were able to terminate their daytime attacks of migraine by between 30 minutes and 6 hours of sleep, while 28 (56%) found that a complete night of "particularly deep" sleep would relieve their headache. These observations suggest the possible efficacy of sedation for migraine or status migrainosus.

It has been the experience of most clinicians that many patients with an attack of migraine (or even of muscle contraction headache) respond well to a simple barbiturate-induced period of sleep. These patients often do not require either vasoconstrictive or analgesic agents. In the decade of the 1960s, this author had good results treating patients with prolonged (24–72 hours) pentobarbital-induced sleep periods. Some clinicians find that vasoactive agents, such as ergotamine and isometheptene, are more effective for treating migraine when combined with a sedative, such as a dichloralphenazone or barbiturate.

On the other hand, there is the paradox mentioned at the beginning: some patients develop an attack of migraine after a night of sedated sleep. Many even anticipate the night with some degree of dread, or fear that they will be awakened from sleep by a headache.

The existence of a temporal relationship between sleep and migraine has long been reported in the literature. One of the best descriptions is by Bing (5), who stated: "Sometimes it (migraine) descends upon the patient like a bolt from the blue, when the latter goes to bed with a free head and in a general state of well-being in the evening, and wakes up in the morning with a bad headache."

Migraine can also occur during the middle of the patient's nocturnal sleep period, and it frequently follows brief periods of diurnal sleep, that is, naps. Some attacks of nocturnal headache are reported to occur during dreams. The aura of such an attack of classic migraine is occasionally incorporated into the dream's content, a dream which is then interrupted by a severe headache.

RELATIONSHIP BETWEEN STAGE OF SLEEP AND HEADACHE

In the late 1940s, Gans (6, 7) recognized the relationship between sleep and migraine, and when he selectively deprived patients of nocturnal "deep sleep," reported a decrease in both frequency and severity of the migraine attacks. He stated: "As soon as he (the patient) showed the faintest sign of falling into deep sleep (unnatural body posture, sinking back of the head, or snoring) he was gently touched, whereupon he immediately returned to the superficial sleep level." The precise stages of sleep which were "rationed" is not known, as he did not use electroencephalographic monitoring; however, this procedure may have had the effect of decreasing both slow wave (stages 3 and 4) and rapid eye movement (REM) sleep.

Over the past several years the author and his co-workers have studied this phenomenon in several ways. The first of the studies (8) was done to investigate whether it was during a specific stage of sleep that patients were aroused with nocturnal migraine. The patients were studied using standard nocturnal sleep study techniques. For 45 nights we studied three patients with common migraine (two for 7 nights, and 1 for 6 nights), three patients with cluster headaches (two for 6 nights, and one for 7 nights), and one with psychogenic headache (6 nights). During this time we were able to record 19 headaches (9 cluster, 8 common migraine, 2 psychogenic). In the patients with cluster and common migraine, the 17 awakenings with headache came either during rapid eye movement (REM stage) sleep or immediately following this stage (11 from REM, 4 within 3 minutes following REM, and 2 between 3 and 9 minutes following REM). The two episodes

of psychogenic headache occurred more than 29 minutes after awakening, and were considered not to be directly related to sleep.

Kayed et al (9) studied one case of chronic paroxysmal hemicrania for 4 nights, which enabled them to observe 18 attacks. Seventeen of these 18 awakenings with attacks of chronic paroxysmal hemicrania occurred during the REM period. The only one which was not associated with REM may have been caused by movement, which is a precipitant of some of the patient's diurnal attacks.

Hsu et al (10), as part of their study of early morning migraine, recorded 19 patients with common migraine for 33 nights. They found that 34% of the time that a patient awakened during, or within 10 minutes after, a REM period (32 occasions), he developed a headache. The four non-REM awakenings occurred in patients who were allowed to continue their medication. While this study is interesting, it only included one night for adaptation to the sleep laboratory and the study night (which would be considered by many authors a first night and recovery night) and, therefore, the sleep Hsu et al studied was not the same as normal sleep.

Additional evidence to support the relationship between the REM period and migraine is provided by the sleep-shift study performed by Dexter and Riley (11). In it, a patient with REM-related migraine shifted her sleep period by 7 hours (from a 2300- to 0630-hour sleep period to a 1600- to 2400-hour sleep period). During the 4th week of this process, the patient was studied for eight consecutive evenings, and she showed six arousals from REM with headache symptoms. These findings lend support to the hypothesis that migraine is triggered by REM physiology and that it is not locked to the 24-hour circadian rhythm. Since recent literature (12) suggests that the REM cycle, in a suppressed form, continues throughout the daytime hours, it may be that this study only documented the appearance of REM which would have also precipitated headaches if the patient were not asleep.

When Gans (6, 7) first reported improvement of headache by the disruption of sleep he was unable to document either the depth of the sleep or its stages. Since any procedure which regularly disrupts sleep is inherently stressful, this provides us with another paradox: if stress is a precipitator of migraine, then why does the stress of sleep disruption not increase its frequency?

In 1979 we did three studies in which we tried to unravel this phenomenon reported by Gans (6, 7). In the first one (11), patients with a history of frequent arousals from daytime naps by severe migrainous headaches were allowed to sleep in the sleep laboratory for 3–5 days, starting each day at 1300 hours. They were only monitored for sleep stages and for the reporting of headaches.

Of 17 nap periods monitored, 16 were associated with sleep, though one with only a brief period of stage I sleep. All five patients had at least one nap period followed by a complaint of headache within 1 hour after arousal. Eight of the 17 nap periods eventuated in headache, while 9 of the nap periods did not lead to headache. In all naps which were headache-free, only stage I and stage II sleep were recorded. In all naps which were associated with headache upon arousal (or within 1 hour after it), periods of stages III, IV, or REM sleep were recorded.

The second study (13) followed a group of patients who complained of frequent morning awakenings with severe headache, but only occasional midsleep periods of arousal with headache. This study showed that there was a relationship between an increase in the total slow wave and REM sleep (total stage III + IV + REM) and a tendency to awaken with headache symptoms; indeed, this finding was predictive. A second part of that study showed that pharmacological reduction of deep sleep (stage III + stage IV + REM), using dextroamphetamine or imipramine, reduced the headache symptoms significantly.

While there is some confusion about which stage of sleep (stage IV or REM) is the "deepest" stage of sleep, these findings do help to explain Gan's observations, and do demonstrate the relationship he described between decreasing deep sleep and the improvement of the symptoms of migraine.

BIOGENIC AMINES

Since Kimball et al (14) first described the effects of reserpine enhancement of migraine symptoms, and Curran et al (15) described the urinary changes of 5-hydroxyindoleacetic acid alteration in patients with migraine, the biogenic amine theories of the mechanism of migraine have been the most popular and have remained the most viable despite a lack of complete corroboration for them.

The alteration in three of these biogenic amines, serotonin, epinephrine, and norepinephrine, have been studied in patients with sleep-related headache. Dexter and Riley (11) have studied changing levels of serotonin in both daytime naps and in nocturnal sleep periods. The daytime nap studies, performed on asymptomatic medical student controls, revealed that platelet-bound serotonin stayed relatively stable during nap periods composed of only stages I and II sleep. However, those nap periods which contained stages III-IV and REM sleep had wide variation of platelet bound serotonin. Actual headache patients were not evaluated in this study however.

Findings during napping were similar to the findings from nocturnal sleep studies, which showed very wide variation of platelet bound serotonin during sleep, with no differences seen between normal subjects and patients who awakened with attacks of migraine. This nocturnal study did show a significant relationship between the onset of REM and the decrease in platelet-bound serotonin. In 47 20-minute intervals in which platelet bound-serotonin declined, 30 (or 64%) were associated with the onset of REM. This finding complimented the previous data. The inability to show a difference between normal controls and migraineurs does not eliminate the possibility that serotonin is involved in the mechanism of migraine. However, it does serve to question the idea that an alteration of serotonin release is the major factor causing migraine, and instead suggests that the genetic basis of migraine may involve the target organ affected by serotonin, or that it may, on the other hand, be completely unrelated to serotonin.

The adrenergic biogenic amines (catecholamines) were studied in a similar fashion by Hsu et al (10), who found that, during sleep, patients showed a significantly higher total plasma catecholamine level (epinephrine and norepinephrine) in periods which were preceded by headache, with most of the increase being in the norepinephrine fraction. However, during this study tryptophan levels were not altered following headache onset.

NONMIGRAINOUS HEADACHES AND SLEEP

The relationship between muscle contraction headache and sleep has not been explored. While there may be some relationship, we have been unable to document any primary muscle contraction headache patients who have nocturnal arousals or morning awakenings with headache. The patients with muscle contraction headaches whom we studied had their headache begin more than 20 minutes after they awakened.

In the past, one of the most common headache syndromes relating to sleep has been seen in patients with hypertension. These headaches are reported to improve when the hypertension is controlled. However, this has been recently confused as well by the recognition that morning headache is frequently associated with an obstructive sleep apnea syndrome (16). In one group of 50 patients, 52% had hypertension. Headaches of patients with sleep apnea syndrome observed by this author are similar to hypertensive headaches in that they tend to clear up fairly rapidly on their own, or with the use of simple analgesics after awakening. While there are still many unknown factors about the pathophysiology of this type of headache, the outstanding mechanisms that must be considered are hypoxia and transient hypertension.

The headache associated with increased intracranial pressure is also present upon awakening and is also responsive to simple analgesics. It is often seen in cases of brain tumor. It is clinically important that these diagnoses be considered in nocturnal headaches, as pain may not be their most serious consequences.

ROLE OF THE AUTONOMIC NERVOUS SYSTEM

Recent studies on the relationship between the autonomic nervous system and migraine may help clarify both the pathophysiology of migraine and also the confusing paradoxes noted in studies of sleep and migraine. From a review of the existing data, a possible hypothesis may be stated as follows: Migraine may occur from an inability of the brain to dampen the central and peripheral autonomic nervous system's response to changes mediated through the reticular activating system of the brainstem. Over the past half century there has been a well-accepted relationship between autonomic nervous system function and migraine (and possibly muscle contraction) headaches. Early experiments on the effects of epinephrine were, and remain, quite convincing. The relationship commonly seen between depression and headache, and the possible role of serotonin in depression, is also suggestive. Recent investigations into the central autonomic system and its potential control of small arteriolar tone has given rise to a new and broader view of the mechanism of migraine (17).

The central adrenergic system was demonstrated by Swanson and Hartman (18) to originate from diffuse areas of the pons and medulla and from a well-localized area, the locus ceruleus. From these areas the system projects anteriorly to terminate both synaptically and as free boutons. The locus ceruleus has been investigated most, because of its precise localization. It has been found by Raichle et al (17) to be serving a function analogous to the peripheral sympathetic system in its ability to effect both cerebral blood flow and vascular permeability.

With these observations it may well be that humoral changes reflect peripheral effects of ongoing central neurogenic activity. Although these peripheral mechanisms may be significant, they may only reflect secondary changes or responses to primary central nervous system changes, which Lance (19) has postulated. Since this system is anatomically and biochemically closely associated with the mechanisms of the sleep-wake cycle, as summarized by Jouvet (20), it could be associated with the onset of migraine and the arousal with headache during the REM phase of sleep.

While many areas of confusion still remain about how headache syndromes relate to the physiology of the sleep-wake cycle, there are some consistent findings: (a) Nocturnal arousals with attacks of common migraine, cluster, and chronic paroxysmal hermicrania are related to the appearance of REM sleep. (b) In many headache patients, sleep is a convenient and effective therapy for an acute attack. (c) In some patients, common migraine may improve with sleep restriction and/or with sleep pattern alteration. The next few years will probably give us a better understanding of the details of this process as a result of ongoing studies, both clinical and research.

REFERENCES

1. Liveing E: *On Megrim, Sick-Headache, and Some Allied Disorders.* London, Churchill, 1873.

2. Gowers WR: *A Manual of Diseases of the Nervous System.* London, Churchill, 1888, p 790.

3. Wilkinson M, Williams K, Leyton M: Observations on the treatment of an acute attack of migraine. *Res Clin Studies Headache* 6:141–146, 1978.

4. Blau JN: Resolution of migraine attacks: sleep and the recovery phase. *J Neurol Neurosurg Psychiatry* 45:223–226, 1982.

5. Bing R: *Lehrbuch der Nervendrankheiten.* Basel, Switzerland, B. Schwabe, 1945.

6. Gans M: The interrelationship of sleep and migraine. *Acta Med Orient* 2:97, 1943.

7. Gans M: Treating migraine by "sleep rationing." *J Nerv Ment Dis* 113:405, 1951.

8. Dexter JD, Weitzman ED: The relationship of nocturnal headaches to sleep stage patterns. *Neurology* 20:513–518, 1970.

9. Kayed K, Godtlibsen OB, Sjaastad O: Chronic paroxysmal hemicrania IV: "REM sleep locked" nocturnal headache attacks. *Sleep* 1:91–95, 1978.

10. Hsu LKG, Crisp AH, Kalucy RS, Koval J: Early morning migraine: nocturnal plasma levels of catecholamines, tryptophan, glucose and free fatty acids and sleep encephalographs. *Lancet* 1:447–450, 1977.

11. Dexter JD, Riley TL. Studies in nocturnal migraine. *Headache* 15:51–62, 1975.

12. Othemer E, Hayden MP, Segelbaum R: Encephalic cycles during sleep and wakefulness in humans: A 24-hour pattern. *Science* 164:164–447, 1969.

13. Dexter JD: The relationship between stage III + IV + REM sleep and arousals with migraine. *Headache* 19:364–369, 1979.

14. Kimball RW, Friedman AP, Vallejo E: Effect of serotonin in migraine patients. *Neurology (Minneap)* 10:107, 1960.

15. Curran DA, Hinterberger H, Lance JW: Total plasma serotonin, 5-hydroxyindoleacetic acid and p-hydroxy-m-methoxymandelic acid excretion in normal and migrainous subjects. *Brain* 88:997, 1965.

16. Guilleminault C, van den Hoed J, Mitler MM: Clinical overview of the sleep apnea syndromes. In Guilleminault C, Dement WC (eds): *Sleep Apnea Syndromes.* New York, Alan R. Liss, 1978, vol 11, p 5.

17. Raichle ME, Hartman BK, Eichling JO, Sharpe LG: Central nonadrenergic regulation of cerebral blood flow and vascular permeability. *Proc Natl Acad Sci USA* 72:3626, 1975.

18. Swanson LW, Hartman BK: The central adrenergic system. An immunofluorescence study of the location of cell bodies and their efferent connections in the rat utilizing dopamine-B-hydroxylase as a marker. *J Comp Neurol* 163:467–506, 1975.

19. Lance J: Mechanism and management of headaches. In *Mechanism and Management of Headache,* ed 4. London, Butterworth Scientific, 1982, p 162.

20. Jouvet M: Biogenic amines and the states of sleep. *Science* 163:32, 1969.

CHAPTER TWENTY FOUR

Depression and Headache: A Pharmacological Perspective

SEYMOUR DIAMOND, M.D.

Depression is an entity which has plagued mankind for centuries and will surely continue to do so in the future. In Shakespeare's *Tragedies,* he described the symptoms of depression, in Macbeth, Lady Macbeth, and Hamlet, with surprising clinical accuracy (1). It has been estimated that, in family practice in the United Kingdom (2), depression is the fourth most frequently diagnosed disorder. In the United States it ranks 12th (3).

I have, in previous work, referred to depression as the great masquerader of modern medicine, its role similar to the earlier role of syphilis (4). The manifestations of depression are often subtle, and the diagnosis is frequently missed. Most physicians are probably able to recognize the classically depressed patient. This is the patient who walks into the office with a certain look of sadness, and whose speech and movements are slow. This depressed person exhibits little interest in anything, and sighs frequently (5). However, since the majority of depressed patients do not adhere to the classic model, their diagnosis will require some investigation by the physician.

The depressed patient often presents with a wide variety of complaints which can be categorized as physical, emotional, and psychic (cognitive). The physical complaints include chronic pain and/or headaches, sleep disturbances (typically severe insomnia and early awakening), appetite changes, anorexia and weight loss, amenorrhea, and a decrease in sexual activity, ranging at times to impotence in the males or frigidity in the female. Emotional complaints include feeling "blue," and anxiety. Finally, psychic complaints may be comprised of statements such as "Morning is the worst time of the day," suicidal thoughts, death wishes, and rumination over the past, present, and future. (Tables 24.1–24.3).

The physician must obtain a thorough history, which should include a detailed psychiatric inventory discussing the patient's marital relationship, occupation, social relationships, life stresses, personality traits, habits, methods of handling tension situations, and sexual problems (6).

Depression can be classified into three major categories. First, the normal grief related to illness or death, which we have all probably experienced. Second, a reactive depression, which may be associated with physical illness or the use of medications, or may occur in association with psychiatric illness. These are often self-limited and usually respond well to the tricyclic drugs. Finally, the third type of depression is the endogenous or primary depression. This may be unipolar (recurrent depression only) or bipolar (depres-

TABLE 24.1.
PHYSICAL COMPLAINTS

COMPLAINT	% OF PATIENTS
Sleep disturbances	97
Early awakening	87
Headache	84
Dyspnea	76
Loss of weight	74
Trouble getting to sleep	73
Weakness and fatigue	70
Urinary frequency	70
"Spells"—dizziness	70
Appetite disturbances	70
Decreased libido	63
Cardiovascular disturbances	60
Sexual disturbances	60
Palpitations	59
Paresthesias	53
Nausea	48
Menstrual changes	41

sion alternating with mania). It is patients in this last category that are more likely to manifest the symptoms of depression already mentioned (Fig. 24.1) (7).

A headache secondary to depression is usually considered a muscle contraction headache. This headache is a steady non-pulsatile ache, often distributed in a bandlike pattern around the head. It may be described as viselike, a steady pressure, a weight, a soreness, or a distinct cramplike sensation. The headache is often capricious, bizarre, and follows no definite pattern as to location, although the occipital portion of the skull is frequently affected. Its duration is a distinguish-ing feature. A depressed person will often describe his headache as lasting for years or throughout his life. A depressive headache is usually dull and generalized, characteristically worse in the morning and in the evening. This diurnal variation is the most distinct character-istic of the headache and has provided a cor-rect diagnosis of severe depression when other features have been inconspicuous.

Certain details about the headache may indicate an underlying depression. These headaches usually appear at regular intervals in relation to daily life events, occurring on weekends, Sundays, holidays, and on the first days of vacation or after exams. The periods from 4:00 pm to 8:00 pm and from 4:00 am to 8:00 am show the greatest occurrence of "ner-vous type" headache. These are usually the periods of the greatest and, sometimes, the most silent family crises. Headache may occur early in the morning when the depressed pa-tient awakens and his fantasies of conflict with family members or colleagues at work are ac-tivated. In discussion with the depressed pa-tient, we find that the headaches often occur when the patient leaves the relatively quiet atmosphere of the office for a weekend at home. The headache often coincides with in-terpersonal situations in which the sufferer feels compelled to appear comfortable, re-laxed, and agreeable, although he is strug-gling to repress his resentment towards some-one whom he is expected to love and respect.

People with depressive illness may de-velop bodily symptoms and, conversely, peo-ple with painful organic diseases tend to be-come depressed. It should be noted that too little attention is given to the depressive as-

TABLE 24.2.
EMOTIONAL COMPLAINTS

COMPLAINT	% OF PATIENTS
Blue; low spirits; sadness	90
Crying	80
Feelings of guilt, hopelessness, unworthiness, unreality	65
Anxious or irritable	65
Anxiety	60

TABLE 24.3.
PSYCHIC (COGNITIVE) COMPLAINTS

COMPLAINT	% OF PATIENTS
"Morning is the worst time of day"	95
Poor concentration	91
No interest; no ambition	75
Indecisiveness	75
Poor memory	71
Fear of insanity, physical disease, death; rumination over past, present, future	50
Suicidal thoughts; death wishes	35

pects of chronic pain and its treatment. The physical complaints dominate the situation so that the underlying depression tends to be overlooked. Because most patients will consult the doctor for bodily disturbances, a careful questioning of patients with chronic pain is essential. If these complaints include fatigue, tiredness, a heavy feeling, sleep or appetite disturbances, or sexual dysfunction they are frequently clues to an underlying depression.

Two factors often provide insight that the patient may be depressed. First, the physician should determine if there is a prior history of depression in the patient or his family. The patient should be questioned if he has noticed similar symptoms in relatives or himself. Many will indicate previous occurrences of these symptoms. The patient may describe obscure symptoms which were actually depressive equivalents. Second, the patient may relate the onset of his symptoms to a particular event. The depressive attacks may follow a wide variety of events which the patient perceives as traumatic or feels as a personal loss. The event may be out of proportion to the severity of the resultant depression. A patient may note that the symptoms followed some form of bodily injury, illness, injection, sur-

gery, or even a diagnostic test. He may emphasize that his symptoms result from this event. The incident to which the patient attributes the headaches or other depressive equivalent is not compatible in degree with the resultant illness; it should not be as overwhelming as perceived. The patient often feels weakened or maimed by the event. If not subsequent to an illness or accident, depression may follow some change in role, position, or socioeconomic status. Loss of a loved one often triggers normal depressed states. It can also initiate a malignant depression beyond the scope of the loss. The patient's history will reveal the loss to have an important or a peculiar significance for him.

Although recognizing that these statistics were gathered at a headache clinic, we have found that 84% of depressed patients indicated that headache was one of their complaints or their only complaint. In Table 24.1 the most frequently listed complaint with depression is sleep disturbance (8). Ninety-seven percent of the patients that I or my colleagues examined presented this complaint. In younger patients, variation in sleep is less consistent, and the older individual typically experiences more difficulty with sleep. Sleep

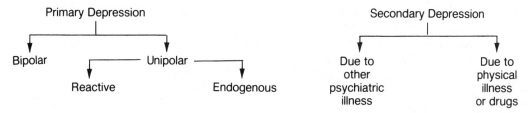

Figure 24.1. *Depressive disorders.*

TABLE 24.4.

CLUES THAT ILLNESS MAY BE SECONDARY
TO DEPRESSION

1. Multiple complaints that do not fit a recognizable picture;
2. Development of new symptoms as soon as others are helped;
3. Bad cooperation with treatment;
4. Symptoms that occur only in the presence of a certain individual, in a particular place, or at a certain time of year;
5. History of psychiatric problems; and
6. The physician is confused and feels out of control of the patient.

disturbances may manifest themselves as hypersomnia, insomnia, early awakening, or disturbing dreams. Early awakening is one of the most common sleep disturbances.

Characteristic of depressed patients are signs and symptoms affecting various bodily functions. If a multitude of somatic complaints exists, depression should be suspected (Table 24.4) (7).

The emotional complaints characteristic of depression may vary (Table 24.2) (8). Also, emotional changes can fluctuate over the course of the illness. During the examination, if the patient feels despondent or cries the physician will naturally consider depression. Yet some people are unable to cry, but wish they could. Although the patient may have accomplished much in life, such as a successful career, the impression he creates with his physician does not reflect his awareness of this. The clue to depression here is the introversion of the patient. Emotionally his mind is centered on himself and his illness. He repeatedly reviews his mistakes and misdeeds and deprecates himself. Feelings of inadequacy and incompetence are common and persistent in these people; they look to the future with despair. Phobias and fears of a variable nature are common, such as fear of insanity, of being alone in the house, of changing jobs, or of moving. Irritability and hostility are frequent emotional symptoms.

The patient may present a multitude of psychic complaints (Table 24.3) (8). An impairment in concentration or memory, loss of interest, difficulty in making decisions, and despondency occur frequently in depression. These may produce thoughts of suicide, ideas of reference, and delusions.

To the depressed patient, everything is an effort. Some experience complete psychomotor retardation, and have difficulty eating, sleeping, thinking, and dressing themselves. Daily tasks become major chores. Older people can have serious memory defects ("pseudodementia"). They may have delusions of cancer or other incurable illnesses. The physician cannot dispute these ideas. They also may become fanatic about religion, riddled with guilt, or develop delusions of poverty. If wealthy, they may become miserly.

Although some authors feel that pseudodementia occurs rarely (9), other experienced clinicians indicate that up to 15% of elderly patients referred for evaluation of dementia are depressed and that depression frequently presents as apparent dementia (10). When the depressed patient is extremely apathetic, hopeless, or negative and will not cooperate with mental status testing, or if his thinking is slowed, dementia may be incorrectly diagnosed. In addition, many patients with chronic brain syndromes are also depressed, and display loss of interest in usual activities, apathy, emotional withdrawal, sleep disturbances and, possibly, suicidal thoughts. The points listed on Table 24.5 (11) usually distinguish dementia from pseudodementia (10, 12–15).

Certain drugs (Table 24.6) can produce depressive reactions in susceptible patients or may cause an increase in an existing depressive state (7). A depressed patient may resemble an anxious patient, and be mistakenly treated with ataractics or neuroleptics. Under treatment with such tranquilizing drugs, a regression may indicate that the diagnosis was incorrect.

Some anxiety is present in all depressive states, but its intensity varies from subject to subject (Table 24.7) (16). Certain severe pain disorders, such as trigeminal neuralgia and

TABLE 24.5.
DIFFERENTIATING DEMENTIA FROM DEPRESSION

DEMENTIA	PSEUDODEMENTIA
Cognitive deterioration is well established before depression develops (although the patient may not be consciously aware of being demented)	The patient is significantly depressed before complaints of memory loss and difficulty in concentrating begin
Affect is labile and shallow	Depressive feelings are severe, pervasive, and easily communicated to the examiner
Negative past history and family history of psychiatric disorder	Past history or family history of affective disorder and related conditions
Symptoms fluctuate	Symptoms do not fluctuate
Loss of function is relatively consistent (e.g., memory and calculating ability are equally lost)	Mental status abnormalities are inconsistent; e.g., the patient cannot perform serial subtractions but is able to handle complex calculations related to his business
Symptoms worse at night	Symptoms may be worse in the morning
Guilt and lowered self-esteem not prominent	Guilt and lowered self-esteem obvious
Vegetative signs not prominent	Vegetative signs may be present
Patient attempts to answer mental status questions but is unable to do so and becomes more frustrated and depressed	Patient does not try to answer even simple questions and becomes annoyed and withdrawn when more questions are asked

the thalamic syndrome, can result in an occurrence of a secondary depression, which may be severe, and the patient may consider suicide. Although somatic symptoms and headaches are often symptoms of depression, it should be reiterated that a depression can result from chronic organic illness.

The biochemical determinants of depression have been researched heavily for the past 30 years. Much of our present knowledge comes from work completed in the mid-1950s (17). During that time, it was observed that tubercular patients treated with iproniazid developed euphoric states. It was later learned that iproniazid is a monoamine oxidase inhibitor and produces increasing levels of norepinephrine and serotonin in the brain and body tissue. At about this time it was observed that a small percentage of patients being treated for hypertension with rauwolfian alkaloids such as reserpine developed severe depression indistinguishable from endogenous depression. These alkaloids were noted

TABLE 24.6.
DRUG CATEGORIES WHICH MAY BE ASSOCIATED WITH SECONDARY DEPRESSION

Analgesics and anti-inflammatory agents
Antibiotics
Anticonvulsants
Antihistamines
Antihypertensives
Antiparkinsonian drugs
Cardiac drugs
Chemotherapeutic drugs
Hormones
Immunosuppressives
Sedatives and tranquilizers
Others—alcohol, caffeine, and "recreational" drugs

TABLE 24.7.
DIFFERENTIAL DIAGNOSIS OF ANXIETY AND DEPRESSION

Depression
  Persistently depressed mood
  Diurnal variation
  Early morning awakening
  Psychomotor retardation
Anxiety
  Panic attacks
  Severe agoraphobia
  Marked depersonalization, derealization, or perceptual distortions

to deplete the brain of both of these biogenic amines. These observations evolved into the current psychophysiological theory of depression, which considers it to be an illness involving defects in the production of multiple neurotransmitters.

The importance of antidepressant drugs in pain control in large measure results from their effects on the synthesis and metabolism of serotonin (5-hydroxtryptamine) and norepinephrine. It has been found that neurons containing serotonin and norepinephrine are part of the brain's analgesia system (18, 19). A descending serotonin pathway in the dorsal spine cord, originating in the raphe nucleus, and an interlacing of norepinephrine and opioid producing neurons in the locus ceruleus are of particular interest to pain researchers (18). Drugs altering the synthesis or uptake of serotonin and/or norepinephrine, which includes virtually all antidepressant agents, would be expected to play a role in the brain's regulation of pain. Serotonin antagonists have been known to influence both opiate- and stimulation-induced analgesia (20). In animals, tricyclics produce analgesia either directly (21) or through potentiation of opiates (22).

These discoveries provide only a beginning in our understanding of the etiology and control of pain. However, enough information has been gained to formulate preliminary hypotheses and guidelines concerning the use of antidepressants in pain management.

The most popular biological theories of depression hold that the disorder is associated with depletion of brain monoamine neurotransmitters such as serotonin and norepinephrine. Determining which of these two substances is most important in depression is controversial. Evidence is available to support both the norepinephrine and serotonin hypotheses (23). Other neurotransmitters, such as dopamine and endorphin, may also be involved in depression (24). The recent discovery of endogenous, opiate-like substances in the brain, the endorphins and the enkephalins, has significantly advanced our understanding of pain. Recent findings suggest that

pain transmission in the central nervous system is controlled by an endorphin-mediated analgesia system which can be activated by several exogenous agents and actions, including opioid substances, electrical stimulation, acupuncture, and even placebo (25–29). Detailed reviews of biological theories of depression are fairly abundant in the literature.

Researchers are investigating biochemical methods to measure depression. One of the larger areas of interest concerns the measurement of 3-methoxy-4-hydroxyphenylethyleneglycol (MHPG) in the urine. MHPG is the main metabolite of norepinephrine in the central nervous system, and a patient's urinary levels may reflect his level of norepinephrine metabolism (30–32). There is some controversy, however, over the precise amount of urinary MHPG that is derived from the central nervous system. It has been noted that there are subgroups of depressed patients who have decreased MHPG in the urine, while other groups of depressed patients have normal or increased levels of MHPG. It has been suggested that perhaps two types of depression exist, one in which norepinephrine metabolism is disrupted and serotonin and dopamine systems are normal, and, one in which serotonin metabolism is disrupted but norepinephrine and dopamine metabolism is normal. One study found a statistically significant correlation between the presence of three symptoms of depression, namely, guilt, agitation, and diurnal variation, and a high MHPG level. Thus, the MHPG level may be valuable in selecting appropriate drug therapy.

Studies revealed that low MHPG depressives have a better response to imipramine and desipramine, and a poorer response to amitriptyline and nortriptyline. In contrast, high MHPG patients responded more effectively to amitriptyline or nortriptyline. Maas (30) argued that low MHPG patients had low norepinephrine but normal serotonin and that high MHPG patients had a low serotonin but normal norepinephrine suppression.

The results of earlier studies which showed that low MHPG patients respond favorably to drugs that exert potent effects on noradrenergic systems, including nortriptyline, maprotiline, imipramine, and desipramine, have been duplicated (33–35). Since amitriptyline is not simply serotonergic, but rather exerts potent effects on both acetylcholine and norepinephrine activity, the results of studies using amitriptyline have been inconsistent. Its clinical action is similar to that of current tricyclics and tetracyclics.

In recent research, the possibility of three distinct subgroups of depressive disorders has been noted. The groups are differentiated on the basis of low, intermediate, and high MHPG levels (33, 34, 36). Patients with low MHPG, who may have decreased norepinephrine synthesis or release, demonstrated a clear response to imipramine or maprotiline. Normal norepinephrine metabolism is believed to occur in patients with intermediate MHPG levels, and they are therefore poor responders to maprotiline or imipramine. However, this intermediate group may manifest some other neurochemical abnormality. Patients with high MHPG who have intermediate responses to the two drugs may have high norepinephrine output due to subsensitive postsynaptic receptors and/or increased acetylcholine activity.

To explain the disparate results from other studies, a three-group paradigm should be formulated. Low MHPG patients have demonstrated relatively low levels of cerebrospinal fluid 5-hydroxyindoleacetic acid (5-HIAA) in recent studies. A low norepinephrine versus low serotonin hypothesis would be disputed with these observations (35).

Even though the exact mechanisms of action may not be certain, there is a clear contrast in the clinical profiles of these drugs. Clinical observations suggest that noradrenergic drugs (e.g., protriptyline and desipramine) contain more stimulant properties than amitriptyline, trimipramine, and doxepin (the latter possessing more sedative properties). Maprotiline is an exception since it often manifests qualities of a stimulant but has also been considered an aid to help patients sleep, and may possess an anxiolytic potential.

The heterocyclic agents which sedate can also exert considerable effect on both serotonin reuptake and on histamine receptors (37). Their sedating ability results from these actions. The finding of two types of histamine receptors, H_1 and H_2, complicates the issue of histamine blockade. One set (H_1) appears to be related to sedation and weight gain, while H_2 receptors control gastric acid secretion. In vitro, the effect of tricyclics on H_2 receptors suggests that, in a manner similar to cimetidine, some tricyclics may be successful in the treatment of ulcer disease. Early clinical studies have suggested this and other "H_2" indications for certain tricyclics (Table 24.8) (38).

Another test gaining popularity in treatment of depression is the dexamethasone

TABLE 24.8.
RELATIVE EFFECTS OF TRICYCLICS ON BLOCKING ACETYLCHOLINE AND HISTAMINE RECEPTORS (H_1 AND H_2)

	ACETYLCHOLINE	**H_1**	**H_2**
Imipramine	$++$[a]	$+$	$\pm$
Desipramine	$+$	$\pm$	$\pm$
Amitriptyline	$+++$	$++$	$++$
Nortriptyline	$+$	$+$	$\pm$
Protriptyline	$+++$	0	0
Doxepin	$++$	$+++$	$+$
Trimipramine	$++$	$++$	?

[a] 0 = inactive; $\pm$, weak inhibitor/noninhibitor; $+$, weak inhibitor; $++$, moderate inhibitor; $+++$, strong inhibitor.

suppression test (39–41). This test was developed in 1960 for the study of Cushing's syndrome. Basically, the test involves administering a small amount of dexamethasone to the patient at midnight and then measuring serum cortisol levels the following day. In a normal person, feedback mechanisms lead to decreased production of cortisol. In a patient with Cushing's syndrome, there is "nonsuppression," that is, cortisol levels are not diminished the following day. It has been found that a subgroup of patients with an endogenous depression also exhibits nonsuppression. However, unlike Cushing's syndrome, most of these patients show normal suppression in the morning and nonsuppression can only be elicited later in the day. Approximately 45% of endogenously depressed individuals have an abnormal dexamethasone suppression test. Since the test is 96% specific for endogenous depression, only 4 to 7% of patients with other psychiatric disorders including schizophrenia, mania, personality disorders and minor or neurotic depression, will have an abnormal dexamethasone suppression test. If a patient has an abnormal response to the test, the physician must be sure that an organic illness is not causing the abnormal result. These include Cushing's syndrome, pregnancy, and uncontrolled diabetes. He must also review the medications the patient is taking since many drugs will alter the results. Currently, the most useful value of the dexamethasone suppression test (DST) is for monitoring the patient's response to therapy. Normalization of the DST seems to correlate with an improved clinical picture. Patients with an abnormal DST appear more likely to suffer from recurrent depressions than do those patients who exhibit normal suppression. Studies are underway to determine if a patient's response to the DST can be used as a guide for drug therapy. Preliminary work indicates that the nonsuppressors have a better response to treatment. The relationship between the pituitary-adrenal axis and depression is unknown at the present time. The limbic system and cholinergic pathways have been implicated, but further research is required.

Another diagnostic test is the thyroid stimulating hormone (TSH) response to thyrotropin-releasing hormone (TRH). It has been noted that a large percentage of endogenously depressed patients have a blunted TSH response to the administration of TRH. The mechanism for this blunted response is unknown, and the clinical value of this test has yet to be demonstrated.

This research serves as the foundation of our current drug therapies for depression, which primarily use tricyclics and monoamine oxidase inhibitors. Drugs in both of these categories function by increasing the amount of biogenic amines available to the patient's receptor sites. Monoamine oxidase inhibitors (MAOIs) accomplish this action by decreasing the rate of in vivo destruction of biogenic amines. The tricyclic action decreases presynaptic cellular reuptake of the biogenic amines (Table 24.8) (38).

Tricyclics are usually the drugs of choice for headaches caused by depression. This group includes amitriptyline, imipramine, desipramine, nortriptyline, doxepin, and protriptyline. The efficacy of these drugs has been shown in numerous studies (42–46). The tricyclics are considered more effective in endogenous depression and less beneficial when the depressed patient has many accompanying neurotic traits.

The choice of which tricyclic to use is never a simple one since each drug has unique characteristics (Table 24.9) (47). Amitriptyline typically has a powerful sedating effect. Doxepin is equally sedating, but has the least anticholinergic effect in the group. Imipramine is more sedating than desipramine, and nortriptyline falls somewhere in between those two. Protriptyline and desipramine are usually only minimally sedating. MHPG levels can be used as a guide to treatment since patients with a low pretreatment MHPG level respond most favorably to imipramine and desipramine while patients with a normal or high urinary MHPG level respond more fa-

TABLE 24.9.
EFFECTS OF TRICYCLIC ANTIDEPRESSANTS

DRUG	SEROTONIN INHIBITION	NOREPINEPHRINE INHIBITION	DOPAMINE INHIBITION	SEDATIVE EFFECTS	ANTICHOLINERGIC EFFECTS
Amitriptyline	Moderate	Weak	Inactive	Strong	Strong
Desipramine	Weak	Potent	Inactive	Mild	Moderate
Doxepin	Moderate	Moderate	Inactive	Strong	Strong
Imipramine	Fairly potent	Moderate	Inactive	Moderate	Strong
Nortriptyline	Weak	Fairly potent	Inactive	Mild	Moderate
Protriptyline	Weak	Fairly potent	Inactive	None	Strong

vorably to amitriptyline. It should be noted that amitriptyline exerts its greatest effect in blocking the reuptake of serotonin, while desipramine and imipramine function largely by blocking the reuptake of norepinephrine. The dexamethasone suppression test can also be a useful guide to treatment, with the nonsuppressors responding more favorably to desipramine and imipramine, the suppressors responding more favorably to amitriptyline and clomipramine.

Amitriptyline is probably the most widely used antidepressant in office practice. Its common side effects include weakness, fatigue, drowsiness, dizziness, dryness of the mouth, blurred vision, constipation, and muscle tremors. Amitriptyline rarely has to be discontinued due to side effects, as most of them subside if the drug is continued.

MAO inhibitors (MAOIs) are generally considered to be second line drugs for depression. They are not considered as efficacious as the tricyclics and are known to have more drug interactions. A patient on a MAOI must follow a special diet and avoid foods with tyramine (Table 24.10). The most commonly used MAOI is phenelzine sulfate (Nardil) (48). MAO inhibitors block the oxidative deamination of numerous monoamines, including epinephrine, norepinephrine, serotonin, and dopamine. According to prevailing theories, the amounts of these substances present in the brain and elsewhere is increased by the MAOIs, and the depression created by their deficiency is ameliorated or cured. Despite the precautions and fears with

which physicians approach the use of monoamine oxidase inhibitors, they are often found effective when the tricyclics fail. In studies comparing tricyclics and MAOIs (49), the MAOIs tended to exert a stronger antianxiety action while the tricyclics were more effective in reversing weight loss and improving sleep.

Combination therapy, using a tricyclic and an MAOI simultaneously, was previously considered *verboten* in practice. There had been isolated reports of hypertensive, hyperpyretic crises leading to death due to such combined therapy. Standard practice has been to initiate therapy with a tricyclic. If no improvement is noted within 4 to 6 weeks, the drug is discontinued, and after waiting 10 days to 2 weeks an MAOI may be started. But the two drugs were never given together.

In 1971, Schuckit et al (50) reviewed 25 reported cases of morbidity presumed to be secondary to such combined therapy. The results of that study indicated that the risks of combination therapy had been greatly exaggerated. Many of the complications reported could be attributed to drug overdose, while others could be related to the concomitant use of other drugs which act on the central nervous system. In the remaining cases, the tricyclic involved was imipramine, and the MAOIs included iproniazid, tranylcypromine, isocarboxazid, pargyline, and phenelzine. Currently, the author and certain other researchers believe that the combination of a tricyclic and an MAOI may be of value for the depressed patient refractive to all previous therapy. It should be used with caution.

TABLE 24.10.
DIET FOR THE HEADACHE PATIENT ON MAO INHIBITORS[a]

FOOD GROUP	FOODS ALLOWED	FOODS TO AVOID
Beverages	Decaffeinated coffee, colas containing no caffeine. Caffeine sources to be limited to 2 cups daily include coffee, tea, colas	Alcoholic beverages, wines, ale, beer
Milk	Homogenized, skim, 2%	Chocolate, buttermilk
Dairy products	Cottage cheese, cream cheese, American cheese, Velveeta, or synthetic cheese. Yogurt in 1/2 cup portions or less	Aged and processed cheese: includes cheddar, Swiss, Mozzarella, Parmesan, Romano, Brick, Brie, Camembert, Gouda, Gruyere, Emmentaler, Stilton, Provolone, Roquefort, blue and cheese-containing foods (pizza, macaroni, and cheese), yogurt, and sour cream
Meat and meat substitutes	Fresh prepared meats, eggs	Aged, canned, cured, or processed meats, those containing nitrates or nitrites, commercial meat extracts, pickled or dried herring, chicken livers, sausage, salami, pepperoni, bologna, frankfurters, pates, peanuts and peanut butter, marinated meats; any prepared with meat tenderizers, soy sauce, or yeast extracts.
Bread and bread substitutes	All except those on avoid list. Commercial bread.	Homemade yeast breads, fresh coffee cake, doughnuts, yeast and yeast extracts, sourdough breads, breads and crackers containing cheese, any containing chocolate or nuts.
Fruits	All except those to avoid. Citrus fruits (oranges, grapefruit, pineapple, lemon, lime) are limited to 1/2 cup serving per day	Canned figs, raisins, papaya, passion fruit, avocado, red plum, 1/2 banana allowed per day
Vegetables	All except those on avoid list	Italian broad beans, Fava beans, lima, navy and pea pods, sauerkraut, onions except for flavoring
Desserts	All except fresh yeast, raised desserts, or those containing chocolate	Any with chocolate
Miscellaneous	White vinegar, commercial salad dressings in small amounts	Brewer's yeast, chocolate, soy sauce, monosodium glutamate, meat tenderizers, papaya products, Accent, Lawry's and other seasoned salts, soup cubes, canned soups, frozen TV dinners. Some snack items and instant foods contain items to be avoided. Read all labels.

[a] Tyramine content may vary among brand names available in the market because of preparation, processing or storage. It is best to eat only freshly prepared foods to avoid the risk of eating foods that may have been aged, fermented, pickled or marinated. Tenderizers, monosodium glutamate, nitrate or nitrite compounds are likely to be provoking agents. It is important to read labels carefully when shopping and ask questions when eating out.

The efficacy of combination therapy has yet to be shown statistically. However, a recent study has shown that amitriptyline may actually *prevent* hypertensive crises when given in conjunction with a MAO inhibitor (51).

Whereas MAO inhibitors increase the availability of monoamines by decreasing monoamine oxidase concentrations, tricyclics accomplish this by inhibiting the reuptake of monoamines at receptor sites. Fluoxetine, a pure serotonin uptake blocker, has been shown to produce direct analgesia in rats (19). Zimelidine, also a serotonin uptake inhibitor, relieves pain caused by central nervous system and neuronal lesions (52); such pain is unlikely to be secondary to depression.

Fluoxetine and zimelidine are bicyclic agents and have not yet been marketed in the United States. They are mentioned because their action is similar to that of amitriptyline. It is difficult to determine whether an antidepressant's capacity for inhibiting serotonin uptake is a major factor in producing its analgesic effect, and whether the majority of antidepressant drugs used to produce analgesia are simply potent blockers of serotonin uptake.

Three antidepressants, all nontricyclics, have received recent FDA approval. Maprotiline, a potent norepinephrine uptake inhibitor, is a tetracyclic compound and is chemically and pharmacologically related to the tricyclics. It does not alter serotonin concentrations. Clinical trials have shown this drug to be as effective an antidepressant as the standard tricyclics. Its overall side effect profile is said to be lower than that of the tricyclics, but it does have some anticholinergic and cardiovascular side effects (52). Thus, maprotiline may offer some advantages over tricyclics, but patients taking it must be closely monitored for adverse effects.

Amoxapine, another antidepressant, inhibits both serotonin and norepinephrine uptake and also blocks dopamine receptor activity (23). This agent is a demethylated neuroleptic and thus carries a potential for extrapyramidal effects, particularly with long-term use (54). Like maprotiline, amoxapine produces anticholinergic effects that are somewhat milder than those produced by tricyclics (23). In some patients, amoxapine may cause galactorrhea, seizures, and cardiac problems (54). Amoxapine has not been consistently effective in treating depression. According to one investigator (23), amoxapine offers no real advantages over established antidepressants, because it "may in fact introduce some new problems of safety and tolerance."

The most recently approved antidepressant, trazodone, is a triazolopyradine derivative that selectively blocks serotonin uptake and has some α-adrenergic activity. Its anticholinergic and cardiovascular side effect profiles are very low; the most frequently reported adverse effect is drowsiness (23). Trazodone's antidepressant effect is comparable to that of the tricyclics. Its onset of action is relatively rapid (55–57). Trazodone has been shown to be useful in a broad range of depressive subtypes, including with anxious and agitated depressions (58). Cole and colleagues (59) found that so-called "treatment-resistant depressives" respond well to trazodone therapy.

Several other new antidepressants are being tested in this country and will become available over the next few years. Not enough information is available to begin using antidepressants as direct analgesics in routine medical practice. However, when pain is the predominant presenting symptom of depression, in cases where depression is the definitive diagnosis and no organic cause is found for the patient's accompanying pain, antidepressant therapy is a rational initial therapy. The majority of these cases will involve headache.

It must be reiterated that treatment must be comprehensive. A proportion of depressed patients will require concomitant psychotherapy, a position in no way incompatible with pharmacological approaches. The therapeutic rationale for both types of treatment must be carefully explained to the patient, with the physician providing as much information to the patient as possible without frightening him or confusing him in a way that sets back treatment goals. Simon (60) reported a high incidence of suicide among headache sufferers who are unsuccessfully treated, due to feelings of isolation produced by their unalleviated symptoms. Parnell and Cooperstock (61), in their extensive survey, reviewed many critical comments from migraine sufferers regarding the prescribing of tranquilizers. The patients considered this practice as evidencing a lack of understanding of migraine on the part of their physicians. The same reaction could occur with antidepressant therapy if the treatment rationale and the potential side effects are not clearly and properly explained.

Even though pain may be secondary to depression, the pain is quite real, and it is often more obvious to the patient than is the depression. The physician should be cognizant of this factor throughout treatment.

When antidepressant therapy is indicated, the choice of drug will depend on the amount and severity of each drug's side effects, the likelihood of such side effects significantly interfering with the patient's usual habits and life style, and the potential for serious complications. If the pain consists solely or primarily of muscle contraction headaches, an antidepressant with demonstrated anxiolytic effect would probably be the drug of choice.

Combinations of antidepressants and neuroleptic (antipsychotic drugs) have been used, with success, in managing both headache and pain with an organic etiology. However, it would seem prudent to restrict the use of such combinations to intractable or intolerable pain. In everyday family practice, the use of neuroleptics, especially in combination with other drugs, is a fairly extreme and complex treatment approach.

In many cases of frank or suspected depression, psychotherapy is a helpful adjunct to drug treatment. Also, various behavioral manipulations, such as biofeedback and relaxation training, can be valuable and can be continued after the antidepressant medication is stopped.

Many patients with chronic pain abuse drugs due to frustration rather than to personality factors conducive to addiction problems. Before any treatment is initiated, this possibility must be considered and carefully investigated. Excessive drug use by these patients usually involves analgesic preparations. The physician must support the patient in discontinuing the habituating drugs before initiating antidepressant or another therapy. Hospitalization may be indicated for the patient habituated to drugs.

In evaluating any patient, it is essential to differentiate acute from chronic pain. With our current knowledge, antidepressant therapy only seems to be appropriate for chronic pain. Depressed patients rarely consult a physician until pain becomes chronic. The patient seeking medical treatment for acute pain is more likely to have an organic dysfunction requiring immediate medical intervention. This distinction can usually be determined from a careful and adequate history.

The exact mechanism by which depression causes muscle contraction headache has not been determined. EMG recordings have indicated that the muscles of the face, scalp, and neck are usually extremely contracted during a tension headache (62). Often, these patients are unable to relax and have the characteristic features of a furrowed brow and clenched teeth. Vascular factors are also considered to play a role in the etiology of this pain. In contrast to the patient with migraine, the tension headache sufferer may not be getting adequate blood flow to his head secondary to the constriction of the arteries by the contracted muscles. Finally, it has been proposed that one segment of the pain's etiology may be a functional disorder of the nervous system (63). Dalessio suggests that these patients are unable to suppress sensory input from normal or minimally damaged tissue and that the brain misinterprets these incoming signals, thus leading to a chronic pain syndrome. In other words, the patient develops an altered perception of normal sensation, a "hyperalgesia."

To confirm the diagnosis of an exclusively depressive headache, organic causes of head pain must be ruled out. (Of course, depression can accentuate pain from organic conditions as well.) These include cervical spondylosis, discogenic bony anomalies of the occipitocervical joints, basilar invagination, chronic mastoiditis, malocclusion of the temporomandibular joint and, possibly, a posterior fossa lesion (64).

Currently, treatment of tension headaches is often focused on the underlying depression when this is present. In 1964, Lance and Curran (65) demonstrated the effectiveness of amitriptyline in the tension sufferer. His results indicated that greater than 50% of his patients became either headache-free or substantially improved on amitriptyline. The success rate was greater than 80% in his patients over the age of 60. Lance was unable to correlate the response of the patient to the presence or absence of depressive symptoms.

Follow-up studies have confirmed the efficacy of amitriptyline in the treatment of depressive headaches (66, 67). The most frequent cause for treatment failure is undertreatment. It must be emphasized to the patient that an immediate effect does not occur and that he must give the drug adequate time to work. Usually a 4- to 6-week trial period should be completed before treatment is considered unsuccessful.

In patients with a history of analgesic abuse, certain guidelines should be followed. Injections of stress-relieving medications are contraindicated in order to break the pattern of chronic abuse. Drugs should be prescribed on a fixed time schedule, and multiple drug therapy should be reduced to a minimum. Analgesics should be reduced slowly, and patients should be encouraged to continue their daily activities and keep busy to avoid focusing on head pain. Finally, and most importantly, the patient should receive a detailed explanation of the goals and reasons for the therapy. Unless the patient comprehends these goals, the treatment will be fruitless.

Biofeedback has been shown to be useful in the treatment of muscle contraction headaches. Biofeedback is a rapidly expanding therapy with a growing number of clinical applications.

Depression headaches are also often seen in patients suffering from migraine (68, 69). A patient with severe migraines over a long period of time may develop a depression as a result of the chronic pain. Often this depression will manifest itself as a muscle contraction headache. The patient will give a history of intermittent severe headaches for many years with a more recent onset of a mild daily headache.

In 1975, Couch et al (70) showed a weak but significant relationship between migraine and depression. A high correlation was found between depression and migraine associated with paresis, sensory disturbance, difficulty with speech, and loss of consciousness. They postulated that a subgroup may exist in whom depression and migraine are linked and that this subgroup may be identified by the presence of these focal neurological signs mentioned.

It has been shown that the antidepressants sometimes play a role in the treatment of migraine. Couch and Hassanein in 1979 (71) completed a study comparing amitriptyline to placebo in the prophylaxis of migraine. They found statistically significant improvement with the use of amitriptyline. The patients who responded best to amitriptyline were the nondepressed subjects with severe headaches and depressed subjects with less severe migraine. They propose that the antimigrainous effect of amitriptyline is separate from its antidepressant effect. It is unknown if this effect is due to its blocking the reuptake of serotonin and, to a lesser degree, of norepinephrine at the nerve endings, or is due to its anticholinergic, antihistaminic, and antiserotonergic actions.

Anthony and Lance (72) have shown the effectiveness of the MAOIs, specifically phenelzine, for treating migraine. They were able to reduce the frequency of headaches to less than one-half that of the preceding year in 20 of 25 patients. However, there was no correlation between headache improvement and serotonin levels. They concluded that the MAOIs are useful in treatment of migraine, but must be considered a therapy for refractory patients and prescribed with extreme caution.

In conclusion, it should be emphasized that depression is probably the single most prevalent cause of headache, and that more than anything, successful treatment requires recognition of the condition by the physician.

REFERENCES

1. Andreasen NJC: The artist as scientist. Psychiatric diagnosis in Shakespeare's Tragedies. *JAMA* 235(17):1868, 1976.

2. Hodgkins K: Educational implications of the Virginia study. *J Fam Pract* 3:1, 1976.

3. Marsland DW, Wood M, Mayo F: Content of family practice. *J Fam Pract* 3:1, 1976.

4. Diamond S: The masks of depression. *Clin Med* 72:1629, 1965.

5. The Great Pretender. *Emerg Med* 3:21–27, August 1971.

6. Diamond S, Dalessio DJ: *The Practicing Physician's Approach to Headache,* ed 2. Baltimore, Williams & Wilkins, 1978.

7. Avant RF: Diagnosis and management of depression in the office setting. *Proceedings of the Symposium Update on Antidepressants: Pharmacology and Clinical Uses. Fam Pract Recert* 5 (suppl)(1):41–48, 1983.

8. Diamond S: Depressive headaches. *Headache* 4(3):255–259, 1964.

9. Shraberg D: The myth of pseudodementia. *Am J Psychiatry* 135:601–603, 1978.

10. Wells CE: Pseudodementia. Am J Psychiatry 136:895–905, 1979.

11. Dubovsky S: Psychiatric problems in primary practice. In *Psychiatric Problems in Neurological Practice,* no. 5. Philadelphia, Roche Products, 1982.

12. Wells CE: *Dementia.* Philadelphia, F.A. Davis, 1971.

13. Shraberg D: An overview of neuropsychiatric disturbances in the elderly. *J Am Geriatr Soc* 28:422–425, 1980.

14. Dubovsky SL, Weissberg MP: *Clinical Psychiatry in Primary Care* ed 2. Baltimore, Williams & Wilkins, 1982.

15. Post F: Dementia, depression and pseudodementia. In Benson DF, Blumer D (eds): *Psychiatric Aspects of Neurologic Disease.* New York, Grune & Stratton, 1975, pp 99–120.

16. Pohl R: Therapy and management of the anxious/depressed patient. Proceedings of the Symposium Update on Antidepressants: Pharmacology and Clinical Uses. *Fam Pract Recertif* 5(suppl)(1):53, 1983.

17. Maas J: The biology of depression: where we stand. *Psychiatry,* 1973.

18. Diamond, S: Depression and headache. *Headache* 23:122–126, 1983.

19. Messing RB, Phebus L, et al: Analgesic effect of fluoxetine HCl (Lilly 110140), a specific uptake inhibitor for serotonergic neurons. *Psychopharmacol Commun* 1:511–521, 1975.

20. Messing RB, Lytle LD: Serotonin-containing neurons; their possible role in pain and analgesia. *Pain* 4:1–21, 1977.

21. Saarnivaara L, Mattila MJ: Comparison of tricyclic antidepressants in rabbits: Antinociception and potentiation of the noradrenalin pressor responses. Psychopharmacologia 35:221–236, 1974.

22. Malseed RT, Goldstein FJ: Enhancement of morphine analgesia by tricyclic antidepressants. Neuropharmacology 18:827–829, 1979.

23. Feighner JP: Pharmacological management of depression. *Fam Pract Recertif* 4(suppl) (1):13–24, 1982.

24. Fawcett J: Depression at the biochemical level. Psychiatr Ann 109 (suppl):362–368, 1980.

25. Fields HL: Pain. II. New approaches to management. Ann Neurol 9:101–106, 1981.

26. Basbaum AI, Fields HL: Endogenous pain control mechanisms: review and hypothesis. Ann Neurol 4:451–462, 1978.

27. Fields HL, Basbaum AI: Brainstem control of spinal pain transmission neurons. Annu Rev Physiol 40:193–221, 1978.

28. Mayer DJ, Price DD: Central nervous system mechanisms of analgesia. Pain 2:379–404, 1976.

29. Snyder SH, Childers SR: Opiate receptors and opioid peptides. Annu Rev Neurosci 2:35–64, 1979.

30. Maas J: Biogenic amines and depression. Arch Gen Psychiatry 32:1357–1361, 1975.

31. Cobbin D, et al: Urinary MHPG levels and tricyclic antidepressant drug selection. Arch Gen Psychiatry 36:1111–1115, 1979.

32. Blackwell B: MHPG in depression. *Psychiatr Opinion,* July-August, 1979.

33. Schatzberg AF, et al: Toward a biochemical classification of depressive disorders. III: Pretreatment urinary MHPG levels as predictors of response to treatment with maprotiline. Psychopharmacology 75:34–38, 1981.

34. Schatzberg AF, et al: Toward a biochemical classification of depressive disorders. IV. Pretreatment urinary MHPG levels as predictors of antidepressant response to imipramine. *Commun Psychopharmacol* 4:441–445, 1980.

35. Maas JW, et al: Pretreatment neurotransmitter metabolites and response to imipramine or amitriptyline treatment. *Psychol Med* 12:37–43, 1982.

36. Schatzberg AF, et al: Toward a biochemical classification of depressive disorders. V. Heterogeneity of unipolar depressions. Am J Psychiatry 139:471–475, 1982.

37. Richelson E: Tricyclic antidepressants: Interactions with histamine and muscarinic acetylcholine receptors. In Enna SJ, Malick JB, Richelson E (eds): *Antidepressants: Neurochemical, Behavioral and Clinical Perspectives.* New York, Raven Press, 1981.

38. Schatzberg AF, Cole JO: Basic pharmacology and clinical effects of antidepressants. Proceedings of the Symposium Update on Antidepressants: Pharmacology and Clinical Uses. *Fam Pract Recertif* 5(suppl)(1):11, 1983.

39. Carroll BJ, et al: A specific laboratory test for the diagnosis of melancholia. Arch Gen Psychiatry 38:15–22, 1981.

40. Brown W: The dexamethasone suppression test: Clinical application. Psychosomatics 22:951–955, 1981.

41. Gold M, et al: Diagnosis of depression in the 1980's. JAMA 245:1562–1564, 1981.

42. Ayd Jr, FJ: Amitriptyline (Elavil) therapy for depressive reactions. *Psychosomatics,* November-December, 1980.

43. Diamond S, Baltes B: The office treatment of mixed anxiety and depression with combination therapy. *Psychosomatics* 10:360–365, 1969.

44. Diamond S: Use of amitriptyline hydrochloride in general practice. ILL Med J 123:347–348, 1963.

45. Diamond S: Double-bind controlled study of amitriptyline-perphenazine combination in medical office patients with depression and anxiety. Psychosomatics 7:371–375, 1966.

46. Ayd Jr, FJ: Recognizing and treating depressed patients. Mod Med 39(24):80–86, 1971.

47. Diamond S. (consultant): Nine experts review a FP's depression regimen. Patient Care 11:42–77, 1977.

48. Robinson DS, et al: The monoamine oxidase inhibitor, phenelzine, in the treatment of depressive-anxiety states. A controlled clinical trial. *Arch Gen Psychiatry* 29:407–413, 1973.

49. Ravaris C, et al: Phenelzine and amitriptyline in the treatment of depression. A comparison of present and past studies. Arch Gen Psychiatry 37:1075–1080, 1980.

50. Schuckit M, et al: Tricyclic antidepressants and monoamine oxidase inhibitors. Arch Gen Psychiatry 24:509–514, 1971.

51. Pare CMB, Hallstrom C, Kline N, Cooper TB: Amitriptyline will prevent the "cheese" reaction of monoamine oxidase inhibitors? Lancet 2(8291):183–186, 1982.

52. Taub A: Relief of post-herpetic neuralgia with psychotropic drugs. J Neurosurg 39:235–239, 1973.

53. Loque J, Sachais B, Feigner J: Comparisons of maprotiline with imipramine in severe depression: a multicenter controlled trial. J Clin Pharmacol 19:64–74, 1979.

54. Ayd F: Trazodone: A unique new broad-spectrum antidepressant. Int Drug Ther Newsletter 14:33–40, 1979.

55. Fabre L, McLendon D, Gainey A: Trazodone efficacy in depression: a double-blind comparison with imipramine and placebo in day-hospital type patients. Curr Ther Res 25:825–834, 1979.

56. Ban TA, Lehman HE, Amin M, et al: Comprehensive clinical studies with trazodone. Curr Ther Res 15(suppl):540–551, 1973.

57. Angoli A, Piccione M, Casachia M, et al: Trazodone vs desipramine: a double-blind study on the rapidity of the antidepressant effect. *Mod Probl Pharmacopsychiatry* 9:1974.

58. Kellams JJ, Klapper MH, Small JG: Trazodone, a new antidepressant: efficacy and safety in endogenous depression. J Clin Psychiatry 40:390–395, 1979.

59. Cole JO, Schatzberg AF, Sniffin C, et al: Trazodone in treatment-resistant depression: an open study. J Clin Psychopharmacol 6(suppl):49–54S, 1981.

60. Simon W: Symptoms and suicide. Psychiatr Q 43:327–339, January 1969.

61. Parnell P, Cooperstock R: Tranquilizers and mood elevators in the treatment of migraine: an analysis of the Migraine Foundation questionnaire. Headache 19:78–89, 1979.

62. Lance JW: *Mechanism and Management of Headache.* London, Butterworth, 1978.

63. Dalessio DJ: Some reflections on the etiologic role of depression in head pain. *Headache* 8:28–31, 1968.

64. Friedman AP: Muscle contraction headache. Am Fam Physician 20(5):109–113, 1979.

65. Lance JW, Curran DA: Treatment of chronic tension headache. Lancet 1:1236–1239, 1964.

66. Diamond S: Psychogenic headaches with mixed anxiety and depression. Ill Med J 147:268–269, 1975.

67. Diamond S, Baltes B: Chronic tension headache treated with amitriptyline, a double-blind study. Headache 11:110–116, 1971.

68. Diamond S: The psychiatric aspects of headache. In Cochrane AL: *Background to Migraine.* New York, Springer-Verlag, 1970.

69. Cox D, Thomas D: Relationships between headaches and depression. Headache 21:261–263, 1981.

70. Couch J, et al: Evaluation of the relationship between migraine headache and depression. Headache 15:41–50, 1975.

71. Couch J, Hassanein R: Amitriptyline in migraine prophylaxis. Arch Neurol 38:695–699, 1979.

72. Anthony M, Lance JW: Monoamine oxidase inhibition in the treatment of migraine. Arch Neurol 21:263–268, 1969.

CHAPTER TWENTY FIVE

Cyclical Migraine: Its Relationship to Depression and Its Treatment with Lithium

JOSE L. MEDINA, M.D.

Migraine is usually classified as classical or nonclassical, depending on whether focal neurological manifestations are present or absent during the attacks. This classification is important from a pathogenetic point of view, but it does not usually alter decisions about therapy.

A more practical classification uses the temporal pattern of migraine as its basis. In this manner migraine can be classified as menstrual migraine, a migraine that occurs around the menses; weekend migraine, a migraine that occurs on weekends; sporadic migraine, a migraine that happens once or twice a month; frequent migraine, which occurs weekly or almost weekly; and finally, cyclical migraine, which is the subject of this chapter. The importance of this temporal classification of migraine is that it allows one to use prophylactic therapy in a more considered manner. One should use daily prophylactic medication in patients with frequent migraine and can use it in the other types of migraine during the headache-prone periods. One would normally not use prophylactic therapy in sporadic migraine.

Cyclical migraine (1, 2) is characterized by its occurrence in numerous episodes, each lasting for several weeks, separated by head-ache-free intervals, also of several weeks duration. I first became aware of this pattern in 1976, from observation within several weeks of each other of two patients who fit this pattern (3). One of them reported unusual mood changes a few days before the group of migraines started. In reviewing the literature, it was noted that Sacks (4) had described a 55-year-old patient with 5- to 6-week bouts of common migraine every year. He did not mention any mood changes.

PATIENT CHARACTERISTICS

The author has kept records on 37 patients with cyclical migraine, 29 women and 9 men, with ages ranging from 22 to 55 (mean = 33.4). A family history of migraine was present in 22. The incidence of this type of headache is low.

CHARACTERISTICS OF THE HEADACHE

The headaches have all the characteristics typical of migraine. They usually shifted from one side of the head to the other during the same cycle, and did not waken any patients from sound sleep. The average duration of the headaches was 19 hours. Table 25.1 summarizes the characteristics of the headaches. From this description, it is apparent that these are ordinary migraine. What makes cyclical migraine unique is its occurrence in cycles.

HEADACHE CYCLE

Headaches characteristically occurred in groups separated by periods free, or relatively free, of headache. The length of the cycle varied to between 2 and 20 weeks (average, 5.8 weeks), while the cycle frequency ranged from 1 to 12 per year (mean = 4.5). During the cycles, patients had between one and seven headaches per week (mean = 3). A frequent symptom was a constant, low-intensity, unilateral or bilateral headache between attacks. This occurred in 17 patients.

Fifteen patients noted that their headache cycles occurred during specific seasons. In six, headache groups tended to occur during the spring or fall; in four, during spring and summer; in one, during fall; and in four, during the winter.

Three women patients observed that the beginning of their cycles often coincided with menstrual periods. However, many menstrual periods were not followed by headaches.

DEPRESSION

During the cycles, 29 patients complained of depression; in six, the affective changes occurred 2–3 days before each cycle of headaches started. These patients usually described a lack of energy, fatigue, irritability, poor concentration, memory loss, anorexia, loss of interest in hobbies, decreased libido, constipation, and insomnia. Many of these

TABLE 25.1.
CHARACTERISTICS OF THE HEADACHES

	NO. OF PATIENTS		NO. OF PATIENTS
Location		*Aura Manifestations*	
Unilateral	23	Scintillating scotoma	11
Bilateral	14	Hemiparesthesias	5
Quality		Visual distortions	1
Throbbing	26	Word-finding difficulties	1
Pressure-like	6	Vertigo	3
Sharp	4	Metallic taste	1
Burning	1	*Associated Symptoms*	
Intensity		Nausea	31
Severe	31	Photophobia	23
Moderate	3	Audiosensitivity	19
Area Affected		Vomiting	15
Frontal	33	Congested nose	3
Temporal	22	Tearing	2
Occipital	14	Dysarthria	2
Parietal	10	Drowsiness	1
Face	3	Horner's syndrome	1
Neck	2	Diarrhea	1
Type of Migraine		Paleness	1
Nonclassical	20		
Classical	17		

symptoms are those seen in primary depression.

In 10 patients, a more detailed account of psychiatric symptoms which accompanied headache cycles was obtained. Nine of these ten showed significant pessimism about the future. They all complained of sadness, and nine felt like weeping, all of the time, for no apparent reason. Four patients believed that they let other people down. Four patients wished to die, but did not attempt suicide. All of them observed that making decisions during this period was unusually difficult. Seven stopped practicing their hobbies during the time they had headaches. The frequency of sexual intercourse was decreased in six patients. All of the 10 patients felt irritable, tense, and touchy. Five patients reported particular difficulty remembering things because of poor ability to concentrate. Seven described a very low energy level and continuous feelings of fatigue. Six patients complained of lack of self-confidence and poor self-esteem. Insomnia was present in six patients, constipation in three, and anorexia in two.

Some of these patients expressed their feelings during these periods well: "During the headache periods, I am fatigued; I do not feel like myself; and I feel crummy." Another patient gave the following account: "It seems that everything is against me, and I feel like quitting my job." Another reported: "During my sick weeks, I feel like I will fail at everything I do." One patient, who is a very efficient secretary, described unusual symptoms during her cycles: she would constantly reverse numbers and letters. This occurred both during and in between the headache attacks. Her boss would be amazed at those phenomena when she would hand him messages so he could return the day's calls, and she was almost fired for that reason. After the cycles were controlled, her spatial orientation returned to normal.

During remission periods, patients had few or no headaches. Twenty patients were completely free of headaches, while 17 complained of occasional minor ones. These minor headaches were once or twice a month,

were mild in intensity, and short in duration. During the period of headache relief, the patients also noted a disappearance of their depression, and return of their moods to a normal level. Only four patients felt full of energy and overly confident. One stated: "I feel I will succeed in everything I do, and nothing can interfere with my success." Another one said, "During the good periods, I am my old self and full of energy."

One of the most intriguing questions raised by these observations is what makes migraine become cyclic. As yet, there is no answer. About half the patients have had the same characteristic pattern since their migraines began, and the other half have had sporadic migraines for a few years before the cyclic migraine started.

DIFFERENTIAL DIAGNOSIS

The diagnosis of cyclic migraine should be based on the following criteria: (a) the presence of classic or nonclassic migraine; (b) the headaches' occurrence in cycles lasting at least 2 weeks; (c) multiple, clearly separated attacks of migraine during the cycle; and (d) evidence of previous cycles of headache interspersed with intervals free or relatively free of headaches.

Several conditions can be mistaken for cyclic migraine. One of them is periodic cluster headache, which bears many similarities to cyclic migraine. However, there are also many differences (5): (a) Cluster headaches are more often seen in males, cyclic migraine more often in females. (b) Cyclic migraine is long-lasting, with a duration of 6 hours to 2 days; cluster headache usually last less than 2 hours. (c) Cluster headache is invariably unilateral and does not shift from side to side during the same cycle; cyclic migraine can be either bilateral or unilateral, and shifts from side to side during the same cycle. (d) Cyclic migraine is often preceded by a scintillating scotoma or other focal neurologic aura; cluster headache, as a rule, is not associated with an aura.

Cluster headache variant differs from cyclic migraine because of the presence of continuous headaches with frequent, short-duration, localized headaches that occur many times per day, and also because the former has frequent jabs of pain. No cyclic depression has been noted during cluster headache variant.

One type of prolonged migraine presents with very infrequent attacks, 3–6 per year, but each attack is a continuous headache which lasts about a week or two. This headache differs from cyclic migraine because of its continuous nature; these patients do not have a pattern of clearly separated migraine attacks.

Cyclic migraine should also be differentiated from ergotamine headaches (6). Ergotamine headaches are frequent, daily, or almost daily, throbbing, predominantly unilateral headaches that respond quickly to ergotamine. A rebound headache occurs again several hours later or within the next couple of days. The patient takes ergotamine very frequently, usually exceeding the recommended weekly allowance. In many instances, this excess results in signs of ergotism: decreased peripheral pulses, coldness of the limbs, and trophic changes in the skin. In ergotamine headaches, there are no cycles to the headaches.

Finally, other periodic headaches may occur in subclinical manic-depressive illness (7). These are usually mild, dull, generalized headaches which resemble muscle contraction headaches more than migraine. Nevertheless, both this type of headache and cyclical migraine respond to lithium carbonate.

TREATMENT

Attacks of cyclic migraine respond, as does any migraine attack, to ergotamine tartrate. However, this drug is a bad choice for cyclic migraine, because attacks are frequent and the patient will therefore tend to take the drug more than twice a week. Since some metabolites of ergotamine have a half-life of 35 hours

(8), it will tend to accumulate, provoking ergotamine headaches, and compounding the problem. Symptomatic treatment with a combination of analgesic and antiemetic medications may be sufficient. The best treatment is prevention of the headache.

The drug that most consistently controls cyclic migraine is lithium carbonate. As a rule, the patient needs 300 mg or less of lithium carbonate t.i.d. One does not need to reach high blood levels to achieve remission of headaches. Twenty-five of the 28 cyclic migraine patients, treated with an average dose of 900 mg per day of lithium carbonate, improved. Nine had complete remission; seven had a 75% reduction in the length of headaches; and nine patients had a 50–75% reduction in headache duration. Side effects were mild because the lithium blood levels were kept low (mean blood level was 0.5 mEq/liter). In only one patient did we need to stop medication due to side effects (personality changes).

As can be seen, lithium carbonate is very effective in this disorder. It usually controls cyclic migraine within the 1st or 2nd week of treatment. Nevertheless, it should be administered with proper care. Therapy, once initiated, should be continued for at least 1 month beyond the anticipated duration of the cycle, because the headaches may otherwise return. This was the case in two patients who stopped the drug prematurely. Unfortunately, some patients have such frequent cycles, or cycles of such long duration, with such short headache-free periods, that they may need continuous lithium treatment.

The amount of lithium required by patients with cyclical migraine is less than that needed to control manic-depressive illness. In the last 10 patients seen with cyclic migraine, the author never used more than 600 mg of lithium per day, and still had excellent results. This effectiveness was summarized by a patient: "I do not get headaches during these weeks as long as I do not forget to take my lithium pills."

However, the decision to administer lithium carbonate on a maintenance basis for many months should not be taken lightly, because of the danger of kidney disease (9). Therefore, in these instances other remedies can be tried. Unfortunately, alternative medications are generally less effective than lithium. For example, in a study I conducted, only one of six patients showed a mild response to propranolol. Four of nine patients responded, to some degree, to tricyclic antidepressants. One patient responded to Sansert, but preferred lithium. Two patients responded to Naproxen. Nevertheless, Naproxen, tricyclic antidepressants, or β-blockers should be tried before administering lithium carbonate on a maintenance basis for long periods. If use of lithium carbonate is necessary on a continuous basis, the author recommends using it for no longer than a year. It should be noted, though, that regular usage of maintenance lithium is standard practice in psychiatry for patients with manic-depressive disease. Usually, after the first 2 months, patients can titrate their own dosage, and many only need 300 mg of lithium carbonate daily or every other day. This small amount may be enough to keep headaches under control. Periodic determination of lithium blood levels should be done in all patients.

In conclusion, here is a disorder in which headaches follow a cyclical and fairly predictable pattern, are accompanied in almost all cases by an affective disturbance—depression—and respond to the medication developed as the primary treatment for manic-depressive illness worldwide. This raises most intriguing questions about the relationship of this disorder to manic-depressive disease.

REFERENCES

1. Medina JL, Diamond S: Cyclical migraine. *Arch Neurol* 38:343–344, 1981.
2. Medina JL: Cyclic migraine: a disorder responsive to lithium carbonate. *Psychosomatics* 23:625–637, 1982.
3. Medina JL, Diamond S: The clinical link between migraine and cluster headache. *Arch Neurol* 34:470–472, 1977.
4. Sacks UW: *Migraine: The Evaluation of a Common Disorder.* New York, University of California Press, 1970.
5. Ekbom K: The clinical comparison of cluster headache and migraine. *Acta Neurol Scand (Suppl)* 41:1–48, 1970.
6. Anderson PG: Ergotamine headache. *Headache* 15:118–121, 1975.
7. Freedman A, Kaplan H, Sadock BJ: *Comprehensive Textbook of Psychiatry.* Baltimore, Williams & Wilkins, 1967, pp 676–705.
8. Meier J, Schreier E: Human plasma levels of some antimigraine drugs. *Headache* 16:96–104, 1976.
9. Neu G, Manschreck TC, Flores JM: Renal damage with long-term use of lithium carbonate. *J Clin Psychiatry* 40:460–463, 1979

Medication Compliance among Headache Patients[1]

CHAPTER TWENTY SIX

RUSSELL C. PACKARD, M.D.
PATRICK O'CONNELL, M.D.

Medication is a major, often primary treatment modality used in the management of headache. However, even the most thorough and well-designed therapeutic regimen with appropriate medication will fail without patient compliance. It is difficult to identify patients who do not take their medications as prescribed, but it has been generally noted that 30–50% of patients make some error with their medication (1) or neglect their treatment (2).

Within recent years, noncompliance or the inability to stay in treatment or adhere to a treatment regimen has been recognized as a major health care problem. Noncompliance rates as high as 90% have been reported for various medical treatments (3). This chapter will review a recent study conducted by the authors to evaluate medication compliance among headache patients, and also explores some of the psychodynamic and personality factors involved in compliance.

EVALUATING COMPLIANCE

During 1985, 100 consecutive new outpatients presenting to our headache clinic were interviewed extensively in regard to their use of prescribed medication. Only patients who

had seen at least one previous physician and received at least one previous prescription were included. Age, sex, educational level, and headache diagnosis were also determined. Patients were reevaluated over a 3-month period for compliance, noncompliance, or any change in their medicine usage.

The interview was obviously critically important to obtaining this information. Some information, however, was obtained by a headache history form used routinely in the clinic, which has a list of 40 commonly used headache analgesics and prophylactic medications for patients to identify as to their previous/present use and effectiveness. History was then specifically obtained as to whether they were still taking medication, how they were taking it, dosage, timing, whether it was helpful or not, and any side effects or problems they were having. Patients were also asked if they ever forgot to take their medicine, missed doses, took extra doses, or used any other medicine.

There are no generally accepted standards of criteria for establishing abuse or

---

[1]Data from this chapter were presented in part at the Annual Meeting of the American Association for the Study of Headache in Chicago, June, 1986.

overuse of medication. Criteria offered by Diamond and Dalessio (4) were followed in part in determining medication overuse, such as daily use of analgesics or the ingestion of more than 100 simple analgesic tablets per month; recurring use of 10 mg or more of ergotamine tartrate or its derivatives per week; use everyday or every other day of ergotamine tartrate; daily or almost daily use of compounds containing barbiturates, other sedatives, or tranquilizing substances. The patients were often queried as to whether they carried medications with them, whether they placed them in strategic locations around the house, office, or car, or whether they were taken ritualistically, that is, at the time of awakening, retiring, or at certain other times of the day.

Patients were followed in the study for at least 3 months after their initial presentation. Those requiring continued medication were carefully instructed in the importance of proper use, specific goals of medication treatment, expected or delayed actions, and common side effects, and were instructed to call or return if they experienced untoward side effects. Explanations were also given as to basic mechanisms of the medication, such as relieving scalp muscle contraction or stabilizing blood vessels, etc.

Fifty-two patients were initially determined to be noncompliant with prescribed medication while 48 were compliant. The age range of compliant patients was 19–71 (average age 35). Noncompliant patients' ages ranged from 16 to 61 with an average of 34. Although 81 of the 100 patients presenting were female, the ratios of males and females for compliance or noncompliance were almost identical. Forty-two patients were referred by physicians, and 58 came self-referred. No significant difference was noted between compliance and noncompliance from these two groups. Educational levels attained by both compliant and noncompliant patients similarly showed little difference.

Headache diagnoses of compliant and noncompliant patients are shown in Table 26.1. The most frequent presenting headache type in general was the vascular headache type with 41% of the entire group. Mixed headache syndrome accounted for 25%, and posttraumatic headaches of various types accounted for 20%. Headache diagnosis did not differentiate compliant or noncompliant patients.

Some headache types were combined together somewhat loosely, i.e., the rare or occasional benign exertional vascular headache or "atypical" vascular headache were included under the category of vascular headache for the purposes of this study because there was no statistical change or difference by separating them out. Similarly, deriving different diagnostic subgroups of posttraumatic headaches did not alter the findings. Cluster and chronic paroxysmal nocturnal hemicrania (CPNH) were combined, but

TABLE 26.1.
HEADACHE DIAGNOSTIC CATEGORIES

NONCOMPLIANT (*N* = 52)		COMPLIANT (*N* = 48)	
Vascular	21	Vascular	20
Mixed	14	Mixed	11
Posttraumatic	10	Posttraumatic	10
Mixed	7	Mixed	7
Vascular	2	Vascular	1
Muscular	1	Muscular	2
Muscle contraction	4	Muscle contraction	3
Cluster/CPNH	2	Cluster/CPNH	3
Occipital neuralgia	1	Occipital neuralgia	1
	52		48

only one case of CPNH was identified, and the patient was compliant.

Reasons for noncompliance varied widely and are listed in Table 26.2. A number of patients (31) had more than one reason or complaint accounting for noncompliance that could not clearly be differentiated into one main reason, i.e., "I stopped taking the medicine because it wasn't working and the side effects bothered me," or "I guess I took more than I was supposed to take and I also took it with anything over the counter that I could find." When these situations occurred, both reasons were recorded. The most frequent problems noted were combining prescribed medication with other medicine (prescribed or over the counter), taking more or less than the prescribed amounts of daily prophylactic medication (with occasional patients using prophylactic medications on a prn basis). Analgesic overuse or abuse occurred frequently, as did stopping medication on their own because of side effects or several other factors, as noted in the table listing.

Several patients delayed taking medication at the first sign of headache until the headache was bad or because they were afraid to take it for fear of sleepiness on the job or because they were mothers caring for young children. A few patients looked up medication in *Physicians Desk Reference* and stopped taking them for fear of side effects or misunderstanding, i.e., "Why was I getting an antidepressant for migraine?" A number of patients filled their prescription, but never took it or had received a prescription and never filled it at all.

On follow-up over a 3-month period, all patients requiring medication were given careful instructions (oral and/or written) and explanations for proper medication use. Of the initial 52 noncompliant patients, 24 (46%) took medication as prescribed. Twenty-four continued to be noncompliant, and four were lost to follow-up. Although almost half of the noncompliant patients became compliant, almost half continued to be noncompliant (see Table 26.3). Of the initial 48 compliant pa-

TABLE 26.2.
REASONS FOR NONCOMPLIANCE

NO. OF PATIENTS	REASONS
12	Combined medication (prescription or nonprescription)
11	Overuse/abuse of analgesics (including nonprescription)
10	Took less than prescribed dose of prophylactic medications (missed doses regularly, "forgot" to take, or used prn)
8	Took more than prescribed dose of prophylactic medications
8	Delayed taking until headache was bad (6) or they were afraid (2)
7	Stopped taking—side effects
7	Stopped taking—not working
6	Stopped taking—ran out
3	Stopped taking—cost
3	Stopped—looked it up, spouse threw away, pharmacist said "dangerous."
3	Filled prescription; never took—looked it up, feared addiction, couldn't read.
3	Never filled prescription—didn't like medications
2	Borrowed medications from others on regular basis
2	Didn't know what they were taking (not taking "right").

TABLE 26.3.
FOLLOW-UP EVALUATIONS

NO. OF NONCOMPLIANT PATIENTS: (52)		NO. OF COMPLIANT PATIENTS (48)	
24	Became compliant	30	Remained compliant
24	Continued noncompliant	6	No follow-up necessary
4	Lost to follow-up	5	Long standing drug/ETOH Problems
		5	Became noncompliant
		2	Lost to follow-up

tients, 6 did not require follow-up, 2 were lost to follow-up, 30 remained compliant, and 20 were discovered to be noncompliant. Five of these patients had clearly been noncompliant at the time of the initial interview, but had falsified or minimized their background use of medication and/or alcohol. Three were medication abusers, and two were suffering from significant alcoholism or using alcohol for pain relief. Ironically, one alcoholic patient refused prescribed medication because of fear of addiction. Only one of these patients was successfully rehabilitated.

DISCUSSION

In the third edition of *The Diagnostic and Statistical Manual of the American Psychiatric Association,* noncompliance with medical treatment refers to behavior judged unrelated to a mental disorder, such as concern that treatment may be worse than the illness itself (5). This description may be oversimplified and may not apply well to situations in which noncompliance may be emotionally motivated due to denial of illness, or to patients who continually manage their medical conditions inconsistently and/or even destructively. Although the present study did not specifically address psychodynamic or personality factors in noncompliance, a recent study has noted that some patients who consistently and/or deliberately refuse to follow medical advice often meet criteria for a borderline personality disorder (6).

The present study points out the impor-

tance of obtaining an accurate detailed history in regard to medication usage. Although identifying patients who do not take their medication as prescribed has been described as difficult (1, 2), it was rather surprising how detailed attention to drug-taking history elicited remarkably honest and candid information from patients. Specific questions helpful in obtaining this information have been presented previously. Also, asking about seldom-reported side effects, such as weight gain, sexual function, or constipation, will often lead to shy confessions of difficulty. If this area of treatment is not thoroughly evaluated, important medication information may be simply passed off or missed entirely. This could lead to appropriate medications being eliminated from future consideration, continued unexplained treatment failures, or poor results.

Obtaining an accurate history of drug overuse or abuse has been reported as especially difficult (7). This was an area of concern in our study because 5% of the patients did have drug or alcohol abuse problems that were initially well concealed or denied. Patients who were overusing medication in general were more vague about medication use and reluctant to give exact amounts consumed. Another major headache clinic reported that at least one-half of patients seeking help for headaches indulge in overuse of medication to relieve their distress (8). Some of these patients are reluctant or ashamed to discuss their reliance on drugs. Others may be frightened that their medication will be taken away if they admit to the extent of their use. Some believe, naively, that only prescribed medication need be reported and may restrain from reporting or discussing their use of over-the-counter analgesics (9). Over-the-counter analgesic history must be specifically asked about, especially since these medications are frequently combined with other prescribed medicine and some may contain similar ingredients, such as aspirin, acetaminophen, or antiinflammatories.

Unfortunately, no single factor proves generally useful as a predictor of compliance, given the complexity and variety of individual defenses and coping styles. Age, sex, educational level, and headache diagnosis generally do not predict compliance. Even patients who continually keep their clinic appointments are not necessarily compliant (10). Some patients may respond positively to details about their treatment, whereas others shun them; some patients respond to scares with increased denial, whereas others are well served by confrontation. Among the many factors associated with poor compliance are failure to understand the purpose of medication or treatment, problems in relating to authorities, and complacency (10).

Forgetfulness is a frequently cited reason for noncompliance, but it is really not an explanation. It may be a rationalization to cover unconscious or partly conscious concerns about the patient's health status, his diagnosis, or various concerns about medicine. There may be unspoken fears of adverse side effects, addiction, or loss of independence. The use of a daily prophylactic medication may not be understood or appreciated when the patient goes through a headache-free period or when a headache develops while taking a medication supposedly given to prevent it. Many patients have magical expectations that medication will completely get rid of their headache, or cure them. It is not unusual for patients' expectations to differ considerably from physicians' (11). Well-intentioned friends and relatives may also infuence or undermine adherence to a treatment regimen. Complex dosing regimens, unpleasant side effects, and poor communication, explanations, or directions from the physician or his

office staff may also reduce compliance (17).

Rather than asking how a patient's noncompliance can be overridden, it makes more sense for the clinician to inquire how noncompliance can be prevented in the first place, and how it can be managed clinically once it has occurred (13). It is first of all important to realize that a patient may become noncompliant for valid and important reasons. Some side effects may truly be undesirable or even dangerous. Patients should be enlisted as participants in their treatment and encouraged to report problems so that appropriate adjustments and changes can be made.

Useful recommendations to assist compliance among headache patients include: establishing a doctor-patient relationship with a sense of working together on the compliance problem; providing sufficient time for questions and explanations at office visits; offering a clear and understandable treatment plan; clarifying expectations and goals of treatment; explaining any delay in onset of action of some drugs (antidepressants); adapting dosages to patient routines; enlisting the aid of family members; discussing common side effects in advance; and monitoring compliance and offering assistance to those patients who have problems. Even a patient's noncompliance can be useful for determining underlying psychodynamic factors involved in the treatment process, such as possible primary gain a headache may represent by defending against underlying anger or depression or secondary gain of continued attention from one's physician and/or family. These psychodynamic factors and the role of personality traits in compliance will now be explored in further detail.

PERSONALITY TRAITS AND PSYCHODYNAMIC ISSUES IN PRESCRIBING PRACTICES

In *Being and Time,* Heidegger (14) states that the nature of human existence is "being-with"—being with the people and things of one's world. As Stone described in *The Internal World of the Infant* (15), this is apparent almost from the first moments if not days of existence, as evidenced by the infant's intense interest in his surroundings and especially in his caretakers. For Stone, autism is not an intrinsic feature of human existence, certainly not the first phase as some theorists would have it. One is from the very start exploring relationships and affectively reacting to them. Inherent, however, in being with others is the frightful risk of losing one's sense of self in theirs, of falling prey to their way of conceiving reality—not to mention the risk of actually falling prey to them physically (11). This conflict between the wish for freedom and the need to control and defend oneself in the world is thus one cardinal feature, among several others, of human existence. By the time a patient arrives at the physician's office, his personal modes or mechanisms of control and defense are automatic and unconscious. Varying portions of his existence are already compromised, having been unsurped or distorted by important figures in his life. These are also the seeds of transference and countertransference, the perceptions of others and ways of relating to them that are colored by prior experience.

Thus, when a patient decides to come to a physician for treatment, a relationship commences the moment he arrives at that decision, that is, even before he actually sees the physician. It is a function of past experience and future anticipation, conscious and unconscious factors. When the relationships begins in fact, it is therefore not only immediate and "real," but also reflects the patient's degree of comfort with his dependent needs, his need to retain control, his prior experience with physicians and medications, and inculcated and acquired cultural expectations.

Consciously, the relationship develops in the context of a balance of comfort with dependent needs and the desire to retain control—for both physician and patient. Unconsciously, needs out of awareness and the defenses to keep them that way color—or sometimes dominate—the relationship.

Traditionally, medicine has sanctioned a dominant, giving role for the physician and a passive, receptive one for the patient. Things go relatively smoothly and predictably when physician and patient fit these stereotypical roles. The physician expects to be in control, and the patient expects to be "treated," to have hands laid on and to be given medication. (Perhaps some physicians even choose the profession because it meets such needs, just as there are patients who seem to be unduly comfortable with the patient role.) When this fails to occur, the patient senses that he has been shortchanged, and symptoms may remain little affected.

Over the past decade or two, however, this traditional orientation and power balance have been in flux. The entrance upon the medical scene of third party payers with their relatively sudden and aggressive assumption of dominance has begun to seriously complicate and erode traditional expectations. These factors, often ignored by both patients and physicians, may significantly influence and alter patient expectations and response to treatment and medication.

Generally speaking, however, physicians want our patients to take their medicines, and, barring prior mishap, they do too; unconsciously, however a patient's apparent willingness to cooperate may be compromised or even vitiated by unconscious needs and defenses. In our prescribing practices, therefore, it behooves us to take these unconscious needs and defenses into consideration—the patient's and ours (as much as we can be aware of ours).

The issues of cooperation and resistance between physician and patient can be viewed in terms of transference and countertransference, positive and negative.

Transference-based attitudes and feelings of the physician toward the patient, whether conscious or unconscious, are referred to as countertranference. They are a composite of past experiences with important persons in his life. When they are positive in character and tone, they are sometimes not only consistent with his role, but also conducive to it. If, however, the patient evokes negative attitudes and feelings, resistance in the patient is fostered, and treatment founders instead. Either way, it may result in reactions to medication which are inexplicable on strictly pharmacologic grounds.

When the same sort of misperception occurs in patients, it is referred to as transference. Negative transference must be detected and dealt with, either by open exploration and interpretation, or by coopting the patient's defenses.

Unconscious issues of cooperation between physician and patient can also be approached from another important vantage point: personality defenses. The various personality disorders: histrionic, compulsive, paranoid, passive-aggressive, etc., allow patients to preserve their dependence on others in different ways, which are often outside of awareness. These different defensive styles also have implications for the issue of medication compliance and the best ways to deal with its absence.

In prescribing for histrionic patients, for example, one should keep in mind that in part their defense is a matter of unconscious role playing of an exaggerated version of the culture's current definition of idealized femininity and masculinity. For a male patient, therefore, one might want to emphasize that the goal of medication is to restore his independence as soon as possible. For the histrionic female, the goal might be portrayed in terms of her concerns about appearance and feelings of femininity and desirability, that is, what the medication might do to restore her feeling of femininity and attractiveness. The histrionic patient may deal with unconscious sexual or aggressive conflicts and anxieties via the "sick role." As with the psychosomatic patient discussed briefly below, psychotherapy is best combined with medication.

One aspect of the compulsive defense is a matter of trying to please others by attempting to be "good," to be precise, to do things just right. "Rituals" are therefore most apt to engage the patient's energies.

The passive-aggressive patient, on the other hand, is stubborn and resistant in trying to preserve his autonomy. Instead of effectively preserving it, however, he is committed unconsciously to doing the opposite of what he is expected to do. The physician should therefore, not be authoritarian when giving him instructions about taking medications, and should leave as many of the details as are safely possible to the patient.

The psychosomatic patient can be expressing deeply hidden dependent conflicts via somatic pathology and, therefore, can be poorly responsive to medication. Psychotherapy may become a must.

The overtly dependent patient is bereft of the disguise of a formal "mechanism of defense" against these needs. The physician can all too easily indulge such a patient's dependence by casting the giving of medication as though it were a "gift." But care is needed to avoid inducing psychological dependence on the medication, such that it would be difficult to give up if this is later indicated.

The narcissistic patient has disavowed or disowned the unpleasant or negative aspects of his personality, and to make matters worse, has aggrandized what he considers idealized traits, and made them part of his ego ideal. Because he does not wish to see his defects, recognizing the need for him to take medication is sometimes particularly onerous. To complicate the issue, he may have an unconscious need to defeat the therapist, giving rise to a negative therapeutic reaction, or outcome. When this is the clinical situation, one might suggest, therefore, that the need for medication is only temporary—that the patient might manage without it, but that he would certainly feel and function much better with it. Even so, it will probably prove to be touch and go with the narcissist.

The paranoid patient projects the negative and aggressive aspects of his personality onto others, leaving him suspicious as well as grandiose and abrasive. It may be very difficult or impossible to overcome his fear of medication, or of being "poisoned." One might paradoxically emphasize both the healing aspects and the side effects of the medication prescribed. It is paramount to be scrupulously truthful with the paranoid patient, and to avoid being overly reassuring or informal.

We believe the avoidant patient will present little problem in accepting medication prescribed. Although very timorous and reticent, he is still eager to establish a relationship with someone who cares. Focusing on medication gives him a chance to develop a relationship with his physician at a pace that he can manage comfortably.

The schizoid patient is basically fearful of closeness—so much so that he has dissociated his lonely and dependent feelings. He is, therefore, prone to focus on medication to avoid the human aspects of and feelings inherent in a doctor/patient relationship. Unless the physician intrudes affectively, these patients are likely to be compliant about taking prescribed medications.

According to some theories, the antisocial or psychopathic patient has, from his earliest moments, never enjoyed a human relationship. It is an existential possibility that has long ago been either denied him or been sealed off by him because of the extreme danger that he feels it poses. He lives for himself alone, and for the pleasure of the moment, and will use or abuse medication as much for its euphoriant as for its ameliorative effects. His use of medication may bear little relationship to his real therapeutic need for it. The physician will have to carefully supervise the patient and ration out the medications and, preferably, terminate their use as soon as is clinically feasible. The patient may even sell his prescription rather than use it.

These are some of the many examples of using a knowledge of personality traits to shape one's prescribing practices.

It may be added that, in some patients, the medication may take on a symbolic meaning, e.g., representing the physician. Taking the medication is tantamount to incorporating the physician, identifying with him in a very special and intimate way. Simply carrying the medication or even just the unfilled prescription, on their person may be a way in

fantasy, albeit very dependent, of keeping the physician close by.

Reactions to medication and side effects also play their role in the transference and countertransference or unconscious relationship with the prescribing physician. If the reactions and/or the side effects are ameliorative, the physician's prestige will be enhanced; if negative, damaged. Correspondingly, the physician may see the patient as a "good" patient, or as a resistant one.

In prescribing medications the overall therapeutic goal must be kept in mind, and their use kept within that framework. The use of medications tends to focus therapy on reality rather than unconscious issues. It may well be that medication is especially important at the outset of therapy, when the patient is too anxious, depressed, or confused to explore issues for insight.

Particular mention should be made of the use of placebo. DeWald (16) cautions that placebo use has a relatively high potential for being discovered by the patient. The result is a disastrous undermining of trust precluding any further useful therapy with the same therapist and/or such danger of loss of face that the patient must then hang on to his symptoms for dear life. If placebos must be used, some authors suggest that they at least be pharmacologically active substances to avoid such outcomes.

Finally, some hazards inherent in drug therapy can be listed for the patient; these include: addiction, suicidal attempts or gestures, failure to follow instructions, taking too much or too little of medications prescribed, and excessive sedation with further weakening of any ego deficits. For the physician they may include: combatting side effects with additional medications that compound drug problems, the use of medication to avoid dealing with the patient's other more pressing therapeutic needs, or using medication unconsciously to keep the patient at a distance or avoid dealing with him as a person (16).

In summary, compliance and the overall results of pharmacotherapy depend upon a complex combination of desired physiological effects, side effects, and psychological factors involving both patient and physician, and unconscious cultural and transference/countertransference influences.

REFERENCES

1. Berkow R (ed): *The Merck Manual*, ed 14, vol 1, *General Medicine* 14th ed. Rahway, NJ, Merck, Sharp & Dohme laboratories. 1982,

2. Kaplan HI, Sadock BJ: *Comprehensive Textbook of Psychiatry*. ed 4. Baltimore. Williams & Wilkins, 1985.

3. Zisook S, Gammon E: Medical noncompliance. *Int J Psychiatry Med* 10:291–303, 1980–1981.

4. Diamond S, Dalessio DJ: *The Practicing Physicians Approach to Headache*, ed 3. Baltimore, Williams & Wilkins, 1982.

5. *Diagnostic and Statistical Manual of Mental Disorders*, ed 3. Washington D.C., American Psychiatric Association, 1980.

6. Boehnert CE, Popkin MK: Psychological issues in the treatment of severely noncompliant diabetics. *Psychosomatics* 27:11–20, 1986.

7. Murray TG, Goldberg M: Analgesic abuse and renal disease. *Annu Rev Med* 26:537–550, 1975.

8. Saper JR: Drug overuse among patients with headache. *Symposium on Headache. Neurologic Clin* 1:465–477, 1983.

9. Saper JR: *Headache Disorders: Current Concepts and Treatment Strategies*. Boston, Wright-PSG Publishers. 1983.

10. Pasnau RO: *Consultation—Liason Psychiatry*. New York, Grune & Stratton. 1975.

11. Packard RC: Emotional aspects of headache. *Symposium on Headache. Neurologic Clin* 1:445–456, 1983.

12. Bernstein JG (ed): Clinical aspects of refusal. In *Clinical Psychopharmacology*. ed 2. Boston, John Wright-PSG, 1984.

13. Appelbaum PS, Gutheil TG: Clinical aspects of treatment refusal. *Compr Psychiatry* 23:560–566. 1982.

14. Heidegger M: *Being and Time*, ed 7. New York, Harper & Row. 1962.

15. Stone DW: *Interpersonal World of the Infant*. New York, Basic Books, 1985.

16. DeWald PA: *Psychotherapy: A Dynamic Approach*, ed 2. New York, Basic Books, 1973.

CHAPTER TWENTY SEVEN

Drugs and Headache: Misuse and Dependency

NINAN T. MATHEW, M.D., F.R.C.P. (C)

Chronic headaches have to be viewed as a major public health problem. They result in loss of productivity, increased health care dependency, billions of dollars spent on ineffective and often harmful over-the-counter (and prescription) medications, habituation to medications, and secondary problems in family, social, and sexual life.

Chronic recurrent headache, like other chronic pain, can be associated with a number of psychological complications. Psychological factors which might bear on the management and prognosis of chronic recurrent headaches include depression, neuroticism, chronic "headache" behavior, drug dependency, and increased use of health care facilities (1).

Misuse, overuse, and dependency on medications, both prescription and nonprescription (over-the-counter), stem from many factors. These include:

1. Frequency and severity of the headaches
2. Associated depression, anxiety, and neuroticism
3. Associated chronic sick behavior
4. Iatrogenic rebound headache phenomenon from certain drugs, such as ergotamine and caffeine
5. Attempts to counteract drug-induced complications, such as sleeplessness, dizziness, nausea, and depression, etc.

In spite of the fact that scientific knowledge about the pharmacology of drugs used in the treatment of headache has increased over the last few decades, in clinical practice, a great many misconceptions about the relief of headache pain still persist, and most drugs are chosen empirically. The reasons for this discrepancy include the lack of an experimental model for headache, or, for that matter, for chronic pain, and the difficulty in conducting clinical studies using analgesics. The latter reason stems from difficulties in adjusting dosage level, difficulties in proper selection of patients and in choice of appropriate control groups, the difficulty in ruling out placebo effects, and the impossibility of objectively measuring headache intensity.

There are also many things which suggest that acute headache pain, such as that associated with migraine, is different from other forms of pain. Ergotamine, though usually effective in relieving the pain of a migraine headache, is totally ineffective in reducing other types of acute pain. Other pharmacologic agents, such as β-adrenergic blocking drugs, methysergide, and calcium channel-blocking drugs have prophylactic value in headache treatment, but are not particularly effective in other forms of chronic pain.

Before going into the details of the type of drug overuse and dependency seen in headache populations, certain terms should be defined in order to avoid confusion in the subsequent discussion. The World Health Organization has defined addiction as, "A behavioral pattern of overwhelming involvement with obtaining and using a drug." In this definition addiction is a form of "drug abuse," defined as the use of any drug in a manner that elicits social disapproval. Both addiction and drug abuse refer to voluntary behaviors, and are not to be confused with drug tolerance (decreased effectiveness of a given dose after repeated doses) and physical dependence (withdrawal symptoms when a drug is discontinued), which refer to pharmacological effects. A prescription medication that can be used "as needed" (prn) automatically implies that the patient has been provided with medical and social approval to use that drug. In fact, such patients are given permission to obtain drugs for pain whether they need analgesic protection or not. Ordering "prn" prescriptions for pain medication in emotionally unstable patients or in overtly neurotic patients can quickly lead to a conditioned pain and drug-seeking behavior pattern unrelated to actual nociception (2). Drug overuse is thereby afforded social legitimacy through the physician's "headache prescription."

The physician himself may be responsible for creating a dependency on medication or for encouraging misuse of medications. Certain physicians, based on their convictions and practice, deny patients adequate pain control by only ordering analgesics in insufficient dosages or by insisting upon unduly long intervals between dosages. This results in inadequate pain relief, and encourages the patient to seek other prescriptions or to use multiple drugs for pain relief. Physicians afraid of causing addiction to a particular drug sometimes choose to prescribe many different drugs for the same patient, each in less than optimal doses. In doing so, they may unknowingly actually put the patient on the road to multiple drug addiction, as cross-tolerance builds up.

Obtaining an accurate history of overuse is difficult. There are many reasons for this. Some patients are ashamed of their reliance on medications, and are therefore unwilling to divulge it. Others may be frightened that their medications will be taken away if they admit the extent of their use. Still others naively believe that only prescription medications need be reported, and therefore refrain from mentioning their use of over-the-counter analgesics unless these are specifically asked about.

There are no set standards for establishing the presence of medication abuse in headache patients. The author's own practice is to consider the following criteria, modified from Saper (3):

1. Daily analgesic ingestion, or use of more than 100 analgesic tablets per month.
2. Recurrent use of 8 mg or more of ergotamine tartrate or its derivatives per week.
3. Daily, or almost daily, use of compounds containing barbiturates, sedatives, or tranquilizing substances.
4. "Ritualistic" administration of analgesics (that is, upon awakening, retiring, or at other specified times of the day) in the hope of thereby averting headache attacks which have not yet begun.

In cases where a history of excessive medication use is suspected but cannot be obtained from the patient it may be necessary to obtain blood and urine samples to test for analgesic and tranquilizing compounds.

NONNARCOTIC ANALGESICS

The most commonly used nonnarcotic analgesics are aspirin and acetaminophen. Many over-the-counter analgesic preparations contain aspirin or acetaminophen along with caffeine and, occasionally, phenacetin. "Sinus headache" medications combine these agents with antihistamines and decongestants.

ASPIRIN

Aspirin and other salicylates have been shown to inhibit the synthesis of prostaglandins, which are involved in complex interreactions with various neurotransmitters within the still poorly understood pain-modulating system. Adverse reactions to aspirin are well known, and include gastrointestinal symptoms, gastric distress, change in prothrombin time and platelet aggregation, and symptoms of neurotoxicity such as tinnitus, dizziness, and confusion. The most dangerous factor about aspirin is its easy availability. Many chronic headache patients develop compulsive needs to take large quantities of aspirin, which then produce the various symptoms described above. Unknown to them, and often to their physicians, these patients develop symptoms of gastric distress or neurotoxicity, become frightened, and as a result increasingly behave in a fashion that reflects their feeling of being chronically sick.

The most commonly reported symptom from aspirin use is minor gastrointestinal upset, which is seen in 2–10% of patients taking aspirin occasionally. An estimated 30–50% of patients taking excessive aspirin (10 or more tablets a day) experience significant gastric upset (4). Aspirin may directly irritate the mucosal lining, or, through its inhibiting effects on prostaglandins, may result in a reduction of mucin and an increase in gastric acid secretion. Occult blood is present in the stool of most patients taking moderate to high dosages of aspirin, an effect clinically significant in women who regularly have abundant menstrual bleeding. It is estimated that 6–8 aspirin tablets a day will result in 2–4 ml of blood in the stool. Greater daily intake can cause 30 ml or more of blood loss per day. Over two-thirds of patients regularly overusing analgesics have reduced red blood cell production (5). Hemoglobin levels below 12 g, which rise to normal when aspirin intake is discontinued, is common in analgesic overusers, and suggests both blood loss and suppression of hematopoietic processes (6).

A number of other side effects and drug interactions need to be recognized. Use of large amounts of aspirin for long periods may result in transient, mild elevations of serum glutamic-oxaloacetic transaminase (SGOT) and serum glutamic-pyruvic transaminase (SGPT), particularly in children (7). Aspirin may aggravate preexisting liver disease, but does not generally cause liver damage in healthy adults. Interactions with other medications include enhancement of the effect of antihypoglycemics, interference with the action of uricosuric agents, inhibition of the effect of spironolactone, and precipitation of hemorrhage when combined with anticoagulant therapy. Corticosteroids reduce the level of plasma salicylate. Administration of aspirin in patients using nonsteroidal antiinflammatory agents will sometimes aggravate gastric irritation.

Occasionally, impairment of central nervous system function includes mild to moderate mental changes, such as depression. Salicylates may also produce nausea and vomiting as a result of stimulating medullary chemoreceptors. Mild respiratory alkalosis may be present at therapeutic doses, and endocrinological disturbances, including effects on secretion of adrenal steroids, have been reported (8).

Hypersensitivity reactions to aspirin have to be kept in mind as well. These include erythematous skin reactions and severe asthmatic attacks. A patient who is sensitive to aspirin may also be more likely to react with hypersensitivity to nonsteroidal antiinflammatory agents and related substances (4).

CAFFEINE

Even though caffeine is known to potentiate the analgesic effects of many analgesics and also, by increasing gastric absorption, to potentiate the effect of ergotamine, excessive use of caffeine-containing over-the-counter medications can lead to various side effects which adversely affect the prognosis of chronic headache patients.

Caffeine is a powerful stimulant. It raises the heart rate and enhances the force of cardiac and skeletal muscle contractions. Caffeine increases gastric secretion, causes diuresis, relaxes smooth muscles (particularly in the bronchi), and affects the basal metabolic rate (9–11). As a powerful CNS stimulant, caffeine may enhance intellectual effort, but it is likely to impair recently acquired motor skills involving delicate muscular coordination. Furthermore, the stimulant effects of caffeine may be followed by depression. The amount of caffeine ingested by the general population is rather high due to significant coffee, tea, and soft drink consumption (Table 27.1). Many nonprescription as well as prescription medications contain caffeine. Untoward reactions may occur following ingestion of approximately 1 g of caffeine per day. Typically, patients taking large daily amounts of caffeine do not experience toxic symptoms for years. For most adults, 300–500 mg of caffeine per day represents an excessive load. Tolerance develops, however, and chronic use of up to 900 mg (approximately equal to nine cups of coffee per day) is common. Levels in the blood peak 30–45 minutes after oral ingestion of caffeine (12).

The symptoms of caffeinism may be divided into three categories:

1. Mood disturbances
2. Sleep disturbances
3. Effects of withdrawal

Mood disturbances associated with caffeinism include anxiety, jitteriness, tremulousness, agitation, irritability, muscle twitching, lightheadedness, palpitations, and gastrointestinal distress. Greden has reported several patients, initially diagnosed as suffering from anxiety neurosis, who were instead experiencing caffeine intoxication (9–11).

Sleep disturbances include delayed sleep onset and frequent nighttime awakening. Caffeine counteracts the hypnotic influence of barbiturates, leading to increased need for and dependence upon sedative medications if these are being used.

Caffeine withdrawal symptoms include headache, grogginess, malaise, drowsiness, lethargy, rhinorrhea, yawning, irritability, depression, and even nausea (12). Headache associated with caffeine can be consequent to either toxicity (too much) or to withdrawal (too little). Caffeine withdrawal headache occurs about 8 to 16 hours following abstinence from chronic overindulgence. It is characterized as a generalized throbbing discomfort, usually occurring in the morning upon awakening, and promptly relieved by more caffeine. It is not uncommon for patients to take excessive caffeine-containing analgesics during the day and wake up around 4:00 or 5:00 AM with excruciating head pain, which in turn is relieved by a few more caffeine-containing analgesic tablets. Accompanying symptoms include fatigue, grogginess, cloudy thinking, and lessening of ambition. Compared to controls, regular excessive users of caffeine-containing substances demonstrated elevated muscle tension levels and other symptoms of anxiety 3 or more hours after the sudden discontinuance of such medicines (13). This suggests that anxiety symptoms may be a consequence of both toxicity to caffeine and of withdrawal from it.

TABLE 27.1.
CAFFEINE CONTENT OF FOOD

SOURCE	ESTIMATED CAFFEINE (MG)
Brewed coffee (cup)	100–150
Instant coffee (cup)	85–100
Tea (cup)	60–75
Decaffeinated coffee (cup)	2–4
Cola (8 oz)	40–60
Cocoa (cup)	40–55
Chocolate bar	25

PHENACETIN

The problems are compounded when aspirin is combined with phenacetin and caffeine, as is the case in the numerous "APC" preparations. The potential complications of phenacetin are well-known. Due to its lack of safety for long-term use, the Food and Drug Administration has recently withdrawn phenacetin from many of the over-the-counter medications; however, in major medical centers, pa-

TABLE 27.2.
CAFFEINE CONTENT OF COMMON DRUGS

DRUG	MG	DRUG	MG
APC	32	Anacin	32
Cafergot	100	Bromo seltzer	32
Darvon compound	32	Cope	32
Fiorinal	40	Midol	32
Migral	50	Vanquish	60
Wigraine	100	Excedrin	66
Pre-Mens	30		

tients with phenacetin nephropathy are still seen. The predominant manifestations of this nephropathy are hematuria and, in extreme cases, chronic renal failure. Phenacetin and its metabolites are believed to induce oxidative tissue damage in the renal papillae, and concomitant ingestion of salicylates probably potentiates this process (14). Long-term use of aspirin alone does not appear to be nephrotoxic (15). Eighty-five per cent of patients with analgesic nephropathy are women 35 years or older who have a long history of headaches or backaches, for which they had been taking large amounts of analgesics, usually a total of about 1 g per day for 1–3 years (14). It is important to note that patients with impending analgesic renal damage are asymptomatic early in the course of the illness. Hypertension is present in about 50–70%, and intravenous pyelographic studies often demonstrate reduced renal size and caliceal deformities (14). Renal damage can be reversed in most instances if such drugs are discontinued early, though when patients continue to use phenacetin containing analgesics they go on to develop progressive renal damage. Sclerosis of the lower urinary tract capillaries is pathognomonic of the condition (16). Renal tumors have also been reported as a complication of analgesic nephropathy (17).

ANALGESIC/SEDATIVE WITHDRAWAL SYNDROME

Symptoms induced by sudden withdrawal from analgesic preparations containing barbiturates include agitation, confusion, impairment of memory, euphoria, hallucinations, paranoid ideation, nausea, vomiting, and increased headache. The importance of early recognition of such addiction, and the frequency of this withdrawal syndrome, has been emphasized by Preskorn et al (18). They reported withdrawal symptoms in patients overusing Fiorinal (which contains a barbiturate, aspirin, and caffeine), for a period of 6 months to 2 years. In the author's experience, Fiorinal is one of the most commonly overused medications in headache treatment. Sudden discontinuance after prolonged use can result in marked distress.

A number of vague central nervous system effects are noticed in patients undergoing withdrawal from analgesic/sedative combinations. These include fine tremors, enhanced sensory perception, muscle cramps, hyperreflexia, insomnia, agitation, and intense headaches. As a result, withdrawal from these medications should be done gradually. In some cases, the patients must be hospitalized so that these untoward effects can be counteracted with proper supportive measures. When the patient has engaged in sustained high dose sedative abuse, temporary substitution of a different sedative is sometimes required. Naturally, it is quite important to simultaneously institute proper prophylactic antiheadache treatment, so as to prevent these patients from returning to reliance upon analgesics.

Diazepam (Valium) is another medication which is frequently overused in chronic headache treatment. Valium has to be withdrawn gradually to avoid a plethora of symptoms, which can even include generalized seizures.

REFRACTORY HEADACHE AND ANALGESIC/SEDATIVE ABUSE

It has been the experience of many clinicians who have carefully followed headache patients over a long period of time that excessive use of analgesics and analgesic/sedative combinations on a daily basis interferes with effective prophylactic treatment. This applies both to the treatment of migraine with medications such as β-blockers, and to the treatment of muscle contraction headaches with tricyclic antidepressants. Once the analgesics and sedatives are entirely withdrawn, and following a period of readjustment, prophylactic medications again become effective. There is no proper explanation of the mechanism behind this shift. It is possible that prostaglandin, endorphin, or neurotransmitter systems may be interfered with by the analgesic/sedative combinations, and that this in turn nullifies the effect of prophylactic antimigraine agents. Complex interactions between these medications and receptors in vascular smooth muscle, as well as in other tissues, is also a possible mechanism.

ERGOTAMINE ABUSE

Unrestricted use of ergotamine is often associated with habituation, increased headaches, and withdrawal symptoms closely mimicking acute migraine attacks (19). Headache symptoms linked to ergotamine abuse are referred to as "ergotamine headaches" (20). Ergotamine headaches appear to occur in 4–11% of patients being treated for headaches in neurological units (21, 22). These headaches are typically daily, dull, and characterized by constant occipital pressure spreading forward along both parietal bones (23). The headaches characteristically become worse following ergotamine withdrawal. These patients

also frequently complain of coldness in their extremities. A detailed study found that even small doses of ergotamine tartrate taken regularly can cause both a continuous headache and withdrawal symptoms if the drug is discontinued (20).

Reports of more serious problems from ergotamine therapy have also appeared in the literature. Classical ergotism, involving gangrenous vascular complications of the fingers, toes, and tips of the nose, are rare nowadays, but they are well-documented in the older medical literature (24). However, it is apparent that even though classic signs of ergotism may not develop, the continuous use of ergotamine in weekly doses of more than 7–10 mg may be dangerous (25). It can cause subclinical ergotism, marked by disturbances in the peripheral circulation and by changes in the cardiovascular and neuromuscular systems, and by changes in EEGs (25, 26).

Among the signs and symptoms of ergotism are mental aberrations (lassitude, confusion, and mood disturbances), seizures, muscle cramps, ocular changes (midriasis), cataracts, papillitis, amblyopia, retinal hemorrhage, glaucoma, temperature disturbances, and brain ischemia; but the most frequent signs are of peripheral vasoconstriction, with reduced pulses and distal ischemia. In addition, paresthesias, localized edema, itching, substernal distress, emesis, and bradycardia may occur.

The other important characteristic of ergotamine headaches is that appropriate preventive medications do not succeed in preventing what otherwise appears to be a typical vascular headache. Ergotamine abuse headaches characteristically respond only to more ergotamine.

Patients vary in regard to their tolerance of ergotamine preparations (27). Individual clinical response to ergotamine varies widely. The severity (and even the existence) of withdrawal symptoms also does not seem to directly correlate with the dose and the duration of ergotamine abuse (19). Large individual differences in the systemic availability of equivalent doses have also been reported

(28, 29). Ala-Hurula et al (20) reported that the duration and severity of withdrawal symptoms did not correlate with either dosages or plasma levels of ergotamine. In only 4 of their 21 patients (who were followed for 3–6 months) were headache symptoms unimproved after ergotamine withdrawal.

In most cases, headache symptoms get considerably, though temporarily, worse after the patient stops abusing ergotamine. In some cases the symptoms, often indistinguishable from migrainous headaches, may be severe enough to make ergotamine discontinuation impossible (22). In spite of these difficulties, and in spite of a marked relapse rate, termination of ergotamine abuse is widely regarded as beneficial for patients (30).

Patients with cluster headache, many of whom also take excessive amounts of ergotamine tartrate, seem less vulnerable to this syndrome.

Although the plasma half-life of ergotamine is roughly 95 minutes (31), a slow tissue half-life—34 hours (32)—and a later peaking may in part explain the development of toxicity and rebound in patients taking ergotamine tartrate only a few times per week. Because the addictive potential of ergotamine may be enhanced by renal disease, malnutrition, vascular disease, heavy smoking, pregnancy, and birth control pills, patients with these conditions should be warned to reduce or avoid ergots. The physician should periodically review the amount and the frequency of ergotamine use to avoid ergotamine headaches or other toxic effects. For the symptomatic management of migraine headaches, clinical experience dictates restricting ergotamine use to two or three times per week.

OTHER MEDICATIONS WHOSE PROLONGED USE POSES POTENTIAL HAZARDS

Methysergide (Sansert) effectively controls migraine in 60–70% of patients. Because of this success rate, many patients rely on methysergide prophylaxis. Prolonged use of methysergide is occasionally associated with the severe and serious complications of retroperitoneal fibrosis, pulmonary fibrosis, or cardiac fibrosis. Obstructive uropathy with hydronephosis and subsequent renal failure have also been reported to follow prolonged methysergide use. Because of these experiences, methysergide is preferably prescribed for only 4 months at a time, with a sufficient methysergide-free interval insisted upon before this treatment is resumed.

Patients with chronic cluster headache who respond to corticosteroids may find the drug difficult to discontinue: their headaches reoccur when they try. The physician thus has the responsibility of restricting the corticosteriod dosage to prevent long-term side effects, such as osteoporosis, cataract formation, aseptic necrosis of the hip, gastritis, gastric ulcer formation, or gastric bleeding. Other, alternative drugs may have to be found, although this is not easy in many cases.

TREATMENT OF MEDICATION OVERUSE

It is a general observation that patients who have become habituated or who are dependent on analgesic/hypnotic/ergotamine combinations also show a high incidence of depression, neuroticism, and chronic headache behavior, factors which have to be taken into consideration when dealing with these patients. Hospitalization in a headache or pain unit may be the most effective way to withdraw these patients from their medications. The withdrawal is often best done gradually, using substitute medications in certain cases. Hospitalization also allows time to explore the psychological and behavioral patterns of these patients, patterns which are often found to have a major influence in perpetuating the patient's headaches. Our inpatient program includes psychometric evaluation (using self-rating depression scales, anxiety scales, pain behavioral analysis, and the Minnesota Multiphasic Personality Inventory) and daily observations by physicians and psychologists, as well as by nurses. Besides gradual replacement of medications to which the patients are habituated with prophylactic medications, the patients learning of biofeedback therapy and relaxation exercises is an integral part of his recovery program. In addition, behavioral therapy or traditional psychotherapy by a trained psychologist or psychiatrist is essential. It addresses such issues as nonassertiveness, depression, and problems in interpersonal relationships. "Headache behavior," headache as a form of communication, its controlling, punishing, and protective values, are only a few of the issues which must be considered to see if they are relevant to the particular patient. With such a combined approach, the majority of these patients can be rehabilitated, and headache frequency can be reduced to tolerable levels. A professional and supportive environment in an inpatient unit makes an immense difference. Educating the patient and his family about the importance of their reactions to him and on the effect of the patients' behavior on his overall prognosis is also important.

REFERENCES

1. Mathew NT: New horizons in the management of headache: the headache clinic. In Packard RC (ed): *Neurologic Clinics*, vol 1, no 2. Philadelphia, WB Saunders, 1983.

2. Brena SF: Drugs and pain: use and misuse. In Brena SF, Chapman SL (eds): *Management of Patients with Chronic Pain*, ed 1. New York, Spectrum Publications, 1983.

3. Saper JR: Drug overuse among patients with headache. In Packard RC (ed): *Neurologic Clinics*, vol 1, no 2. Philadelphia, WB Saunders, 1983.

4. Beaver WT, Kantor TG, Levy G: On guard for aspirin's harmful effects. *Patient Care* 13:48–83, 1979.

5. Murray TG, Goldberg M: Analgesic abuse and renal disease. *Annu Rev Med* 26:537–550, 1975.

6. Saper JR: *Headache Disorders: Current Concepts and Treatment Strategies.* Littleton, MA, Wright-PSG Publishers, 1983.

7. Moertel CG, Ahmann DL, Taylor WF, et al: Relief of pain by oral medication: a controlled evaluation of analgesic combinations. *JAMA* 299:55–59, 1974.

8. Woodbury DM, Fingl E: Analgesics, antipyretics, antiinflammatory agents, and drugs employed in the therapy of gout. In Goodman, LS, Gilman AL (eds): *The Pharmacological Basis of Therapeutics,* ed 5. New York, Macmillan, 1975.

9. Greden JF: Coffee, tea, and you. *The Sciences,* Jan. 1979, pp. 6–11.

10. Greden JF: Anxiety of caffeinism: a diagnostic dilemma. *Am J Psychiatry* 131:1089–1092, 1974.

11. Greden JF, Fontaine M, Lubetsky K, et al: Anxiety and depression with associated caffeinism among psychiatric patients. *Am J Psychiatry* 135:963–966, 1978.

12. Ritchie JM: Central nervous system stimulants. In Goodman LS, Gilman AL (eds): *The Pharmacological Basis of Therapeutics,* ed 5. New York, Macmillan, 1975.

13. Shite BC, Lincoln CA, Pearce NW, et al: Anxiety and muscle tension as 3 consequences of caffeine withdrawal. *Science* 209:1547–1548, 1980.

14. Goldberg M, Murray TG: Analgesic associated nephropathy. *N Engl J Med* 299:716–717, 1978.

15. Emkey RD, Mills JA: Aspirin and analgesic nephropathy. *JAMA* 247:55–57, 1982.

16. Mihatsch MJ, Zollinger JU, Torhorst J: Pathognomonic lesions of analgesic nephropathy, letter. *N Engl J Med* 300:1275–1276, 1979.

17. Bama DS, Aronson A, Merrill JP, Graham P: Headache and analgesic nephropathy and tumors. *Headache,* 19:358–363, 1979.

18. Preskorn SH, Schwin RL, McKnelly WV: Analgesic abuse and the barbiturate abstinence syndrome. *JAMA* 244:369–370, 1980.

19. Rowsell AR, Neylan C, Wilkinson M: Ergotamine induced headaches in migrainous patients. *Headache* 13:65–67, 1973.

20. Ala-Hurula V, Myllyla V, Hokkanen E: Ergotamine abuse: results of ergotamine discontinuation, with special reference to the plasma concentrations. *Cephalalgia* 2:189–195, 1982.

21. Wainscott G, Volans G, Wilkinson M: Ergotamine-induced headaches. *Br Med J* 2:724, 1974.

22. Anderson PG: Ergotamine headache. *Headache* 15:118–121, 1975.

23. Lippman CW: Characteristic headache resulting from prolonged use of ergot derivatives. *J Nerv Ment Dis* 121:270–273, 1955.

24. Harrison TE: Ergotaminism. *JACEP* 7:162–169, 1978.

25. Diege-Petersen H, Lassen NA, Noer J, Ton-

nesen KH, Olesen J: Subclinical ergotism. *Lancet* 2:65–66, 1977.

26. Hokkanen E, Waltimo O, Kallanranta T: Toxic effects of ergotamine used for migraine. *Headache* 18:95–98, 1978.

27. Horton BT, Peters GA: Clinical manifestations of excessive use of ergotamine preparations and management of withdrawal effect: report of 52 cases. *Headache* 2:214–227, 1963.

28. Ala-Hurula V, Myllyla VV, Arvela P, Heikkila J, Karki N, Hokkanen E: Systemic availability of ergotamine tartrate after oral, rectal and intramuscular administration. *Eur J Clin Pharmacol* 15:51–55, 1979.

29. Ala-Hurula V, Myllyla VV, Arvela P, Karki N, Hokkanen E: Systemic availability of ergotamine tartrate after three successive doses and during continuous medication. *Eur J Clin Pharmacol* 16:355–360, 1979.

30. Tfelt-Hansen P, Aebelholt-Krabbe A: Ergotamine abuse. Do patients benefit from withdrawal? *Cephalalgia* 1:29–32, 1981.

31. Wilkinson M, Orton D: Some observations on the use of ergotamine tartrate. *Headache* 21:159, 1980.

32. Meier J, Schreier E: Human plasma levels of some antimigraine drugs. *Headache* 16:96–104, 1976.

SECTION FIVE

Treatment

CHAPTER TWENTY EIGHT

An Overview of Treatment Options for the Psychologically Influenced Headache Patient

JANE ROBERTS GILL, M.S.W., C.S.W.

The goal of this chapter is to increase physicians' awareness that psychotherapy is more than a homogeneous undifferentiated treatment for the emotionally distressed headache patient. It offers different solutions for different problems, just as the general physician has many treatment options for treating back pain. In this chapter, I shall attempt to provide a brief overview of the major types of therapy available to treat patients' psychosocial problems when these impinge upon or contribute to headaches.

Physicians are fully cognizant that depression, disturbance in interpersonal relationships, and acute or prolonged emotional trauma need treatment if their patients' headaches are to be relieved. But should they refer the patient for biofeedback or for psychoanalysis? Would a psychiatrist, psychologist, clinical social worker or some other qualified mental health professional provide the most appropriate and most effective treatment? Or, should the primary physician decide to treat the patient's emotional difficulties himself?

Selection of appropriate therapy and therapist depend on the type of problem the patient has and the type of human being the patient is; these can be determined by careful listening and observation. Can the patient talk about feelings and interpersonal relationships? Is he aware of, and sensitive to, his own and other peoples' feelings? Does he react with warmth and humor? Or is he a person who cannot describe important people in his life, becomes puzzled when asked about his own feelings, and is oblivious to his effect upon the feelings of others? These very different types of people may have similar types of headaches. Each, however, is likely to respond better to quite different types of psychotherapy.

Effectiveness of therapy depends on the appropriateness of the referral, the way in which the referral is made, the clinical skills of the therapist, the matchup between the two people who will be working together and, as will be elaborated on in this chapter, the appropriateness of the particular therapy for the particular patient. The primary physician needs to make clear to his patient why he believes a referral for psychotherapy might help, and why he has selected a particular therapist and type of treatment. It also benefits the transition if he makes clear his confidence in the psychotherapist's competence. In this way, the primary doctor/patient relationship helps the patient begin psychotherapy with a positive attitude and expectations.

There are three major categories of psychotherapy: behavioral, somatic, and psychodynamic.

BEHAVIORAL TREATMENT

Behavior Therapy is most often provided by psychologists trained in learning theory. It emphasizes how problems can be understood and treated when viewed as the long-term effects of learned responses to positive or negative stimuli. It is useful for patients with limited insight into their feelings, but who like to think logically. As its name implies, behavior therapy's strongest suit is in treating patients whose primary problem is a form of disordered and self-defeating behavior. Patients can be helped to recognize which behaviors either produce headaches directly, or, more commonly, lead to feeling states which frequently eventuate in headache. Through analysis of the contingencies which maintain these behaviors, a plan can be devised that allows the patient to unlearn maladaptive behaviors and acquire better ones. It should be emphasized that pain *per se* is not a behavior.

Cognitive Therapy involves talking with a therapist about those thoughts which accompany headaches in order to attempt to block the illogical ones which add to the distress of head pain. The therapy is concerned with learned ideas, expectations, prematurely or illogically formed conclusions, and with their effect on behavior. It does not specifically deal with the unconscious.

SOMATIC THERAPIES

For purposes of this chapter, this term will include the relaxation therapies, although they are not always so characterized. Somatic therapists attempt to increase the patient's awareness of the functioning of, his own body and how it responds to strains. Therapy is directed towards helping the patient learn to modify physical responses in positive ways.

Relaxation Techniques are designed to help patients reduce physical tension which may be contributing to their pain. Progressive Relaxation, Autogenic Training, and Meditation are some of the best known techniques, and each in some fashion teaches the patient to be more at ease physically. Relaxation techniques are particularly useful with patients who have difficulty recognizing feelings and who tense up physically in reaction to emotional stressors. These approaches do not attempt to discover why a patient becomes tense in a particular circumstance, nor to find out whether there is an underlying cause for his headaches. Relaxation techniques help some patients to reduce their use of medications.

Hypnosis is used by highly trained psychiatrists and psychologists to produce relaxation and, on a deeper level, to reduce the patient's attention to sensations of pain. It is often an effective way to reduce the need for pain medication with problems such as headache. A number of patients cannot be hypnotized, however, perhaps because they fear losing control. Such patients respond better to one of the relaxation therapies which allows them to maintain control. Patients who can be hypnotized do not always obtain complete relief of pain, but can usually reduce the intensity of their pain to a more tolerable level. For example, a young woman who was increasingly disabled by Atypical Cluster Headaches obtained some relief from their severity with the use of self-hypnosis. She was able to induce a sense of "removing herself from her body" and then, as a dispassionate observer, to reflect upon the dreadful agony her body "over there in the bed" must endure. She then reported experiencing only mild discomfort.

Biofeedback is a therapeutic modality which is used somewhat differently by therapists with different training. Psychodynamically trained clinicians use it to provide a bridge between somatic manifestations of distress and psychodynamic treatment. To them, biofeedback is a tool rather than a treatment, one comparable to using an electrocardiogram to learn about the patient's physiological reactions, rather than to treat them. Biofeedback makes both patient and therapist aware of changes that take place in reaction to certain feelings. A patient might notice that each time he speaks of his father's recent death, the instrument indicates a physical reaction related to it. Adler and Adler (personal communication, June 1983) point out that "biofeedback has the ability simultaneously to show the psychological and physiological aspects of the disordered functioning that constitutes disease to both therapist and patient, and unambiguously to demonstrate their synchronization. This facilitates the patient's introspection about his problem."

PSYCHODYNAMIC THERAPIES

Psychodynamic psychotherapy is provided primarily by psychiatrists, psychologists, and specifically trained clinical or psychiatric social workers. Emotional conflicts or trauma which may have produced or contributed to somatic symptoms such as headache are evaluated as are present day underlying problems which generate current psychological and psychophysiological distress. The patient may not recognize that these problems are relevant to his headaches. Psychodynamic psychotherapists consider pain which comes from strong and unresolved difficulties in the patient's unconscious, as well as from sources of dysphoric emotion of which the patient is fully aware. The efficacy of these therapies is based upon the patient's ability to relate his feelings to his life experiences, and ultimately to understand the nature of important relationships, past and present.

Supportive Therapy is one of the most useful types of treatment for headache patients. It may be provided by the primary physician, or by a mental health professional.

Supportive treatment ranges from kindly discussion of the problem with the patient, to an attempt to help him recognize and use his own coping strategies more effectively. It encourages the patient to use adult strengths he has already acquired to fullest advantage.

Time-Limited or Goal-Directed Therapy focuses on a particular emotional conflict which affects the patient's headaches. It attempts to help him better define the problem, and find the most constructive way to deal with it. Short-term treatment may help the patient recognize other areas of difficulty which he wishes to continue exploring with the therapist.

Long-Term Treatment attempts to increase the patient's self-esteem and rapport with others by helping him to understand his own and others' motivations. It aims at changing neurotic, depressive, or anxiety-provoked defensive patterns that interfere with healthy functioning. This type of treatment can be extremely useful for patients in whom longstanding psychosocial problems trigger headaches.

Psychoanalysis is a long-term treatment designed to change ego structure by using the patient's capacity for insight to help him understand and modify his defensive patterns. Psychoanalysis has less of a role in treating somatic problems than it does in fully elucidating them.

AN IMPORTANT FACTOR IN DETERMINING PATIENT-THERAPY MATCHUP

People vary enormously in their capacity to recognize when they are having feelings and in their ability to describe precisely what it is they are feeling. Many people prefer not to express feelings openly, while some others have never fully learned what feelings are. The ability to identify feelings develops gradually, from the time of birth onwards. It begins in the subtle, nonverbal interactions between mother (or mothering person) and child.

Later, as language develops, and as the child gains an increasing capacity to distinguish between self and others, he also learns how members of his extended family, friends, and neighbors express feelings. A child who grows up without adequately learning about how to sense feelings in those closest to him is as emotionally handicapped as a blind child is visually handicapped. If the child is intelligent, he may perceive that people expect emotional responses from him, and may learn to simulate appropriate feelings.

Clinical clues which alert physicians to this type of emotionally handicapped patient are an imitative quality to his affect and to his response when asked how he feels. There is usually a history of severe early deprivation. A further warning note is sounded by the patient's trouble in describing more than superficial personality characteristics of people with whom he is supposedly in close contact. For example: A 22-year-old, three-times-married woman consulted her doctor about a band-like headache which had become severe after she and her husband returned to the spot where she was gang-raped at age 17. She was unable to describe any feelings about the event. Her husband's description, on the other hand, conveyed the fear and shock one would expect that she felt. The psychological history revealed that her mother had been hospitalized with chronic schizophrenia shortly after the patient's birth. She had no adequate mothering throughout infancy and early childhood, but was continually shifted from one household to another. During a recent hospital admission she learned that she was pregnant. She was totally unable to describe how she felt about having a baby; instead, she merely looked blank when the question was posed. Several days later, after she had talked with her husband, she had learned to imitate the expected enthusiastic response. Her ability to learn to go through the motions of feeling enabled her to make a more adequate surface adaptation to life. Such a patient's headache problems are not amenable to psychodynamic therapy, but are

better treated by supportive therapy and medications, often best provided by the primary physician.

In marked contrast to this emotionally starved young woman is another patient, one who illustrates how someone referred for headaches may make use of several types of psychodynamic treatment. She presented with a history of occasional migraine headaches beginning in adolescence. Ever since her marriage necessitated a move to an unfamiliar city, the headaches increased in severity and frequency. The move required her to leave both an excellent job, one in which she was a valued employee, and her family. She spoke with intense feelings about what each of the members of her family meant to her. The patient was troubled that, because her husband's family came from a lower social stratum than her own, she felt her mother had not given full approval to the marriage. Except when she was away at college, the patient had always lived with her identical twin, and now felt deprived of her support. As a result the patient now felt quite alone, conflicted about her marriage, and deprived of her close friends. She was initially referred for supportive psychodynamic therapy, which focused on uncovering headache precipitants and teaching her how to better cope with them. Nevertheless, her insightfulness, intelligence, and sensitivity soon led her to begin to question the implications of much that had occurred in her life; therapy then shifted to long-term treatment to resolve or modify maladaptive patterns in her close relationships. Psychodynamic therapy has not only helped her to recognize interpersonal precipitants to her headaches, but also to develop into a more self-confident person. Her headaches have decreased markedly as a result.

Most headache patients will use only one of the psychodynamic therapies. Which one is the most apropos depends on the patient's sensitivity and personal goals, the therapist's skills, and the assessment as to whether the patient will benefit more from support of his underlying strengths, or from uncovering and modifying neurotic patterns.

After careful observation and attentive listening to his patient to learn how physical, social, and emotional factors intertwine to produce headaches, the physician may refer him for behavioral, somatic, or psychodynamic therapy. This brief survey of treatment options has presented an overview of the orientations, methods, and goals of different psychological treatment modalities.

CHAPTER TWENTY NINE

The Patient with Acute Migraine: Definitive Support

MARCIA WILKINSON, D.M., F.R.C.P.

Migraine is an ill-defined, self-limiting recurring condition which may cause intermittent discomfort to the sufferer for many years. The majority of attacks occur without warning, at times which may be inconvenient and socially embarrassing. There are no signs of migraine that can be objectively measured and, as with other types of pain, its severity can only be assessed by the patient. The medical practitioner must rely solely on a subjective description of symptoms to make a diagnosis. The clinical definition of migraine has been the subject of dispute for many centuries and remains so today. The World Federation of Neurology (1) has provided one of the better definitions, but even it has its disadvantages:

Migraine is a familial disorder characterized by recurrent attacks of headache widely variable in intensity, frequency and duration. Attacks are commonly unilateral and are usually associated with anorexia, nausea and vomiting. In some cases they are preceded by or associated with neurological and mood disturbances. All the above characteristics are not necessarily present in each attack or in each patient.

Patients who suffer from migraine are typically very worried about their attacks, as most of them have had at least several particularly unpleasant headaches at particularly inconvenient times, and they cannot be certain that it will not recur when they are least expecting it. In an effort to deal directly with acute attacks when they occur, the City of London Migraine Clinic was started in May 1970 (2).

DEVELOPMENT AND SERVICES OF THE CLINIC

For several reasons it was felt that there should be a clinic in the City of London itself where patients could go for help when they had an acute headache. This central location was necessary because no migraine sufferer would willingly travel for more than half an hour once his symptoms started. Although only about 25,000 people live in London proper, nearly three-quarters of a million people go there to work each day; there is no other place in England where such a large number of people are gathered together under stressful conditions.

The present clinic is in a delightful Georgian home, built about 1760, on four floors, with an oval staircase. Its structure is unusual because on the ground floor there is only a narrow hallway, the rest of the space taken up by an arch through which the coach and horses used to go to the mews at the back. Despite its central location, the area is secluded and quiet.

The Clinic has evolved to offer two types of service: an emergency service for those coming during an acute attack, in which case a patient can come anytime the Clinic is open; and patients seen by appointment, for consultations with their family doctor, in which case a letter of referral is required. It is rare. for facilities that treat patients by appointment only to see many patients in the throes of an acute attack. In its first 13 years the City of

London clinic treated 4,500 patients for acute attacks, and 20,000 for routine consultations, and it is on the basis of this experience that the present treatment at the Clinic is provided.

Over the last 10 years a number of headache clinics have been started worldwide (3, 4). Most of them treat acute as well as recurrent headache problems. The concept that an acute headache requires a specialist's treatment is a relatively new idea, and its implementation in the form of special clinics has shed light on the best methods for treating an acute attack. The City of London Migraine Clinic was the first free-standing facility to give such emergency treatment. Most clinics are in major teaching hospitals; these provide excellent services, as full investigatory facilities are available on the spot should the patient require them.

It is from such centers that much of the new knowledge about treatment of acute migraine has come. Recent interest has centered on the use of ergotamine (5) and in the use of ergotamine combined with aspirin or paracetamol (acetaminophen) (6, 7) in the acute attack; but perhaps the greatest interest has been directed toward the value of using metoclopramide (often this must be given intramuscularly) (8–10) and the newer domperidone (11) to treat the nausea and vomiting which accompanies migraine. A rather simple treatment combining rest, an antinauseant, and a mild analgesic and, in some cases, a small dose of ergotamine, has been found effective in all clinics in Europe (12, 13).

The type of patient coming to a clinic depends upon the population characteristics of the district it serves. The most successful units have generally been in big cities where there is a large commuter population. Having treatment available close by, and being allowed to rest in a clinic, is much better than having to keep on working in a noisy office. In an urban population, it is mostly office workers who come to such a clinic; but these include all types, from secretaries to managing directors. In the past, it has sometimes been true that many men did not wish to admit to having migraine, as they regarded it as a "neurotic female" type of illness; but over the last few years, opinion is changing, and about one-third of the patients seen with an acute headache today are men.

EVALUATION OF THE PATIENT

Once the diagnosis of migraine has been established, the doctor should reassure the patient that there is no serious intracranial pathology. The fear, expressed or hidden, that recurrent, severe headaches are due to tumor is widespread, and each patient should be specifically reassured on this point. Before this reassurance can be given the doctor must have taken a full history and done a complete examination—in other words, he must have a sound basis for the reassurance. Very often, the effect of removing this fear is great enough to either partially or completely relieve the headaches. Because it has been suggested that migraine may be a distorted protective response to a real or imagined threat to the brain, trigger factors must also be discussed with the patient.

Many patients with severe headaches demand not only to be examined, but also to be fully investigated as well. The full investigational program includes skull x-rays, CT scan, electroencephalogram, psychological assessment and, sometimes, a cerebral angiogram. To do all these is usually both costly and unnecessary as, unless there is a history of a change in headache pattern, a focal neurological disturbance, or some abnormal physical signs, it is extremely rare to find major intracranial pathology. If one investigation is to be done, a CT scan is probably the one of choice, as it is noninvasive and gives a good deal of information. But even this is normal in most headache cases. A full neurological evaluation should be done on anyone who develops headaches for the first time over the age of 50. A study at the City of London Migraine Clinic showed that less than 2% of migraineurs developed their first headache after the age of 50.

The best way to treat migraine is to prevent attacks from occurring in the first place; it is therefore important to eliminate factors which may initiate an attack. There are many of these, and stress is one of them. Anyone who works in a city office is daily subjected to many stressors. There is the effort of getting to work—most London commuters have journeys which vary from 1 to 3 hours in duration. Traveling may be difficult, particularly in the winter, when there may be delays of the buses or trains due to fog and ice. Many migraine sufferers have a history of travel sickness as a child and, although most of them grow out of it, a bumpy, unpleasant, and late journey may trigger off an attack. The noise of clattering typewriters and the need to get things off in time are additional stressors.

A new factor is the video or computer screen. Some jobs now involve working at a screen for several hours a day, and some migraine sufferers find this difficult. Office lighting is sometimes bad, and ill-fitted neon lights may flicker. Food is sometimes a migraine trigger and "fast food," often greasy and overcooked, may provoke an attack. Other people bring cheese sandwiches to work, or eat a bar of chocolate at lunchtime instead of having a proper meal, and this too may induce an attack.

Much has been written about the weekend "release" headache, occurring when the strain of the week is theoretically over, but some women may get headaches on weekends because Saturday is their busiest day. During the weekend, shopping and housework must be done, and women must see to the needs of their families, as well as enjoy themselves. Other women develop headaches on Monday mornings, when everyone has left the house for work or school.

Alcohol is a common trigger, and most parties are held on a Friday or Saturday. This, combined with a late night out and the noise of a disco, may cause an attack. A lower percentage of migraine sufferers smoke or drink than in the population as a whole, and this may be because both are potential migraine triggers. An excess of positive ions in the atmosphere is thought by some to bring on an attack; many offices and airports have now installed negative ionization machines.

TREATMENT OF THE ACUTE ATTACK

A patient's decision to come to a clinic for his bout with migraine indicates that he considers himself in need of help, and the first thing for him to know (12) is that he is going to get it. The reception must be both friendly and businesslike, with the least possible time spent in registration and other formalities. Above all, the patient must not be expected to wait an hour or two before he is dealt with, as may happen in some busy hospital emergency departments. As soon as possible, he should be taken to a quiet room and be allowed to lie down, with enough blankets to keep him warm. The City of London Migraine Clinic has a special room in which there are comfortable beds, not hospital or examination couches, and the room is kept quiet and dark. The clinic is fortunate to be situated in one of the London squares where, although it is only a quarter mile from St. Paul's Cathedral, there is very little traffic noise, and what there is, the Georgian shutters are very effective in keeping down. It is also within easy walking distance of many offices.

Once the patient has been made comfortable by the Sister in charge, he is seen by the doctor, who prescribes appropriate treatment as discussed previously: rest, an antinauseant, and analgesics. About one-third of the patients are given a small dose of ergotamine tartrate.

REST AND SLEEP

Rest and sleep are an essential part of the recovery process, and many patients find that they do not get better until they have slept. For most people who are working, this means waiting until they get home and are able to get to bed; but if a facility where they can sleep is offered in the clinic, it hastens the recovery process. The staff at the City of London Migraine Clinic found that patients recovered much more quickly if they were able to sleep than if they only rested or dozed (14). Some sufferers get over their attack if they are able to sleep for even a short period, lasting as little as 10–15 minutes.

In 1976, a study of 310 patients attending the Clinic attempted to discover what factors affected the rate and completeness of their recovery from an acute attack. Significant factors were found to be the length of time the headache had been present before arrival at the clinic, and whether the patient was able to sleep soundly. Patients who arrived early in the attack had significantly fewer headaches in the next 7 days than did those whose headache had lasted 24 hours before their coming. Patients who slept, with a sedative where indicated, recovered more quickly than those who did not sleep, but the depth of sleep did not appear to affect the rate of recovery.

Because sleep is a necessary part of the recovery process, drugs containing caffeine should be avoided when possible. Most preparations of ergotamine contain 50 or 100 mg of caffeine to promote ergotamine absorption, but it is better to give a caffeine-free preparation if possible. Some people like to try to work off their migraine, and for this purpose take large doses of caffeine and ergotamine. This type of action is usually self-defeating, because although the caffeine and ergotamine may allow the patient to carry on for a short time, the headache will usually persist or recur, and further nausea may develop as a result of excess ergotamine intake. Furthermore, overdose of ergotamine tartrate is one of the commonest causes of migraine lasting more than 24 hours. In 4 years at the City of London Migraine Clinic, 256 cases were referred for ergotamine poisoning.

To help the patient get the needed sleep, it may be necessary to give a small dose of one of the short-acting benzodiazepines. Neither large doses of benzodiazepines nor barbiturates should be used because of the dangers of habituation and the hangover effects. The mean time that patients need to stay in the clinic is just over 3 hours. The goal should be for the patients to have recovered both from the migraine and the effects of treatment in that time. Any drug, such as a barbiturate, whose action lasts for many hours, should therefore be avoided.

A migraine attack rarely prevents the sufferer from carrying out an important duty, such as making a meeting, giving a lecture, or sitting at an examination, but it is the fear of such a thing happening that worries people. Once an attack has started, medication should be taken as soon as possible. Patients should be instructed in proper use and timing of their medication.

Patients coming to the clinic are typically anxious and upset, and want a refuge from all the day-to-day trials that beset them. They are relieved when they find that there are people who are interested in their condition and are prepared to do something about it. Often, they are worried about business or family appointments, and if they know that the clinic staff will put through a call to their place of work, or to their family, it relieves this anxiety, and they can then relax and obtain full benefit from treatment. They are encouraged to stay until sufficiently recovered to return to work or go home. If they are still feeling badly by closing time, arrangements are made for them to be taken home by a friend or relative, or other transport is arranged. As most patients come to the clinic either in the second half of the morning or at lunchtime, it is only rarely that they are not feeling better when the clinic closes, however. On the occasions when this does occur, the patient can be admitted to the hospital for the night.

USE OF ANALGESICS

Headache is the main symptom of migraine, and all patients coming for treatment want relief from pain. Analgesics are often best combined with a medication for nausea and vomiting, as these may be the most distressing of symptoms when they occur.

The very fact that the patient is coming into a calming atmosphere where treatment is available helps; the knowledge that in a short time he will be given something for his distress is itself a relief. The soothing atmosphere alone, however, is apparently not enough to fully do the job. In the early days of the clinic, a trial was done in which some patients were given sterile water instead of an antinauseant, and in a subsequent trial some were given a placebo tablet instead of an analgesic. Although there was modest improvement in both of these groups of patients, in neither case was the result as good as when a real antinauseant or analgesic was used.

Under clinic circumstances it has never been necessary to give painkillers other than aspirin or paracetamol (acetominophen) (13). In particular, narcotics or barbiturates have not been used. Even with such simple analgesics as aspirin and paracetamol, single doses are usually effective within a few minutes of administration, especially if these drugs are given in a soluble or effervescent form. Their action reaches its peak after 1 or 2 hours and fades within about 6 hours. This is an ideal time span, as the mean patient stay is about 3 hours. Although the simple analgesics are very effective if taken at the time of the attack, they should not be used regularly, as their continued use may give rise to a chronic pain syndrome.

The use of relatively quick-acting analgesics ensures that there is no "hangover" period, as is seen with narcotics or barbiturates. The half-life of phenobarbitone is 24–96 hours, while that of sodium amytal is 14–42 hours. In the United Kingdom, benzodiazepines have supplanted barbiturates for most purposes, but barbiturates are still used in preparations such as Bellergal (phenobarbitone, 20 mg; belladonna alkaloids, 100 μg; ergotamine tartrate, 300 μg). In the United States, Fiorinal, which contains 50 mg of barbiturate, is still used.

Some clinicians favor large doses of these and other drugs to ensure that the patient is "knocked out" and sleeps for a considerable period. The best treatment is one which not only alleviates symptoms, but also which preferably allows the patient to go to sleep with a minimum of side effects. This is why simple analgesics, a small dose of ergotamine tartrate and, if necessary, one of the short-acting benzodiazepines should be used. At times, ergotamine tartrate is not absorbed well orally because of nausea (14). In these cases it may be given effectively by suppository (15).

STATUS MIGRAINOSUS

Headaches which persist for 3 days or more have been called "status migrainosus;" but the only patients seen at the City of London Migraine Clinic with headaches persisting for more than 3 days have either been taking too much ergotamine or have tension or some other type of headache in addition to their migraine.

Although the term status migrainosus has been used for many years, it does not seem to the author to describe an actual clinical entity. Gowers (16) makes no reference to it, nor does Wolff in his classic work on headaches, nor do Raskin and Appenzeller (17). Brain (18) describes a condition which he calls "status hemicranialis." This is a headache preceded by visual symptoms which may occur more than once a day for a period of days, i.e., repeated, separate attacks.

More recently, Sacks (19) described a patient who experienced daily migraines which were at first confluent with one another—this condition he calls "migraine status." Later on, he describes the treatment of "Status Migrainosus," a term which he puts in quotes. He defines the term "status" as the occurrence of confluent or continuous attacks of paroxysmal illness, whether epileptic, asthmatic, or migrainous in nature.

True migraine status must be treated as a medical emergency. The patient is likely to have suffered excruciating headache for several days without a pause, to be prostrated from incessant vomiting, and to be seriously dehydrated. Sacks recommends:

The first acts of the physician must be reassurance and protective seclusion, for the intensity of the patient's anxiety and the agitated movements of relatives milling around in a well-intentioned but intensely irritating manner are likely to be important factors in perpetuating the state. The patient will be in need of massive medication; parenteral barbiturates, codeine or morphine, antiemetic drugs and frequently strong tranquilizers. Ergotamine is not indicated in this situation, and is prone to aggravate rather than ameliorate the symptoms . . . Attacks of migraine in their nature, tend to be of limited duration but attacks of migraine status are nearly always associated with intense hidden emotional stresses, the desperate quality of the symptoms reflecting the intensity of the underlying emotional substitute.

In other words, it is the intense emotional reaction which takes over from the migraine attack. Taverner (20) describes a condition wherein severe and prolonged or frequently repeated migraine attacks may amount to status migrainosus.

Lance (21) has another definition. He states that "uncommonly patients may progress to 'status migrainosus' when they awaken each day with a recrudescence of their migraine headache" and later defines status migrainosus as "daily, severe headaches persisting in spite of hospital admission."

The most recent study is that of Couch and Diamond (22), and here they use the term to cover several conditions:

1. A continuous severe headache over a prolonged period

or

2. Frequent severe headaches of the migraine type which are severe enough to cause the patient great discomfort and disability.

It would seem, therefore, that there may not be a clinical entity of "status migrainosus";

and, significantly, the ad hoc committee for classification of headache did not include it in their definition.

Occasionally, a true migraine attack may last for 3 days if untreated, but the majority of patients labeled as having status migrainosus seem to have another type of headache, or they have migraine in combination with another type of headache, or they suffer from ergotamine tartrate poisoning. If a patient suffering from a status migrainosus picture is seen, a careful history should be taken and a full examination done to establish the exact clinical situation.

It must be recognized that there is no such thing as a "cure" for migraine, but that it is relatively easy to give relief from a particular headache. Migraine is not a killing disorder, but a severe attack is not merely disturbing but disabling, and deserves the full attention of the attending doctor.

REFERENCES

1. World Federation of Neurology: *Background to Migraine,* A.L. Cochrane (ed) London, Wm. Heinemann, 1970.
2. Wilkinson M: *Background to Migraine, 4th Migraine Symposium,* JN Cumings (ed.) London, Wm. Heinemann, 1971, pp 8–13.
3. Olesen J, Aebelholt A, Veilis B: The Copenhagen Acute Headache Clinic: organisation, patient material, treatment results. *Headache* 19:223–227, 1979.
4. Houdal H, Syversen GB, Rosenthaler J: Ergotamine in plasma & CSF after I.M. and rectal administration to humans. *Cephalalgia* 2:145–151, 1982.
5. Volans GN: Absorption of effervescent aspirin during migraine *Br Med J* 2:265–268, 1974.
6. Ross-Lee L, Heazlewood V, Tyrer JH, Eadie MJ: Aspirin treatment of migraine attacks-plasma drug level data. *Cephalalgia* 2:9–15, 1982.
7. Ross-Lee L, Eadie MJ, Tyrer JH: Aspirin treatment of migraine attacks, clinical observations. *Cephalalgia* 2:71–77, 1982.
8. Volans GN: The effect of metoclopramide on the absorption of effervescent aspiring in migraine. *Br J Clin Pharmacol* 257–263, 1975.

9. Slettnes O, Sjaastad O: Metoclopramide during attacks of migraine. In Sicuteri F (ed): *Headache: New Vistas.* Florence, Italy, 1977, pp 201–204.

10. Hakkarainen H, Allonen H: Ergotamine vs metoclopramide vs—their combination in migraine attacks. *Headache* 22:10–13, 1982.

11. Amery WK, Waelkens J: Prevention of the last chance: an alternative pharmacologic treatment of migraine. *Headache* 23:37–39, 1983.

12. Wilkinson M: The treatment of acute migraine attacks. *Headache* 15:291–292, 1976.

13. Wilkinson M: Treatment of the acute migraine attack. *Cephalalgia* 3:61–68, 1983.

14. Wilkinson M, Williams K, Keyton M: Observations on the treatment of an acute attack of migraine. In Friedman AP, Granger M (eds): *Research & Clinical Studies in Headache.* Basel, S. Karger, Vol 6, pp 141–146.

15. Graham AM, Johnson ES, Persaud NP, Turner P, Wilkinson M: The systemic availability of ergotamine tartrate given by three different routes of administration to healthy volunteers. In press, 1987.

16. Gowers WR: *Diseases of the Nervous System, Second Edition.* London, J.A. Churchill, 1893.

17. Raskin NH, Appenzeller O: *Major Problems in Internal Medicine: Headache XIX.* Philadelphia, Saunders, 1980.

18. Brain L: *Diseases of the Nervous System, Sixth Edition.* London, Oxford University Press, 1962.

19. Sacks OW: *Migraine—Evolution of a Common Disorder.* London, Faber & Faber, 1970.

20. Taverner D: Drug treatment of cranial neuralgias. In Vinken PJ, Bruyn GW (eds): *Handbook of Clinical Neurology.* American Elsevier, 1975, vol 5, pp 378–385.

21. Lance JW: *Mechanism & Management of Headache, 3rd Edition.* London, Butterworths, 1979.

22. Couch JR, Diamond S: Status migrainosus: causative and therapeutic aspects. *Headache* 23:94–101, 1983.

CHAPTER THIRTY

Psychotherapy and the Headache Patient

CHARLES S. ADLER, M.D.
SHEILA MORRISSEY ADLER, PH.D.

"Socrates would prescribe no physic for Charmide's headache till first he had eased his troubled mind . . ." (1)

Since the time of Socrates, the importance of including "talk" in the treatment of headache has been recognized. This is most important today when, despite the prominence of psychological factors in chronic headache, only a small percentage of the 10–20% of the general population who suffers from it are ever seen in a setting which addresses emotional issues therapeutically. Such a setting might be with a psychiatrist interested in headache who has kept updated in his neurological training; or, it might be through a collaboration between a mental health professional and a neurologist or some other "treating physician." (In this chapter we will arbitrarily define the "treating" or "primary" physician as one whose specialization is in an area other than psychiatry.) Yet much of this treatment effort will fall directly upon the shoulders of the interested primary physician himself.

Primary physicians see approximately four times as many patients with psychiatric disturbances as do psychiatrists. The figure for patients with clear-cut physical manifestations and subdiagnostic psychological triggers—like many headaches—is probably skewed even more. Migraine patients, for example, are known to not readily seek help for their symptoms (2). We must thus be resourceful to bring effective help to those patients who might not realize the potential for relief available through a current and comprehensive approach to headache—one which may include psychotherapy.

In this chapter we will address the needs of both primary physicians and mental health providers. We begin by looking at the treatments typically used by treating physicians, and move sequentially toward more intricate forms of psychotherapy for headache. The reader is invited to direct his attention to those parts of the chapter which might prove most relevant to his practice.

Although psychological treatment for headache can be either plain or fancy, if it is to be effective it is always founded on the bedrock of the physician's empathic concern for the patient's plight. Following the diagnosis, the most important objective of the first few interviews is the establishment of a good rapport. If this is not secured the patient will sense it, and be unlikely to profit from therapy. If present, it forms the cornerstone of the therapeutic contract, and allows the physician to confront the patient's self-defeating character traits. To develop this rapport, the physician is sometimes required to see beneath a stoical facade or a regressed state that has put off others. Yet to do this effectively he may be best advised to rely upon the compassion which in part motivated him to enter medicine in the first place. Even if other factors require that psychotherapeutic goals be limited, if this empathy is present, and the dignity of the patient's struggle is recognized and communicated, the benefits derived from treatment will be greater than the sum of medications prescribed.

PSYCHIATRIC CARE AND THE TREATING PHYSICIAN

The primary physician often has a special relationship with his patient, one which has both advantages and disadvantages when it comes to treating the emotional aspects of headache. The advantages include: (a) his accrued knowledge of the patient, the patient's family, and their life situation; (b) established trust by virtue of significant previous encounters; (c) the patient's anticipation that the treating physician, because of his organic orientation, will understand the "the pain is real"; (d) he is initially less intimidating to talk to than a mental health professional for many

patients; and, (e) the patient may have greater confidence that his pharmacological needs will be attended to in a familiar manner.

Certain limitations also confront the primary physician working in this area. They include the following. (a) In a nonpsychiatric practice the physician's time is inherently more limited, more expensive due to overhead, and more subject to interruption by emergencies. (b) As specialists in other fields are only trained in the fundamentals of psychiatry, they often have justifiable apprehension about taking on an intensive psychotherapeutic role. The primary physician may also be unsure that talk alone can help, concerned that his professional image will become unclear, or worried that, like unchecked bleeding during surgery, the treatment situation will deteriorate and become uncontrolled in his hands. For example, he may fear that his interventions will simply release sorrow or dependency needs of critical proportions.

Castelnuevo-Tedesco (17), who has been teaching medical psychotherapy to primary physicians for years, recommends certain guidelines. First is that the primary physician only treat patients with mild-to-moderate emotional disturbance, based not on diagnosis but on degree of disruption of social and

TABLE 30.1.
PSYCHOTHERAPY FOR THE TREATMENT-RESISTANT HEADACHE PATIENT

Selinsky (3)	"The migrainous syndrome can be materially benefited by psychotherapy . . . only two or three of these 200 patients whom I examined have possibly ever been approached previously from this therapeutic viewpoint."
Sperling (4)	"In the thirteen to sixteen years of followup of the twenty-three migraine patients (14 adults, 9 children) I found that their treatment was a complete success. There has been no recurrence of the migraine headache in any of these cases to date. So far as I am aware such results have not been obtained with any other method of treatment."
Wolff (5)	"Of the fourteen subjects in this series who presented themselves as patients and who made an effort to deal with their problems, twelve secured relief in the sense that the attacks became fewer and less severe . . . in five persons who had had attacks at two-week intervals the episodes were reduced to three or four a year."

TABLE 30.1 (*Continued*)

Kolb (6)	"Psychotherapy is indicated certainly for all those patients in whom control of episodic headache may not be accomplished through pharmacologic treatment and in whom, in addition to headache, personality disorders play a predominant role in a general social maladaptation."
Knopf (7)	". . . the factor of "emotional disturbances" and "mental strain" . . . is no longer something that has to be accepted as inevitable and unchangeable . . . In the future it will not be enough to state that those factors have a contributing or perhaps causative influence, but psychotherapy will have to be made available as one of the means to combat this illness."
Karpman (8)	"Casual headaches are very common and may be ignored, but persistent headaches require definite attention . . . such headaches, including migraines, often respond satisfactorily to psychotherapy."
Hunter (9)	"[Describing results of psychotherapy for the treatment of migraine.] The most impressive feature was the overall reduction of interval medication. No relation was observed between duration of migraine and therapeutic result. Table IV shows that in 94% there was a significant improvement in migraine, in 86% in psychiatric disturbance, and in 97% a significant reduction of drug intake."
Howarth (10)	"[Describing results of study] Of the remaining 59 patients, 39 were individuals in whom stress factors had been found and within this group it was seen that where the stress factors were relieved all the patients showed improvement. Where stress factors continued to operate, which was in 20 patients, only 12 showed improvement. This was a difference significant at the 1% level (x = 7.6, p less than 0.01, 1 d.f.). (Tension headache.)"
Fromm-Reichmann (11)	". . . about the analytic therapy of migraine: five of my patients became practically cured; two got decided relief as to the number and intensity of their attacks; one remained practically uninfluenced."
Friedman (12)	"Nevertheless, an understanding of the underlying psychologic factors plays an important part in the management of migraine, for in the ability of the patient to handle emotional tension lies the most satisfactory means of preventing the attacks in the majority of the cases. (Migraine.)"
Friedman (13)	"It must be emphasized that the most effective prescription in treating chronic muscle contraction headache is dynamic psychotherapy, which tries to find the source of conflicts within the personality of the patient. (Tension headache.)"
Drake and Ebaugh (14)	"The treatment of choice in tension headache is a combination of psychotherapy and drug therapy. Psychotherapy is a more effective prophylactic than pharmaco-therapy. The number of therapeutic agents recommended for the treatment of tension headache indicates the unsatisfactory status of drug therapy alone for this condition. (Tension headache.)"
Alvarez (15)	"No treatment of migraine is satisfactory that does not make a careful appraisal of the personality of the migraine sufferer along with the management of the purely medical aspects of the problem."
Featherstone and Beitman (16)	"Psychotherapy may be quite helpful, since those who improved had a much higher entrance into psychotherapy than those who did not improve. (Marital migraine.)"

economic functioning. Naturally, this excludes the most serious emotional problems and far-reaching treatment goals. He has found that weekly 20-minute appointments are usually adequate for this purpose, and recommends that if after 10 such sessions progress has not been significant, psychiatric referral be considered.

He suggests that treatment focus on the one individual with whom the patient is having greatest difficulty in the present, and that it should avoid technical jargon. The physician's best techniques are usually the same ones he would use when helping a friend with a problem. Even giving direct "advice" is often beneficial if it stems from an objective understanding of the patient and his situation. Treating physicians usually have better instincts about how to help people with interpersonal problems than they give themselves credit for, and they do best when they rely on these as their primary psychotherapeutic tools. A large part of good clinical medicine is good listening, and in this the primary physician has had considerable training and practice.

Help should always be provided in a fashion that is congruent with the physician's personality. As every psychiatric resident at some point discovers, it is both awkward and unproductive to imitate a therapeutic style that doesn't really suit him. Suggestions in this chapter should not, therefore, be taken rigidly. Each physician will discover through trial and error how he works best with his patients' psychosocial needs, and which types of psychologically influenced patients he is most comfortable and successful with. One should never underestimate the value or validity of these self-taught lessons.

If he decides to take on a patient with more challenging psychological problems, it is recommended that the physician arrange to meet with a psychiatrist for formal collaboration. Such consultation improves one's ability to listen with his "third ear" for the remarkably recurrent themes related by headache patients. In time, the treating physician may feel excitement from recognizing clues to problems in the course of what had previously seemed like "chatter." In addition, he will come to more quickly recognize which patients have problems beyond his expertise, and will develop an effective and tactful style of referring them for more intensive treatment.

For the patient who ultimately requires referral for intensive psychotherapy, the time spent by the primary physician in attempting to handle the problem himself will have been time well spent. It will have oriented the patient to general concepts of psychiatric treatment, given him a feel for what to expect in psychotherapy, and given him a head start in learning about his specific problems. This makes it more likely that he will follow through with the referral and will stick with the treatment.

When to refer is not always clear-cut. Sometimes the physician knows he has reached this point because the patient's headaches get worse and are joined by other physical symptoms; sometimes he knows because new psychiatric symptoms appear, such as agitation, suicidal ruminations, or inappropriate behavior; sometimes it will be signaled by nothing more than the gradual but definite feeling that one is in over his head.

The method and timing of referral is important. One must convey to the patient that referral is not a sign that the primary physician has given up, and that his active involvement will continue. It reduces the patient's anxiety if the referral is made for a specific rather than a vague reason, when it is possible to give one.

In the authors' experience, headache patients often bring energy and motivation to psychotherapy, and make good use of it. It is important to find a psychiatrist who shares this optimism, one who is also sensitive to pitfalls in the psychotherapy of patients with physical problems. A personal conversation to explain the primary physician's perspective on the problem is important to supplement any written communications.

DEFINING TREATMENT GOALS

At the start of treatment it is important to consider its goals as clearly as possible, in collaboration with the headache patient. This is particularly true in short-term, highly focused treatment, because if this therapy wanders, it is soon over without accomplishing its purpose.

In a perfect world, reasonable therapeutic goals would be perfectly clear after the initial evaluation. In fact, goals are often somewhat hazy at the start of treatment. This is inevitable, as clarification of the patient's problems and needs continues throughout therapy, and his motivations and capacity to deal with psychological issues often become clear only after there has been an opportunity to observe his responses to interpretations and to the therapy process. The patient may also have hidden expectations of therapy; he may not even be aware of some of them. These hidden expectations often come to light as therapy proceeds.

The agreement between physician and patient to interact with each other in a certain way with the aim of accomplishing specific tasks is termed the "therapeutic contract." It defines the mission of the treatment and the responsibilities each of the parties has in pursuing it. Although this should be enunciated as clearly as possible, the physician need not reveal perceptions of the patient if to do so would be countertherapeutic; indeed, getting the patient to be able to hear and accept certain things about himself is often a major therapeutic goal in itself. For example, a wife who consciously feels only devotion towards her husband and is quite unconscious of her anger at him or of its relationship to her headaches might have treatment goals expressed in general terms. She need not be told that an aim of treatment is to understand her fury at her husband.

The wish for cure is often an unspoken expectation of the patient. It is sometimes helpful to remind him that the degree of symptom relief obtainable depends partly upon the natural history of the syndrome and partly upon the strength of the patient's genetic predisposition. If the prognosis is uncertain, it is better here to err on the side of optimism, better still on the side of silence. Still, because pain is the acknowledged reason that the headache patient visits the physician in the first place, its amelioration must be the starting point when defining goals. Thus, the physician should make clear that the psychotherapeutic work will be aimed at easing the effect of psychological disturbances upon the physiology, thereby reducing the tendency of such responses to eventuate in headache. Feasible goals may include diminution of headache intensity and frequency, modulation of the way in which pain is attended to, and reduction or elimination of disability accompanying pain. An example of a more specific goal might be: "One of our aims will be to see why you feel such unbearable tension at staff meetings; that will help us figure out how to prevent the headaches that follow them."

Goal-setting statements may be specific or general. Long-term uncovering therapy is usually facilitated by setting less specific goals. Headache exacerbation may be the most prominent symptom of a generally inefficient manner of relating to the world, one which also needs to be understood to make other areas of the patient's life symptom free and fulfilling.

Factors to consider when setting goals for therapy include: the patient's age; his psychological-mindedness and motivation for treatment; the level of his psychopathology and its duration; the presence of strong situational triggers (a good prognostic sign); the attitudes toward treatment, from supportive to destructive, of important family members; the patient's history of taking on, meeting, and surmounting challenges similar to psychotherapy in the past; the patient's experience, if any, with previous psychotherapists; and, even, unfortunately, his ability to afford treatment.

Sometimes the initial interview reveals that the most critical stimulus initiating the headache is an overwhelming reality situation rather than an intrapsychic difficulty. Here, the goal of therapy may simply be to help the patient cope effectively with his problems. A patient is often relieved and reassured when an authority figure specifically recognizes how much stress he has been trying to fend off; what is evident to his friends may be inapparent to the patient.

A patient starting psychodynamic psychotherapy should be prepared for the sometimes difficult nature of what he is about to undertake, as treatment occasionally brings up feelings he would rather not confront. He should be told that coming to grips with discomfiting feelings will reduce their ability to interminably or recurrently nibble away at his emotional well-being in ways that exacerbate headache.

THREE LEVELS OF PSYCHOLOGICAL ASSISTANCE

Like snowflakes, patients are only indistinguishable from far away. Treating a patient on the basis of his diagnosis alone does not afford full recognition of his uniqueness. Thus, a treatment successful with one patient may fail miserably with another, even though they share the same diagnosis. Therefore, although psychological treatment of headache can range from the concrete to the abstract, it is the type which most closely fits the specific needs of the patient which is "best"—all other criteria are moot.

Generally, three levels of therapy for the emotional aspects of headache can be identified, none of which is inherently better than the other—each has patients for whom it fits just right. Although these three categories can be theoretically defined and bounded, in practice their borders are more porous. A patient's mental state is as dynamic as his physiological one, and his changing needs demand that the therapist shift the fulcrum of therapeutic technique to meet these needs.

The first level is that of support, education, and helping the patient to rearrange some of the external contingencies in his life. The second level involves dynamic psychotherapy of limited depth, length, or objectives. The third level involves long-term psychotherapy or psychoanalysis which aims at creating major, permanent changes in the patient's psyche or character.

All physicians should be able to provide the first level of help. Many primary physicians may be interested in providing the second level of help, either alone or in collaboration with a mental health professional. The third level of treatment is performed only by specialists.

SIMPLE SUPPORT

Almost all headache patients can benefit from the techniques of simple support. The physician's tools are his availability, predictability, patience, interest, knowledge, empathy, and authority; these are powerful tools, never to be underestimated. Considering the discouraging odyssey headache patients have often traveled, reassuring the patient that the doctor will stick with him as long as his distress remains unsolved is the cornerstone of such support. The techniques of simple support can be represented by the acronym MERVE: *Medicate, Educate, Regulate, Ventilate, Exonerate.*

MEDICATE

The presence of medication at the top of the list is not meant to imply that it is the most important element in supportive care. Obviously, the first consideration in prescribing drugs is whether their pharmachological actions will be helpful. Nevertheless, when—and even whether—drugs are prescribed for a particular patient is determined *in part* by the symbolism drugs have for the patient. For example, tranquilizers given in the first session may indicate to a patient that the physician feels the case is too hopeless to treat any other way, or that he is not interested in finding out which situations cause the headaches. Conversely, the giving of drugs may be viewed as a sign of the physician's interest, with the drugs themselves then becoming a valued talisman symbolizing that interest.

Thus, although medication alone is rarely sufficient therapy for a chronic painful illness, when prescribed for well-chosen reasons it can convey to the patient that the physician takes the patient's suffering seriously, and is interested in helping with all the tools at his disposal. This necessarily implies that the rationale for taking this route is communicated to the patient in private conference, rather than leaving him to read it from the prescription slip in the hallway following the appointment. The art of prescribing dovetails with other aspects of the physician/patient relationship, as patients feel a sense of contact with the doctor through the doctor's medicine. Good feelings about the physician make his pills work better.

The psychoactive drugs typically used for emotional aspects of headache can be divided into sedative/hypnotic and antidepressant categories. Psychostimulants, such as dextroamphetamine, currently have no indications in the treatment of headache, and neuroleptics are used but rarely.

Ataraxic medications, such as benzodiazepines, can be useful in situational crises or periods of decompensation. Hypnotics may be given for several nights in sequence to break into a pattern of insomnia, or may be used every third night over a slightly longer period.

The applications of antidepressants to headaches is covered in detail in Chapters 13 and 24. When they are given for depressive symptoms, these drugs are typically more effective if vegetative signs (insomnia, weight loss, constipation, impotence, trouble concentrating, decreased psychomotor behavior) are present, and are less likely to help if the depressive posture is a longstanding characterologic response to life's inevitable disappointments. If the treating physician encounters unsatisfactory results with such a drug regimen, however, it is commonly because

the dosage is too small or the trial time too short.[1]

EDUCATE

The patient with chronic illness often has a distorted perception of his body, especially of the afflicted part. Even intelligent and otherwise sophisticated patients are not immune to these misperceptions; as a result, a useful screening technique is to inquire about what the patient understands to happen during his headaches, prior to offering an explanation (which might otherwise not cover and relieve his specific worry). Educational methods using illustrations can help counter fantasies of frightening anatomic and physiologic transformations during a headache if these are uncovered. In addition, the physician needs to describe the effect of stress on bodily functions and on the pathways for headache in particular, so the patient can appreciate that the connection between stress and pain is physiological rather than mystical.

Blau (18) has documented the need for the physician to directly ask the patient about any fears or fantasies. He describes extensive and previously unreported fears or phobias in

---

[1] Just as the psychological is entwined with the somatic in the causation of headaches, the psychotropic and somatic actions of the medications used to treat them also seem to be curiously inseparable. The ability of low-dose tricyclic antidepressants to help headaches in seemingly nondepressed patients is one example. The mechanism for this is not entirely clear. It has been hypothesized that, for tension headache, it may work by inducing vasodilation in the cephalic musculature. Ataraxic drugs such as diazepam also often act as muscle relaxants, and most medications marketed as muscle relaxants are also, to some extent, calming. Patients perceive the fixed combinations of minor analgesics and barbiturates merely as "strong pain killers," unaware that their only difference from over-the-counter preparations is the barbiturate. Narcotics, of course, in addition to being potent analgesics, are potent tranquilizers. This is evidenced by the number of street addicts who pay a great price for a narcotic's ability to help their emotional pain.

50 of 75 outpatients with migraine. These included fears of death, disability, insanity, and "bursting" of the head, as well as of neoplasm. He suspects such fears may increase the patient's discomfort during attacks.

The patient with migraine will likely be aware that constitutional factors play a role in the disorder. It is important to impress upon him that a genetic tendency is not as much like a judge's sentence as it is like a judge's warning. If those inherent proclivities are treated with knowledge and respect, the patient is not doomed to suffer the endless cycle of migraine his father endured.

When all other treatments finally prove to be of limited help, the patient needs to "learn to live with his pain" or, more accurately, in spite of it. The physician can encourage him to figure out how to do this. He can assist the patient in fashioning a philosophy for dealing with pain through discussions about the meaning of pain in one's life, the difference between handicap and disability, and the relevance of attitude. Sometimes the patient's family also needs to be educated about the patient's headaches about their treatment and even, on some unfortunate occasions, about their reality.

REGULATE

A headache patient's life should be led·at a reasonable rate with a comfortable, predictable rhythm. It may be necessary for the physician to emphasize the correlation between certain activities which the patient can control, such as skipping meals, and the physiologic response that eventuates in headache. The physician can also discuss how a balanced program of regular exercise can discharge tensions, modulate aggression, and reduce the patient's susceptibility to external stressors.[2]

If the patient repeatedly reports or it is repeatedly observed that other "priorities" defeat his wish to avoid things that lower his threshold for headache—for example, drinking at parties or staying up too late—the phy-

sician should challenge the patient to puzzle out his motivation for behaviors which treat his body with such disregard.

VENTILATE

Many patients with headache have built up large stores of anger, resentment, or grief, and have no one with whom they can talk to "get it off their chest." Here, it can be enough for the physician to provide a nonjudgmental atmosphere in which the patient is given an opportunity to share his fears, ventilate his anger, and be coached through periods of discouragement. This often results in reduction of tensions, and will sometimes even lead the patient to spontaneously abreact a particularly difficult experience which is affecting his headaches. The physician need not indicate that he agrees with all of the patient's perceptions and hostilities, but by remaining silently interested he is not really doing so. Instead, he gives the patient a chance to say how *he* saw what happened and how *he* felt about it. This is especially valuable with the patient who seems to be burdened with great wellsprings of inner pressure.

EXONERATE

Because the headache patient is frequently ruled by an overzealous superego, he may

---

[2] This is especially true with migraine and cluster headache patients. Meals should be eaten at regular intervals and, especially with migraineurs, should not be skipped. Patients susceptible to dietary triggers of migraine can be given reference material on practical ways to avoid the specific foods they have found relevant to their headaches. Periods of rest during the day, though not napping, are important for the patient to schedule, even if he has not learned a formal relaxation technique. Having the patient chart his daily activities for several weeks may help both physician and patient to determine which situations are most likely to precede headaches. Patients who develop migraine on weekends should be encouraged not to "sleep in," and to schedule some activities which approximate the more active pace of the weekday.

need the doctor's help in challenging it. If the physician becomes aware that this harsh conscience is causing a patient to have unrealistic and self-punitive attitudes about perceived past failures or past misdeeds he should try to reduce them. When the patient is himself incapable of abdicating certain intolerable responsibilities, the physician may need to use his medical authority to permit the patient to do so without feeling guilty. With selected patients, one way to challenge this superego is to issue old fashioned "doctor's orders" prohibiting the patient from overtaxing himself in specific areas where he has set unreasonably high expectations. When the patient is too anxious or ashamed to face his family with his limitations, it is sometimes helpful to have a conference to advise the family that it is not in the interest of the patient's health to continue certain duties.

PSYCHODYNAMIC PSYCHOTHERAPY

THE CONTINUUM

In the first part of this chapter we refer to two types of psychological assistance, supportive and psychodynamic, which can be further divided into three segments on a treatment continuum. The first segment has been covered under "simple support." The major factors distinguishing the second from the third segments of this continuum are the intensity of the therapy and extent of its goals. Naturally, this implies some differences in technique; but the basic understanding of the patient from which these techniques are derived does not change. Methods of treatment in the second segment emphasize understanding the interaction between life events and consciously accessible feeling states, as well as the patient's attempts to cope with both. Treatment in the third segment puts more emphasis on understanding the role of unconscious or unrecognized motives in the patient's feelings, behavior, and symptoms.

In this treatment continuum, the role of the therapist is that of navigator, continually maneuvering the discussion along the optimal channel between the shoals of premature interpretation and the reefs of too little challenge. Because they differ primarily in degree, the process and the techniques of segments 2 and 3 will be considered together.

THE PROCESS

In the sanctuary of the doctor's office, the patient has a chance to evaluate the realities of the situations he faces and the appropriateness of his reactions to them. Because the patient needs to relate his entire history in a relatively short time, he is helped to see its continuity, and the connections between past and present attitudes he has held toward life are made more vivid. When viewing his life in chronological perspective, patterns become apparent that are missed in just living it day to day.

Because the patient knows the relevant aspects of his own story better than anyone, the physician does not need to lead him every step of the way. It is truly striking how well patients who feel they are being listened to compassionately guide their own self-reflections to create a favorable therapeutic experience. Headache patients especially do better when their part in the therapy is active rather than passive, with the therapist acting as a "consultant" during these self-reflections.

If the patient's characteristic responses to events and people in his life are inappropriate, he is encouraged to consider whether he is reacting to events in the present on the basis of relationships and conditions that existed in the past. Then, doctor and patient work together to discover if there are specific correlations between events and feelings of the past and reactions in the present. If this proves to be the case, the patient is reminded or helped to see that, although his options for feeling and acting were limited when he came up against important problems when he was younger, his current capacity to understand and influence situations is far greater.

Even though the patient may not learn all of the relevant analogs to his current ways of reacting, he will often feel better simply through this discovery: *there are reasons; a certain type of logic regulates how he feels and what he does.* The patient is typically relieved when he recognizes that many of his emotional symptoms are the result of specific causes in the course of his development, rather than the random aftereffects of misfortune.

As he is listening, the physician tries to construct in his mind's eye an overall model of the patient's life and feelings, complete with an image of the characters and motivations of the principal players. In successive sessions, as in successive acts of a play, new characters are introduced, the therapist's view of the old ones becomes clearer and more enriched, and the pattern of relationships and points of the drama start falling into place.

As the therapist tracks the patient's story, he listens for emotional reactions to events or their absence as closely as he listens to the description of the events themselves. He ponders what emotions and motivations accompany behavioral descriptions, and whether these are consciously accessible or have been mischievously diverted by the patient's defenses.

If, as the patient talks, he seems to be unaware of what he is feeling—as evidenced by a dissociation between affect and mannerisms—the therapist will usually point this out. To do this accurately, the therapist must synthesize his abilities to listen and observe with his intuition and compassion.

It is important that the physician allow himself the gratification of listening to the patient's story with the same active curiosity he has when reading a novel or watching a play. Because many conflicts can aggravate chronic headaches or be aggravated by them, the best way to truly understand the patient's specific problem is to listen carefully to his story on a rational and an intuitive level. The most relevant problem can exist far beyond what is

usually inquired about. It can range from something as simple as envy of a co-worker to a frustrated yearning for existential meaning in life.

It is within this context that the patient talks about his headaches and brings up things he considers stressful or otherwise important, whether the connection with headache is clear or not. Recurring patterns of cognition, emotion, and behavior start to reveal themselves as therapy proceeds. The physician tries to discern situational and emotional patterns that precede or accompany headache, and to identify the particular elements within them that are most distressing for the patient.

These recurrent emotional themes or patterns of behavior should generally be pointed out, including those that occur in the relationship with the therapist. The aim of such interpretations is not merely to discourage self-defeating behavior, but to arouse the patient's curiosity about his motivation for that behavior. It is helpful to ask oneself how the headaches could be seen as an adaptive innovation designed by unconscious defenses to solve a specific problem or to restore the patient's psychic equilibrium.

Whenever a common theme is observed to precede headaches (which can be by as much as 3 days in migraine), the patient's attention is drawn to it. The therapist then attempts to further characterize the common denominator, and to refine his understanding of why it is so important. These insights are then referred back to when trying to reconstruct the events leading up to headaches reported in subsequent sessions.

It is generally acknowledged that intellectual understanding of symptom dynamics is by itself rarely sufficient to effect long-term character change. As most psychological problems spring from troubled or conflicting motivations rather than from intellectual or educational shortcomings, they rarely can be repaired through intellect alone. This has particular pertinence to headache patients, many of whom already overemphasize the use of intellect to the detriment of adequate contact with their fears, hurts, and needs. Thus it is important for the patient to actually experience and acknowledge his states of conflicting and competing emotions while still maintaining an observant attitude. Intellect and cognition play an important part in therapeutic insight, but alone do not comprise it. The visceral insight process is facilitated as the patient sees that the physician is not discomfited when strong feelings arise.

Over the course of more extended therapy the patient can expect to have periods when things are going well, periods when progress seems stuck at a plateau, even periods when his situation seems temporarily worse. This is the normal pattern of progress towards better functioning.

As in other areas of medicine, there may be brief relapses even after "successful" treatment. These can usually be handled by "booster sessions." In short, the patient returns for several sessions and is helped through a period of added difficulty. Like an actual booster shot, the earlier therapeutic experiences and insights are typically reawakened by these sessions, which both strengthens and speeds up their therapeutic effect.

Additional factors in the psychotherapy process are pace, resistance, and transference.

Pace

Therapy for each patient has its own inherent rate and rhythm. The optimal rate at which therapy can proceed is determined by following the patient's lead, by careful observation of the patient's responses and, finally, by trained intuition and analysis. Elements that must be factored into this equation include: longevity of symptoms, the patient's emotional sensibility, his "ego strength" and capacity to use insight, the extent to which his social milieu can accommodate revisions and, finally, the extent to which the patient's headaches have become enmeshed in serving the needs of his character bureaucracy. Important in this regard are headaches that have become necessary for justifying pivotal life decisions or failures, as these may need to be relinquished at a slower pace. The inertia of the emotional status quo necessitates that even under ideal conditions there are limits to how rapidly permanent psychological change can be effected.

Once the patient develops confidence that the therapist will not pressure him impatiently or insensitively and that he will be allowed a measure of control in the therapy process, feelings of trust and security start to solidify. The doctor and his office become valued symbols of sanctuary within which the patient can retreat to rethink and reflect. The therapist also becomes an objective friend who can be trusted to act in the relationship without hidden personal motives. Under this protective umbrella, the patient feels safer to think about the implications of what he says without having to "watch what he says" for fear of unraveling someone's aggression. Such a situation may even confer temporary immunity from the patient's own aggressive attitudes and impulses toward himself while he reappraises his reactions to life.

The therapist who mistakenly feels he is facilitating therapy when he pushes the patient to "get on with it," or "stop wasting time," or "come to the point" does so at some risk. In much the same way that a bony callus forms around a fracture to protect it, psychiatric symptoms may have built up around ancient emotional injuries to stabilize these injuries and reduce the pain they cause. If one tries to shave away such symptoms too fast or to break down such defenses too quickly, various forms of resistance appear which advise the therapist to slow down. If the therapist does not heed these warnings and keeps pushing, either the resistances will increase, forcing therapy into a stalemate, or the patient will leave treatment, or the disrupted defenses will release too much emotion too soon. In this last condition, the original psychological trauma that had previously been contained by headache or other symptoms is prematurely exposed to the patient, leaving him unprotected and vulnerable.

In short, treatment that is pushed rather than guided, and self-knowledge that is thrust upon the patient rather than offered to him may cause a shock wave; the reverberations of that shock wave can include regression, retreat, or exacerbation of both headache and psychiatric symptoms. The patient may develop depression, paranoia, or other symptomatic manifestations of his inability to deal constructively with these painful insights or memories. At these points, doctors are prone to remember the statement of Publius Syrus that "there are some remedies worse than the disease." On the other hand, this capacity of unconscious mechanisms to manufacture additional symptoms when the patient's equilibrium with his past is threatened with faster change than it can accommodate may also be used by the physician as a source of feedback about the effects of his interventions.

Especially with headache patients, the feeling of lack of control that can result from painful material being rooted out too quickly can be a foreign and disquieting experience. During the initial stages of treatment they may want to reassure themselves that the physician will permit them some measure of control over the rate at which historical events and reactions will be uncovered and, within limits, they should be accorded this prerogative. This is one of the keys to successful therapy with headache patients, and its abrogation is one of the most common causes of failure.

Resistance

Resistance is one of the hallmarks of psychotherapy with patients, and headache patients are no exception; they often show even more resistance. At some point in treatment, the therapist may observe that a patient becomes uncomfortable or anxious about certain topics or insights, or expresses reluctance to delve into them further.

Generally, of course, the principal goal of therapy is for the patient to overcome resistance and make peace with truths behind it; nevertheless, achievement of this goal should not be allowed to run roughshod over the clear message from the patient that danger zones are being approached, that, for many possible reasons, sometimes good ones, he is feeling threatened. At these points, the therapist is faced with a choice: either to augment or to challenge the resistance. To make this decision, the therapist must consider the patient's tolerance level for challenge and need for temporary protection from the feelings being resisted. Here, the therapist necessarily will consider the resistance within the context of the patient's life circumstances, and his status in therapy: What can the patient constructively bear? Will kindness to him dictate inquiries honed to reveal to him that piece of the puzzle, that part of the truth which he resists? Or will it instead dictate a temporary refocusing of treatment to shield him from prematurely recognizing these things?

Resistance always involves anxiety; however, the particular feelings or memories which are causing the anxiety varies. A frequent culprit with the headache patient is fear of betraying allegiance to his family. He may even feel guilty on this score just by going along with the idea that something about his past might be contributing to his problems, and might even wonder out loud, "Maybe I'm just feeling sorry for myself. . . . my problems are no worse than what everyone puts up with. . . ." Many a headache patient has been observed to fear that anything but unquestioning family loyalty is treasonous. Just by continuing to look at himself in therapy, the patient often thinks he is being disloyal to his family. When there is such frantic backpedaling and strong resistance, even the most sophisticated patient sometimes needs to be reminded that the point of therapy is not to place blame or find scapegoats.

As therapy continues, the headache patient is frequently seen to come into contact with feelings of anger toward early caretakers, the resistance to which, when present, is often manifested as guilt. As recognition of such anger will generally find its way to consciousness in its own time, the therapist should be especially cautious about applying pressure in this area (19).

Headache patients frequently have a significantly harder time dealing with anger or with situations that would normally trigger anger. When repressed or suppressed for many years, anger may accumulate, with the result that the patient fears his anger is unusually strong or dangerous. If a patient's recognition of an underlying anger enters into his associations in a gradually increasing, seesaw fashion, he may need reassurance that recognizing and even experiencing this anger does not mean he must act on it; it need not destroy his valued relationships. Indeed, a common aim of therapy with headache patients is to eventually allow such anger to diminish, though not, this time, through repression, but as a consequence of identification and acceptance of what has gone before. What the patient recognizes—in a way considerably more profound than it appears superficially—is that he no longer must feel immersed in the contingencies of childhood or their emotional consequences because he is no longer a child. He, in partnership with circumstance, now has the greatest say in shaping the emotional contingencies of life. This perspective on reality also applies when the traumatic situations were encountered after childhood, though these usually leave a less permanent stamp.

Anger occasionally arises towards the therapist, usually initiated by some real, though minor, insensitivity on his part, which becomes exaggerated in the patient's mind. If the patient represses his hurt and anger, as he often will, migraine has been observed to start right within the therapeutic hour (11, 20, 21). When the patient has been helped to identify and directly express his anger in these sessions beginning migraines have been reported to recede, demonstrating for the patient the relevance of unexpressed anger to his headache diathesis. A working through of conflicts that inhibit normal expression of self-assertion is a milestone in the therapy of most chronic headache patients.

Transference

Reduced to its essence, the principle of transference states that a person expects from relationships what he has learned—and mislearned—to expect from relationships. It can also be defined as the reexperiencing of emotional contingencies of the past in adult relationships where they do not actually fit. The most crucial learning of this sort occurs in early childhood, at which time the child's mind observes and absorbs the contingencies of his particular environment; these become translated into the rules he will later anticipate and instill into important adult relationships. Curiously, these expectations eventually become relatively, though not entirely, impervious to modification simply by virtue of having different and better experiences with people later in life. The concept of transference is central to understanding psychodynamics both of headache patients and of patients with other psychologically ·influenced chief complaints.

How are these expectations acquired? A youngster of 6 may learn, for example, to expect that if he tries to "help Mom with lunch," he will be commended for his initiative; or he may learn to expect punishment for disturbing her routine and "making a mess." He may further learn that he can cut his punishment short by adopting an obedient and submissive demeanor; or he might discover that there is absolutely no way to predictably escape punishment. Experience may teach him to expect specific types of punishment as well: one child will routinely get the "silent treatment" while another routinely gets "the switch." By the time they have grown to adulthood, these patients will unconsciously prepare themselves differently, both psychologically and *physiologically,* for these different expected outcomes in relationships with authority figures, with resultant implications for susceptibility to headache type. This example shows how a child extrapolates lessons from innumerable tiny interchanges with his parents and other central figures, such as brothers and sisters. These "lessons" point toward some final assumptions, correct and incorrect, concerning what life with people is all about. The incorrect ones are transference.

Few people ever resurrect the influences that went into these conclusions and judge them afresh from the perspective of an adult. Therefore, the phenomenon of transference is fairly universal. The better the childhood environment and the defenses used to cope with it, the weaker and less deleterious is the influence of transference. But when it does cause trouble, the patient will find himself misinterpreting interpersonal signals and reacting to people in accordance with these misinterpretations. This can disrupt important relationships, even in patients whose functioning is not compromised enough for a psychiatric diagnosis.

The transference can include positive expectations as well as negative ones. "Positive transference" shows up in treatment in the form of a patient's exaggerated or magical expectations of the therapist's power, interest, or ability to cure. Patients sometimes thrive temporarily when bathed in the glow of such an artificially idealized relationship; this is technically referred to as a "transference cure." Although praise from patients is flattering to hear, if it seems to be a regard that the physician has not yet had an opportunity to fully earn, he should recognize it as a case of mistaken identity. Positive transference is also subject to extremely rapid, and equally undeserved, reversal.

When they exist, the negative aspects of transference are most comfortably seen in descriptions of the patient's relationships to family members or workmates. It is here that the patient can also best be helped to see his anachronistic expectations. Less comfortable to observe, but no less real, is if the patient has a transference reaction to the therapist. While it is sometimes necessary to analyze transference feelings, especially negative ones, that arise towards a therapist in psychotherapy, this task is rarely central to treatment, and it is an especially risky business with headache patients. However, it is always im-

portant to quickly identify and correct important, negative, transference-induced feelings about the therapist in order to neutralize their potential to scuttle treatment. It is even more helpful if the therapist can use these misperceptions to better understand the patient and to advance the therapy. In aiding the patient to see his exaggerated response (transference reaction) it helps immeasurably to acknowledge the small kernel of truth that usually initiates the overreaction.

The therapist can often anticipate from the psychosocial history which attitudes and behavior the patient might be hypersensitive to; he can then be particularly careful that he does not realistically aggravate these potential transference expectations. With the migraine patient, for example, this frequently includes having a critical attitude, inhibiting the patient's expressions of assertiveness or annoyance, having expectations of the patient which are unduly high or insufficiently flexible, and conveying a feeling that the patient's illness or troubles are inconveniencing the doctor. For many headache patients, the physician's prescribing habits and promptness for appointments can become battlegrounds, whether identified as such or not. Avoiding the patient's vulnerable areas not only safeguards against hurting him by reopening old wounds, but also allows the therapist a clear view of any transference misperceptions. If, for example, the patient comments, "I was out of ergotamine when a terrible migraine started Saturday morning, but didn't call the office for a refill until Monday because I knew you wouldn't want to be disturbed on weekends. . . .", it is essential for the physician to be perfectly clear that nothing about his interactions with the patient had inhibited him from calling outside office hours. This knowledge increases the physician's confidence when he concludes that one cause of the patient's low self-esteem is an expectation of intolerance from others. Such an encounter occurring early in therapy can alert the therapist to watch for similar transference patterns in the patient's dealings outside the office. He might notice, for example, that this same patient regularly submits himself to minor indignities at the hands of his department chairman. Pointing out analogies between problematic current interpersonal situations and the position the patient felt himself to be in emotionally in the past helps the patient to see not only *what* is misperceived, but *why* it is. After the patient becomes aware of these similarities between then and now he is aided to see the essential—and previously unrecognized—differences between the two.

COMMON TREATMENT ISSUES IN HEADACHE

Certain issues are common in psychodynamic psychotherapy with headache patients. These do not necessarily come as single notes sequentially arranged in time, but rather as point and counterpoint, as melodies weaving through the course of treatment.

Superego and Excessive Expectations

One of these is the need to confront a patient's unreasonable expectations of himself. He will often need to reevaluate both the form and the content of his superego. Helping him evolve a more empathic, less critical view of himself is frequently one of the cornerstones of successful therapy. The benefits of a reality-based reduction in the stridor and inflexibility of these expectations has often been cited.

The patient can be asked to search out and reflect upon those experiences that originally formed the basis of his attitude towards himself. However, this task usually has meaning only after incidents come to light which reveal to the patient's inner ear the shrill and uncompromising tones of his conscience. The patient sees in such incidents that, when compared to the standards of performance held by friends and colleagues, his own lack perspective. The therapist may initially need to point out that inequitable obligations are not simply unreasonable: they are also unfair. A

migraineur, for example, might acknowledge this disparity, yet somehow not "feel right" acting otherwise. The therapist then needs to reinforce the patient's own recognition of this disparity. In time, further examples of the patient's intolerance for his human fallibility inevitably arise, at which point he should be increasingly encouraged to come to grips with his fear of change.

Increasing the Patient's Perspective

If the patient has inappropriate guilt or disappointment about how he handled a situation in his youth, he may not realize that the circumstances he was faced with would have been difficult for almost anyone; when this was true he needs to develop empathy towards his limitations or failures. Thus, the therapist should help the patient gain a realistic perspective on shameful episodes in his personal history if this is lacking. In a similar vein, the patient can often be helped to make peace with the important people in his past and, especially, with his parents when those relationships have been marked by seemingly unresolvable bitterness, anger, submissiveness, or disappointment. For example, if the quality of parenting was limited due to their emotional problems, it often benefits the patient to conceptualize his parents' limitations as a sort of illness, one symptom of which is an inability to provide certain things children need, and to consider that the parent might have been really incapable of behaving differently. This helps the patient view his parents' character traits from a neutral or empathic, rather than solely from a moral or self-involved, vantage point. It also allows the patient to see that if there was a void or an ongoing aggravant in the relationship, the lack may have been in the parent, and may not have been due to some essential inadequacy or failing in the patient himself. In this way the patient neither has to deny a problem nor like it but, by virtue of developing an accurate empathy, may learn to reduce the bitterness, hurt, or lack of self-confidence which can be a consequence of misperceptions about the causes of the troubled relationship. And ultimately, to learn that there is something of value, even in imperfect relationships, something which can be accepted, perhaps even loved.

For many patients, self-punitive tendencies are tied to their incorporation of the expectations of a harsh or domineering parent. This is through the defense of identification with the aggressor. If the patient were to relinquish these aspects of his superego—that is, of his identification—he would be emotionally thrown back in time to the situation that existed before the identification, when he felt vulnerable to the parents' demands, scorn, resentment, emotional isolation, punishments, or condemnation. The feelings evoked by being at the receiving end of these attitudes are in great measure obviated if the patient shares his parent's same strict attitudes toward the childlike impulses within himself. If, as an adult, he starts to remember and have empathy for the feelings of that child, he is again buffeted by the original anxiety, anger, and loneliness. This explains why one sees this curious phenomenon of a patient who is reluctant to give up an intolerant attitude towards himself. Reassessing this defense is one way in which psychotherapy can help the patient maneuver through a difficult period of intensive maturation.

Anxiety

A predominant source of anxiety in headache patients is their fear of not being well thought of in social interchanges, or of failing to perform up to standards. The migraine or tension headache patient may project overly critical aspects of his superego onto others, and may not expect to be viewed in a tolerant manner by them. For the tension headache patient, fear of actual verbal or physical attack is sometimes seen as well, although it may only be experienced as a vague and diffuse foreboding.

While these anxieties are in one sense certainly understandable and even predicta-ble, the portion of the anxiety that springs from the patient's misperception of other's motives, for example, that they would not tolerate his taking a break from responsibilities, is what can be profitably worked on in treatment.

Migraineurs—but especially cluster patients—report anxiety about the headaches striking at just the wrong time, when they are trapped in some situation and unable to take prompt evasive action. The cluster patient may dread having an attack when he is confined and unable to lock himself away in solitude to weather the storm and give vent to the accompanying feelings. During a cluster period many such patients fear an attack starting when they are aboard an airplane, for example. The less able the cluster patient is to refrain from actions that would appear unstable to outsiders, the greater this fear.

Many headache patients structure their lives in a carefully balanced equilibrium; events which require major changes, induce upheavals, or demand flexibility in the face of uncertainty, all threaten this equilibrium in unknown ways, and can cause anxiety. Winds of change are especially threatening to the patient living in a house of cards!

Finally, continual interaction with someone overburdened with aggressive energies can destabilize patients with migraine or tension headaches. They sometimes need the therapist's help to simply—and permanently—extricate themselves from that relationship.

Anger

Feelings that follow insight can run the gamut from disappointment to rage. Because many of the insights alluded to earlier signal a partial separation from the internalized image of an important relationship, they may also trigger feelings of loss. It sometimes happens that anger is finally confronted when the patient recounts, in an affectless tone of voice, a tale of having been treated in a way that would typically evoke both hurt and anger. The therapist might comment, "Most of the time if a child comes home to find that, without his being told, his pet has been 'put to sleep' for convenience, he would not only feel sad, but betrayed." In the reflective silence that follows, the patient may at long last get angry, and may recognize that other sources of anger have been stewing inside him over the years. Because he does not try to push the anger away this time, his physiology does not rebound into a headache, and an important benchmark has been reached.

Sadness

Another common theme in psychotherapy of headache patients is the need to recognize and work through feelings of repressed sadness for the composite small signs of disapproval, disinterest, and disaffection on the part of a relevant caretaking figure. Certain elements in the family experience are recollected with greater frequency by headache patients. These include: little discussion of feelings; a general atmosphere of coldness, minimal empathy, and insensitive discipline; exploitative expectations for achievement at school or in athletics; perfunctory advice at menarche; an immaculately groomed parent who was reluctant to touch or be touched; and persistent favoritism for one of the siblings. One way to make memories of home more vivid is to ask the patient to contrast them with other important relationships, ones in which he remembers a different emotional tone. For example, headache patients often recall contacts with an especially loving grandparent, uncle, or neighbor who provided a counterpoint to the home atmosphere.

Unresolved Grief

A fourth theme that frequently surfaces during psychotherapy of the headache patient is unresolved grief (23). This term refers to present-day symptoms, often subtle and pervasive, which are consequent to bottled up feelings. Sadness predominates, but isn't the only one. These result from the patient not having undergone normal and necessary mourning for an important loss. The loss is usually that of a parent, spouse, child, or sibling through death, divorce, or abandonment. Grief (the emotional component of bereavement) and mourning (the cognitive and behavioral working through of grief) are suppressed or repressed.

Mourning involves the intermittent, involuntary remembering, over a period of months or years, of images and feelings about the lost person, of his attributes, and of experiences shared with him. Many of these rememberings are accompanied by crying spells. This painful but normal process is necessary to relegate the loss to the past, as well as to vividly recover and durably retain the good memories from the relationship.

In unresolved grief the need for mourning is blocked and remains unfinished business. As a result, the patient may be beset by depression, anxieties, or physical symptoms such as headache. These symptoms recur until the process by which grief is unburdened is completed. If mourning is never resumed, the resulting dysphoria and interference with new relationships can last a lifetime. So may the accompanying headaches.

Recognizing unresolved grief is important because it is treatable and, in many patients, will lead to remission. If the therapist gently encourages the patient to review the details of his relationship with the person, even mourning delayed 40 years can be completed, often with surprising rapidity. It helps to remind patients that the brain contains a protective mechanism which, like a circuit breaker, intermittently shuts off the grieving to prevent it from becoming unbearable. This same mechanism continues discharging and dampening surges of memory throughout the mourning process. And, bit by bit, the power of these memories to disrupt the flow of life is neutralized. Therapy here is simple, direct, and rewarding for the therapist. Unresolved grief is, however, an exception to the rule that time alone heals all wounds.

Existential Determinants

Another issue which frequently arises in therapy is the existential meanings that the head pain may have acquired (24). The justification for major decisions in life, such as not accepting a promotion or not going to graduate school, may have been largely based upon an anticipation that continuing headaches would make these ventures too difficult. Over the years, the headaches may even evolve into a major theme around which the patient relates to others: he is known as the man whose life is dominated by migraines. He must perceive the headaches as an indomitable foe to feel that a lifetime fighting them was not a lifetime squandered. An unconscious ambivalence about losing the headaches ensues.

The psychological literature (25) contains accounts of patients blind since birth whose vision was restored in midlife through surgery. Many of these patients, rather than becoming elated, became depressed; some committed suicide. It was hypothesized that this curative operation had made their past suffering and their endurance despite it seem wasted and meaningless. Similar dynamics may be operative in the headache patient past midlife whose treatment lags unaccountably. Thus, the physician should keep evaluating, throughout treatment, not only whether the patient's headaches are better, but whether the patient's life is better.

There is an adage in surgery: "It may be difficult to cut out pain with a knife." It is also difficult to blunt the propensity to pain with a drug. Although the complexity of psychogenic factors which need to be managed when treating psychological aspects of headache may appear intimidating, most will yield ground to the common sense of the compassionate physician.

REFERENCES

1. Moeuch G: *Headache.* Chicago, Yearbook Publishers, 1947, p 187.
2. Bille B: Migraine in children. In Carroll JD, Pfaffenrath V, Sjaastad O (eds): *Migraine and Beta-Blockade.* Molndal, AB Hassle, 1985, pp 110–115.
3. Selinsky H: Psychological study of the migrainous syndrome. *NY Acad Med Bull* 15:757–763, 1939.
4. Sperling M: A further contribution to the psychoanalytic study of migraine and psychogenic headaches. *Int J Psychoanal* 45: 549–557, 1964.
5. Wolff HG: Personality features and reactions of subjects with migraine. *Arch Neurol* 37:895–921, 1937.
6. Kolb LC: Psychiatric aspects of the treatment of headache. *Neurology* 13:34–37, 1963.
7. Knopf O: Preliminary report on personality studies in thirty migraine patients. *J Nerv Ment Dis* 82:270–285, 400–414, 1935.
8. Karpman B: Psychogenic aspects of headache. A symposium. *Clin Psychopathol* 10:1–26, 1949.
9. Hunter RA: Psychotherapy in migraine. *Br Med J* 1:1084–1088, 1960.
10. Howarth E: Personality and stress. *Br J Psychiatry* 3:1193–1197, 1965.
11. Fromm-Reichmann F: Contribution to the psychogenesis of migraine. *Psychoanal Rev* 24:26–33, 1937.
12. Friedman AP, Merritt HH: Migraine. In Friedman AP, Merritt HH (eds): *Headache, Diagnosis and Treatment.* Philadelphia, F.A. Davis, 1959, pp 201–249.
13. Friedman AP: An overview of chronic, recurring headache. *Wisconsin Med J* 71:110–116, 1972.
14. Drake FR: Tension headache: a review. *Am J Med Sci* 232:105–112, 1956.
15. Alvarez WC: The migrainous personality and constitution, the essential features of the disease; a study of 1500 cases. *Am J Med Sci* 213:1–8, 1947.
16. Featherstone HJ, Beitman BD: Marital migraine: a refactory daily headache. *Psychosomatics* 25:30–38, 1984.
17. Castelnuevo-Tedesco P: Psychotherapy for the non-psychiatric physician: theoretical and practical aspects of the twenty-minute hour. In Karasu TM, Steinmuller RI (eds): *Psychotherapeutics in Medicine.* New York, Grune & Stratton, 1978, pp 242–258.
18. Blau JN: Fears aroused in patients with migraine. *Br Med J* 288:1126, 1984.
19. Frazier SH: The psychotherapeutic approach

to patients with headache. *Mod Treatment* 1:1412–1424, 1964.

20. Friedman AP: Migraine: an overview. In: Pierce H: *Modern Topics in Migraine.* London, William Heinemann Medical Books.

21. Kolb LC: Psychiatric and psychogenic factors in headache. In Friedman AP, Merritt HH (eds): *Headache, Diagnosis and Treatment.* Philadelphia, F.A. Davis, 1959, pp 259–298.

22. Grinker RR, Robbins FP: The head and the special senses. In Grinker RR, Robbins FP: *Psy-chosomatic Case Book.* New York, Blakiston, 1954, pp 109–142.

23. Adler CS, Adler SM: Psychiatric treatment of headache. *Panminerva Med* 24:145–149, 1982.

24. Adler CS, Adler SM: Existential deterrents to headache relief past mid-life. *Ad Neurol* 33: 1982.

25. Von Senden M: *Space and Sight: Perception of Space and Shape in the Congenitally Blind Before and After Operation.* London, Methume, 1960.

CHAPTER THIRTY ONE

From Theory to Technique: a Psychotherapeutic Miscellany for Headache

CHARLES S. ADLER, M.D.
SHEILA MORRISSEY ADLER, PH.D.

The therapist's use of treatment approaches which capitalize on the headache patient's characteristic strengths and shelter his common vulnerabilities, as described in previous chapters, is often the key to translating a good theory into a clinical success. The psychologically influenced headache patient benefits most from psychotherapeutic techniques which, though not necessarily complex, are specific to his individual needs. Because even a slight modification of the usual therapeutic approach in this direction can be valuable, this chapter will suggest some pragmatic way in which this can be done.

For example, with posttraumatic headache disorder, one of the most perplexing and difficult to treat in the field of headache, the physician may be best advised to shift his focus from the pessimism of uncertainty to the intellectual challenge it inspires. It is the only condition in which one and the same organ, the brain, experiences the assault, receives the injury, assesses the injury, communicates the injury, and has fantasies about the injury—in short, reacts to the organ's damage with the damaged organ. This interplay is to medicine what Heisenberg's uncertainty principle is to physics. Furthermore, headaches are only one aspect of the post-head trauma syndrome, a condition whose boundaries are confused by intersecting names and overlapping concepts: Posttraumatic headaches, posttraumatic syndrome, posttraumatic neurosis, posttraumatic stress disorder. We will thus devote specific attention to this disorder in the latter part of the chapter.

In this chapter we briefly describe certain discrete points we have found effective in treating headache patients, and that patients have shown us or told us were most helpful. Some are specific to a particular headache diagnosis; other are not, but may be applied to the headache patient regardless of diagnosis. The points which follow should only be viewed as suggestions designed to be modified if needed on a case by case basis.

1. *Be warm but formal.* Migraineurs are often somewhat formal people. They generally respond best when the tone of the interaction allows the physician to be seen as their consultant in the true sense of the word—equal in dignity but more knowledgeable—aiding them in their battle with headache. It is important to be sensitive to the migraine pa-

tient's need to feel in sufficient personal control of many situations. Therapy is usually one such situation.

2. *Establish structure.* Compared to the migraineur, the tension headache patient can often more directly acknowledge that emotionally distressing events are the primary cause of his headaches. He is therefore likely to feel relieved if the therapist maintains a traditional, calming but authoritative role. Greater structure in the relationship reassures the tension headache patient that he will have effective help in controlling anger.

3. *Avoid passivity.* Most headache patients are put off by a passive therapist. They dislike those long silences which many people consider the image of good psychotherapy, but which are often, in fact, a parody of good psychotherapy—and are especially likely to be *poor* psychotherapy for the anxious headache patient. In a similar vein, most headache patients react badly to psychotherapists who remain aloof or who maintain a distant "mystique."

4. *Shelter the patient's self-esteem.* Self-esteem is frequently low in tension headache patients; in migraineurs it is often more vulnerable than it appears. Indeed, because the migraineur often seems self-contained and not in need of help the physician can misapprehend the patient's frailties. To build esteem and help the patient save face one can: (a) acknowledge how difficult it may have been for the patient to come for treatment; (b) acknowledge the patient's occupation or any accomplishments or achievements he shares with you; (c) speak in the "third person" about how others might feel about situations the patient confronts; (d) refer to "research findings" in a way that allows the patient to understand a point without taking it as a personal criticism; (e) talk about how other people typically handle similar situations, leaving it for the patient to conclude that he might consider such a reaction also; and (f) finally, with migraine especially, emphasize that emotional stress is a spark which lights the tinder of migraine rather than its full cause.

5. *Never challenge the authenticity of the patient's pain.* It is presumptuous to think one can "know" better than another what he or she feels, and it is a presumption which often spells disaster for therapy with headache patients. The less the patient must prove the reality of his pain the less defensive he will be in working with the physician. This attitude applies to all types of headache, and whether or not there is psychological overlay.

6. *Harness positive attributes.* Use the patient's characteristic strengths and favorite ways of handling things to therapeutic advantage. Most patients prefer to be active participants in their treatment. This gives them a feeling of control over the rate, rhythm, and content of material which is brought up. Migraineurs, especially, respond well when encouraged to use an intellectual coping style to think about psychophysiological correlations. Encouraging them to read books appropriate to their level of sophistication is particularly useful. One gets further by allowing the patient to see himself as Sherlock Holmes; the clever physician contents himself with being Dr. Watson.

7. *Avoid encouraging regression.* Many psychologically influenced migraineurs have tried to discard childhood's ways prematurely, and are made uncomfortable if pressured to remember these in therapy. Nevertheless, because exploration of childhood is frequently needed to correct a present problem, these remembered experiences must be approached somehow. Fears, fantasies, and memories related to the past should be engaged slowly, with the therapist mindful of the patient's pace and tolerances. In short, the therapist should titrate the patient's confrontation with the past. Sharing the rationale for this approach helps the patient handle the frustration typically required by psychotherapy without feeling as though the pot of emotion is being randomly stirred. Discussions are most productive when the therapist directly relates past feelings and actions to present ones.

8. *Don't rush treatment.* Biology and psychology can only change so fast. Learning

new ways to relate to one's body and social milieu is not a reasonable short-term expectation for the psychologically influenced headache patient. Treatment length should be adjusted to the individual's requirements, and must take into consideration the patient's need to make what he has learned in therapy a part of his basic "sense of self," in a way resilient enough to withstand the inevitable assaults of circumstance. A patient whose therapy has been too short often does well until challenged by crisis, when he may find himself unable to rapidly reconstitute. We have found (1) such a patient is then more likely to become disheartened, and revert to old ways of feeling and interacting. In contrast, patients treated with sufficient therapy to accomplish this internalization can usually ride out such setbacks; they can lose a battle without feeling they have lost the war.

9. *Set reasonable goals session to session.* Generally, therapeutic expectations should be incrementally progressive and gradual, and focused upon a small enough segment of each problem that the patient does not feel overwhelmed by it. Interim assignments can be useful. For example: "Until our next meeting, when this feeling of impatience arises concentrate on answering these questions: What am I feeling? Where or when have I felt this way before? What helped then?"

10. *Reduce unrealistically high expectations.* The patient with migraine is usually overly critical of his need for relief, and feels strongly the pressure to live up to his responsibilities. All too often he comes to therapy prepared to get through this obligatory task just as dutifully as he has gotten through others in life. It is therefore best if the tone of therapy shuns the imperative.

11. *Allow covert dependency as appropriate.* At times, this proves to be especially important for those migraineurs who, on the surface, seem to need covert dependency least. Such patients are rarely comfortable acknowledging needs they perceive as reflecting an inner "weakness." Patients with problem-atic migraines have often been emotionally on their own for so long that the ability to appropriately depend on someone else is often vital to their successful treatment, and it is a privilege that they rarely will abuse. It typically helps the migraineur move toward a flexible sense of trust and independence, rather than into regression. Allowing controlled dependency is also frequently important with cluster patients. Yet with both types of patients it is usually preferable to avoid making interpretations about dependency, especially early in therapy. Therefore be dependable, but don't talk about it; allow the process to remain covert.

12. *Avoid surprise encounters.* While no patient likes to be caught off guard, and it is not always predictable or preventable, the migraineur is often especially disconcerted by the prospect of a sudden lack of control over emotions such as sadness or anger, and defends himself against it energetically. If the clinical picture gives reason to suspect that powerful feelings will eventually surface, the surprise can be ameliorated by discussions which prepare the patient for this in advance. For example: "You have been too busy trying to survive to have had the time to get angry. I expect that sooner or later we are going to come into contact with that anger, and if we do, it will be important to let yourself express it. Then you can get the anger off your chest, and that will leave you feeling better."

13. *Avoid extremes of the treatment spectrum.* Headache patients do best with therapies whose curative elements are balanced between intellectual and affective components; these techniques lead to insight but avoid overintellectualization, and teach the patient to make contact with his feelings, without repeatedly flooding him with them. Reductionist application of otherwise valid theories—applications which, in absolute terms, convert the great complexities of mind to simplified behavior, lack of rational explanation, or formulaic catharsis—rarely help. Thus, the more fervent and one-size-fits-all therapies, however much they convince their propo-

nents of their correctness and efficacy, are un-likely, over the long term, to convince the patient's physiology.

14. *Capitalize upon initial momentum.* Sometimes the chronic headache patient feels he is the only one who takes his headaches seriously enough. An initial meeting of sufficient duration emphasizes to both the patient and his family that the doctor appreciates that the headaches are a significant problem and that treatment may require consideration of all aspects of the patient's situation. While practice realities vary, even 60–90 minutes is reasonable for the first meeting. Additional appointments should follow shortly to capitalize on the momentum that motivated the patient to seek consultation.

15. *First and second childhoods.* An area of particular difficulty for some patients which may be overlooked is that of child rearing. Strains in this area are often denied out of shame, but the responsibilities may be more than the patient feels able to handle. Several things can be done to help the patient, not only in this circumstance, but if, for similar reasons, anxiety or resentment about the task of caring for people is revived by the need to tend to elderly parents.

The chance to express his uncertainties and resentments in the shelter of the doctor's office often eases such a patient's burden. The physician sometimes needs to give the patient permission to get concrete assistance with child rearing. These same patients may have trouble with parents or in-laws who become ill, difficult, or unable to care for themselves. This common source of resentment is all too often suppressed in order to struggle on with dutiful obligations, real and imagined. The situation is aggravated if responsibilities to the parents conflict with duties to spouse and children. Again: help the patient find a practical way to share the load or to reduce it. Can other members of the family take on some of these burdens? Can someone be hired?

16. *Teach the patient about his tension.* It is helpful to teach the migraine, tension, or cluster patient to detect the subtle and early signs that a headache, or a headache cycle in the case of cluster, might be on its way. This means teaching him to become attuned to his body. The migraineur, for example, often impatiently wishes to push aside such sensations when he determines that they are "interfering with his plans." With the help of the therapist, the patient can learn to pinpoint slight mood shifts and other sensory changes that typify his prodromal period. As the nature of the prodrome varies from patient to patient, these details are specifically ascertained for each person using commonly seen elements as guides. The patient can then take corrective action in advance: resting, relaxing, leaving the party early, or taking preventative medication. Biofeedback and other self-regulatory skills are known for their effectiveness in helping a patient become more aware of how he is feeling, and especially of when tension is accumulating. If, despite these attempts to avert it, a headache begins in earnest, the patient needs to immediately initiate activities designed to control it. For the migraineur, this might mean going to bed rather than cooking dinner and ignoring the headache while it builds. For the tension headache patient, this might mean initiating pharmacological or, better still, self-regulatory relaxation measures.

17. *Formal termination is rarely necessary.* It is seldom helpful to formally terminate treatment. The patient may only come in occasionally, or may taper off in frequency of visits, confident that there is an "open door policy" which allows him to return if needed. Patients report that such an open-ended approach encourages them to continue actively integrating what they learned in therapy into their lives.

18. *Treat the "posttraumatic" as well as the headache.* The first job in therapy of a patient suffering from posttraumatic headaches is to clarify what other symptoms accompany head pain, even if he has been referred for headaches. Headache may serve as the title for the overall disorder, or may be the

only aspect of it which seems sufficiently defined for the patient to focus on; however, another aspect of this condition often most disrupts the patient's life. The physician may wish to ask questions which allow the patient to consider that those "soft" neurological problems that frequently seem to accompany the syndrome may also be consequences of the injury. Although not suggesting what the patient *should* feel, he thus helps the patient define how he *does* feel. This process frequently allows the patient to finally refine an elusive sense of dysphoria into its constituent elements, and forms the basis for planning a treatment approach which is not too narrowly focused to serve the patient's actual needs.

19. *Clarify one's use of the word "traumatic."* "Traumatic" in "posttraumatic" can have two quite separate meanings: one is the physical trauma and resultant injury to the tissues of the brain; the other is the psychological "trauma" incurred by the patient during the experience, and recorded by neurons that are not physically damaged. In psychiatry, this latter condition is referred to as the "posttraumatic stress disorder." Symptoms stemming from it are functional, often appear psychological, and usually result from the brain's attempts to "replay" disturbing memories through the patient's consciousness, and thereby diminish their intensity and pathogenicity. Memories of traumatic physical experiences, such as intense pain, can also be reexperienced this way, and this can be confusing for the physician. Conversely, the first type of "trauma"—actual physical injury to brain substance—can also present with signs and symptoms which look and sound psychological, depending upon the functions served by the part of the nervous system which suffered cell damage.

20. *Elucidate organically based "psychological" symptoms for the patient.* Most patients are used to thinking of cognitive/emotional symptoms from a psychological or moral perspective, and this viewpoint is frequently reinforced by others. Many of the posttraumatic symptoms which appear neurotic may however, be organic, and the pa-

tient can be told of this possibility if he has them. Such symptoms may include: (*a*) headache, (*b*) lightheadedness or dizziness, (*c*) trouble concentrating and maintaining vigilance, (*d*) fatigue, (*e*) insomnia, (*f*) memory and attention problems, (*g*) anxiety, (*h*) emotional lability, (*i*) trouble with crisp, novel, or creative thought, (*j*) decreased sexual interest or capacity, (*k*) irritability, (*l*) decreased sensitivity to social norms, (*m*) lack of reserve, that is, the inability to concentrate on multiple tasks simultaneously and, occasionally, (*n*) tearfulness or depression. The patient may need to know as well that these symptoms can act synergistically and "chase" one another: the insomnia may accentuate fatigue; the poor ability to concentrate may intensify memory problems; concern that he will be unable to function up to standards adds to anxiety; the experience of failing at things for reasons he can't explain leads to depression. Such explanations sometimes reassure the patient who was told his neurological examination and laboratory results were normal, and who is understandably puzzled or apprehensive about the origins of his disordered mentation.

21. *Explain why work exacerbates the patient's problems.* Many patients need to understand why symptoms worsen when they return to work or school, especially if the sincerity of their motivation to reenter the work force is being questioned by family members or attorneys or, couched in terms such as "secondary gain," by other medical personnel. One can explain to the patient that it is only at the point when he resumes work that his brain is taxed to function at peak efficiency and is required to interpret events and people with subtlety. If it is incapable of functioning at this level, it stumbles, just as the car back from the shop develops a rattle at full highway speed even though it passed the mechanic's short "test drive" with flying colors. In the same way, social symptoms not obvious in a casual conversation may be brought out by more stressful interpersonal encounters. Sometimes, even when others think the patient is performing well, the patient knows he

is not sharp, not feeling "right," and is not "himself."

22. *Describe the natural history of posttraumatic symptoms.* The patient with organic problems still feels "off" and knows something is amiss. He can be informed that the natural history of such symptoms following accidents is generally time limited. Prepare the patient to expect that improvement might come only gradually. Regular appointments also help. Keep in focus that the posttraumatic headache patient still feels out of focus. The patient whose diffuse neurological impairment looks psychological has, as his most central disorder, *disrupted attention.* The "lenses of the brain," like those of a projector accidentally dropped, no longer focus their images precisely on the screen of consciousness. This characteristically makes people anxious; therefore, although time is the most appropriate first treatment, it should always be supplemented by carefully considered reassurance and support.

23. *Psychotherapeutic treatment implications vary.* At least three types of psychological factors can accentuate the physiological disruption of posttraumatic headaches. The first is the patient's emotional reaction to the organic mental disruption. It is aggravated if organic symptoms are intense, or if the life situation in which he must function is complex. The second factor is the psychological trauma accompanying the physical trauma. For example, the patient may have been in an automobile accident in which others were killed or seriously injured. Third, longstanding psychiatric disturbances can be exacerbated, or latent psychiatric disturbances can be unmasked, by the accident and the subsequent illness. This third effect is more than just a result of pain acting as a nonspecific stressor; mild disordered mental functioning of organic origin can handicap the patient's ego in ways that compromise his ability to get along if he habitually has used only marginally effective psychological defenses. For such a patient, it then becomes impossible to function as before, or to spontaneously adopt new ways of handling stress.

24. *Shelter the injury.* In therapy it is important to discuss with the patient the reality that there are some activities from which he must restrain himself for healing to occur. This may include advising him of a potential hypersensitivity to alcohol, "recreational" or prescription drugs, overwork, or to insufficient sleep. Some complex tasks he previously enjoyed—for example, piloting his private plane—may need to be postponed. A quick return to work or school is not a magic formula, and if applied in a rigid way will cause some patients to fail and develop doubts about their capacities or prognosis. The patient who takes on too great a task and fails may regress, and the anticipation of failure may keep him from trying again.

25. *Avoid specific aversive stimuli.* If the patient was conscious during the accident he should avoid stimuli that remind him of it, as these can directly trigger, in a susceptible patient, unpleasant memories of hallucinatory intensity. These "memories" might be ideational, visual, emotional, or vestibular; they are manifestations of the posttraumatic stress disorder. For example, it may be inadvisable for the patient to drive to work every day on the same route on which the accident occurred, particularly if he regularly tenses up as he approaches the spot.

26. *Explain the homeostatic dynamics of nightmares.* Nightmares directly or symbolically related to the accident are also symptomatic of the posttraumatic stress disorder. Such nightmares represent attempts by brain mechanisms to have the patient reexperience the images, sensations, or other memories of the accident. These usually appear in a fragmented fashion. The purpose of their reappearance during sleep is to reduce the distress caused by such memories. The patient will probably be relieved if educated about these dynamics. Because these dreams are potentially therapeutic, if the patient awakens during one, he should try to relax and not fight the dream images.

27. *The family as a support system.* When the family's anxieties or inability to understand the headache patient's symptoms or

lack of progress cause its members to impede treatment with overprotection or excessive expectations, a visit to the physician by the family as a whole may help clarify things. Family members sometimes need to know that the patient's problems are real and not just willful.

28. *Treat a posttraumatic neurosis as you would any true neurosis.* Whether initiated, uncovered, or accentuated by the head injury, a neurosis is a neurosis, and its roots are usually in the patient's childhood developmental experiences, with subsequent events essentially acting only as triggering or activating mechanisms. Their optimal treatment, therefore, is the psychodynamic and uncovering approaches of traditional psychotherapy. In such therapy, certain themes are seen frequently in posttraumatic headache patients:

a. Changes in role expectations may disrupt defenses.
b. Patients who develop psychiatric complications are more often found to have been in accidents in which the context has psychologically troublesome aspects to it and, therefore, requires discussion.
c. There is often anger at the person responsible for the accident which has caused the patient ongoing pain and disablement.
d. Guilt about others who were injured or killed is a frequent theme when the accident was the patient's fault; but guilt may be present even if it wasn't. It is then known as "survivor guilt."
e. Head injuries are frequently ones which, had conditions been slightly different, might have proved fatal; anxiety from having confronted the tenuousness of one's life may be activated.

29. *Visualize what happened.* At certain times in treatment, the patient's capacity to remember the injury-inducing situation may be blocked. At these points, he may need to recall visual and other phenomena more than verbal or cognitive ones. These memories are sometimes best revived by having the patient temporarily shut his eyes so that he might better "see" what happened and once again experience what he was feeling and thinking at the time.

30. *Abreactive therapies.* The posttraumatic stress disorder has gained public recognition through its frequent appearance in individuals who have had prolonged exposure to combat. Symptoms of the disorder include insomnia, nightmares, anxiety, feelings of social alienation, avoidance of stimuli related to the event, hallucination-like intrusions of memory fragments into consciousness, recurring pain, insecurity, and the spontaneous appearance of emotional and somatic phenomena. As this picture also often accompanies posttraumatic headaches, the experience gained by psychiatry in treating the same disorder incurred in other contexts, including combat, can be used. The abreactive therapies are particularly well adapted to treating the type of symptoms encountered in the posttraumatic stress disorder.

Abreactive techniques facilitate homeostatic mechanisms which may help the patient put traumatic memories in the past. They are especially useful for treating the psychophysiological consequences of head trauma. One of the most complex of these techniques is termed Autogenic Neutralization (2), which was developed from the Autogenic Training method of relaxation. The process capitalizes upon the homeostatic power of brain mechanisms similar to those that guide dreaming, which elaborate a gradually evolving confrontation with traumatic memories and associations.

Hypnosis is a second abreactive method for modifying traumatic memories, and is also quite powerful in skilled hands. The "amytal interview," using any of a number of sedating medications, is a third means of reducing the pathogenic impact of posttraumatic memories by decreasing the anxiety which is keeping them repressed. In conjunction with the patient's suggestibility, each of these therapeutic techniques can effectively lower barriers to repressed memory, as has been found by Kolb.

31. *Discuss the difference between handicap and disability.* A handicap interferes with activities; a disability stops them. The difference between these two often depends on the patient's attitude towards the problem and his optimism that it will be worthwhile to learn to work around it. The patient needs to be helped to think of concrete ways in which he can cope with his most specifically troublesome problems. In the course of his pioneering work on electricity, the 19th century physicist Michael Faraday found his short-term memory slipping due to mercury poisoning of which he was unaware. He simply switched to note-taking and continued his seminal experiments. In a similar manner, one can help the posttraumatic headache patient to find a niche in life which maximizes opportunities to use his remaining assets and minimizes the liability of residual deficits.

CONCLUSION

Problem headache patients often are "problem patients" because psychological factors have been overlooked, misidentified, or incompletely treated. Not all headaches accentuated by psychological problems will have psychological solutions, even in the best of hands. Nevertheless, it will be surprising how many such patients can obtain significant relief when these issues are focused upon in a kindly, knowledgeable, and continuing fashion.

REFERENCES

1. Adler CS, Adler SM: An analysis of therapeutic factors seen in a ten-year study of a psychophysiologically and psychodynamically oriented treatment for migraine. In: Rose FC (ed): *Migraine: Clinical and Research Advances.* Basel, Karger, 1985, pp 186–198.
2. Luthe W: *Autogenic Therapy.* New York, Grune & Stratton, 1973, vol. 6.

CHAPTER THIRTY TWO

Perspectives from a Headache Center with an Inpatient Unit

JOEL R. SAPER, M.D.

Headache ranks between seventh and ninth as the most frequent reason given by patients for medical visits, and accounts for approximately 10 million yearly office appointments with physicians (1–3), a figure which does not include visits to non-M.D. mental health professionals or quasihealth care providers, such as chiropractors, hypnotists, acupuncturists, and others.

Chronic headache is an incompletely understood malady for which a consistently reliable therapy does not exist. This disorder is of such immense magnitude, disabling in impact upon its sufferers, and so historically shrouded in myth, misinformation, and misapplied terminology, that those who suffer from it are rendered particularly vulnerable to ill-trained, at times deceitful, "practitioners" promising relief and cures. Even those seeking the most qualified help are frequently shuttled between legitimate medical providers, each of whom applies the techniques of his or her specialty in an attempt to bring about relief.

In 1945, Dr. Arnold Friedman and his colleagues developed, at Montefiore Hospital in New York, the first hospital-based headache clinic in the United States. During the past 10–15 years, a proliferation of both private and hospital-based headache centers has occurred.

Headache authorities and research and treatment centers for headache are located in Norway, England, Sweden, Italy, Canada, Japan, Denmark, the Netherlands, Israel, Finland, West Germany, Poland, Australia, Austria, South America, and France. Several national and international headache societies exist, among them The American Association for the Study of Headache, the World Federation of Neurology's group on headache and pain, the International Headache Society, the Italian Headache Society, the German Migraine Society, the Scandinavian Migraine Foundation, and the British Migraine Trust. Two major journals for headache disorders are currently published: *Headache,* published in the United States by the American Association for the Study of Headache, and *Cephalalgia: An International Journal of Headache,* published in Norway in conjunction with the International Headache Society.

THE PATIENTS OF A HEADACHE CENTER

GENERALIZATIONS

Two broad headache categories exist: those headaches resulting from disease, whereby headache represents a signal of pathology (secondary headache conditions), and those in which persistent pathological findings are lacking (primary headaches). In the primary category, uncertain physiological circumstances render patients more susceptible to a variety of physiological events, the predominant expression of which is pain.

Headaches which signal disease are usually diagnosed and treated by family physicians and specialists from various fields. Similarly, many of those suffering the primary disorders, manifested by periodic, occasional headache, obtain excellent results through the efforts of family physicians and specialists.

Nonetheless, a large number of patients complain of daily, almost daily, or reliably recurring pain which appears refractory to even the most aggressive and appropriate efforts. To many, if not most, pain has become the dominant theme of life and very often of the lives of their families. Emotional, marital, and socioeconomic distress either preceded the onset of headaches, or is likely as a consequence of them. Patients seek the help of one physician or source of relief after another, suffer from the absence of trusting and supportive doctor-patient relationships, and soon become victims of feelings of isolation, desperation, and helplessness. Depression, resentment, anger, and defensiveness are widespread within this group.

Large numbers of patients have travelled many medical miles in search of help, and most take an excessive amount of analgesics for control of pain. To each new physician they frequently present a thick packet of medical records reflecting a sometimes well-charted, but usually redundant, course among many specialists and subspecialists. They have undergone many procedures: tooth extractions, eye refraction, sinus drainage, septum straightening, turbinate removal, temporomandibular joint correction, psychotherapy, neck tractioning, hysterectomy, immune system desensitization, vertebrae manipulation, and hormone regulation. Patients quote the opinions of family practitioners, dentists, marriage counselors, ophthalmologists, otologists, psychiatrists, psychologists, allergists, chiropractors, neurologists, and gynecologists. They carry diagnoses reflecting not only the best opinion of their most trusted physicians but also a variety of "authoritative" explanations and fad diagnoses clipped from weekly tabloids purchased at grocery store counters.

These patients are the failures of the traditional approaches to headache. As a group, they complain of daily or almost daily pain, use analgesics frequently, and are depressed, defensive, and desperate. It is this group that appears to dominate the population in headache centers. Many verbalize the belief that their journey to the headache center is their "last chance" before ultimately sinking into painful resignation that things will never be better.

SPECIFIC FEATURES OF HEADACHE CENTER PATIENTS

Over half of the patients seeking care at the Michigan Headache and Neurological Institute have daily pain. Most have experienced headaches for over 10 years, usually since childhood or adolescence. Studies on this population (3–6) suggest that most began to experience intermittent migraine during the first 26 years of life. After that age, many patients evolve into a second headache pattern in which there occurs nonmigrainous headache events with superimposed periodic migraine attacks. The majority of patients are women.

Several other features characterize this population. Excessive analgesic use is common, with most patients taking 6–8 or more analgesic tablets a day. Not infrequently, the use of over 20 tablets a day is recorded. Depression with anxiety elements is commonly encountered, as is the presence of sleep disturbance. Stressful family dynamics, and a family history of depression, substance abuse or alcohol overuse—and headaches—are present in many patients.

This group of patients exhibits what this author calls the Chronic Headache Complex (3, 5, 6), which represents a constellation of somatic and emotional distresses believed to reflect both central and peripheral physiological events, often aggravated by psychological disturbances having psychodynamic and situational implications. Although unhappiness is common, the unhappiness does not appear greater in this group than in patients with occasional intermittent headaches (4).

Many of the patients have had psychotherapy prior to coming to the center, and have either failed to benefit or resisted the effort. Because primary and/or secondary psychological distress is present, it is clear that many patients clearly require psychotherapy as part of their treatment. While many seem willing to accept it as *part* of their treatment, some express resentment when psychotherapy is recommended as the primary therapeutic tool for headaches.

Patients frequently vocalize their reluctance to accept the stereotype that comes with the referral to the psychologist or psychiatrist, offering the opinion that both family physicians and mental health professionals are guilty of a bias towards the patient with headache. Many believe that this bias results in less than objective assessment and treatment. More than a few have flatly rejected the referral to the psychotherapist, seeking instead fad, unqualified, or other unconventional forms of treatment, all of which tend to focus on "physical" explanations which are, of course, more acceptable to many patients than are inferences that mental health issues are relevant to headache pathogenesis.

No matter how skilled and tireless, a physician *acting alone* cannot satisfy the needs of many in this population. Most require many hours of professional time, education, psychotherapy, and help with certain aspects of their lives, and deliberate and aggressive medical management. Amelioration of the medical, social, and emotional distress of this group, including issues which often permeate the entire family, cannot for the most part be accomplished by any professional alone. The recognition of this resulted in the development of our institute.

Not all patients exhibit the above features. The remainder of headache patients entering this particular center have a variety of entities, including posttraumatic syndrome, cluster headache, intermittent migraine, acute muscle contraction pain, and primary psychiatric disease with somatic expression.

THE DEVELOPMENT OF A PRIVATE HEADACHE CENTER

As stated, this center, The Michigan Headache and Neurological Institute, was conceived out of the notion that an individual or even a group of physicians alone cannot generally devote sufficient time to or degree of involvement in the lives of many of the patients who seek help for intractable headaches to adequately ameliorate their distress.

The center was founded in 1978 by a primary professional staff that included two Ph.D. psychologists, a clinical nurse specialist in neurosurgery, and myself, a neurologist. The remaining members of the staff, which numbered ten, included three additional RNs, a technician, and clerical personnel.

Over the following 8 years, the staff has more than tripled in size and now includes three neurologists who share medical responsibilities for the outpatient and inpatient population, an associate M.D. anesthesiologist who serves as practicing consultant for general pain disorders, two Ph.D. psychologists, a nurse counselor with a Master's degree, a clinical coordinator (BSRN), and 10 additional nurses.

The two Ph.D. psychologists, together with the counselor with a Master's degree, provide psychodiagnostic and psychotherapeutic services for the outpatient program, offering traditional psychodynamic, behavioral, biofeedback, stress management, and other psychological treatments, in addition to psychodiagnostic and psychophysiological assessments.

The remainder of the staff, now numbering 35, is composed of laboratory technicians (trained in general laboratory and neurodiagnostic techniques), clerical personnel, and the center's administrator.

This program thus provided personnel capable of affording patients a comprehensive headache treatment program, combining in a unified and coordinated group, interdisciplinary assessment and treatment programs for patients with recurring and chronic headache.

THE DEVELOPMENT OF AN INPATIENT HEADACHE UNIT

IDENTIFYING THE NEED

During the first 2 years of this practice, three key observations prompted the belief that the development of an inpatient unit was mandatory if successful treatment were to be realized for many of the patients coming to the center.

The first observation was that the center's population had become increasingly skewed towards patients with daily pain refractory to appropriate outpatient treatments. Aggressive, innovative, and broad therapeutic efforts were required, and outpatient visits, even with multidisciplinary facilities, could not effectively address many of the factors present in a sizable number of patients. Although mental health treatment, substance abuse counseling, and traditional headache therapies can be delivered successfully to many headache patients on an outpatient basis, the complex symptomatic, socioeconomic, and medication overuse fabric of so many patients coming to this center rendered efforts that were not both intensive and daily likely to fail.

The second important observation which prompted development of an inpatient unit was the recognition of how much urgency patients with acute or subacute daily pain commanded. Put somewhat differently, pain does not comply with the traditional standards of urgency when compared to other illnesses generally considered benign and not life-threatening. Many patients with daily painful conditions exhibit an inability to "continue on" week after week in an outpatient treatment setting, frequently making the pace of this type of therapy unacceptable.

A third key observation was that many patients coming to a pain center are so heavily ensconced in excessive drug indulgence that pharmacological dependency, toxicity, and even clear medical risk make outpatient efforts unacceptable and destined to fail.

Several examples illustrate the need for inpatient level care.

Consider the professional, executive, mother, or self-employed patient with daily, intense headache who uses analgesics excessively to maintain his or her functional effectiveness. Predicated upon the necessity to adequately perform with respect to domestic and vocational responsibilities, a patient justifies the use of increasing amounts of analgesics. This often provokes an escalation of headache refractoriness and analgesic-induced adverse reactions. Even when psychological issues are not sufficiently complex to prevent successful pharmacotherapy, appropriate preventative medication will likely fail to effect a beneficial result until the analgesics are withdrawn (3). Discontinuance of analgesics, however, results in increasingly disabling pain. Successful outpatient treatment of this patient may take months. Many patients will not or cannot, despite proper motivation, accept this transition, and choose instead to continue analgesic use.

Many patients with daily pain also suffer from longstanding emotional and substance abuse disorders, in which headache may represent the somatic expression of psychiatric disease or a primary substance abuse problem.

Intermittent outpatient therapy for a patient complaining of daily disabling pain is often unsuccessful because it fails to engage the patient at a sufficient pace and intensity to alter his life circumstances or his responses to them.

Yet another example is the headache patient who also has serious medical disease: cerebrovascular or cardiovascular illness, hepatic disease, renal impairment, or gastrointestinal ulceration. The development of an effective treatment regimen for headache which does not aggravate the medical problem can be difficult and time-consuming. It requires patience and innovativeness, as well as coordinated efforts among several medical disciplines. Many patients simply will not or cannot restrain themselves from excessive use of vasoconstrictors, analgesics, or other contraindicated therapies during the weeks or months during which outpatient treatments are being "tested" for effectiveness.

Many who have headache and a serious medical condition complain that their physicians treat the primary medical illness well, but do so at the expense of ignoring the headache problem, which is commonly overlooked in the overall planning of therapy. For example, certain antihypertensive drugs, particularly those containing hydralazine, reserpine, or thiazide diuretics, can aggravate headache tendencies (3). Antiasthmatic medication containing aminophylline or similar preparations can intensify vascular headache events in patients predisposed to them. Hormones for the treatment of endometriosis or for the prevention of menopausal or postmenopausal consequences, or vasodilating agents for the treatment of vascular occlusive disease, often provoke such devastating headaches that patients will, against medical advice, discontinue treatment.

It is sometimes possible on an outpatient basis to treat the complications arising from excessive therapy for pain, such as gastrointestinal bleeding, ergotism, renal disease, and drug dependency, but it is another problem altogether to simultaneously address the primary headache process which, if left untreated for very long, results in a return to the former therapy and in reemergence of the adverse reactions.

The pharmacological challenges and monitoring demands posed by these dilemmas cannot easily be met by outpatient level care, particularly when patients are focused not on the most serious of their conditions, but on that which is most painful.

THE UNIT

In 1979, the initial elements were conceived for an inpatient headache unit to be devoted primarily to the treatment of intractable headache disorders (7). The process was carried out in close collaboration and cooperation with the administration of a private, university-affiliated, community hospital. Various allied professional groups within the hospital were identified and served as advisors in the development of the broad range of services considered important in treating refractory headache patients.

Over a course of several years, the current 16-bed inpatient unit evolved. The unit is staffed by its own specially trained nursing team that serves both a traditional medical nursing function for the acute medical illnesses that are frequently encountered in the headache population, and a clinical role with headache and pain patients. The unit has its own social workers, and has representatives from physical and occupational therapy, dietetics, pharmacy, and recreation therapy. Consulting psychiatrists, psychologists, internists, family practitioners, and physiatrists, along with other medical specialists, are available upon request. Biofeedback therapy and relaxation programs are employed with most patients.

During the course of hospitalization, which generally averages between ten and fourteen days, patients attend a variety of instructional seminars, and individual, family, and group psychotherapeutic and investigational sessions. Medical rounds are made daily. Patients are provided both acute medical treatment and intensive nonmedical management programs, individually determined, which emphasize behavioral, family, and traditional psychodynamic factors.

Recently, this inpatient unit has been surveyed by the Commission of Accreditation of Rehabilitation Facilities (CARF), and the program was awarded maximum 3-year, accreditation, marking the first time a treatment facility primarily treating headaches has been accredited in accordance with national standards.

THE STRUGGLES: POLITICAL AND OTHERWISE

The development of this unit and its activities has not been without struggle, conflict, and controversy. Several major areas can be identified.

The emotional and physical complexity of the patient population for which the unit was created necessitated treatment approaches that took into account the need to treat a spectrum of potential problems. At any one time these might include substance abuse and intoxication, withdrawal, severe depressive responses, anger and hostility directed at staff, sabotaging and resistant behavior by patients and families and, of course, acute and chronic daily pain and medical illness.

Many patients experience *both* acute and chronic pain. This makes it difficult to generalize about pharmacological therapy. The issue of symptomatic "prn" medication illustrates this point. Most *general* pain programs avoid the use of symptomatic (prn) medications for pain problems. Many pain programs primarily treat chronic pain, and limiting "prn" medication is readily accomplished. It is a more challenging problem when acute pain problems, such as cluster headache, acute migraine, and trigeminal neuralgia, are superimposed upon a chronic, daily pain pattern. Appropriate respect for the intensity of these events is required in order to chart a course towards a successful preventative program, while promoting sufficient patient compliance to allow other features of the program to have therapeutic influence. Nursing responses to acute pain complaints, and program policies toward "prn" medications in some, but not all, patients, required careful and deliberate planning.

Aside from the problems of pain management, political and territorial issues arose. Headaches, after all, are considered within the domain of several specialties, including neurology and mental health. Neurosurgical, otolaryngological, and other subspecialties also claim a primary role in the treatment of some headache patients.

Prior to the development of the inpatient headache unit, two specialty programs existed in this hospital, both of which addressed problems frequently encountered in the headache population: an "open" mental health unit and a formal substance abuse treatment program, which had been formed several years earlier. Both were well managed and highly regarded in the community as providing effective treatment for two problems encountered in many chronic headache and pain patients.

Both programs, through their directors, medical staffs, and nursing staffs, expressed concern regarding the overlapping of services and the competing demand for hospital resources. Sincere concerns were raised regarding the ability of a program directed by a neurologist (this author) to manage the dilemmas of psychiatric and substance abuse present in so many of the patients admitted to the inpatient headache unit. Prior to the existence of a headache center, and based upon traditional perspectives regarding the treatment of headache patients, many seeking help for a primary complaint of headache would have been viewed as patients most appropriately triaged to a psychotherapist, mental health unit, or substance abuse program.

Adding to the problems were issues regarding the administration of certain medications for the treatment of pain that heretofore had been used primarily in the treatment of specific psychiatric illnesses. Current pharmacological management of pain employs the use of agents such as tricyclic antidepressants, monoamine oxidase inhibitors, lithium carbonate, and phenothiazines. The administration of these medications for headache troubled various hospital professionals, particularly mental health nursing personnel, most of whom were not aware of the application of these medications to pain. Several openly expressed concern and criticism that these medications were being inappropriately administered, since the diagnosis for which the nurses felt these medications were primarily indicated could not be established in the headache patients.

Each of the three programs espoused a somewhat different approach to the treatment of what were at times similar or overlapping problems. The concern raised by our colleagues was genuine. To some of them, the legitimacy of a pain treatment program required substantiation.

Many of these struggles impacted on our patients directly. A percentage of patients entering the headache unit were considered candidates for aggressive mental health unit care, and with their permission were transferred to the mental health unit as part of their long-term headache management. Several patients, early in the development of the headache unit, encountered conflicting and troublesome differences in staff attitudes towards "pain patients" and in their approaches to pain. This prompted defiance on the patients' part, and resistance towards working on mental health issues. Many signed out against medical advice. Differing program philosophies created stress among patients, and strains between program staffs as well.

In time, frank communications were initiated via a series of direct meetings between individual physicians, administrators, and allied staffs, and were supplemented with intensified inservice training. The apparent willingness of the physicians involved to cooperate, and their basic respect for each other's professional territories, augmented by the liaison role assumed by an innovative hospital administrator of all three programs, were essential components in the solution of these problems.

The major political struggles, in retrospect, seemed to arise from issues of autonomy of the headache unit, an autonomy that was essential for the staff to practice in accord with the philosophy towards head pain of those who directed the unit. It was thus necessary for the headache unit to have its own nursing staff, mental health professionals, and allied services. That this would generate legitimate concern by members of the existing mental health and substance abuse programs regarding territorial delineations, supervisory activities, and general qualifications was understandable. A basic motivation to work together and a respect for the experience and commitment of the various staffs, together with a committed effort by hospital adminis-

tration, led to amelioration of these differences over the course of 2 years.

ADMISSION CRITERIA TO THE UNIT

Admission to the headache unit is restricted to patients who fulfill one or more of the following criteria:

1. Daily and continuous pain, intractable and unresponsive to appropriate outpatient treatment.
2. Pain accompanied by excessive medication use, to the extent that alleviation of both the pain and the medication overuse cannot be achieved without aggressive inpatient level intervention.
3. Pain accompanied by serious adverse reactions or complications to an extent that continued outpatient therapy would aggravate these conditions.
4. Pain in the presence of significant medical disease such that appropriate treatment of pain symptoms might aggravate or induce further illness.
5. Pain in the presence of sufficient emotional disturbances such that successful management by other than inpatient level intervention was unlikely.

FINAL THOUGHTS

It is the author's personal opinion that most patients with chronic, intractable headache experience a basic biological predisposition to headache having both central (brain) and peripheral implications. The central influences most likely involve hypothalamic, limbic, and rostral brainstem mechanisms, mediated by neuroamines and peptides, relevant to the supposed pathogenesis of chronic pain, migraine, depression, and sleep disturbances (3). In addition, frequently, but not necessarily, preexistent or secondary psychological or social disturbances exist. For those patients who seek center-based help, many either refuse to see psychological issues as important, or have already sought the help of mental health professionals who have not, despite the traditional nature of the therapy, succeeded in ameliorating the pain, the accompanying pain behavior, or the other allied distresses. Many patients have substance abuse problems and family and social dynamics which either contribute to the headache problem or sabotage efforts at treating it. In some, pain has become a form of communication, protection, or has taken on another valued role requiring that efforts to eliminate the symptom take these complexities into account.

Some patients who appear to possess appropriate motivation are nevertheless unwilling to accept the link between medical and psychological symptomatology. Referrals to psychiatrists or psychologists by family physicians or others are frequently seen as inappropriate or punitive, reflecting an attitude, according to the patient, that he or she is unstable, and that the pain is "in my head." The advantage of a treatment center, which may also focus on mental health issues when relevant, is that it provides an important umbrella of "legitimacy" to the headaches which promotes the psychotherapeutic process. In the minds of many patients, referral to a mental health provider for primary therapy for headache confirms the opposite. Some patients appear to seek in a headache center alternative answers, treatments, or reassurance from "medical" personnel that serious disease is not present. Many seem willing to eventually undergo mental health treatment, but their willingness to do so is predicated upon the satisfaction of issues of legitimacy, and exclusion of medical or neurological disease. Many find much more acceptable the balance between mental health and traditional medical therapies that are encountered in the centers.

An organized multidisciplinary and broadly based assessment and treatment program are necessary for many headache patients. Patients must trust the system and perceive a commitment on the part of the professional staff. The members of the staff must recognize that patients attending such a center present a challenging set of dynamics, requiring both time and patience. Many patients have expressed fear that failure to respond to treatment would mean an eventual rejection, and were gratified to learn that lack of progress would not bring with it a reluctance to continue the effort.

Appropriate pharmacotherapy seems particularly important. Nonmedicinal interventions such as biofeedback, behavioral modification, traditional psychotherapy, marital counseling, dietary management, and exercise are important as either adjunctive or primary interventions. However, many if not most patients with intractable headache require at least some pharmacotherapy, particularly early in the course of treatment and sometimes on a chronic basis as well.

The population with chronic headache may well have suffered, in addition to their pain, rejection and bias by even a well-meaning traditional medical community. Patients with this illness must receive legitimate respect and appreciation for the complexity of their illness as well as a commitment by their health professionals toward its amelioration. They must not, as is frequently the case, be thrust into the laps of quasilegitimate practictioners who appeal to the needs of this rejected, often medically naive population, nor be forced to suffer the indifference shown by many in the traditional health care community.

Packard's observations confirm (8) that the headache patient wants and needs much more than simple headache relief. He needs to understand the headache problem in terms which are comprehensible and logical and to see evidence that his headaches will command the same legitimate commitment and effort afforded other major medical illnesses. This is especially true when the chronic pain severely impairs the patients' quality of life, as is so often the case.

Despite the many limitations in our understanding of chronic headache and the people who suffer from it, most patients who suffer from even intractable headache disorders are capable of being helped to an extent that brings acceptable relief of pain and normalization of many of life's activities. Unfortunately, not all patients can be satisfactorily helped at this time. For some, it is because their condition exceeds current knowledge (3). For others the need to be sick or the fear to be well can defeat even the most committed effort of those from whom help is sought. For others, it is because the application of therapy has been ill-timed, poorly conceived, or inappropriately delivered.

Persistent, qualified, and compassionate attempts will, however, bring recognizable and satisfying relief to most sufferers of recurring headaches. Although the chronic headache patient is prone to isolation and despair, the belief that someone actually cares, understands, and is trying to help will plant the seed of hope, from which many successful therapies eventually grow.

REFERENCES

1. Cypress BK: Headache as the reason for office visits. National ambulatory case survey: U.S. 1977–1978. Advance data, from Vital and Health Statistics of National Center for Health Statistics, 1981; 67:1–7.

2. Diehr P, Wood RW, Bar V, et al: Acute headaches: Presenting symptoms and diagnostic rules to identify patients with tension and migraine headache. *J Chron Dis* 341:147–158, 1981.

3. Saper JR, *Headache disorders: Current Concepts and Treatment Strategies.* Littleton, MA, John Wright-PSG Publishers, 1983.

4. Saper JR, Winters M: Chronic "mixed" headaches: profile and analysis of 100 consecutive patients experiencing daily headaches (abstr). *Headache* 22:145–146, 1982.

5. Saper JR: Changing perspectives on chronic headache. *Clin J Pain* 2:19–28, 1986.

6. Saper JR: Chronic headache complex. *Aches and Pains* 4(5):20–23, 1983.

7. Van Meter M, Saper JR: An inpatient headache unit: development, direction, and struggles (abstr). *Headache* 21:126, 1981.

8. Packard RC: What does the headache patient want? *Headache* 19:370–374, 1979.

9. Van Meter M, Saper JR, Ross M: Inpatient treatment of intractable headaches—An outcome study (abstr). *Headache* 23(3):144, 1983.

ADDITIONAL SUGGESTED READINGS

Saper JR: Ergotamine tartrate dependency: Features and possible mechanisms. *Clin Neuropharmacol* 9(3):244–256, 1986.

Saper JR: The chronic pain syndrome (newsletter). *Topics Pain Management* 1(5):17, 19, 1985.

Saper JR: Inpatient units for intractable headache (newsletter). *Topics in Pain Management* 1(6):23, 1985.

Saper JR: Analgesic rebound: pain killers inducing treatment refractoriness (newsletter). *Topics in Pain Management* 1(8):29, 32, 1986.

CHAPTER THIRTY THREE

The Psychological Use of Biofeedback and Other Self-Regulatory Techniques in Headache Treatment

CHARLES S. ADLER M.D.
SHEILA MORRISSEY ADLER, Ph.D.
RUSSELL C. PACKARD, M.D.

Learning of any sort requires feedback of information. Percussion of a chest involves the use of feedback; so does becoming proficient at a video game. Table manners may be acquired simply through the feedback of a "certain look" from one's parents; in learning to play the piano, one correlates the feel of his fingers on the keyboard with the resultant sound, and continually adjusts his motor activities until it sounds "musical" (1). Thus, learning is often little more than repeated, increasingly sophisticated trial and error; and all trial and error is ultimately dependent upon feedback.

Feedback has been defined as a process by which a "system" controls and corrects itself by reviewing results of past performance (2). The science of feedback is called cybernetics, and it was developed in part to create the engineering technology that could guide missiles into space. The human body is a "system" with an exquisite degree of self-regulatory capacity for which it relies upon feedback mechanisms, most of them entirely automatic. Body temperature, breathing and heart rate, eye coordination, and balance are examples. Even so high level a phenomenon as an attorney's questioning a witness in court relies upon feedback principles. The attorney asks the questions, listens intently for the response, and depending upon the effect of his first question, either pursues that line of argument or takes a different tack.

The term "*bio*" feedback is used when the body's natural feedback mechanisms are intentionally augmented with mechanical instruments in order to teach an individual how to guide or modify a part of his physiology in a beneficial direction. Sometimes this involves intensifying the person's awareness of a bodily process of which he is already partially aware, such as the state of contraction of his frontalis muscle. Sometimes it involves making him aware of a process that he normally has no knowledge of whatsoever, such as his pulse amplitude. To do this an electronic instrument is used to record information about a continuously changing physiological process. The information is then displayed to the patient in an intensified form, and through one of the major routes of sensory input: sight, hearing, or touch. This enables the person to use trial-and-error experimentation with the feedback to discover how what he thinks, feels, or does influences that bodily function, and to learn which mental initiatives move him in a predetermined and desirable direction. Whether he is trying to learn to relax his jaw muscles or to warm his hands, he finds that certain self-generated thoughts, associations, or behaviors move the feedback (and therefore his physiology) in the right direction (therefore he repeats them) whereas others either do nothing or move him in the wrong direction, and are eventually discarded. In time he will usually learn to alter the feedback quickly and even automatically, much as the pianist's fingers eventually become quick, smooth, precise, and nearly automatic. With the help of such techniques, patients often become able to influence those physiological processes which have, through malfunction, become the final pathway in the pathogenesis of headache.

Studies conducted during the 1960s introduced to medicine an evolving technology which provided a means to teach patients volitional control over physiological functions that were previously believed to be involuntary. This was the formal beginning of what we today call "biofeedback," although its roots can be traced to a much earlier time. Because most of this work was couched in conditioning terminology, it will be important to review the theoretical basis for conditioning, termed "learning theory," before moving on to its specific clinical application to headache.

For many years it was accepted as dogma that changes in that part of the physiology governed by the autonomic nervous system—heart rate, electrodermal response, blood pressure, and the like—could only be brought about reflexively. Classical, or "Pavlovian," conditioning was viewed as the mechanism through which such "visceral learning" occurred. In classical conditioning,

any physiological change that can be elicited involuntarily by one stimulus can be conditioned to be set off by a different stimulus. The new response is termed a "classically conditioned reflex"; Pavlov's dogs (3) salivating in response to the dinner bell are the best known examples.

In the process of becoming classically conditioned, a person is essentially passive, responding automatically and reflexively to what is done to him. For example: he is given a painful shock which automatically increases his heart rate; if the shock is consistently preceded by a tone, in time the tone will begin to elicit that same response, in a predictable, even lawful, fashion. The event usually bypasses motivation; it little matters what the person wants to do or not do. Rather, the response is involuntary, triggered initially by the shock and subsequently by the tone alone. An entirely different mechanism, however, is involved in learning volitional behavior.

The model known as "instrumental," or "operant," conditioning involves reinforcing the organism after it produces a desired response. In laboratory research, the rate and consistency with which a hungry animal presses a lever can be controlled by rewarding him with food each time he does so; or, he can be "taught" to stop pressing the lever by consistently stopping the food. Either pleasure or relief from pain is made contingent upon the animal initiating the desired volitional action. The reward, or "reinforcer," in operant conditioning is anything which makes it worthwhile for the organism to choose to do something which was, in any case, already well within its capabilities. Human operant conditioning, for example, involves systematically providing some desired reward: money, privileges, praise, or encouragement. Thus, while Pavlovian conditioning involves only reflexive, involuntary physiological changes in the organism, operant conditioning can theoretically be used to alter any item of behavior under volitional control.

Since man appears to have been curious about the relationship between his mind and his body since the start of recorded history (and to have evolved changing views of it throughout the course of that history) just where "biofeedback" can be said to have started depends upon how deeply one wishes to trace the roots. Meditative techniques for relieving physical illness were practiced in the ancient Greek temples of Aesclepius, and it could be argued that the first "biofeedback" was performed by the mythical Greek god Narcissus, who used the mirror-like capacity of a lake to reflect upon his own image (4). Work in the first half of this century documented the effects of thoughts and emotions upon different realms of physiology in man. However, it was not until the mid-1960s that a series of investigators at different institutions in the United States began a concerted drive to determine the effects of sharing this information with the patients on a continuing basis, to see whether they could influence it. Interest of the public was aroused when Basmajian (5) showed that subjects could use feedback to learn to differentially contract a single motor unit, and when Kamiya (6) showed that subjects could learn to produce increased α- rhythm, using feedback from an electroencephalograph.

A number of investigators tried to see whether they could also apply the operant conditioning model to modify visceral activity. In 1967, Kimmel (9) documented that subjects could acquire some control of their electrodermal response. Patients' ability to control their heart rates was documented by Shapiro et al in 1970 (7). In 1972, Engel (8) was able to teach patients to vary their heart rates to modulate certain cardiac arrhythmias. When the patient raised his heart rate even slightly in this study, a signal light (the "reinforcer") turned on.

These studies on operant control of autonomic functions initially elicited considerable controversy. A number of scientists were unwilling to accept the results as proof that it was possible to acquire direct cortical control over autonomic activity. Rather, they argued, the subjects had merely learned to change their physiological responses either (a) by using im-

agery to take advantage of classically acquired conditioned reflexes or, (b) by means of covert muscular activity. In a now-classic paper published in 1969, Miller (10) reported several experiments that he and his co-workers had carried out on curarized animals—thereby eliminating the possibility of muscular mediation. These studies showed that a variety of autonomic responses could be modified by means of operant conditioning. Rats, for example, could learn to vary heart rate and blood pressure independently of each other, or to alter intestinal motility. The specificity of these responses was so great that the investigators could train rats to increase blood flow in one ear while simultaneously decreasing it in the other. Subsequent studies (11) laid to rest any lingering doubts about the possibility of achieving operant control over autonomic processes, and a major effort to convert this new paradigm into a useful therapeutic modality began.

BIOFEEDBACK AND RELAXATION

A fundamental tenet of biofeedback (and other self-regulatory therapies) is that man has greater potential to influence his body than he makes use of. The very same biological mechanisms capable of producing harmful effects when stimulated by excessive stress are presumed capable of using those same neural and hormonal pathways to facilitate health instead. Indeed, the almost universal experience of people working in this area is that most people can learn a simple means of relaxation which, if they practice it regularly, will reinforce their resistance to stress-induced illness. However, although there is consensus about the helpfulness of self-regulation, there is less unanimity about why it works.

The form of this debate usually centers around the importance of specific, as opposed to nonspecific, therapeutic factors in treatment. One point of view has it that the "wisdom of the body" is a natural function inherent in its biology, and that the brain knows how to work towards efficient self-repair of dysfunction; and that it does this best when it is regularly put into a calmed state. Just as a fracture supported by a cast will knit together, and just as a properly bandaged laceration will automatically stop hemorrhaging, protect itself against infection, and close the wound, the nervous system, when temporarily buffered against the strains of the environment, will automatically go about its maintenance.

An alternative point of view is that the body is not always wise, and its mechanisms are sometimes actually misguided or archaic . . . otherwise, why has it not been able to repair itself? This viewpoint presses for specific external corrective interventions for the precisely analyzed excess or deficiency that defines each disease state. Its advocates are less impressed with the psychological aspects of relaxation, and may even feel that the relaxed state is incidental, rather than essential, to any repair that takes place. They might correctly point out that many lacerations exsanguinate without a tourniquet, become infected without antibiotics, or scar without sutures.

Both points of view are valid, but not necessarily equally valid for each application of biofeedback, or for each patient, any more than is the theoretician who emphasizes the need for an empathic doctor/patient relationship and a good bedside manner more or less correct than the one who wishes to find the precise diagnosis and treat it with the precise drug. In most applications of biofeedback, both factors will play at least some part. Thus, time has shown the controversy about whether the beneficial effects of biofeedback are the result of relaxation alone, or whether the learning is more specific, to be a question whose answer varies with the illness and even with the patient; but for many conditions, including headache, generalized relaxation techniques are often equally effective.

In 1970, the first author, along with Budzynski and Stoyva (12), first demonstrated that patients trained with frontal muscle biofeedback would experience fewer tension headaches. While the effect of EMG feedback was initially viewed as being site specific, it soon became apparent that its influence also generalized to other body areas. As the level of their frontalis muscle tension decreased, individuals usually became progressively more muscularly relaxed in general. This was evidenced both by falling levels of tension in other muscle groups and by the patients' verbal reports. These findings contributed to the 'rediscovery' of other relaxation techniques, ones which had been developed in earlier times.

Although the history of relaxation training goes back to antiquity, where it formed one component of various religious and meditative disciplines, its more systematic and scientific study began with the work of Schultz (13) in 1932 and Jacabson in 1938 (14). Schultz and Luthe (15) developed the self-regulatory method known as Autogenic Training.

Autogenic Training has been used widely in Europe, Japan, and other parts of the world. The technique has many similarities to self-hypnosis. In it, the patient learns how to effectively concentrate on a series of phrases, known as "standard formulae," which then induce calmness, relaxation, and specific bodily and mental changes. The formulae include autosuggestions for heaviness and warmth of the arms and legs, coolness of the forehead, evenness of respiration, and so on. This procedure requires the patient to practice his formulae regularly. It has been shown (16) to effect predictable neurophysiological changes which can have profound salutary effects on a wide range of psychologically influenced physical disorders, including headaches. A popular method for learning relaxation, Autogenic Training is easily mastered by most patients. Individuals who strongly resist disciplined routines or who are made uncomfortable by passivity may find this technique more difficult. Autogenic Neutralization, a more advanced but related method (16), has been shown to augment the patient's innate homeostatic reparative capacities to a far greater degree.

The work of Jacobson (14) on Progressive Relaxation emphasizes another aspect of relaxation, one which focuses exclusively on teaching deep and widespread muscular relaxation. This technique involves the sequential contraction and relaxation of different muscle groups, with the patient concentrating intently on pinpointing the sensations that accompany muscular contraction and its absence. Eventually, the patient learns how to omit the contraction step and merely focuses upon reestablishing the sensations that accompany muscular release. The formal training process takes a fair amount of time, but has frequently been abbreviated in recent years for purposes of systematic desensitization. Progressive Relaxation is often combined with Autogenic Training phrases; however, as the mental state in the former is active and in the latter passive, they should only be used sequentially.

Other general techniques include the Relaxation Response (17), the Quieting Reflex, Yoga, and Transcendental Meditation, procedures which have aroused considerable popular interest. There has also been a resurgence of interest in the ethical use of hypnosis (18) for psychosomatic conditions. This is an important development, because hypnosis is a powerful and versatile tool, one whose methods and capacities have evolved over a long history. It can be used to alter the way in which pain is attended to or, in a more advanced usage, for highly trained individuals to make contact with unconscious material relevant to certain patient's headaches.

How is the appropriate general relaxation therapy selected for a given patient? Unfortunately, the choice will usually be made for reasons more pragmatic than abstract: what is available in the area or the preferred approach of the local professional most competent to treat patients with self-regulatory therapies. Fortunately, as is the case in choosing between benzodiazepines, the distinctions are usually not critical ones. If they are persistent, most people can learn to relax well with any one of the competing systems.

The term "biofeedback" is at times used to refer to all general relaxation and self-regulatory therapies. It is more accurate to view biofeedback as only one branch of those therapies. Relaxation and self-regulation are not synonymous, and biofeedback is not primarily a general relaxation therapy, at least not when it is used alone: its procedures tend to be specific, specialized, or anatomically localized. It can aid generalized relaxation training, but usually does not replace it.

In the treatment of headache, the most effective approach has been to use biofeedback therapies to assist general relaxation. The two approaches are complementary, and teach the patient how to modulate physiological functions that interfere with relaxation or that set off headaches. Supplementing basic relaxation training with biofeedback can also show patients how their thoughts and feelings are related to their physiology.

In the context of a more generalized form of relaxation training, biofeedback is usually an advanced technique called in as a "specialist." Its advantage of being able to be precise and specific is not always utilized in general relaxation training, and at times may even be a disadvantage. In the end, the biofeedback is simply a concept (feedback) aided by a tool (the instrument) applied to biological systems. As there are many instruments, it is actually a kit of tools.

A number of studies have addressed whether general relaxation techniques and biofeedback procedures are equally effective. As biofeedback for headache is best used in combination with other relaxation therapies, these compare and contrast studies, even when well done—they rarely are—are usually of dubious practical relevance.[1] Such studies typically use a biofeedback group, a

---

[1] Because most studies of this type use too few patients, or treat the patients for too short a period to expect true change, or don't treat according to criteria, one should not rely heavily on their findings. Criteria that make a patient appropriate for one self-regulatory treatment rather than another include more than the diagnosis. That results of such studies are contradictory is no surprise. Ensuring that any of these classical techniques are learned and implemented well is more important than the differences between them.

nonbiofeedback relaxation group, and a no-treatment control group. For example, Haynes et al (19) compared the effectiveness of frontal EMG feedback to a passive relaxation program. Both patient groups showed significant reduction in tension headache, compared to that of untreated controls, but the feedback group did not differ significantly from the relaxation group.

However, another study by Haynes et al (20) showed that EMG feedback lowered tension in frontal muscles more quickly than did passive relaxation, or a tense-relax program. Other studies suggested that such feedback often produce faster and deeper relaxation than verbal relaxation routines alone (12, 21).

WHAT HAPPENS IN A TYPICAL BIOFEEDBACK SESSION

To clarify just what is meant by biofeedback, perhaps we can briefly trace a patient's progress through a "typical" session. The patient will generally settle back into a comfortable chair or recliner in an office free of unfamiliar distraction.

If a patient is dubious of his ability to learn any self-regulation, it may be instructive to use analogies to other nonverbal learning experiences which he has mastered, both voluntary and autonomic, that now seem reflexive but were once learned deliberately and laboriously: learning to walk, to use a fork, to control his bladder, or to postpone tears until an appropriate time. This may make the patient more confident about undertaking treatment. Because he will be expected to encounter plateaus or even temporary setbacks in his progress, he should be informed that such fluctuations are normal when learning any major skill, whether playing the piano or raising one's peripheral temperature.

Biofeedback instruments come in all sizes and all degrees of sophistication, ranging from small portable units for supplemental practice at home, to devices the size of a small ham radio that are most appropriate for general clinical use, to elaborate and expensive research instruments that most resemble the cockpit of a jetliner. This should not obscure the fact that the fundamental process in biofeedback is as simple as the taking of one's own pulse. The best instrumentation is the one sufficient to get the job done least obtrusively, as the machine is in essence merely a facilitator of a dialogue between a patient's conscious mind and his physiology.

Start feedback with a parameter over which the patient has greater control, to provide him with a nonfrustrating introduction to the process. A good rule of thumb is to move from the more general task to the more specific one and from the easier to the more difficult, always keeping the goal easy enough that the patient feels that his overall efforts during the session have been successful.

The patient's innate ability to perceive what is going on within his body is enhanced by the feedback in four ways: (a) he can become aware of a process he was entirely unaware of before, such as the electrical conductivity of his skin; (b) a weak or vague sensation is put in a more useable form (a scale of colored lights replacing a muddled sense of muscular tension), or (c) a more intensely vivid form (such as a clear crescendo or decrescendo of sound); (d) the original sensations are paired with a varying numerical "score," allowing the person to actually quantify a sensation. Computer electronics have lately enabled this feedback to be presented in a more creative or engaging fashion, such as by using a visual display of a hare racing with a tortoise; if the patient can modify his physiology enough, the electronics will ensure that the tortoise wins the race.

Recording equipment is attached lightly to the area of interest and connected to the biofeedback instrument with fine wires. This is frequently followed by brief practice of one of the standard methods of general relaxation.

We usually start with Progressive Relaxation to give the patient a preliminary familiarity with the gross sensations of tension and relaxation and an early feeling of achievement. Shortly thereafter (and practiced separately), autogenic exercises are taught. These provide the patient with shorthand cues for initiating a relaxed state when needed. One or two formulae are introduced at each session, and are first practiced in the presence of the therapist.

Pre-session measurements may next be taken to help assess progress. The patient then remains quiet and concentrates on attempting to influence the feedback in the desired direction. He might be told to "do whatever you find works to make the tone go down." He is advised that this will generally work best if he experiments with altering the feedback by using a passive or neutral, rather than an active striving, or goal-directed manner of thinking. The patient then tries things (e.g., tensing his forehead and then "letting go"); he tracks the shifting feedback; he sees what works to trigger change in either direction; selects those initiatives that move it in the desired direction; and further defines what it is about the state of mind that works best. He may conjure up images to move him towards a particular goal, such as memories of the sun warming his hands to achieve that end. Eventually, such intermediary images will become redundant. Indeed, he will eventually find the feedback itself unnecessary as he learns to enter at will into the mental state that changes his physiology in the desired direction.

In the first few sessions the patient learns quite graphically that only he is in charge of changes in his body that, when they occur in other settings, may lead him down the path towards symptoms. Indeed, he inevitably discovers that no outside event can "get to" his physiology without his acting as an intermediary, wittingly or unwittingly. This helps the patient regain hope that it will eventually be possible to better modulate his reactions to life's vagaries. It also helps the patient to reclaim feelings of greater responsibility for what happens in his body than may be inspired by those forms of medical care in which one is the passive recipient of the decisions and interventions of others. The expectation in almost all biofeedback applications is that, as a result of having established stronger trade routes for contact between the patient's

conscious awareness and his sometimes unruly physiology, he will become attuned to early cues of impending physical distress, and will frequently sense when things are starting to go wrong before they flower into full-blown symptoms. There is also the expectation that, if the patient *can* be helped, it will be both prophylactically and in aborting individual symptom episodes.

Although the division of time in the session should be modified according to individual needs, time for discussion is always allotted at both the beginning of treatment and after the feedback. Towards the end of the session, the patient is asked to share any correlations he made during it, with the feedback left silently running to gauge physiological reactions to the discussion.

Initial recordings of the level of physiological activation typically improve over a course of therapy. However, these are less valid indicators of true progress than are such things as the patient's increasing awareness of impending somatic tensions at home and work, his ability to use the techniques to quiet himself in those settings and especially to avert or decrease symptoms there, and his reporting of decreased medication usage. It is helpful for the patient to know he can return in the future for one or two "booster sessions" if he has let his practice lapse, and if stressful events in his life have again taken the driver's seat. "Successful" patients generally continue practicing their biofeedback techniques at home, either on a regular or an intermittent basis, and they increase their use of it during periods of added tension.

BIOFEEDBACK IN HEADACHE TREATMENT—GENERAL CONSIDERATIONS

HEADACHE DIAGNOSIS AND PATIENT SELECTION

The prime diagnostic indications for self-regulatory treatment of headache are tension, migraine, and mixed headaches. It is also sometimes beneficial with posttraumatic headaches. The Ad Hoc Committee on the Classification of Headache (22) drew a clear distinction between "muscle contraction (tension) headache" and "vascular headache of the migraine type." Although this is the classification currently most in favor, some subsequent studies have failed to confirm this dichotomy, either by looking at presenting symptomatology (23–25), or on the basis of psychophysiological findings (26). Several authors currently believe that these two types of headache are the extreme ends of a continuum (26–28).

Historically, muscle contraction headache patients have been treated with EMG biofeedback from the frontal region, while migraineurs have been treated with temperature feedback from the hands. More recently, temporal artery pulse amplitude feedback has also been used for the latter group. These are still the most generally useful forms of feedback for these diagnoses (29). In those migraine patients where scalp muscle tension is also high, there is evidence that EMG feedback is a useful addition to treatment (21). Several authors routinely treat headaches with a combined EMG-thermal feedback approach, usually in combination with autogenic phrases and/or Progressive Relaxation. This combination is especially suitable for patients who have mixed tension-vascular headaches (30). One usually begins with EMG feedback, as it is easier for the patient to understand and feel some control over. The two types of feedback are sometimes useful for treating certain posttraumatic headache patients, especially those whose symptoms time alone has not helped.

Biofeedback has not proven effective thus far for treating cluster headache (31, 32), although the spontaneously fluctuating nature of the disorder makes the ultimate long-term utility of biofeedback here undetermined. Biofeedback is also usually less successful with menstrual migraine (33, 34); it can, however, be helpful for treating those women whose migraine continues throughout their pregnancy, as this is a time when pharmacologic therapies are necessarily limited.

Headache diagnosis is only one of the relevant factors affecting patient selection for self-regulatory therapies. Motivation, personality, tolerance for medications, desire to avoid medications, frequency and severity of attacks, overall tension level, and willingness to practice between sessions are some additional factors to take into consideration.

Certain types of patients prove particularly well matched with biofeedback. For example, the patient who doesn't believe that his worries have any relationship to his physical symptoms can expect to receive some education from the biofeedback. The patient who tends to intellectualize and rationalize to resist any honest recognition of feelings may find that his verbal fortress has been simply bypassed. At the opposite end of that spectrum is the action-oriented, alexithymic patient, who somatizes feelings and needs assistance in reinterpreting his bodily sensations; biofeedback's concreteness and immediacy may prove a less frustrating way for him to do this than verbal therapy. Finally, the patient who trusts mechanical devices more than people, and who is not motivated to change that preference, may find himself most comfortable with this form of symptom control.

As with most new treatments, patients who have failed to improve with previous approaches swell the ranks of the newly referred until, for many, the new treatment proves as disappointing as the old. Patients with high motivation and ego strength, the type that tend to do better in other therapies are, not surprisingly, also the ones most likely to be helped with self-regulatory techniques.

CLINICAL STUDIES AND PLACEBO RESPONSE

The numerous clinical and research studies scientifically justifying biofeedback vary greatly in quality. Many of these studies, unfortunately, adhere to stereotyped protocols which gain little support from their unsophisticated hypotheses and flimsy treatment, despite the overbearing statistical analyses that sometimes accompany them. Such studies make it difficult for the clinician to discern what he should or should not do or can and cannot believe. Moreover, many studies neither incorporate a sufficient understanding of the complexity of human anxiety, nor sufficiently distinguish between student volunteers and psychiatric patients. In some, professionals well experienced in relaxation procedures do not instruct the patients. In others, patients are not trained to a set criterion of demonstrated ability, but instead, are arbitrarily assigned to treatment lasting a predetermined number of sessions. Long-term follow-up of results may be lacking, except for a paper-and-pencil questionnaire. In short, many studies have left us with more information than knowledge (35).

Haber et al (36), who reviewed self-control procedures and biofeedback as treatments for headache, found that studies suffered from a variety of methodological shortcomings. Few experiments had an adequate design, and few demonstrated that subjects actually acquired control of the targeted response. Despite these faults, most studies found biofeedback useful in treating migraine, tension, and mixed headaches.

It is common knowledge that some headache patients respond, at least for awhile, to placebo. A study by Cox et al (37) examined the possibility that, as patients tend to seek professional help when their headaches are becoming worse, many interventions might spuriously appear to be effective, if the exacerbation soon peaks and the headaches recede naturally, whatever is or is not done. Chronic tension headache patients were separated into three groups: frontal EMG feedback, general relaxation procedure, and placebo (a capsule which they were told was a time-release muscle relaxant). Both treatment groups reduced their headaches significantly more than the placebo group, a difference still present at a 4-month follow-up.

Wickramasekera (38) replicated the finding that biofeedback needed to be truly contingent to achieve clinical results. His study included a false feedback period, and he reported that while patients did not improve when given the random feedback, they improved dramatically when given access to true feedback. A placebo effect was not seen.

Only one study used false feedback in a fashion somewhat analogous to an active placebo. Otis et al (39) arranged for each patient in their study to receive accurate feedback when trapezius muscle tension was increasing, but false feedback when trapezius tension was decreasing. Such a procedure allowed the patient to "test" the feedback: if he contracted his trapezius, the feedback tone changed instantly. Subjects in this experiment learned to tense the muscle, but not to relax it. Nonetheless, two-thirds showed reduced headaches by the end of the study, while a no-treatment control group failed to show any improvement.

Biofeedback is not "just placebo"; however, the nature and usefulness of the placebo have drawn the attention of many workers in the field, as the relaxing qualities of the self-regulatory therapies in many ways intentionally recruit the same innate biological pathways that placebos activate automatically. Although the effect of placebo has been eliminated from certain applications of biofeedback, it is not always possible to design experiments that can do this for one simple reason: there is nothing that feels like relaxation but actually isn't. On the other hand, the mechanisms that account for a placebo's beneficial effects are powerful, biochemical, universal, and specific. It can be thought of as an innate biological reflex, one which typically accounts for 60% of an analgesic's relief, whether that be aspirin or morphine. Thus, to the extent that biofeedback can predictably supplement its specific physiological effects with the synergistic action of a placebo this can be considered a benefit to patients, however frustrating to theoreticians.

EFFECT OF MEDICATION

Most headache patients treated with biofeedback are also taking some form of medication.

Some have pursued a nondrug therapy because medication has produced too many side effects or because it relieves too few headache symptoms. Even when medications are working, biofeedback can still be used as an adjunctive technique, one which may facilitate a reduction in the prescribed dosage.

Pharmacotherapy is often an indicated concomitant with self-regulatory treatments, and a modified form of it is appropriate to continue following treatment. The two approaches can even complement or potentiate each other's effects, especially in initial stages of treatment. Diazepam plus EMG feedback was found to be more useful for reducing the anxiety of psychiatric patients than was either one used alone (40), and EEG feedback training potentiated the effects of Ritalin on hyperkinetic children (41). At other times, self-regulatory techniques can stand in for drugs when necessary. Many clinical situations can be found in which sedatives are either risky or contraindicated, and yet the patient needs to be calmed. Common ones include the chronically suicidal patient, the ex-addict, the patient allergic to available compounds, the patient whose religious beliefs forbid the use of medications, and the patient who thinks of medication as an unacceptable "crutch."

It has been reported that certain medications have the potential to occasionally alter biofeedback's effectiveness. Patients using propanolol sometimes exhibit variability in their ability to learn peripheral temperature control by means of thermal feedback. A similar difficulty was seen during EMG training of patients taking amitriptyline (42). The great majority of patients can eventually reach training criteria even if receiving these medications. However, for those who find the biofeedback unduly frustrating and nonproductive, a trial without medications is worth considering.

AGE

Self-regulation can be used for patients of any age. Children and adolescents often take to biofeedback with enthusiasm, and many experience it as a form of game. In fact, children have been found to learn autonomic self-regulation as much as five times faster than adults (4, 43). Significant reduction in the need for medications has also been reported among children with headache who have been trained with biofeedback (44).

As might be expected, older patients often require more time to master biofeedback techniques; yet, treatment should not be withheld because of age alone. Age is not an absolute barrier to the use of biofeedback. Elderly people may take a bit longer to learn the self-regulation, but they usually can. This is despite the findings of Blanchard et al (45) that, in their experience, only 18% of patients 60 years and older were improved with biofeedback clinically, and none of the five tension headache patients in that age range improved. It is most important to be mindful of other factors in the elderly that can influence diagnosis or treatment: a higher prevalence of organic disease, frequent degenerative changes in the cervical spine, multiple medication regimens, and psychological factors such as loss-induced depression, a restricted life style, or fear of dying. If the older patient seems blocked in progressing with self-regulation, one of these factors is quite often the cause.

FREQUENCY AND NUMBER OF SESSIONS

Sessions are usually once or twice a week to begin with, tapering off to less frequent appointments once the basics have been mastered. Seeing patients twice a week encourages them to practice at home, which is essential for success in the long run. Treatment length varies significantly from patient to patient, as it is clearly modifiable by many factors, including patient variables, illness variables, experience of the therapist, and therapeutic goals. Most patients, however, can learn basic relaxation skills that can be maintained in 10–15 sessions lasting 45 minutes. The number of sessions is typically increased when psychotherapeutic measures are integrated into the treatment, something which is indicated more often than not (46). Patients with psychogenic posttraumatic headaches, or patients whose headaches have proven longstanding and refractory, may also require longer treatment.

Patients are generally able to maneuver the feedback signals in the quiet of the doctor's office sooner than they are able to effectively apply these skills to their dysfunctional physiology during tension-producing episodes outside the office. With self-regulation, as with psychotherapy and tricyclic antidepressants, sufficient treatment time is required for the improvements to take hold and become integrated into the patient's way of life. Many patients have given up in discouragement because they did not know they could expect better results if they practiced more frequently and kept working at it for several months. All self-regulatory therapies are sensitive to this "dosage requirement."

As in other areas of medicine, this therapy can be terminated when the patient has reliably learned the relaxation technique he has come to learn, and has obtained the maximum possible relief from headaches. Allotting a fixed number of sessions for learning of self-regulatory skills is therefore not a reasonable approach and, in fact, is, from a biological or clinical perspective, inherently arbitrary.

CONTRAINDICATIONS AND CAUTIONS

The primary caution is that biofeedback techniques will be overvalued, and not viewed as tools but as a comprehensive treatment. Another precaution: apply these techniques only after more acute medical or psychiatric problems have been treated. It is also assumed that the biofeedback therapist will be fully trained in the disorder being treated and qualified in the technical details of biofeedback, or that the therapist will be under the direct supervision of a professional so qualified.

In general, self-regulatory techniques have few serious contraindications or side effects. The patient has nothing chemically added to his body to which he can be allergic; no potentially incorrect interpretations are being insisted upon; and the interventions are less invasive than having one's temperature taken. Actually, there are so few serious dangers associated with these techniques that the incautious professional can be lulled into not concerning himself enough about the ones that are.

Temporary distortions of body image may occur during relaxation, and on occasion these have been reported to exacerbate hallucinatory activity in schizophrenics (47). For this and other reasons, biofeedback is contraindicated in acute schizophrenia. The insulin requirements in insulin-dependent diabetics may drop with successful treatment, causing the patient to become hypoglycemic if his dosage is not monitored. For a similar reason, antihypertensive medications may also need readjustment. Patients who are extremely depressed, hypochondriacal, or suffering from an obsessive-compulsive disorder generally do poorly.

COST EFFECTIVENESS

A number of clinicians question the value of biofeedback for headache patients because of its expense. Cost may also be a matter of practical concern for patients. At times this has led to attempts to shortcut teaching of relaxation by using less effective self-instruction techniques. One reason these don't work as well is that the patient concludes that if the professional doesn't truly take the learning of relaxation seriously, why should he?

A recent study (48) compared medical expenses reported to have been incurred by 45 headache patients both "before" and "after" various combinations of relaxation and biofeedback training. Expenditures for headache treatment in the 2 years "before" treatment averaged $995; for the 2 years "after," the comparable average was $52 (48). Within the limitations of the study, the conclusions speak for themselves.

BIOFEEDBACK FOR TENSION HEADACHE

Treatment of the muscle contraction or tension headache has been one of the most thoroughly studied, accepted, and applied uses of EMG biofeedback. On the surface, the rationale for such treatment is so simple it appears elegant: specific muscles are causing pain because they are in prolonged spasm; with the help of biofeedback the patient will see how to relax them and reverse the pathogenetic process. This view, though correct, considers only one level of reality. What is not considered is this: if spastic muscles hurt, why does the patient contract them in the first place? The answer is usually unknown to both the patient and his physician. The mechanisms and psychodynamic aspects of muscle contraction headache are discussed elsewhere in this book.

The electrical activity generated by a muscle or muscle group is an indirect but reliable measure of its state of contraction in electromyographic (EMG) biofeedback. Surface electrodes are attached to the frontal region or, alternately, over selected muscle groups of the face, neck, shoulders, and arms, as EMG activity in these areas are often a sensitive indicator of overall relaxation. As any distressed muscle group can be selectively targeted for feedback, the technique is capable of a good measure of patient-specific flexibility. Some patients require nuchal feedback more than frontal. Full procedural techniques are beyond the scope of this chapter, but can be readily found in excellent references on biofeedback (49).

Several studies have indicated that tension headaches are accompanied by increased tension in the frontalis muscle. Thus, the frontal EMG recordings of patients during a tension headache are usually significantly higher than comparable scores for patients not experiencing such headaches. Hutchings

and Reinking (50), in 1976, found dramatically elevated baseline frontalis EMG levels in 18 patients with severe tension headaches when compared to nonheadache controls.

In 1970, Budzynski and Stoyva (12) found that, as a group, patients prone to tension headaches have significantly higher frontalis EMG readings than individuals not so affected. In 1973 they went on to publish the first controlled study using EMG feedback for tension headache (51). It compared three groups, each comprised of six patients. In the 2 weeks before treatment, all patients were monitored to determine pretraining EMG levels. The first group received accurate frontal EMG feedback; the second group received false feedback; and the third group was simply monitored for an equivalent period. Patients were given relaxation instructions to practice at home, and had 16 30-minute treatment sessions over an 8-week period.

The primary findings were:

(a) That EMG feedback training resulted in a significant decrease in frontal EMG in the group which received true feedback, but not in the control group which received false feedback.

(b) Four of the six patients in the treatment group showed a large decrease in headaches; subjects in the other groups had considerably less improvement.

(c) The degree to which the resting frontal EMG dropped in the treated group correlated highly with the patient's clinical improvement. Four of the six patients in the biofeedback treatment group had maintained their gains after 18 months.

(d) There was a significant reduction in use of headache medications and tranquilizers by patients who received accurate feedback when compared to that of the controls

Subsequently, most tension headache studies have reported a 50–70% reduction in frequency and severity of headaches using a roughly similar protocol (41–43). Typically included was a 3- to 6-month follow-up of patients. However, an investigation by Adler and Adler (52), in which they combined psychotherapy with EMG feedback, obtained an 88% improvement rate, one which was maintained at the time of a follow-up 5 years later. These findings suggest that EMG feedback is indeed a specific therapy for tension headache, and that its value is enhanced by combining it with psychotherapy.

Summarizing the data, both controlled and uncontrolled studies reach the same conclusion: EMG biofeedback is of benefit in the treatment of tension headache. Recent studies continue to demonstrate that EMG biofeedback leads to a clinically and statistically significant reduction in tension headache activity (53, 54). While some researchers find a strong relationship between the degree of baseline EMG reduction and clinical improvement, others do not. Although quantifications of pain is clearly difficult, headaches are usually reduced by more than 50%.

It is important to note that most non-biofeedback self-regulatory procedures—Autogenic Therapy, self-hypnosis, and Progressive Relaxation, for example—are also effective in reducing tension headache. Biofeedback sometimes promotes a faster drop in both EMG levels and headache activity, however, and it is more acceptable to some patients and necessary for certain others. It may be especially useful when the patient is quite out of touch with his state of muscular contraction and is, for whatever reason, unable to use the simpler techniques to remedy that situation.

BIOFEEDBACK FOR MIGRAINE HEADACHE

The use of biofeedback for migraine headaches was first suggested by Elmer Green in 1972 after a serendipitous finding at the Menninger Clinic: a subject being trained with thermal feedback aborted her beginning migraine headache as soon as her hand temperature increased. This encouraged Sargent et al (55) to further experiment with what they termed "autogenic feedback training." Schultz (12), and then others, had earlier reported that many patients could alleviate migraine attacks by using autogenic standard exercises, which include the thought of warm extremities. The Menninger group combined the autogenic phrases with thermal feedback from the upper limbs to teach patients to warm their extremities. "Passive concentration"—the *sine qua non* of autogenic therapy—was used to induce specific physiological changes, such as warmth in the hands. They found that hand temperature was directly related to blood flow, as measured with a plethysmograph. Results of this first Menninger group (55) study were: 63% of 20 migraineurs were evaluated as improved; in their second study, 74% of 63 migraine sufferers improved (53) as measured by decreased headache severity and analgesic use. In a follow-up evaluation, Solbach and Sargent (56) found that 74% of 55 subjects had a significant reduction in headache activity 2 years after the study ended.

Thermal feedback of peripheral skin temperature is usually recorded from the fingers, toes, or forehead by thermisters gently taped to these areas. In most applications, including for migraine, the aim is to learn to warm the extremities. Warm extremities imply that there has been a relaxation of the muscular walls of the arterioles, thereby permitting increased blood flow to the skin of the arms and legs. In order to accomplish this, the patient must discover how to decrease his sympathetic vascular tone, as this controls the constriction of skin arterioles. The changes in peripheral temperature are, in other words, simply surface reflections of a pattern of decreased sympathetic activity. Therefore, by learning to increase the blood flow to his extremities, a patient is concomitantly learning to reduce the sympathetic output to his cephalic vasculature. With time and practice, most people can learn to increase their peripheral temperature by 10–15°F, and occasionally by more than 25°F.

The rationale for using "hand-warming" techniques in migraine rests on the assumption that migraineurs have an inherent vasomotor instability, and that the headache phase of each episode is associated with peripheral vasoconstriction and cephalic vasodilation. Elliott (57) has in fact shown impaired reflex vasodilation in the limbs of migraineurs compared to controls.

Many studies have confirmed the effectiveness of biofeedback in helping large numbers of patients learn to diminish the frequency of their migraine headaches (54, 58). A sophisticated study by Mathew et al (59) showed that changes in cerebrovascular flow rates (as measured by xenon inhalation) accompanied successful thermal biofeedback, and was coincident with the acute cessation of a beginning migraine headache.

As the headache phase of migraine is associated with dilated extracranial arteries, it has been suggested that directly teaching patients to reduce their temporal artery pulsations might thereby block this symptomatic vasodilation and prevent the headaches. (In the initial biofeedback studies, patients were also trained to cool their foreheads.) Koppman et al (60) were able to teach nine migraineurs to dilate and vasoconstrict their temporal arteries with the use of reflectance photoplethysmographic feedback. Friar and Beatty (61), using temporal artery feedback, reported significant improvement in migraine symptoms and a decrease in medication use among their patients. Gauthier et al (62) found hand warming and temporal artery pulse volume reduction feedback equally effective.

In summary, treatment of migraine with biofeedback can be helpful if the training is not abridged, if relevant psychological issues are not ignored, and if some form of relaxation practice is continued in the years following treatment (63). Generalized relaxation procedures are also helpful for many patients with migraine. Whether to use these techniques with a particular patient is partly determined by his headache frequency, his motivation, and his responsiveness to other treatments. The severity of his headaches and their disruptive influence on his functioning are also important considerations. Patients with infrequent migraines may prefer to rely on medication for symptomatic treatment. As noted previously, biofeedback can be particularly useful to treat children with migraine.

OUTCOME OF BIOFEEDBACK TREATMENT

LONG-TERM OUTCOME

In 1976, a 5-year follow-up study of 58 patients by Adler and Adler (52) reported that overall, major improvement (75–100% remission) occurred in 86% of patients at the end of this period. Forty-two percent of patients had either no headaches or only very occasional ones. The authors felt the combination of psychotherapy and biofeedback was the essential factor in this success rate. A subsequent 10-year follow-up (64) of 53 migraine patients by these same authors using matched controls further demonstrated the long-term usefulness of self-regulation in this disorder. The criterion was for patients to raise their temperature predictably to 95°F and to then be able to maintain this while visualizing a personally stressful situation. Headaches decreased from a mean of 36/year to a mean of 5.8/year. The improvement was significantly ($p = 0.01$) enhanced by the addition of psychotherapy, even if this only consisted of a few sessions of learning to identify their emotions at times.

In a 4-year retrospective study of 693 patients, Diamond and Montrose (54) found that many variables affected outcome, including sex, diagnosis, number of follow-up sessions, personality, and other psychological factors. Females were generally more successful than males, and patients below 30 years of age had greater overall success. In a 5-year retrospective study of survey results from 413 biofeedback patients, Diamond (65) reported in 1979 that up to 90% of patients believed biofeedback helped them relax; 40% believed biofeedback produced permanent reduction in headache frequency or severity; 30% found temporary or intermittent relief; and approximately 30% reported no improvement.

TRANSFER OF SELF-REGULATORY SKILLS

For a successful outcome, the patient must find some practical way to transfer the various self-regulation skills into the daily routine of his life. If he does not, headaches will return before long. Unfortunately, this phase of biofeedback treatment is often neglected. A major factor promoting the successful transfer of these skills is the patient's commitment to doing regular home practice. This generally requires that he take a "relaxation break" at least twice daily for 15 minutes or more. Patients are more likely to actually do this if they are helped to formally schedule practical places and times for it. If a patient repeatedly neglects to do home practice, it is a sign of resistance, and should not be ignored. It may indicate that something in the therapy or in the transference is being overlooked, or it may be the patient's way of announcing that he has greater need of the therapist's psychotherapeutic skills than of the relaxation.

Patients should also begin to identify physiological cues that signal an impending headache. The signs preceding a tension headache, for example, might include buildup of muscle tightness in the neck and shoulders, or a slight feeling of pressure in the brow. As soon as he becomes aware of such cues, the patient should begin relaxation practice to keep it from turning into a headache. Eventually, this sequence typically becomes an overlearned habit, and sinks below the patient's level of awareness. In like fashion, the migraine patient should become increasingly aware of when his hands are too cool, and of other phenomena which accompany his own characteristic prodrome; he can then use this information as a signal that he had best begin hand warming. Doing this is more difficult in those cases of common migraine, where in such forewarnings are minimal or absent; these patients may be best advised to simply initiate hand warming at frequent intervals throughout the day. Stroebel (66) recommends that patients perform a 10-second warmth exercise roughly 30 times a day.

Another way to facilitate transfer of learning is to have the patient visualize stress situations relevant to his own life circumstances, and to maintain his relaxed state during these visualizations to inhibit backsliding. Sufficient follow-up sessions should also be encouraged.

NONSPECIFIC BENEFITS OF BIOFEEDBACK

The need to learn some simple way to intermittently return to a normal or lowered level of arousal is not a luxury for mankind, but is as basic as the need for adequate sleep, nutrition, and exercise. Many people can achieve this through reading, music, gardening, walking, or some other personally devised way to pace themselves. It is surprising how often chronic or recalcitrant headache patients lack this ability. Some cannot let down even during sleep. Conversely, once they do learn how to relax, the benefits may generalize to many areas of their lives.

Important, nonspecific benefits of both biofeedback and relaxation training have been observed in clinical practice (35). These include:

(a) When the patient has fears or misconceptions about psychologists or psychiatrists, ambivalence about trusting one, or confusion about whether his problem could be in part psychological, the time required to learn relaxation allows the patient to get to know the therapist and to reappraise the situation. Because biofeedback is viewed as a "medical" procedure, it allows the patient to save face during this introductory period. For the same reason, many physicians feel more comfortable referring patients for biofeedback than for psychotherapy. It can provide a gentle introduction to psychological treatment for many unsophisticated, alexithymic, or simply apprehensive patients.

(b) The patient with longstanding problems may feel both helplessness and hopelessness. Biofeedback can cut into these feeling states, as patients are often relieved to find that, even though they may be unable to change all the stressors in their life, they can at least influence their reactions, and in that way gain some autonomy from these stressors.

(c) The patient learning to regulate his physiology with biofeedback finds he must dissociate the part of himself which *observes* (his "observing ego") from the part of himself that *experiences* sensation and initiates change. Because he must carefully attend to his sensations to correlate them with the feedback he must, in essence, observe himself. In this role, he learns to develop a passive or even curious and detached attitude towards his symptoms. This helps him to put emotional distance between his sense of "selfhood" and his dysfunctional physiology. It is also an introduction to the self-observant attitude needed in psychotherapy, if this eventually becomes necessary.

(d) As a result of focusing on his body, the patient may become more aware of its needs for rest, crying, touching, etc. He sometimes also recognizes ways in which he has ignored those needs in the past.

(e) New information contributing to the diagnosis of either psychiatric or somatic conditions may come to light during the course of biofeedback. As his physical activity becomes quieted during a session the patient may, for the first time, become aware of underlying resentments, or of other feelings. If, on the other hand, the patient changes his physiology but his symptoms persist, the accuracy of the original medical diagnosis may need re-evaluation.

PSYCHIATRIC ASPECTS OF BIOFEEDBACK TREATMENT

Another issue which has direct bearing on whether biofeedback procedures will be effective is the extent to which the treatment deals with psychological issues. Many helping professionals think of biofeedback only as "training," while others consider it an instrument-aided form of psychotherapy (67, 68). Whatever the therapist's personal theoretical outlook, psychological issues are empirically present and relevant in many patients. In their 5-year follow-up study of chronic headache patients, Adler and Adler (52) noted that 80% of the subjects required some degree of psychological intervention, and most of the patients who did poorly with biofeedback had not received it. Their 10-year controlled follow-up of migraineurs further supports the contention that relaxation-assisted thermal feedback's long-term usefulness for treatment migraine is significantly enhanced by psychodynamic psychotherapy specifically adapted to the migraineur (46). Patients who received such therapy were found to have fared better at the end of 10 years with respect to headache reduction ($p = 0.01$), and were also found to have continued practicing their self-regulation more than did the matched controls.

A relaxed state may also free up forgotten memories associated with emotionally charged situations (69). Traditional psychotherapy can then be used to deal with this material if needed. Biofeedback is an especially sensitive way to reflect back the patient's physical reaction to such emotional topics when they arise during treatment. If, when the patient is relaxed, an intruding emotion or a conflict-related thought enters his mind, the biofeedback may rapidly shift in the direction of anxiety. Frontal EMG is sensitive to these cognitions if they arise when the frontalis muscle is relatively relaxed. The "surging" frontal EMG pattern caused by intrusion of such thoughts is familiar to therapists experienced in the use of biofeedback. On the other hand, in the presence of a high frontal EMG, the patient's physical reaction to such thoughts may go unnoticed (70). Therefore, thermal and electrodermal (GSR) biofeedback are even more useful in this regard. Depending upon their innate reactivity, particular patients will respond better to one or the other modality.

In the "dialogue" between mind and body, the biofeedback instrument can serve the role of honest broker by pointing out which memories, thoughts, or associations seem to trigger trouble. It does this much as a metal detector swept over the surface of a field will pinpoint buried metal. The patient is often entirely unaware of the troublesome nature of a particular theme; he can use this capacity of the biofeedback to learn more about himself and about what sorts of things trouble him. He may see that his muscles tighten up every time his thoughts drift in the direction of his son-in-law, the one who has yet to evidence the ambition to be financially autonomous. This capacity of the feedback allows it to be a most helpful aid in psychotherapy.

We have termed this signaling of the patient's reaction in the direction of tension to specific thoughts or memories that are hit upon during trial-and-error attempts to alter the feedback "Biofeedback-psychotherapy" (35, 47, 49, 69, 71). Its use is compatible with the psychotherapeutic needs of a number of patients who are unable to discover which topics are triggering their headaches. It allows them to recognize specific thoughts as relevant to their physical discomfort. The patient usually becomes curious when the same thought or image regularly elicits the physical concomitants of anxiety on a feedback instrument, and will bring these observations up for discussion; the significance of these associations to his problems can then be explored.

Although much of the earliest work in biofeedback was performed by experimental psychologists and physiologists whose clinical orientation leaned towards behavior therapy, it has more recently drawn the interest of psychoanalytically-oriented therapists as well (72). The simplicity of biofeedback's basic premise allows it to find application in many theoretical persuasions.

After self-regulatory treatment has started, personality variables continue to play a role. Patients with histrionic personality disorders, for example, often become restless during sessions and neglect practice between sessions. Sometimes they appear bored, but at other times become frightened. A formal approach in a well-lighted room in helpful. In contrast, the obsessive-compulsive patient is typically diligent about home practice and, rather than becoming frustrated that he has to work with the feedback, becomes frustrated that he can't work with it well enough to appease his own perfectionistic expectations. He compares one day's "performance" with the previous one's, and often experiences feedback signals as criticism rather than information. These difficulties are sometimes minimized by using a low sensitivity setting on the instrument, so success at the assigned task appears easier, or by substituting the therapist's supportive verbal feedback about the direction of physiological change for auditory or visual feedback. Any such characterologic styles of confronting new situations can cause treatment to fail, but only if they are pronounced in the patient or ignored by the therapist.

In summary, biofeedback will be most helpful if one expects more of his patient than visceral gymnastics, and more of the therapy than a simplified or abbreviated approach to complex human problems. Each part of the physiology is in homeostatic equilibrium with the patient's entire psychosocial milieu. The patient in acute head pain will not be able to concentrate on learning biofeedback; a man who was mugged on Monday will not be truly relaxed on Tuesday, no matter what his hand temperature is. To use biofeedback most effectively, the effect of these contexts on the physiology should be accounted for in the treatment plan, which should be a comprehensive plan for the rehabilitation, not only of a disordered part, but also of its owner, using pharmacotherapy or other medical care in conjunction with self-regulation. Put another way: biofeedback alone is never a sufficient treatment for headache. But when used properly, and in conjunction with other treatment modalities, it is a good tool, and may allow the patient to gain some "leverage" over his unruly physiology.

REFERENCES

1. Adler CS, Adler SM: Biofeedback. In *Encyclopedia Britannica Medical and Health Annual, 1986.* Chicago, Encyclopedia Britannica, Inc., 1986, pp 377–382.

2. Kroger WS: *Clinical and Experimental Hypnosis in medicine, Dentistry, and Psychology.* Philadelphia, Lippincott, 1977.

3. Pavlov IP: *The Work of the Digestive Glands.* London, Charles Griffin & Company Ltd., 1902.

4. Adler CS, Adler SM: Biofeedback. In Karasu TB (ed): *The Psychiatric Therapies,* The American Psychiatric Association Commission on Psychiatric Therapies. Washington, D.C., American Psychiatric Association, 1984, pp 587–618.

5. Basmajian JV: Conscious control of individual motor units. *Science* 141:440–441, 1963.

6. Kamiya J: Operant control of the EEG alpha rhythm and some of its reported effects on consciousness. In Hart CT (ed): *Altered States of Consciousness: A Book of Readings.* New York, Wiley, 1969, pp 507–517.

7. Shapiro D, Tursky B, Schwartz GE: Differentiation of heart rate and systolic blood pressure in man by operant conditioning. *Psychosom Med* 32:417–423, 1970.

8. Engel BT: Operant conditioning of cardiac function: a status report. *Psychophysiology* 9:161–177, 1972.

9. Kimmel HD: Instrumental conditioning of autonomically mediated behavior. *Psychol Bull* 67:337–345, 1967.

10. Miller NE: Learning of visceral and glandular responses. *Science* 163:434–445, 1969.

11. Pickering TG, Brucker B, Frankel HL, et al: Mechanisms of learned voluntary control of blood pressure in patients with generalized body paralysis. In Beatty J, Legewie H (eds): *Biofeedback and Behavior.* New York, Plenum, 1977.

12. Budzynski TH, Stoyva JM, Adler CS: Feedback-induced muscle relaxation: application to tension headache. *Behav Ther Exp Psychol* 1:205–211, 1970.

13. Schultz JH: *Das Autogene Training.* Leipzig, G. Thieme, 1932.

14. Jacobson E: *Progressive Relaxation,* ed 3. Chicago, University Press, 1938.

15. Schultz JH, Luthe W: *Autogenic Training: A Psychophysiological Approach in Psychotherapy.* New York, Grune & Stratton, 1959.

16. Luthe W (ed): *Autogenic Therapy.* New York, Grune & Stratton, 1969, vols 1–6.

17. Benson H, Klipper MZ: *The Relaxation Response.* New York, Morrow, 1975.

18. Rossi EL (ed): *The Collected Papers of Milton Erickson, vols 1–4.* New York, Irvington, 1980.

19. Haynes SN, Griffin P, Mooney D, Parise M: Electromyographic biofeedback and relaxation instructions in the treatment of muscle contraction headache. *Behav Ther* 6:672–678, 1975.

20. Haynes SN, Moseley D, McGowan WT: Relaxation training and biofeedback in the reduction of frontalis muscle tension. *Psychophysiology* 12:547–552, 1975.

21. Coursey RD: Electromyograph feedback as a relaxation technique. *J Consult Clin Psychol* 43:825–834, 1975.

22. Ad Hoc Committee on the Classification of Headache: Classification of Headache *JAMA* 179:717–718, 1962.

23. Ziegler DK, Hassanein R, Hassanein K: Headache syndromes suggested by factor analysis of symptom variables in a headache prone population. *J Chron Dis* 25:353–363, 1972.

24. Bakal DA, Kaganov JA: Symptom characteristics of chronic and non-chronic headache sufferers. *Headache* 19:285–289, 1979.

25. Waters WE: Review of the epidemiology of migraine in adults. *Danish Med Bull* 22:86–88, 1975.

26. Bakal DA, Kaganov JA: Muscle contraction and migraine headache: psychophysiologic comparison. *Headache* 17:208–215, 1977.

27. Philips C: Tension headache: theoretical problems. *Behav Res Ther* 16:249–261, 1978.

28. Martin PR, Mathews AM: Tension headache: psychophysiological investigation and treatment. *J Psychosom Res* 22:389–399, 1978.

29. Billings RF, Thomas MR, et al: Differential efficacy of biofeedback in headache. *Headache* 24:211–215, 1984.

30. Diamond S, Dalessio DJ: *The Practicing Phy-*

sician's Approach to Headache, ed 2. Baltimore, Williams & Wilkins, 1978, pp 136–137.

31. Kudrow L: *Cluster Headache: Mechanisms and Management.* London, Oxford University Press, 1980.

32. Saper JR: *Headache Disorders: Current Concepts and Treatment Strategies.* Boston, John Wright-PSG, 1978, p 110.

33. Solbach P, Sargent J, Coyne L: Menstrual migraine headache: results of a controlled, experimental, outcome study of non-drug treatments. *Headache* 24:75–78, 1984.

34. Szekely B, Botwin D, Eidelman BH, et al: Nonpharmacological treatment of menstrual headache: relaxation-biofeedback behavior therapy and person-centered insight therapy. *Headache* 26:86–92, 1986.

35. Adler CS, Adler SM: A psychodynamic perspective on self-regulation in the treatment of psychosomatic disorders. In Cheren S: *Psychosomatic Medicine: Theory, Physiology, and Practice.* New York, International Universities Press, 1987.

36. Haber JD, Thompson KJ, et al: Physiological self-control and the biofeedback treatment of headache. *Headache* 23:174–178, 1983.

37. Cox DJ, Freundlich A, Meyer RG: Differential effectiveness of electromyographic feedback, verbal relaxation instructions and medication placebo. *J Consult Clin Psychol* 43:892–898, 1975.

38. Wickramasekera I: Electromyographic feedback training and tension headache: preliminary observations. *Am J Clin Hypn* 15:83–85, 1972.

39. Otis LS, McCormick NL, Lukas JS: Voluntary control of tension headaches. Proceedings of the Biofeedback Research Society Fifth Annual Meeting, Colorado Springs, CO, 1974, p 23.

40. LaValle YJ, Lamontagne Y, Pinard G, et al: Effects of EMG feedback, diazepam, and their combination on chronic anxiety. *J Psychosom Res* 21:65–71, 1977.

41. Shouse M, Lubar J: Operant conditioning of EEG rhythms and Ritalin in the treatment of hyperkinesis. *Biofeedback Self Regul* 4:299–312, 1979.

42. Jay GW, Renelli D, Mead T: The effects of propranolol and amitriptyline on vascular and EMG biofeedback training. *Headache* 24:59–69, 1984.

43. Diamond S, Franklin M: Biofeedback—choice of treatment in childhood migraine. In *Therapy in Psychosomatic Medicine,* vol 4, Autogenic Therapy. Rome, Edizioni L. Pozzi, 1977.

44. Werder D, Sargent J: A study of childhood headache using biofeedback as a treatment alternative. *Headache* 24:122–126, 1984.

45. Blanchard EB, Andrasik F, et al: Biofeedback and relaxation treatments for headache in the elderly: a caution and a challenge. *Biofeedback Self Regul* 10:69–72, 1985.

46. Adler CS, Adler SM: An analysis of therapeutic factors seen in a ten-year study of a psychophysiologically and psychodynamically oriented treatment for migraine. In Rose C (ed): *Migraine: Proceedings of the 5th Int. Migraine Symposium,* Basel, Karger, 1985, pp 186–196.

47. Adler CS, Adler SM: *Biofeedback and Psychotherapy* (audio cassette). New York, Bio-Monitoring Applications, 1975.

48. Blanchard EB, Jaccard J, Andrasik F, et al: Reduction in headache patients' medical expenses associated with biofeedback and relaxation treatments. *Biofeedback Self Regul* 10:63–68, 1985.

49. Basmajian VJ (ed): *Biofeedback—Principles and Practice for Clinicians,* ed 1. Baltimore, Williams & Wilkins, 1979.

50. Hutchings DF, Reinking RH: Tension headaches: what form of therapy is most effective? *Biofeedback Self Regul* 1:183–190, 1976.

51. Budzynski TH, Stoyva JM, Adler CS, et al: EMG biofeedback and tension headache: a controlled-outcome study. *Psychosom Med* 35:484–496, 1973.

52. Adler CS, Adler SM: Biofeedback psychotherapy for the treatment of headaches: a 5-year follow-up. *Headache* 16:189, 1976.

53. Reading C: Psychophysiological reactivity in migraine following biofeedback. *Headache* 24:70–74, 1984.

54. Diamond S, Montrose D: The value of biofeedback in the treatment of chronic headache: a four-year retrospective study. *Headache* 24:5–18, 1984.

55. Sargent JD, Green EE, Walters ED: Preliminary report on the use of autogenic feedback training in the treatment of migraine and tension headaches. *Psychosom Med* 35(2):129–135, 1973.

56. Solbach P, Sargent JD: A follow-up evaluation of the Menninger pilot migraine study using thermal training. Biofeedback Society of America Annual Meeting, Orlando, FL, 1977.

57. Elliott K, Frewin DB, Downey JA: Reflex vasomotor responses in the hands of patients suffering from migraine. *Headache* 13:188–196, 1974.

58. Diamond S, Diamond-Falk J, DeVeno T: Biofeedback in the treatment of vascular headache. *Biofeedback Self Regul* 3:385–408, 1978.

59. Mathew R, Larsen V, Dobbins K, et al: Biofeedback control of skin temperature and cerebral blood flow in migraine. *Headache* 20:19–28, 1980.

60. Koppman JW, McDonald RO, Kunzel MG: Voluntary regulation of temporal artery diameter by migraine patients. *Headache* 14:133–138, 1974.

61. Friar LR, Beatty J: Migraine—management by trained control of vasoconstriction. *J Consult Clin Psychol* 44:46–53, 1976.

62. Gauthier J, Lacroix R, et al: Biofeedback control of migraine headaches—a comparison of two approaches. *Biofeedback Self Regul* 10:139–159, 1985.

63. Adler CS, Adler SM: Strategies in general psychiatry, and biofeedback and psychosomatic disorders. In Basmajian JV (ed): *Biofeedback: Principles and Practice for Clinicians,* ed 2. Baltimore, Williams & Wilkins, 1983, pp 239–273.

64. Adler CS, Adler SM: Physiological feedback and psychotherapeutic intervention for migraine: a ten year followup. In Sjastaad O, Pfaffenrath V, Lundberg PO (eds): *Updating in Headache.* Heidelberg, Springer-Verlag, 1985.

65. Diamond S: Biofeedback and headache. *Headache* 19:180–184, 1979.

66. Stroebel C: *The Quieting Reflex.* New York, G.P. Putnam's Sons, 1982.

67. Frank JD: Biofeedback and the placebo effect. *Biofeedback Self Regul* 7: 1982.

68. Lazarus R: A cognitively oriented psychologist looks at biofeedback. *Am Psychol* 30:553–561, 1975.

69. Adler CS, Adler SM: Interface with the unconscious in biofeedback. Presented at the American Academy of Psychoanalysis, Toronto, Canada, 1977.

70. Budzynski TH: Biofeedback strategies in headache treatment. In Basmajian JV (ed): *Biofeedback—Principles and Practice for Clinicians,* ed 1. Baltimore, Williams & Wilkins, 1979, pp 137–138.

71. Nemiah JC, Michaels R, Horowitz MV, Karasu TB, Greenspan KM, Adler CS, Sedlacek K: Commentary on Glucksman: Physiologic changes and clinical events during psychotherapy. *Integr Psychiatry* 3:175–184, 1985.

72. Glucksman ML: Physiologic changes and clinical events during psychotherapy. *Integr Psychiatry* 3:168–184, 1985.

Index

Page numbers followed by *t*, *f*, and *n* indicate tables, figures, and notes, respectively.

Abandonment, and cluster headache, 229
Abreactive therapies, for post-traumatic stress disorder, 338
Acetaminophen, 290
  for migraine, 310
Acetylsalicylic acid, impaired absorption of, during migraine, 245
Addiction, definition of, 290
Adolescence, of headache patient, 165
Affective disorders, 261*f*. *See also* Depression
Aggression
  control of, 217
  in family, and tension headache, 117
  and headache, 50
  and migraine headache, 44–45, 144, 148, 152, 154, 169
  and tension headache, 117
Alcmaeon, 9
Alcohol, as headache trigger, 308
Alcoholism, 127
Alexander, Franz, 18
  observations on personality and migraine headache, 137*t*
  work on migraine headache, 152
Alexia, 183
  with agraphia, migrainous, 190
Alexithymia, 50–51, 126, 230*n*
Allergies, 82
  and headache, 65
Alvarez, Walter
  observations on personality and migraine headache, 137*t*
  work on migraine headache, 151
Ambition, and migraine headache, 150, 160, 166
Ambivalence, and migraine headache, 160
Aminophylline, 344
Amitriptyline, 68
  for depressive headache, 266–267, 271
  for dysthymic pain disorder, 129
  effects of, 267*t*, 267
    on blocking acetylcholine and histamine receptors, 265*t*
  on MHPG levels, 264
  on noradrenergic system, 265
  and MAOI, to prevent hypertensive crisis, 269
  for migraine headache, 271
  for muscle contraction headache, 204
  side effects of, 267
  for tension headache, 271
Amnesia. *See also* Migrainous transient global amnesia
  after migraine psychosis, 190
  retrograde, and migraine headache, 188–189
Amoxapine, mode of action, 269
Amyl nitrite
  effect on migraine headache, 246
  effect on neurological accompaniments of migraine, 241, 241*f*
Amytal interview, for post-traumatic stress disorder, 338–339
Analgesics, 68
  abuse
    by headache patients, 290
    by pain patients, 271
  for migraine treatment, 309–310
  nonnarcotic, 290–293
  overuse, 341
  renal damage from, 293
  ritualistic administration of, 290
Analgesic/sedative abuse, and refractory headache, 294
Analgesic/sedative withdrawal syndrome, 293–294
Anergia, 126
Aneurysms, 66
Anger
  and cluster headache, 224, 230
  and headache, 76, 120, 324–325
  and migraine headache, 154, 160, 170–171, 177–178
  psychotherapeutic approach to, 328–329, 334
  repressed, in children, 90
  and tension headache, 114, 116–117
Angiography, 66
Angry headache, 95

Anhedonia, 126
Anniversary reaction, 75
Anterior cerebral artery infarctions, 190
Anticipatory anxiety, management of, 89
Antidepressants. *See also specific drug;* Tricyclic antidepressants
  combination therapy, for dysthymic pain disorder, 129
  as direct analgesics, 269
  in headache treatment, 319, 319n
  for migraine headache, 271
  and neuroleptics, combinations of, 270
  in pain control, 124–125, 128, 264
  side effects, 129
Antiemetics, for treatment of migraine, 309–310, 311
Antihypertensives, 344
Antisocial personality, and medication compliance, 287
Anxiety
  and caffeine use, 292
  chronic, 113
  and cluster headache, 328
  and conversion headache, 195–196
  in depression, 262
  and headache, 67, 199, 341
  and migraine headache, 160, 162, 172, 328
  psychotherapeutic approach to, 328
  as result of headaches, 82
  in tension headache, 117–118, 121, 328
  vs. depression, 263t
APC preparations, 292–293
Appreciation, migraineurs' desire for, 178
Aretaeus of Cappadocia, 10
Aristotle, 8
Aromatic amino acid decarboxylase, 251
Arthritis, of neck, 65
Asclepius, 8–9
Aspirin, 290–291
  adverse reactions to, 291
  combined with phenacetin and caffeine, 292–293
  effect on liver, 291
  hypersensitivity reactions to, 291
  interactions with other drugs, 291
  for migraine, 310
Association, process of, 17n
Assyrians, headache treatments, 7
Asthenopic scotoma, 187
Asthma medication, 344
Ataraxic medications, 319, 319n
Atherosclerotic vascular disease, 66
Attention, disrupted, in post-traumatic stress disorder, 337

Attitude, 45
Atypical facial neuralgia, 80
Autogenic neutralization, 338, 352
  for post-traumatic headache, 205
Autogenic therapy, in tension headache, 361
Autogenic training, 302, 352–353
Autoimmune disease, 82
Autonomic nervous system, and migraine headache, 257–258. *See also* Migraine headache, autonomic accompaniments
Autoscopy, 14
Avicenna, 11
Avoidant personality, and medication compliance, 287

Babylonians, headache treatments, 7
Barbiturate
  contraindication in migraine, 309
  for migraine headache, 254, 310–311
Basilar/posterior cerebral artery system, 190
Behavioral therapy, 296, 302
  for pain therapy, 124, 128
  for post-traumatic headache, 205
Behavior modification. *See* Behavioral therapy
Bellergal, 310
Benzodiazepines
  in headache treatment, 319
  for migraine treatment, 309–310
Berkley, Bishop, 13
β-adrenergic blocking drugs, 289
Bickerstaff's basilar artery migraine, 188
Biofeedback, 19, 335
  and age of patient, 358
  definition of, 349
  effect of medication, 357–358
  EMG technique, 356. *See also* Electromyographic feedback
  for headache, 302–303, 353–360
    cautions, 359
    clinical studies of, 356–357
    contraindications, 359
    cost effectiveness, 359–360
    frequency and number of sessions, 358–359
    and headache diagnosis, 355–356
    patient selection, 355–356
  for migraine headache, 355–356, 361–362
  nonspecific benefits of, 363–364
  origins of, 351
  outcome of treatment, long-term, 362–363
  in pain management, 128
  as placebo, 357
  for post-traumatic headache, 205, 355–356
  process of, 349–350

psychiatric aspects of, 364–366
and relaxation, 351–354
for tension headache, 271, 355–356, 360–361
terminology, 350
thermal technique, 356
typical session, 354–355
Biofeedback-psychotherapy, 365
Biogenic amines, and headache, 256–257
Biological clock, 213–214
Blood pressure, 61
Body, migraineurs' attitude toward, 154, 160
Body image, and migraine headache, 187
Borderline personality disorder, 283
in children, 86–87
diagnosis of, 89
treatment, 89
Bradyphrenia, 183
Brain tumor, 257
headache caused by, 60
patients' worry about, 59, 66, 307
symptoms, 82
Breast cancer, metastatic, 82
Briquet's syndrome, 199
Bruxism, 65
BUSS scale, 145

Caffeine, 290–292
content
of common drugs, 293t
of food, 292t
and headache, 61
in medications for migraine, contraindications, 309
overuse, by cluster headache patients, 224
side effects, 291–292
stimulant effect of, 291–292
withdrawal symptoms, 292
Caffeinism, symptoms of, 292
Calcium channel-blocking drugs, 289
Carbon dioxide, effect in migraine headache, 241, 246, 247
Carroll, Lewis, 187
Catechol-O-methyltransferase, 243
Celsus, Cornelius, 10
Cenesthopathia, 187
Cephalagia, 10
Cephalalgia: An International Journal of Headache, 340
Cephalea, 10
Cerebral blood flow, changes in, during migraine headache, 241–242, 247
Cerebral neoplasm. *See* Brain tumor
Cervical disc disease, 65

Character. *See also* Personality
definition of, 46, 48
and headache, 46, 48–51
treatment implications, 51
Character disorder, 48. *See also* Personality disorder; *specific disorder*
Cheirooral syndrome. *See* Digitolingual syndrome
Child rearing, and headache patient, 165–166, 335
Children. *See also* Borderline personality disorder, in children; Depression, major, in children; Psychological factors affecting physical condition, in children
diagnostic criteria for psychological problems in, 88–90
headache in
DSM-III diagnoses most frequently associated with, 91
prevalence, 84
psychopathology, 84
studies of, 90
with migraine, 90
personality traits observed in, 162n
psychiatric evaluation of, 85, 91
treatment considerations, 88–90
Choice, conversion of conflict to, 47
Chronic headache complex, 341–342
Chronic muscle contraction headache. *See* Tension headache
Chronic paroxysmal hemicrania, 255
and sleep-wake cycle, 258
Chronic tension headache syndrome. *See also* Tension headache
definition of, 112
Cimetidine, effect on histamine receptors, 265
City of London Migraine Clinic, 306
development of, 306–307
services of, 306–307
Classical conditioning. *See* Conditioning
Clinic. *See* Headache clinic; Migraine clinic
Clomipramine, effects of, 267
Cluster headache, 119, 295, 335
addiction-proneness of patients, 210–211, 211t, 223–224
and anger. *See* Anger
attack, 224–225
autonomic signs of, 61
biofeedback and, 356
chronic, 207, 211
clinical picture of, 207–208
and conversion reaction, 225–227
corticosteroid therapy, 295
defenses used by patient, 48

Cluster headache—*continued*
   and denial, 219–220
   and dependency issues, 222–223, 334. *See also* Dependency
   and depression, 227–229
   early case history of, 14–15
   episodic, 207, 211
   hereditary factors in, 228
   husband-wife relationship with, 37
   lead-in to headache, 224
   after letdown period, 214, 231
   and life style, 212, 217–219, 320, 320n
   MMPI findings, 145
   neuroticism among patients with, 211t, 211
   and passivity, 222–223
   patient's attempts at resolution of loss and separation, 220–222
   patients' reaction to, 226–227
   patients' statements about feelings and behavior during, 226t
   periodic, 277
   and personality, 208, 212, 214–217, 219, 219n
   personality testing in, 208–210
   and psychic conflicts, 214–217
   psychological conditions preceding, 231
   psychological factors, 212–213
   resistance to psychotherapy in, 232
   sleep studies in, 255
   and sleep-wake cycle, 227, 258
   and stress, 46
   and superstition, 228
   timing of, 213–214
   treatment considerations, 232–233
   treatment-resistant patients with, 210–211
   typical case history, 228–232
   variants, vs. cyclical migraine, 278
Cognitive therapy, 302
Combined migraine/tension headache, 121
Compliance. *See* Medication compliance
Compulsive character defenses, and headache, 217
Compulsive personality disorder
   DSM-III criteria, 140n
   and medication compliance, 286
   and migraineurs' personality, comparison of, 140
Computer screen, and headache, 308
Conditioning
   classical, 350
   instrumental, 350
   operant, 350

   in modifying visceral activity, 351
   reinforcer in, 350
   Pavlovian, 350
Conflict
   definition of, 46
   and headache, 46–48
   treatment implications, 51
Confrontation, usefulness with headache patient, 74
Consciousness, 5
Conversion, in headache patient, 49t
Conversion disorder, 195
Conversion headache, 112, 116
   clinical approach to, 195–198
   defenses used by patient, 48
   definition of, 194
   differential diagnosis, 198–199
   duration of pain in, 197
   nature of headache, 196
   patient's affect, compared to description of pain, 196
   quality and location of headache, 196
   terminology for, 194–195
   treatment of, 199–200
Conversion reaction, 18, 45, 80, 81, 196, 204
   and cluster headache, 225–227
Conversion V on MMPI, 145, 208, 209, 225–226
Corticosteroids, prolonged use, hazards of, 295
Countertransference, 285–286
   and medication compliance, 287–288
Crisis
   definition of, 46
   and headache, 46–47
   treatment implications, 51
Criticism
   and headache, 76
   migraineurs' reaction to, 150
Crookshank, F.G., work on migraine headache, 146
Crying, physicians' reaction to, and therapeutic alliance, 38–39
CT scan, 62, 66, 97, 307
Culture, and psychosomatics, 5–6
Cushing's syndrome, 266
Cybernetics, 349
Cyclic adenosine monophosphate, plasma level during migraine, 243
Cyclical migraine, 275
   and depression, 276–277
   differential diagnosis, 277
   headache characteristics in, 275–276, 276t

headache cycle, 276
patient characteristics, 275
psychiatric symptoms, 277
treatment of, 278–279
Dalsgaard-Nielsen, T., observations on personality and migraine headache, 137t
Darwin, Charles, as migraineur, 15
Daudet, Alphonse, *La Doulou*, 26
Death
ancient Egyptians' view of, 7
primitive views of, 5
Defenses, 42, 48, 174, 285–286
seen in headache patients, 48, 49t, 115, 120, 138, 155, 215
Delirium, brain areas involved in, 190
Della Porta, Gian Battista, 13
Delusions, 262
in schizophrenia, 80
Dementia
depression presenting as, 262
vs. depression, 263t
vs. pseudodementia, 262–263
Denial, 114
and cluster headache, 219–220
use by headache patient, 49t
Dependency
and cluster headache, 222–223, 334
and headache, 198, 215–217, 334
and tension headache, 118
Dependent personality, and medication compliance, 286
Depression, 259, 341
and aspirin use, 291
biochemical determinants, 263
biological theories of, 264
bipolar, 260
and caffeine use, 292
as cause of headaches, 79
classification of, 259
clues that secondary to illness, 262t
and cluster headache, 227–229
and cyclical migraine, 276–277
drug therapies for, 266
emotional complaints in, 259, 260t, 262
endogenous, 259–260
Galen's account of, 10
and headache, 114, 257
headache as sole symptom of, 199
headache secondary to, 260
history in, 261
in children, 87–89
masked, 113, 126, 128

and migraine headache, 171, 271
and pain, 53
physical complaints in, 259, 260t
physical signs in, 36
psychic complaints in, 259, 261t, 262
psychoneurotic, 114
psychophysiological theory of, 264
reactive, 259
as result of headaches, 81
subgroups of, MHPG levels in, 265
and tension headache, 121, 124, 260
treatment, 269–270
treatment-resistant, 269
unipolar, 127, 259–260
vs. anxiety, 263t
vs. dementia, 263t
Depressive headache, 112, 266–267
diagnosis, 271
Descartes, René, contributions to psychosomatics, 13
Desipramine
for dysthymic pain disorder, 129
effects of, 267t, 267
on blocking acetylcholine and histamine receptors, 265t
on MHPG levels, 264
on noradrenergic system, 265
for headache caused by depression, 266–267
Dexamethasone suppression test, 127, 265–267
Dextroamphetamine, 319
Diagnosis, 27, 29
Diagnostic and Statistical Manual of Mental Disorders, third edition, 195
psychological factors affecting physical condition, 4
Diagnostic myths, 64–67
reasons for perpetuation of, 66–67
Diagnostic procedures, and patient, 96–97
Diagnostic tests, 62t
Diary, patients' use of, 77
Diazepam, 319n
overuse, 293–294
plus EMG feedback, 358
Dichloralphenazone, for migraine headache, 254
Digitolingual syndrome, 239, 239f, 249
Disability, vs. handicap, 339
Dodgson, Charles L., 187
Dopamine
in depression, 264
effect of MAO inhibitors, 267
Dopamine-β-hydroxylase, during migraine attack, 243

Doppelganger, 187
Doxepin
  for dysthymic pain disorder, 129
  effects of, 267*t*
    on blocking acetylcholine and histamine receptors, 265*t*
  for headache caused by depression, 266–267
  for tension headache, 122, 204
Draper, G. *See* Touraine, G., and Draper, G.
Dreams. *See also* Nightmares
  patients' recall of, and type of headache, 220
Drives, 41–42
Drug abuse, 290
  obtaining history of, 283–284
  by pain patients, 270
Drug dependence, 290
Drug overuse, 290
  obtaining history of, 283–284, 290
  by pain patients, 343
Drugs. *See also* Medication
  depressive reactions to, 262, 263*t*
  symbolism for patient, 318–319
Drug tolerance, 290
DSM III. *See Diagnostic and Statistical Manual of Mental Disorders*
Dunbar, Flanders, 18
Dyclobenzaprine, for muscle contraction headache, 204
Dysmorphesthesia, 187
Dysphrenic migraine, 183, 186*t*, 186–187
Dysthymic pain disorder
  clinical features of, 125*t*, 125–126
  definition of, 125
  pain of, 125
  psychodynamic features, 126*t*, 126–127
  treatment, 128–130
    success of, 129

Egypt, dynastic, headache treatment in, 7
Eisenbud, J., case study reported by, 43–44
Electrodermal (GSR) biofeedback, sensitivity to conflict-related cognitions, 365
Electromyographic (EMG) feedback, 19, 352, 354, 356
  sensitivity to conflict-related cognitions, 364–365
  in tension headache, 360
Eliot, George, 183
Elkinton, Russell, self-report of migraine headaches, 160, 166–167, 173–174
Emancipation, and migraine headache, 160
EMG feedback. *See* Electromyographic feedback
Emotional stress. *See* Stress

Empathy, 54, 74
  as diagnostic tool, 73
  and headache treatment, 158, 314
  patient's need to develop, 327
Endorphin, in depression, 264
Enkephalins, 264
Enlightenment, age of, headache treatment in, 14–15
Epinephrine
  alterations, in sleep-related headache, 256–257
  effect of MAO inhibitors, 267
Ergomania, 126
Ergotamine (tartrate), 68, 289
  abuse, 290, 294–295
  effect in migraine headache, 240, 241*f*, 247
  impaired absorption during migraine, 245
  for migraine headache, 254, 278, 295, 307
  overdose. *See also* Ergotism
    as cause of migraine, 309
  plasma half-life, 295
  poisoning, 311. *See also* Ergotism
  preparations, caffeine content, 309
  suppository form, 310
  tissue half-life, 295
  tolerance, variations in, 294
Ergotamine-acetaminophen combination, in treatment of migraine, 307
Ergotamine headache, 278, 294–295
Ergotism, 278, 294
  signs and symptoms of, 294
Examination. *See* Physical examination
Exercise, in regulating headaches, 320
Exorcism, 12
Expectations of self, and headache, 75–76
Eyes, examination of, 61
Eye strain, 64–65
Eysenck Personality Inventory, 145

Facial muscles, 42
Factitious disorder, 195
Failure, migraineurs' reaction to, 173
Familial hemiplegic migraine, 189
Family
  of migraineurs, 161–162
  as support system, for post-traumatic stress disorder patient, 337–338
Family conflict, as cause of headache, 79–80
Family history, 60, 74–75
  and headache, 341
  questions important to, 38
Family loyalty, of headache patient, 324
Family psychodynamics, 74–75

Fantasies, unconscious, in genesis of migraine headache, 153–154
Father
　cluster headache patient's relationship with, 220–221, 230
　female migraineurs' view of, 172n
Feedback, definition of, 349
Feelings, expression of
　and patient-therapy match-up, 303–304
　and therapeutic alliance, 38–39
Fever, 61
Fight-or-flight preparations, 114
Fiorinal, 310
　withdrawal, 293
First headache, in psychiatric history, 75
Fleiss, Wilhelm, 17–18
Fluoxetine, mode of action, 269
Follow-up, of headache patient, 99
Forbes, John, 183
Fortification spectra. See Scotoma
Frazier, Shervert
　observations on personality and migraine headache, 135t
　work on migraine headache, 155
Free fatty acids, plasma level, 243
　during migraine, 250
Frequent migraine, 275
Freud, Sigmund, 17–19
Frieburg Personality Inventory, 210
Friedman, Arnold
　observations on personality and migraine headache, 135t
　work on migraine headache, 151–152, 178–179
Fromm-Reichmann, Freida
　observations on personality and migraine headache, 137t
　work on migraine headache, 148–149
Frustration
　migraineurs' reaction to, 150, 177
　reaction to, and headache, 75
Furmansky, A.R., work on migraine headache, 155, 168

Galen, 10
Gender roles, and migraine headache, 167–168
Goal-directed therapy, 303
Goldman, Emma, 26
Goody-goody, 147
Gowers, W.R., 16–17
Grace, W.J., 18
Graham, D.T., 19

Graham, John R., 160n. See also Elkinton, R.
　observations on personality and migraine headache, 137t
　work on migraine headache, 152–153
Greeks, ancient, headache treatments, 8–10
Grief, 259
　and pain, 96
　recording, in psychiatric history, 76
　unresolved, psychotherapeutic approach to, 329
Grief reaction, prolonged, 114
Guilt
　and headache, 50, 324
　and migraine headache, 152, 155, 171

Hallucinations
　of environmental reduplication, 190
　facilitated, 8
　in migraine headache, 187, 190
　in schizophrenia, 80
Handicap, vs. disability, 339
Hand temperature feedback, in migraine headache, 361–362
Hangman's noose, 10
Head, personal significance of, 42–43, 94
Headache
　acute, 10
　　patient characteristics and treatment, 69
　caffeine-associated, 292
　central influences in, 346
　in children. See Children
　chronic, 10
　　patient characteristics and treatment, 69
　　Willis' case history of, 14
　chronic recurrent, psychological complications, 289
　as common complaint, 22
　congenital insensitivity to, 25
　and depression, 261
　differential diagnosis, 59–61
　explanation of cause, importance of, 33
　within family, 48–50
　folk remedies for, 10
　geographic distribution of prevalence rates, 340
　history of understanding of, 3
　and increased intracranial pressure, 257
　as indicator of depression, 260
　interpretation of, 95–96
　intractable, 348
　misconceptions about, 64
　and multiple personality disorder, 101–102
　　case histories, 102–106

Headache—*continued*
treatment of, 108
types of headache experienced by patients, 106–107
mythology of
causes, 64
minimizing, 69
nonmigrainous, and sleep, 257
organic causes, 271
patients' descriptions of, 95
physician's approach to, 94
prevalence of, 340
primary, 340
psychogenic component, 67–68
psychological factors in, 42
contributory, 78–80
elusiveness of, 43
evaluation of, 43
independent, 78, 82
prevalance, 42
relevance of, 42–43
resultant, 78, 80–82
symptomatic, 78, 82
treatability, 43
refractory, and analgesic/sedative abuse, 294
and regulation of attention to painful stimuli, 52–53
secondary, 340
secondary psychological and social disturbances with, 346–347
and serious medical disease, inpatient therapy
for, 343–344
signalling disease, 340–341
significance of, 22–23
treatment of, history of, 4–19
triggers, 308
Headache behavior, 296
Headache clinic, 27–28, 307. *See also* City of
London Migraine Clinic; Migraine clinic
Headache history. *See* History
Headache [journal], 340
Headache-maintaining factors, 81
Headache pain
character of, patient's statement of, 24
description of, 24
existential meaning of, 330
nature of, 23–24
restlessness accompanying, 24
vs. other forms of pain, 289
Headache societies, 340
Headache treatment center, 340
patients, 340–341

specific features of, 341–342
private, development of, 342
Head injury
cerebral circulation after, 202
symptoms after, 201
Health care history, recording, in psychiatric
history, 77
Heautoscopia, 187
Heberden, William, 15
Hebrews, ancient, headache treatments, 7–8
Hemicrania, 10. *See also* Chronic paroxysmal
hemicrania
Hemicrania dysphrenica, 183
Hemoglobin levels, and analgesic overuse, 291
Heterocrania, 10
Hildegard of Bingen, 11
Hippocrates, 8, 9
Histamine receptors, effect of antidepressants on, 265
History, 59. *See also* Family history; Psychiatric
history
essential items of, 60t
questions important to, 37–38
Histrionic personality
and medication compliance, 286
and self-regulatory therapy, 365
Hormones, and headache, 68, 344
Hospitalization, and therapeutic alliance, 39–40
Hostility, migraineurs repression of, 148, 154
Hunter, Richard, work on migraine headache, 153
Huxley, Thomas, 16
Hydralazine, 344
Hydrocollator packs, 122
5-Hydroxyindoleacetic acid, 250
CSF levels, in low MHPG patients, 265
in patients with migraine, 256
Hyperalgesia, 270
Hypersensitivity, 76
Hypertension, 152
and sleep-related headache, 257
Hypertensive headache, 257
Hypnosis, 15, 25, 52
medical, 17
for post-traumatic stress disorder, 338
in treatment of headache, 302
Hypnotics, for insomnia, 319
Hypochondriasis, 195, 199
Hypoglycemia, 82
Hypokalemia, 82
Hypomanic character, 219n
Hypomanic defenses, in headache patient, 49t
Hypothyroidism, 62, 82

Hysteria, during cluster headache attack, 225
Hysterical personality disorder, 198

Identification
  and familial headaches, 49–50
  in migraineurs, 119–120
  with mother, migraineurs', 146–147
  with parent, migraineurs', 172
Identification with the aggressor, 50, 120, 174,
    216, 328
  and cluster headache, 215
  in headache patient, 49t
  and pseudoprogression, 176n
Identity disorder, 86
Identity problems, and tension headache, 118
Illness
  Babylonian and Assyrian view of, 7
  during childhood, in psychiatric history, 76
  views of, in primitive societies, 5
Imipramine
  for depression in children, 89
  for dysthymic pain disorder, 129
  effects of, 267t, 267t, 267
    on blocking acetylcholine and histamine
        receptors, 265t
    on MHPG levels, 264
    on noradrenergic system, 265
  for headache caused by depression, 266–267
  and MAOI, combination therapy, 267
  for muscle contraction headache, 204
  in pain therapy, 124
  for tension headache, 122
Impulsivity, in cluster headache patient, 230
Inpatient headache unit
  admission criteria, 346
  design, 344
  development of, 343–346
    difficulties in, 344–346
    identification of need for, 343–344
  staff, 344
Insight-oriented therapy, 71–72
Insomnia, 126
  management in patient pain, 128–129
  treatment, 319
Instinctual drives. See Drives
Instrumental conditioning. See Conditioning
Insulin, secretion, during migraine, 243
Intellectualization, 333
  in headache patient, 49t
  migraineurs' use of, 174
Interneurons, enkephalinergic, 249–250
Interview, in evaluation of headache, 96
Intracranial hemorrhage, 60

Iproniazid, 267
  mood alteration with, 263
Ischemia, underlying migrainous transient global
    amnesia and acute confusional state, 190
Isocarboxazid, 267
Isometheptene, for migraine headache, 254

Jaynes, Julian, 7
  The Origin of Consciousness in the Break-
      down of the Bicameral Mind, 5
Johnson, Samuel, 13
Jokai, Moritz, 26
Jonckheere, Paul
  case study reported by, 44–45
  observations on personality and migraine
      headache, 135t
  work on migraine headache, 154

Karpman, B., observations on personality and
    migraine headache, 135t
Keres, in Classical Greece, 8
Khouri-Haddad, S.E., observations on personal-
    ity and migraine headache, 137t
Knopf, Olga, work on migraine headache, 147–
    148, 166, 168, 169
Kolb, Lawrence
  observations on personality and migraine
      headache, 137t
  work on migraine headache, 154, 168

La belle indifference, 196, 199, 226
Lance, J.W. See Selby, G., and Lance, J.W.
Learning theory, 350
Leonine facies, 228
Lilliputian perceptions, 186
Linnaeus, Carolus, 14
Lithium carbonate
  combined with antidepressants, for dysthymic
      pain disorder, 129
  for cyclical migraine, 278–279
  maintenance regimen, 278–279
Liveing, E., 16
  work on migraine headache, 146, 254
Locus ceruleus
  in headache, 257–258
  in regulation of pain, 264
London, Jack, 26
Loss
  and cluster headache, 220–222
  recording, in psychiatric history, 76

MacAndrews Scale, 210–211
Macropsia, 186–187
Magical thinking, in cluster headache patient, 228

Male identification, and cluster headache, 217
Malingering, 81, 195, 204
Malocclusion, 65
Manic-depressive illness, subclinical, periodic headaches in, 278
MAO inhibitors. *See* Monoamine oxidase inhibitors
Maprotiline
  for dysthymic pain disorder, 129
  effect on noradrenergic system, 265
  mode of action, 269
Margolin, S.G., 19
Marital conflict, as cause of headache, 79–80
Marriage, in migraine, 166–167
Masochism, 50, 126, 127
Meals, skipped, and headache, 320, 320n
Medication, 62–63. *See also* prn medication
  abuse, by headache patients, 82, 289–290
  dependency on, 289
  for depression in children, 89
  effect on biofeedback, 357–358
  history, 283
  misuse, 289
  myths about, 68–69
  overuse, 281, 289
    treatment of, 295–296
  patients' magical expectations for, 284
  physicians' expectations for, 284
  prophylactic, 294
  reactions to, and physician-patient relationship, 287
  recording, in psychiatric history, 76–77
  side effects, and noncompliance, 282
  in supportive care, 318–319
Medication compliance, 280–288
  evaluating, 280–284
  by headache diagnostic category, 281–282, 281t
  personality factors in, 284–288
  predictors of, 284
  psychodynamic factors in, 284–288
Medication error, prevalence of, 280
Meditation, 302
Menarche, and migraine headache, 148, 168
Menstrual migraine, 60, 168–169, 275
  and self-regulatory therapy, 356
Mental status examination, 71
Mercury toxicity, 82
Mesopotamia, headache treatment in, 6–7
Metamorphopsia, 187, 190
Met-enkephalin, 250
3-Methoxy-4-hydroxyphenylethyleneglycol. *See* MHPG

Methysergide (Sansert), 289
  for cyclical migraine, 279
  prolonged use, hazards of, 295
Metoclopramide, in treatment of migraine, 245, 307
MHPG, urinary
  measurement in depression, 264–265
  used as guide to drug treatment of headache in depression, 266–267
Michigan Headache and Neurological Institute, 341. *See also* Headache treatment center
Microemboli, 82
Micropsia, 186
Middle Ages, headache treatment in, 11–12
Migraine clinic, 27–28. *See also* Headache clinic, City of London Migraine Clinic
Migraine equivalent, 182, 184t–185t, 240
Migraine headache, 68, 69, 112, 113, 237. *See also specific type of migraine*
  altered consciousness in, 187
  and anger. *See* Anger
  attack, 60
    factors affecting recovery from, 309
    sleep in therapy of, 258, 308–309
    treatment of, in clinic, 308–310
  aura. *See also* Migraine headache, neurological accompaniments
    historical description of, 11
  autonomic accompaniments, 239, 242–246, 247f, 248, 250, 257–258
    symptoms of, 60
    signs of, 61
  biofeedback for, 355–356, 361–362
  and childhood home environment, 161–165
  in children, 90
  classical, 133–134, 240f, 248
  classification of, 275
  clinical definition of, 306
  cognitive changes during, 183
  common, 134, 239–240, 240f, 246, 248
    and sleep-wake cycle, 258
  demographic studies of, 133
  depression headache seen with, 271
  developmental issues in, 119–120, 133n, 155, 163
  diagnosis, 181–182
  dissociated, 182
  and dreams, 220
  DSM III category, 4
  and environmental stressors, 138
  evaluation of patient, 307–308
  familial nature of, 60
  Freud's, 18

gastrointestinal symptoms with, 244–245
genetic factors in, 133, 138, 144, 152–153, 161
headache phase, biochemical changes of, 244, 245*f*
Hippocrates' description of, 9
history of, 22
isolated aura, 182
and life style, 320, 320*n*
Liveing's study of, 16
and marital or family conflict, 79
memory disturbances in, 187, 189–190
mental disturbances in, categorization, 183–186
MMPI findings, 145
neurological accompaniments, 239, 241–242, 246
isolated, 240*f*, 248
nineteenth-c. accounts of, 16
objective signs of, 24
observational approach to, 143, 145–155
onset, and timing of stress, 77
organic model of, 181
Pascal's description of, 13
pathogenesis of, 240–251
new theory of, 246
vasoconstriction-cerebral hypoxia-vasodilitation concept, 246*f*
perceptual disorders in, 186
and personality, 108, 134–141, 135*t*-137*t*, 146, 147
and physiology, 133–134, 161
prevalence of, 22
prodromal period, 134
and profession, 133
prolonged, 278
prophylactic therapy, 275
psychic dysfunction during, 182
psychobiological explanation of, 150–151
psychodynamics of
observational studies of, 133
physicians' reluctance to broach issues of, with patient, 131–132
psychological factors in, 60–61, 131–132
prevalance, 42
psychometric approach, 144–145
psychophysiologic mechanism of, 163*n*
Romans' description of, 10
Rorschach studies of, 144
sex ratios, 133
sleep studies in, 255
statistical approach to, 142–143
and stress, 23, 46, 84, 145, 248–251, 308

symptoms of, 239–240
time relationship of, 239*f*
temporal classification of, 275
and tension headache, 121
differences and similarities between patients prone to, 118–119
time relationship to stress, 237, 238*f*
tranquilizer therapy, patients' views on, 270
transient neurological dysfunction in, 182
triggered by head injury, 203
triggers, 149–150, 177
types, taxonomic diagram for, 184*t*-185*t*
visual aura, Hippocrates' description of, 9
volitional and temperamental changes in, 183
Migraine personality, 67, 84, 108, 134, 138, 140, 151
criticisms of theory of, 138–139
Migraine psychoses, 183, 186, 189–190
Migraine sine hemicrania, 182
Migraineurs
adolescence of, 165
in adulthood, 165–169
ambition of, 150, 160, 166
ambivalent attitude toward self, 171–173
characteristics of, 159
childhood of, 161–165
constitution of, 161
coping style, 159–160
defenses used by, 48, 120. *See also* Defenses
descriptions of, 140–141
early environment, 161–164
famous, 4*t*
home environment of, 170–171
insecurity, 160, 164, 169, 173
interpersonal safeguards used by, 176–177
life style, 171–172, 173
loneliness of, 173
and marriage, 166–167
maturation process in, 160
in middle and older age, 169
neuroticism in, 140, 144
parenting by, 165–166
perfectionism in, 139, 150, 160, 173
personality of, 146
physical observations on, 151
physician's manner toward, 332–333
psychologically influenced, 133, 155
developmental perspective on, 158–159
relationship with parents, 149, 161–164
rigidity in, 160
self-selection of, 139
siblings of, 165
strengths of, 159, 179

Migraineurs—*continued*
  and tension, 335
  at work, 166
Migraine-variant, 182
  taxonomic diagram for, 184t-185t
Migrainous acute confusional state, 187, 189, 190
Migrainous transient global amnesia, 187–188, 190
  anatomical substrate of, 188, 188f
Migrainous transient partial amnesia, 189
Migrainous twilight state, 188
Mind/body relationship, 4, 190
  Cartesian concept of, 13
  Homeric view of, 8
  nineteenth-c. view of, 15–16
  Platonic view of, 9
Minnesota Multiphasic Personality Inventory, 78, 113, 143, 208–210
  profiles of headache patients, 145
Mixed headache, 60
  biofeedback for, 355–356
  post-traumatic, 203
  and stress, 46
Monoamine neurotransmitters, 264
Monoamine oxidase, 243
Monoamine oxidase inhibitors, 269
  for depression, 266
  diet for patient on, 268t
  for dysthymic pain disorder, 129
  for migraine headache, 271–272
  mode of action, 267
Morgagni, G.B., 14–15
Mourning, 329
  and cluster headache, 229
  and migraine headache, 176
  recording, in psychiatric history, 76
Multiple personality disorder, 101. *See also* Headache, and multiple personality disorder
  alternate personalities as clues to psychodynamics of main personality, 107–108
  DSM-III criteria, 101
  misdiagnosis of, 101
  physiological and psychological differences among personalities in same patient, 107
Muscle contraction, x-ray appearance of, 62
Muscle contraction headache. *See* Tension headache
Muscle relaxants, 68, 319n
Muscular headache, 112
Myofascial pain dysfunction syndrome, 65–66

Naproxen, for cyclical migraine, 279
Narcissistic personality, and medication compliance, 286
Narcotics, 319n
Nardil, mode of action, 267
Neck
  arthritis of, 65
  examination of, 61
  muscles, spasm of, 112
Neck injury, 203
Neolithic era, headache treatment in, 6
Nephropathy, analgesic, 293
Nerve ending entrapment syndrome, 204–205
Neuralgia, atypical facial, 80
Neurokinin, 240
Neuroleptics, 270, 319
  combined with antidepressants, for dysthymic pain disorder, 129
Neurology, in nineteenth c., 16
Neuropsychological instruments, 78
Neurotic disorder, in children, 90
Neuroticism, in headache patients, 210
Neurotransmitters, in depression, 264
Nightmares, in post-traumatic stress disorder, 337
Night terrors, 220
Nineteenth century, headache treatment in, 15–17
Nocturnal headache, 257
Noncompliance
  causes of, 284
  DSM-III definition of, 283
  by headache diagnostic category, 281–282, 281t
  personality factors in, 283
  prevalence of, 280
  reasons for, 282, 282t
Nonnarcotic analgesics. *See* Analgesics, nonnarcotic
Nonsteroidal antiinflammatory agents, 291
Noradrenaline, plasma level, during migraine attack, 243
Norepinephrine
  alterations in level during sleep-related headache, 256–257
  antidepressants' effect on, 264
  effect of MAO inhibitors, 267
Norpramin, for dysthymic pain disorder, 129
Nortriptyline
  for dysthymic pain disorder, 129
  effects of, 267t
    on blocking acetylcholine and histamine receptors, 265t
    on MHPG levels, 264

on noradrenergic system, 265
for headache caused by depression, 266–267

Objective [term], 5n
Jaynes' use of, 5n
Obsessive-compulsive neurosis, 140
Obsessive-compulsive personality, and self-regulatory therapy, 365
Occipital neuralgia, 203
Occlusive cerbrovascular disease, 66
Operant conditioning. See Conditioning
Optic alloaesthesia, 187
Orbital bruit, 61
Outpatient therapy, for pain patients, 343

Pain, 70. See also Headache pain
acute vs. chronic, 270
assessment of, 92–95
associations with, 93
authenticity of, 333
hospital staff attitudes about, 40
Avicenna's treatment for, 11
Babylonian and Assyrian view of, 7
behavioral therapy for, 124
chronic
antidepressant therapy, 125
depression underlying, 260–261
somatic symptoms associated with, 26
chronic atypical or nonspecific, as depressive disorder, 124–125
chronic noncephalic, comparison with tension headache, 127–128
CNS transmission of, 264
communication of, 26, 53
congenital insensitivity to, 25
control of, 264
in dysthymic pain disorder, 125
experience of, 52, 92
as brain phenomenon, 27
explanation of cause of
patients' ranking of importance of, 31, 31n
physician and patient expectations about, 30, 30t
expression of, 95
infant's expression of, 93
management, 320
and mind/body relationship, 4
nature of, 23
pharmacological management of, 345–346
physician's approach to, 93–94
and pleasure, 25
private signature of, 94

psychodynamics of, 52
of psychogenic origin, 25–27
psychological side effects, 26
public signature of, 94
reciprocal interaction between patient and physician, as definition of, 95–96
response to, 92
Romans' view of, 10
schizophrenic's account of, 80
sensation of, 52
sensitivity to, 24–25
as stimulator of sympathetic nervous system, 248, 248f
symbols associated with, 93
viewed as punishment, 94
Pain-insensitivity, 25
Pain-prone disorder, 125
Pain relief
expectations for
in different clinic populations, 31, 31t, 32
physician vs. patient, 30, 30t
reasonable, 32–33
patients' ranking of importance of, 31, 31n
Pain threshold, differences in, between stress and relaxation, 249
Palinopsia, 187, 190
Paracelsus, 12
Paracetamol. See Acetaminophen
Paranoid personality, and medication compliance, 286–287
Paraphasia, 183
Parents
headache patient's relationship with, 327
migraineurs' relationship with, 149, 161–164
Pargyline, 267
Parturition, and migraine headache, 168
Pascal, Blaise, description of migraine headaches, 13
Passive-aggressive personality, and medication compliance, 286
Passivity, and cluster headache, 222–223
Patient
concerns about cause of headache, 66
expectations about pain relief, studies of, 29–32
expectations about psychotherapy, 317
fears and phobias of, 319–320
increasing perspective of, in psychotherapy, 327–328
reassurance of, 97–99
reporting of headache details, and method of data collection, 32

Patient—*continued*
 treatment-resistant, psychotherapy for, 314*t*-
  315*t*
Peptic ulcer, 224*n*
Perfectionism, and migraine headache, 139
Perseveration, 187
Personality. *See also* Multiple personality disorder
 and bodily functioning, 107
 and cluster headache, 208, 212, 214–217,
  219, 219*n*
 and headache type, in multiple personality
  disorder, 106–107
 and migraine headache, 108, 134–141, 135*t*-
  137*t*, 146, 147
 and self-regulatory therapy, 365
 traits, in headache patients, 118, 145
Personality disorder, 114, 137–138, 201,
 286
Personality style, 134–137
PET scan, 97
Phantom pain, 27
Pharmacotherapy, 347. *See also* Drugs; Medication
Phenacetin, 290, 292–293
 complications of, 292–293
Phenelzine, 267
 for dysthymic pain disorder, 129
 for migraine headache, 271–272
 mode of action, 267
Phenobarbitone, half-life of, 310
Physical examination, in evaluation of headache,
 61–62, 96–97
Physical inadequacy, migraineurs' reaction to,
 150
Physician
 availability, and patients' confidence, 39
 expectations, studies of, 29–32
 primary, 313
  psychotherapy provided by, 318
 style, effect on therapeutic alliance, 37–38
 treating, 313
  and psychiatric care, 314–316
Physician-patient relationship, 29, 34, 313. *See
 also* Therapeutic alliance
 breakdown, 29
 establishment of, 33
 and medication compliance, 284
 psychodynamics, 285
 therapeutic use of, 97
Pineal gland, 13
Pinel, A., 14
Placebo, 40, 97, 119, 287, 357

Platelet
 changes, during migraine, 244, 244*f*
 serotonin content, 244
Plato, 9–10
Platonic dialogues, 9–10
Pleasure, 92
Pliny the Elder, 10
Polysurgery, 114
Positron emission tomography. *See* PET scan
Posterior cerebral artery, 188, 189*f*, 190
Post-traumatic dysautonomic cephalalgia, 203
Post-traumatic headache, 197, 332
 biofeedback for, 205, 355–356
 chronic, definition of, 201
 clinical characteristics, 202–203
 history of, 61
 muscle contraction in, 202
 organicity, 202, 204
 psychological factors, 45–46, 201, 203–204,
  337
 psychotherapy for, themes frequently encountered in, 338
 severity, and severity of head injury, 201
 structural and metabolic factors in, 201–
  202
 treatment of, 204–205
 treatment of accompanying symptoms, 335–
  336
Post-traumatic neurosis, treatment of, 338
Post-traumatic stress disorder, 336
 abreactive therapies, 338
 avoidance of aversive stimuli in, 337
 natural history of symptoms in, 337
 nightmares in, 337
 organic symptoms, 336
 sheltering the injury in, 337
 symptoms of, 338
 synergism of symptoms in, 336
 visualization of injury-inducing situation in,
  338
Preganglionic sympathetic neurons, 250
Pregenital character structure, 153
Pregnancy
 fear of, in migraineurs, 169
 headache in, self-regulatory therapy, 356
 and migraine headache, 148
Primary gain, 81, 196
prn medication, 290, 345
Progressive relaxation, 302, 352–353, 356
 in tension headache, 361
Propranolol
 for cyclical migraine, 279
 for post-traumatic headache, 204

Protriptyline
  effects of, 267t
    on blocking acetylcholine and histamine
      receptors, 265t
  for headache caused by depression, 266–267
Proust, Marcel, 26
Pseudodementia, 262
Pseudoprogression, 48, 119–120, 160, 174–176
  definition of, 174
Psyche, 4
Psychiatric history
  contents, 75–78
  techniques for taking, 72–75
Psychiatric referral
  method and timing of, 98–99, 316
  patients' acceptance of, 342, 347
  and therapeutic alliance, 39
Psychoanalysis, 303, 318
Psychoanalytic psychotherapy, 10
Psychodynamic psychotherapy, 303, 304, 318,
  321–330. See also Transference
  booster sessions, 323
  common treatment issues, 327–330
  and existential determinants, 330
  pace of, 323–324
  process, 321–323
  resistances in, 323–325
Psychodynamics
  definition of, 41
  role in headache, 42–43
Psychogenic headache, 112, 194
Psychogenic illness, 84
Psychogenic pain disorder, 80, 195
Psychological evaluation, 70–71
  physical signs in, 36
  rationale for, 71–72
Psychological factors affecting physical condition,
  in children, 88
  diagnosis of, 89
  treatment of, 89–90
Psychometric tests, 78, 119n, 143
Psychopathic personality, and medication compli-
  ance, 287
Psychophysiological reactions, 45
Psychosis, 199
Psychosomatic orientation, 6n
Psychosomatic personality, and medication com-
  pliance, 286
Psychosomatics, 5–19, 19
  Alexander's work on, 152
  basic tenet of, 53–54
  Sperling's view of, 153
Psychosomatic [term], coinage of, 16

Psychotherapy, 67–68, 270, 286, 296, 342. See
  also Behavioral therapy; Insight-oriented therapy; Psychodynamic psychotherapy; Somatic
  therapy; Transference
  avoiding extremes in, 334–335
  capitalizing on momentum of, 335
  for cluster headache, 232
  for conversion headache, 200
  evaluation of patient's potential for, 71–72
  expectations for, 334
  long-term, 303, 317, 318
  for migraine headache, 153, 155
  pace of, 333–334
  planning, 62
  for post-traumatic headache, 205
  psychoanalytic, 10
  referral for, 301–302
  supportive, for headache patient, 114
  termination, 335
  treatment goals, defining, 317–318
  for treatment-resistant patient, 314t–315t

Quieting reflex, 353

Raphe neurons, serotinergic, 249–251
Raphe unit activity, across sleep-wakefulness
  cycles, 249, 249f
Rapid eye movement (REM) sleep
  and headache, 258
  and migraine headache, 255–256
Rationalization, in headache patient, 49t
Rauwolfian alkaloids, depression with, 263–264
Reaction formation, 120, 166, 174
  in headache patient, 49t
Recognition, migraineurs' desire for, 178
Referral, 301
  psychiatric. See Psychiatric referral
Regression, 120, 174, 333
  and combined headache, 121
  in tension headache patient, 119, 120
  use by headache patient, 49t
Relationships
  and headache, 75
  migraineurs', 170, 175
  and tension headache patient, 120–121
Relaxation, and migraine headache, 248–251
Relaxation response, 353
Relaxation techniques, 302, 335, 352. See also
  Biofeedback, and relaxation
  for headache, 353–354
  nonspecific benefits of, 363–364
  in pain management, 128
Religion, vs. science, 13

REM latency, 127
REM sleep. *See* Rapid eye movement sleep
Renaissance, headache treatment in, 12–13
Repression, 120, 174
    use by headache patient, 49*t*
    use by migraineurs, 154
Resentment, and migraine headache, 160, 164, 170–171, 177–178
Reserpine, 344
    depression with, 263
    enhancement of migraine symptoms, 256
Resistance, in psychotherapy, 323–325
Resort to action, 120
Responsibility, migraineurs' approach to, 150, 160, 173, 178
Rest, in treatment of acute migraine attack, 308–309
Reticular activating system, 237, 238*f*, 248, 257
Rheumatoid arthritis, 152
Ritalin, and EEG feedback, 358
Romans, headache treatments, 10–11
Rorschach Test, 78
    of migraineurs, 144

Sadness, of headache patient, psychotherapeutic approach to, 329, 334
St. Gregory, 12
St. Luke, 10
Sansert. *See* Methysergide
Schizoid personality, and medication compliance, 287
Schizophrenia
    ambulatory, 80
    biofeedback contraindicated in, 359
Schur, M., 18
Schwerbesinnlichkeit, 183
Science, and religion, 13
Scotoma, 10, 13, 182, 239, 239*f*, 247, 248
    effect of amyl nitrite on, 241*f*
Secondary dysphoria-enhancing factors, 81–82
Secondary gain, 81, 198, 336
Secondary headache-maintaining factors, 81
Security, wish for, 172*n*
Sedative, for migraine headache, 254
Selby, G., and Lance, J.W., observations on personality and migraine headache, 137*t*
Self
    awareness of, 5
    migraineurs' sacrifice of, 172, 172*n*
Self-esteem, patient's, sheltering, in psychotherapy, 333
Self-hypnosis
    in tension headache, 361
    in treatment of headache, 302

Self-regulatory skills, transfer of, 363
Selinsky, Herman
    observations on personality and migraine headache, 135*t*
    work on migraine headache, 150–151, 168
Separation
    ambivalence about, 146–147
    and cluster headache, 220–222
Separation anxiety, pathologic, 85–86
Separation anxiety disorder, DSM-III criteria for, 88–89
Serotonin, 244, 245, 250
    alterations, in sleep-related headache, 256–257
    antidepressants' effect on, 264
    brain concentration of, 251
    effect of MAO inhibitors, 267
    reuptake, effect of drugs on, 265
Serum glutamic-oxaloacetic transaminase, effect of aspirin on, 291
Serum glutamic-pyruvic transaminase, effect of aspirin on, 291
Seventeenth century, headache treatment in, 13–14
Sex roles
    and headache, 198, 199
    and migraine headache, 167–168
Sick headache, 60
Sick role, 286
Sinus headache, 65
Sinus headache medications, 290
Sinusitis, acute, 65
Sinus troubles, 65
Skull. *See* Trepanning of skull
Sleep. *See also* Rapid eye movement sleep
    and cluster headache, 227, 255, 258
    and migraine headache, 254–255
    and nonmigrainous headache, 257
    as therapy for migraine, 258, 308–309
Sleep apnea syndrome, 257
Sleep disturbance
    and caffeine use, 292
    and depression, 261–262
    and headache, 341
Sleep stage, and headache, 255–256
Sleep-wake cycle, and headache, 258
Snuff, 12
Social relations, migraineurs', 149
Socrates, 9
Sodium amytal, half-life of, 310
Soma, 4
Somatic therapy, 302–303
Somatization, and cluster headache, 215
Somatization disorder, 79, 195, 199

Somatoform disorder, 195
Soranus of Ephesus, 10
Spatial orientation, disturbances, in cyclical migraine, 277
Sperling, Melitta, work on migraine headache, 153–154
Sporadic migraine, 275
Spreading depression, 242, 246–248, 247f
Spreading oligemia, 247
  during migraine attack, 242
Status hemicranialis, 310
Status migrainosus, 310–311
Stimulants, 319
Stomach, during and after migraine attack, 245, 245f
Stress, 67, 237
  education of patient about, 319
  effect on muscle tone, 237
  and headache, 46–47, 61, 77, 118
  and illness, 18–19
  and migraine headache, 23, 46, 84, 145, 248–251, 308
  and tension headache, 46, 113
Stressors, and headache onset, 77
Stroke, atherothrombotic, 66
Subdural hematoma, 82
Subjective, medicine's approach to, 19–20
Subjective [term], 5n
  Jaynes' use of, 5n
Sublimation, 120
  in headache patient, 49t
  migraineurs' use of, 174
Substance abuse, 343, 347
  and cluster headache, 210–211
Suicidal ideation
  in children, 89
  and cluster headache, 225, 227–228, 229
Suicide attempts, in pain patients and headache patients, 127, 270
Sumer, first recorded treatment of headache from, 6
Superego
  and excessive expectations, psychotherapeutic approach to, 327
  of headache patient, 320–321
  of migraineurs, 154, 155, 160, 172–173, 175
Superficial temporal artery, in migraine headache, 240, 241f
Supportive therapy, 39, 303, 318–321
Suppression, 120
  use by headache patient, 49t, 174
Survivor guilt, 338
Sympathetic nervous system
  activation, by pain, 248, 248f, 250

activity, during migraine, 243–244, 248
Synalgia, 26

Teed, J.L., 16
Teeth grinding, 112
Teichopsia, 13. See also Scotoma
Teleopsia, 187
Temperature feedback, 356
Temporomandibular arthritis, 65–66
Temporomandibular joint disease, 61
Tension, teaching patient about, 335
Tension (muscle contraction) headache
  and aggression, 16, 65, 66, 68, 69, 128, 194, 204, 237, 319n, 335, 356. See Aggression
  and anger. See Anger
  and anxiety. See Anxiety
  biofeedback for, 271, 355–356, 360–361
  caused by depression, mechanisms of, 270
  cause of, 111–112
  childhood history, 116
  chronic, 111
  clinical findings in, 112–114
  compared to post-traumatic headache, 202
  comparison of patients with, and chronic non-cephalic pain patients, 127–128
  defenses used by patient, 48, 120
  definition of, 111–112
  demographics, 112
  and depression, 121, 124, 260
  developmental history of patient, 119–120
  DSM III category, 4
  medications for, 122
  and migraine headache
    differences between patients prone to, 119
    psychological similarities between patients prone to, 118–119
  as modelled headache, 95
  muscle contraction in, 42, 114–116
  pathogenesis, 114–118
  patient's need for structured relationship with physician, 333
  physical findings in, 61
  physical therapy for, 122
  prevalence, 112
  psychodynamics of, 121
  psychological predisposition to, 116
  psychological symptoms of, 113
  psychological triggers of, 118
  psychometric approach to understanding, 144
  self-regulatory techniques for, 122
  signs of, 112
  and sleep, 257
  somatic triggers, 115–116

Tension headache—*continued*
  and stress, 46, 113, 237, 238*f*
  symptoms of, 113
  testing in, 113
  time relationship to stress, 237, 238*f*
  treatment of, 121–122
Thalamic syndrome, secondary depression in, 263
Thematic Apperception Test, 78, 144
Therapeutic alliance, 34–39
  effect of first meeting between patient and physician, 36–38
  emotional aspects of, 38–39
  factors affecting, 35–36
  and office design, 35–36
  physician's role in, 35
Therapeutic contract, 317
Therapeutic myths, 67–69
Therapy. *See also* Psychotherapy
  effectiveness of, 301
  matching patient to, 303–304
  selection of, 301
Thermal feedback
  for migraine headache management, 19, 361–362
  sensitivity to conflict-related cognitions, 365
Thiazide diuretics, 344
β-Thromboglobulin, 244
Thyroid stimulating hormone, response to thyrotropin-releasing hormone, 266
Tilney, F., work on migraine headache, 146
Time-limited therapy, 303
Torture, 25*n*
Touraine, G., and Draper, G.
  observations on personality and migraine headache, 135*t*
  work on migraine headache, 146–147, 165, 166, 168
Tranquilizers, for treatment of migraine, 311
Transcendental meditation, 353
Transference, 177, 285–286, 325–327
  and medication compliance, 287–288
  negative, 326
  positive, 326
Transference cure, 326
Transient global amnesia, 188
Transient migrainous accompaniment, 240
Tranylcypromine, 267
  for dysthymic pain disorder, 129
Trapezius muscles, examination of, 61
Trauma, 336
Trazodone, mode of action, 269

Treatment continuum, 321
Treatment planning, 62–63
Trepanning of skull, 6
Tricyclic antidepressants, 266
  for cyclical migraine, 279
  effects of, 267*t*
    on blocking acetylcholine and histamine receptors, 265*t*
  and MAOI, combination therapy, 267–269
  mode of action, 269
Trigeminal neuralgia, secondary depression in, 262–263
Trigger mechanisms, 61, 77
Trigger points, 112
Trimapramine, effects on blocking acetylcholine and histamine receptors, 265*t*
Tryptophan
  brain concentration of, 250–251
  free plasma level, 243, 250
Tryptophan-5-hydroxylase, 251
Tuberculosis, 53*n*
Tuberculous meningitis, 82
Twentieth century, headache treatment in, 17–19
Type A behavior, 224*n*
Type A personality, 219*n*

Ulrich, work on migraine headache, 146
Unconscious, 17, 41
  mechanisms of, 45

Valium. *See* Diazepam
Vanillic mandelic acid, 243
Van Pallandt, Nina, 26
Vascular headache, 68
  and drug use, 344
  in post-traumatic headache, 203
Vasodilators, and headache, 344
Ventilation, in headache management, 320
Vesalius, 12–13
Video screen, and headache, 308
Virchow, R., 15
Vives, Juan Luis, 17*n*
Von Helmont, 12

Walpole, Hugh, 26
Weber, H., work on migraine headache, 146
Weekend migraine, 275
Weekend "release" headache, 308
Wells, H.G., 26
Whiplash injury, 203, 205

Willis, Thomas, 14
Wolff, Harold G., 19
  observations on personality and migraine
    headache, 135t-137t
  theory of pathogenesis of migraine attack,
    246–247
  work on cluster headache, 213
  work on migraine headache, 149–150, 166–
    169
Wolff, Stuart, 19

Work, and exacerbation of headache patient's
  symptoms, 336–337
Worms, in frontal sinuses, 14

Xenon-133 clearance technique, for measurement of cerebral blood flow, 241–242, 247
X-rays, 62, 97

Yoga, 353

Zimelidine, mode of action, 269